Diagnostic Imaging in Medicine

NATO ASI Series

Advanced Science Institutes Series

A series presenting the results of activities sponsored by the NATO Science Committee, which aims at the dissemination of advanced scientific and technological knowledge, with a view to strengthening links between scientific communities

The series is published by an international board of publishers in conjunction with NATO Scientific Affairs Division

A	Life Sciences	Plenum Publishing Corporation
B	Physics	London and New York
C	Mathematical and Physical Sciences	D. Reidel Publishing Company Dordrecht and Boston
D	Behavioural and Social Sciences	Martinus Nijhoff Publishers Boston/The Hague/Dordrecht/Lancaster
E	Applied Sciences	
F	Computer and Systems Sciences	Springer Verlag Berlin/Heidelberg/New York
G	Ecological Sciences	

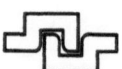

Series E: Applied Sciences – No. 61

Diagnostic Imaging in Medicine

edited by

Richard C. Reba, M.D.

Professor of Radiology and Medicine
Director, Division of Nuclear Medicine
George Washington University Medical Center
901 Twenty-Third Street, N.W.
Washington, D.C. 20037, USA

David J. Goodenough, Ph.D.

Director, Division of Radiation Physics
George Washington University Medical Center
901 Twenty-Third Street, N.W.
Washington, D.C. 20037, USA

Harold F. Davidson, M.S.

Consultant, Office of the Director of Army Research
Department of the Army
Washington, D.C. 20310, USA

1983 Springer-Science+Business Media, B.V.

Proceedings of the NATO Advanced Study Institute on Diagnostic Imaging in Medicine, Il Ciocco, Castelvecchio, Pascoli, Italy, October 10 - 24, 1981

Library of Congress Cataloging in Publication Data

NATO Advanced Study Institute on Diagnostic
    Imaging in Medicine (1981 : Castelvecchio Pascoli,
    Italy)
    Diagnostic imaging in medicine.

    (NATO advanced study institutes series. Series E,
Applied sciences ; v. 61)
    Includes bibliographical references and indexes.
    1. Imaging systems in medicine--Congresses.
2. Diagnosis, Radioscopic--Congresses. I. Reba,
Richard C. II. Goodenough, David J. III. Davidson,
Harold F. IV. Title. V. Series. [DNLM: 1. Radiography
--Congresses. 2. Radionuclide imaging--Congresses.
WN 200 N279d 1981]
RC78.A2N37 1981   616.07'54   82-24552

ISBN 978-94-009-6812-7   ISBN 978-94-009-6810-3 (eBook)
DOI 10.1007/978-94-009-6810-3

Distributors for the United States and Canada: Kluwer Boston, Inc., 190 Old Derby Street, Hingham, MA 02043, USA

Distributors for all other countries: Kluwer Academic Publishers Group, Distribution Center, P.O. Box 322, 3300 AH Dordrecht, The Netherlands

TABLE OF CONTENTS

VI

Acknowledgement

The authors gratefully acknowledge the encouragement and assistance provided by Major General Garrison Rapmund, MC, Commander, United States Army Medical Research and Development Command, Frederick, Md., and Dr. Mario di Lullo, Scientific Affairs Division, NATO, Brussels, Belgium. Without the professional support and encouragement provided by these gracious gentlemen, the Advanced Study Institute on Diagnostic Imaging in Medicine and this book could not have been accomplished. The editors also recognize the contributions of Ms. Diane Hayek to the Conference and this book. Ms. Hayek successfully passed every test of provocation with limitless patience, tolerance and good humor. Finally, we wish to thank the lecturers for the many hours of preparation which went into their lectures, the splendid organization of their written manuscripts, and the way they tirelessly made themselves available for discussion throughout the conference.

Washington, D.C.   November 1, 1982

Richard C. Reba, M.D.
David J. Goodenough, Ph.D.
Harold F. Davidson, M.S.

PREFACE

An Advanced Study Institute on Ultrasonics in Medical Diagnosis was held in Milan, Italy, from 10 to 15 June 1974. This ASI was of a short five-day duration and limited to cardiac diagnosis by ultrasound only. Since that time, the field of diagnostic imaging in medicine has literally exploded with new and improved means of medical diagnosis such as computed tomography, microwaves, nuclear magnetic resonance and other sophisticated techniques. These developments have enabled medical practitioners to make diagnoses with a minimum of danger to the patient, and a maximum of accuracy never before possible, and represent a multi-quantum advance over the early state-of-the-art presented at the 1974 ASI. Since then, several meetings have taken place on these individual topics to bring together experts who presented their latest research results, but none have discussed the entire field of diagnostic imaging in medicine in one meeting nor have they had the teaching character of an Advanced Study Institute.

The art and science of medicine have been altered repeatedly during the eight year interval since the last ASI. Today's clinician must be part technologist and must be enough of an investigator to understand and appreciate the scientific method. The current complex advances in instrumentation and pharmacology have had a marked effect on how medicine is practiced. There was, therefore, an urgent need to bring the entire field of imaging in medicine to one teaching podium where the many advances of the last six or seven years could be reviewed.

In response to this need, the NATO Advanced Study Institute on Diagnostic Imaging in Medicine was held at Il Ciocco, Castelvecchio, Pascoli, Italy, from 10 - 24 October 1981. The contents of this book are derived from the papers presented at this meeting.

The ASI served to bring together scientists and clinicians from diverse disciplines. The papers demonstrate that the interdisciplinary approach to medical diagnosis is a complementary one. The evolutionary progression of the new techniques was described and the utility of the procedures outlined in a series of state-of-the-art lectures given by leading clinical investigators from NATO countries.

Due to the great expansion in non-invasive techniques, clinicians have frequently had difficulty in understanding the greatly improved images. That is, physicians have not been able to integrate and use the information presented by the new techniques because they could not relate the high resolution data to their knowledge of clinical disease. Much of this growth has been possible because of the coupling of detection devices to the digital computer. This activity has provoked clinicians to attempt to exploit and understand fully the capabilities of the physical instruments and the physical scientists that design and operate these systems.

More and more, medical imaging is becoming increasingly involved with chemistry, biochemistry, pharmacology and physiology and is not simply a description of changes in gross anatomy (structure). The new techniques have been refined to a degree that they are now being applied widely in patients. These clinical tests produce data that are capable of being analyzed in a way that will result in a new and improved understanding of human disease. Subjects of the presentations included the following: advances in source and detector technology, accoustical imaging, NMR and microwave imaging, positron and single photon emission tomography, digital radiography and image processing and display techniques. Fundamental lectures describing the theory of the non-invasive procedure preceded presentations describing clinical examinations. Examples of utility and studies of diseases of the abdomen and pelvis, heart and lung, and central nervous system are discussed. Cost-effective and cost-benefit assessment of the new high technology procedures, as well as the use of diagnostic imaging techniques in developing countries, were included.

Washington, D.C.   November 1, 1982

Richard C. Reba, M.D.

SPONSOR'S INTRODUCTION

DIAGNOSTIC IMAGING IN MEDICINE

> Major General Garrison Rapmund
> Medical Corps, United States Army
> and Commander, United States Army
> Medical Research and Development Command

Introduction

The United States Army Medical Department is pleased to sponsor this NATO Advanced Study Institute on Diagnostic Imaging in Medicine.

Diagnostic procedures and equipment available today to assist the physician are enormously improved compared with just a few years ago. The issue for military medicine is, then, how much of this high technology capability is suited to field use? Indeed, we must also ask how much of this high technology is even required forward of the general hospital level of care?

Care of the combat casualty on the high intensity battlefield of the future is going to be extremely difficult at best. Because secure lines of casualty evacuation may not be always available, casualties may not reach definitive care for days. Therefore, physicians and all others who receive casualties in the field will need medical supplies and equipment appropriate for use under these most difficult circumstances, and be thoroughly trained to use them. It is not our goal to package the modern university shock/trauma unit with all its high technology patient support and diagnostic systems and move it to corps and division levels. Rather, our goal is to select from civilian medicine the latest therapeutic principles and technologies which are adaptable to the battlefield environment. Field medical equipment best suited to this environment has seven cardinal characteristics: it should be reliable, easily operated, economic of power requirements, easily maintained, lightweight, rugged and inexpensive. Match these characteristics against modern sophisticated medical equipment and you will quickly

see our problem in applying modern civilian medical capabilities
to field military medicine. And, to make our job more difficult,
to these criteria must be added 'hardening' for operations in a
nuclear and chemical warfare environment. I suspect our NATO
allies assess the situation as we do, so we all share the problem.

Development of new medical equipment just for military field
use can be a very expensive matter. Very rarely has the Army
Medical Department chosen this course in the past, in part because
medical equipment from private civilian medicine generally has done
the job, and in part because funds for equipment development are
severely limited. Can we continue to rely on private industry to
finance the development we need? Personally, I doubt it, unless
there is a strong attainable and unified market to justify the
investment by governments to update field medicine technology.

This NATO Advanced Study Institute offers an opportunity for
all of you, experts and students in the fields of diagnostic radiology, nuclear medicine, and other high technology fields, to consider future applications of these sciences to field military medicine. The seminar atmosphere in these beautiful surroundings
should further unfetter discussions of all possibilities. I
urge you to take fullest advantage of this opportunity. I know
the students will benefit much from this unique experience of
intensive exchange with this assembly of leading world experts.
I hope that you, the experts, will construct during the next two
weeks recommendations for me and for other NATO military medical
planners and equipment developers that will guide the formulation
of new field medical doctrine and the investment in new field
medical equipment.

Part I: Bio-physical Principles of Image Structure and Perception

SPATIAL AND SPATIO-TEMPORAL ANALYSIS
OF BIOLOGICAL FORM AND FUNCTION.

A. COBLENTZ, J.C. PINEAU, R. MOLLARD

Laboratoire d'Anthropologie et d'Ecologie Humaine
45, rue des Saints-Pères 75270 PARIS CEDEX 06

1   INTRODUCTION –

During the last century, the anthropological instrumentation held
an important place in the work of Paul BROCA. Therefore, the anat-
omists and the anthropologists were led to produce a rigorous
technique : the anthropometry. The traditional anthropometrical
techniques made it possible for a quantitative description of the
different segmentary elements.

The bidimensional data measured on the living human body, which
is an irregular shape, supply only one approximate and incomplete
description. Since the dimensions are being measured independently
from one another, it is no longer possible to define between their
relative position in space. Consequently, this data has been insuf-
ficiently measured to quantify in a precise manner the body shape
in terms of volumes, global and segmentary surfaces. It is the same
when we search to situate volume in relation to their surrounding
spaces. The main difficulty lies in the fact that a subject, even
motionless remains a dynamic and a non-static system. The conventional methods of measuring the morphological characteristics
do not supply all the desirable data. The concept of morphology implies a description of the human body's geometry : dimensions, surfaces, volumes. Further, it requires equally the knowledge of the
"dimensional-mass" group linked with the notion of inertial characteristics and with the location of the center of gravity. These
inertial characteristics present a variability linked with the mo-
bilization of segmentary elements and postures of human body. The
concept of morphology as well takes into account the dimension of
time and variations in the course of time.

The use of three dimensional data and the taking into account
of a fourth dimension, time, enabled us to start the research in

this field. These concerns have led us to develop in biometry and biomechanical, methods of measuring the human body and data processing, taking in a better way an account of the biological reality. Steming from static anthropometry, these concepts developed a more elaborate anthropometry : the dynamic anthropometry.

2 CONTRIBUTION OF THE STEREOMETRIC MEASUREMENT IN THE KNOWLEDGE OF THE BIOLOGICAL FORM AND FUNCTION -

In a number of fields, such as anthropology, anatomy, medicine, physiology, etc., the recent developments in the biostereometry by the use of different techniques have allowed us to accomplish considerable progress in our knowledge of the form and function of the human body. This is how, M.W. WITTLE, R.E. HERRON, J.R. CUZZI, and J.E. HUGG (1) analyzed the effects of extended space flight on the bodies of the Skylab astronauts, using biostereometric methods. Stereometric analysis of body shape is performed by obtaining the three dimensional coordinates of a large number of anatomic points on the surface of the body. In using these coordinates the authors have mathematically derived the volume and the surface area of bodily segments and of the body as a whole.

Biostereometry stands out as a very significant evolution in measuring the morphology of human body; it provides not only the values of distances between anatomical points, as in classical anthropometry but, moreover, it describes, with great precision, the spatial location of segmentary elements of the human body with respect to a tri-rectangular reference system (figure n°1).

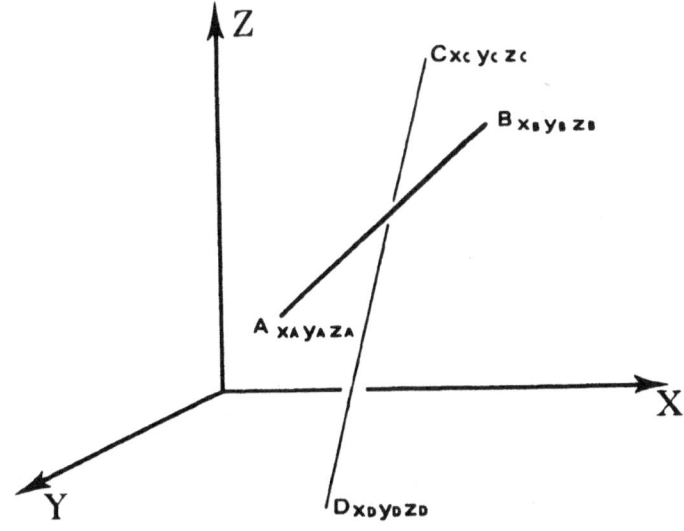

Figure n°1 - Position in space of the segmentary elements of the human body.

4

Each of these anatomical points which are taken into account are
identified by their coordinates X,Y,Z (figure n°2).Thus, with the
help of analytical geometry, it becomes easier to calculate distances
from point to point, from point to segment, from point to plane,
distances between planes, angles of segments or planes, etc.

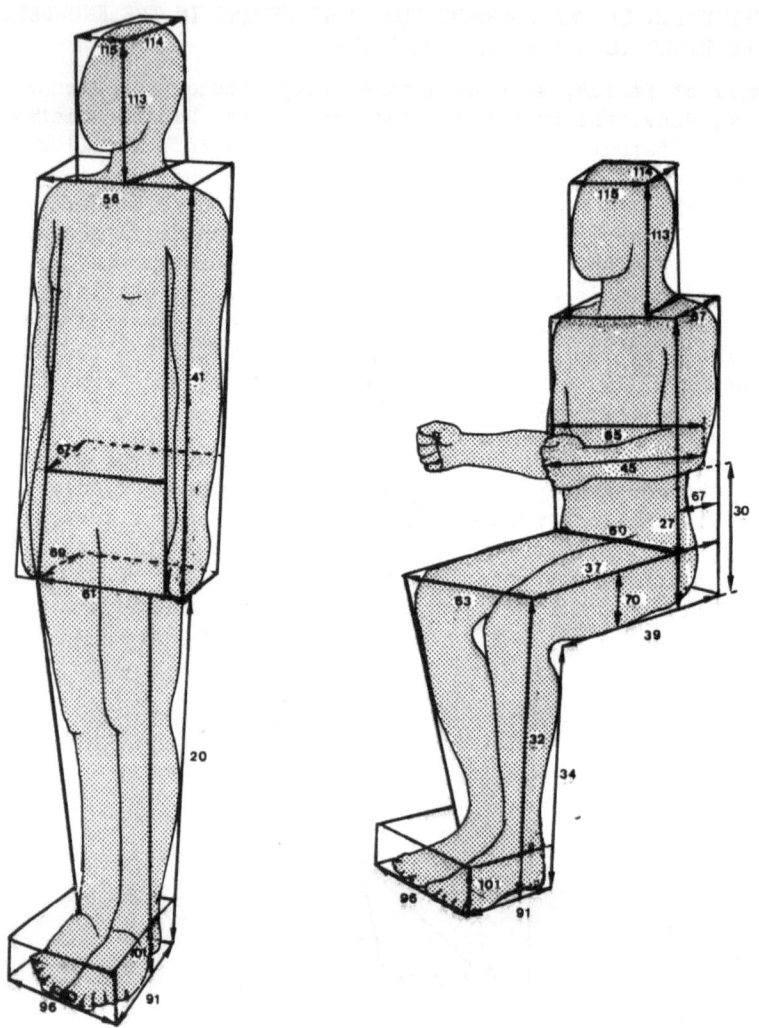

Figure n°2 - Volume of human body : height, breadth, thickness, angles and perimeters.

2.1 Techniques used in stereometry -

From these general principles of the biostereometry two technical
solutions were proposed.

2.1.1 Direct biostereometry with the anthropostereometer :

It has been developed in the Laboratory of Anthropology and Human
Ecology, adapted for the needs in accordance with the desired precision and the analyzed form. This is how we undertook to evaluate
the asymmetries between right and left of the homologous dimensions
of the face of a living person and of a skeletal example on one
hand.

The use of conventional anthropometric techniques does not always enable us to show such a small variation between right and
left sides. The stereometric technique of measurements provides
us with a more precise response. By use of this technique, quasi-
imperceptible differences between right and left sides of the face
of a living person, as well as of a skeleton, can be measured together with variations in the orientation or angulation of anatomical segments in the three-dimensional.

The equipment composes a rigid frame invariably linked with a
tri-rectangular trihedron of reference from which all the anatomical points of the face can be located and defined. They are defined
by their three-dimensional coordinates X,Y,Z,; the median sagittal
plane XOZ being the plane of symmetry for the equipment (figure n°3).

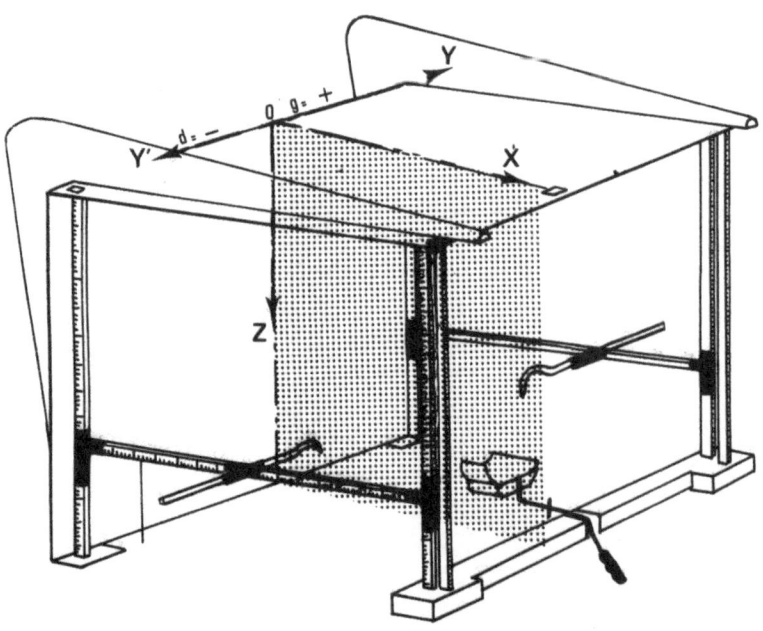

Figure n°3 - Schema of the anthropostereometer seeks to
apply the principles of analytic geometry to anthropometry.

This technique enabled us to detect on a series of dry skulls, the average differences of approximately a millimeter between the two sides of the face which cannot result in an inaccuracy of measurement.

Beyond the morphological study of segmentary anatomical elements, it is possible to approach more functional concepts of posture and gesture. Thus, whatever may be the orientation and functional position of the subject including the segmentary elements (arm, hand, lower limb), they are precisely located in reference to the position in the space which they occupy. It is obvious that such a method becomes valuable in any study of design of equipment and simulation of an operator's post of activity or workplace. Effectively, in such a context, the elements of the man himself (anatomical points) and the elements of the system (commands) are calculated according to a common reference system. We selected the principal of stereometric measurement through the translations by a "data pick elements", following three orthogonal axes of reference. The base of translation elements and data pick off element is composed of a parallelepipedic rack of sufficient dimensions (2,3m. x 2,3m. x 2,5m.) to hold a post of activity (figure n°4).

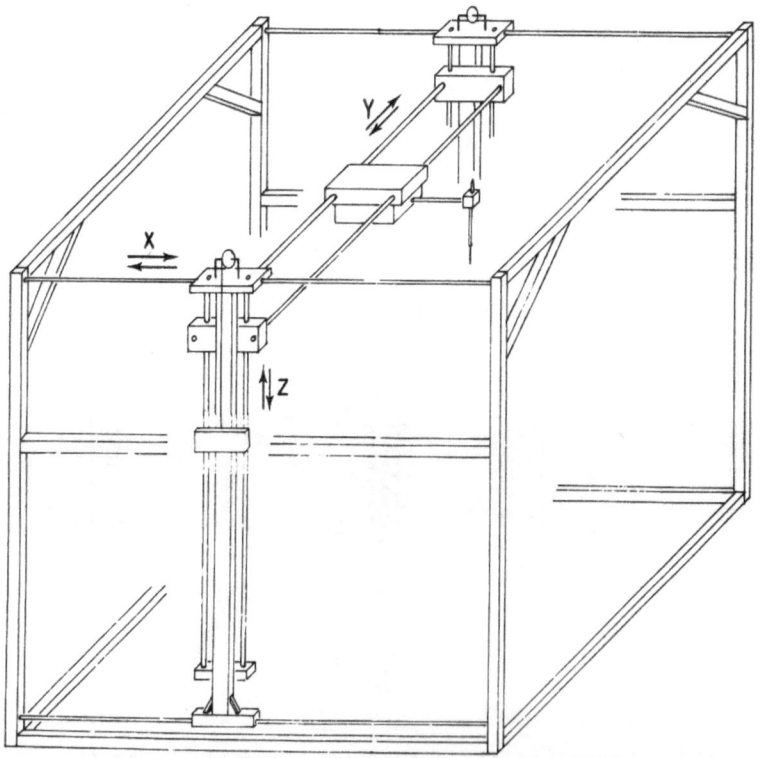

Figure n°4 - Schema of the principal biostereometry.

Three sensors of rectilinear displacements are associated with this mechanical part. They assure the measurements in cartesian coordinates of the posture of the distal extremity of the "data pick element". These sensors are connected to an electronic processing device and in conjunction with a computer base meant for management and information storage (figure n°5).

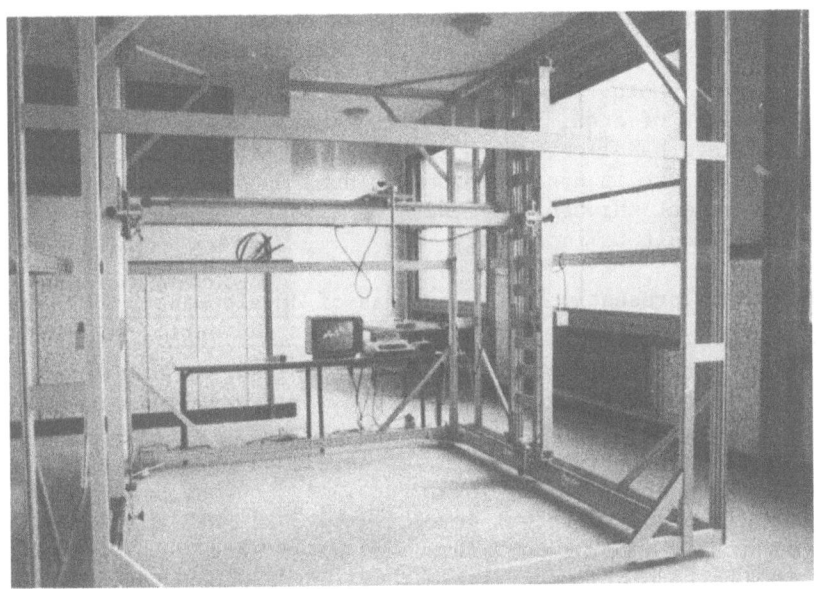

Figure n°5 - The biostereometer.

2.1.2 - The photographic biostereometry with the photogrammetry and the systems of orthogonal shots :

In this case, the acquisition of biostereometric data is no longer made directly from the object, but from photographical or cinematographical pictures of this object.

A technique very much developed at present, providing extremely precise data is represented by the Photogrammetry. B. SHELDON, K.G. HARRY and Col. (3) elaborated a stereophotogrammetric method for the detection of prosthesis loosening in total hip anthroplasty in the medical field as well roentgen stereophotogrammetry. It is used in order to search the effects of medical and surgical treatments of the investigated patients for various reasons : growth distrubances, craniofacial anomalies, disorders of the spine and visceral tumors, etc., G. SELVIK (4).

W. FORBIN, E. HIERHOLZER (5) employ a stereophotogrammetric method for the measurement of body surfaces using a projected grid. The advantage of this method lies in the necessity to evaluate only

one image. The grid slide and the photograph form a sort of
stereo image pair. The grid is projected on the surface to be measured. The coordinates of the grid points in the slide can be calculated by the count, where as those in the photograph have to be
measured.

According to H. TERADA, T. IKEDA (6), the biostereometrical
method using Moire interference fringe, has an advantage in that
the counter fringes on the surface of an object are promptly visible
to the naked eye and are recorded photographically.

Thus, the photogrammetry demands as well the implementation of
many processes of acquisition of data in which heavy interpretation
tends to disturb collection in the field of biostereometry. Furthermore, its use in dynamic biometry demands decomposition modalities of movement through the medium of stroboscopical effects,
equally difficult to implement.

2.2 New means presently in the process of development : opto-elec-
tronical technique - telemetry by laser and optic encoder -

The laser is the basis of most modern techniques in biostereometry.
The laser is a source of coherent light, in other words, strictly
monochromatic, collimated and whose waves are in harmony with
phase betwen them. Its use is being developed more and more
notably in ocular surgery. Thus, the laser contour angiography
is a new technique which was developed by J.M. SHAPIRO (7) for
topographically mapping the retina and optic nerve head of the eye.
A striped pattern of laser light is projected onto the ocular surface through one side of the patient's dilated pupil. Photographs,
taken through the opposite side of the pupil, reveal the topogra-
phy as parallactic displacements of the stripes. A topographic map
is constructed from tracings of the stripes.

A certain number of risks are linked with the same characteristics of laser:
- strength of the laser,
- length of transmission wave,
- method of operation,
- transversal dimensions of beams,
- divergence of beams.

The lesions of the central part of the retina are the most
dangerous. The densities of energy or strength which may lead to
retinal lesions are in the order from 0,1 to 1 J/cm^2 per the im-
pulsive lasers.

In what concerns the biometrical characteristics, the telemetry by laser and optical sensors represent a great improvement.
As a matter of fact, it enables us to locate every point of an
object in space by the location of light spot of the laser beam.

The coordinates X and Y are determined by the Optic Encoder

in accordance with spatial orientation, site and azimuth of the laser beam. The third coordinate Z, measures the distances of points
of the object and the system-camera-laser which is collected from
a value delivered by an optic captor (matrix of diodes coupled to
laser beam) (Figure n°6).

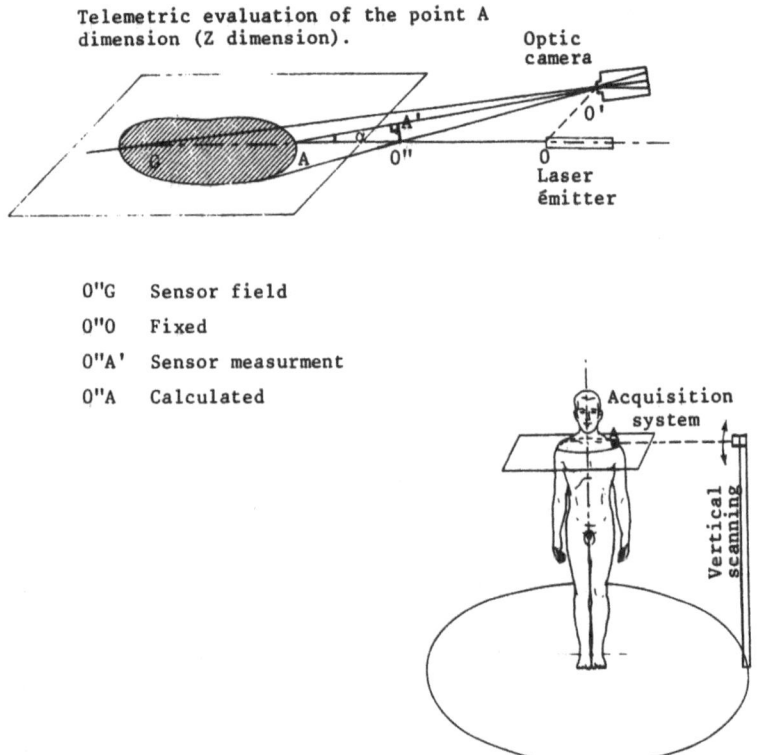

Telemetric evaluation of the point A dimension (Z dimension).

Optic camera

Laser émitter

O"G   Sensor field
O"O   Fixed
O"A' Sensor measurment
O"A   Calculated

Acquisition system

Vertical scanning

Figure n°6 - The principal of the measurement of the human
body by telemetry.

The great advantage of this method in relation to the photogram-
metric method, as mentioned before, is in the absence of intervention
of the human operator, for the phases of the stereorestitution. The
coordinates X, Y, Z by the object are immediately measured and processed by means of computer equipment. The next table shows the
importance of the quality of recorded data according to the techniques used.

DIFFERENT TECHNIQUES	TYPE OF MEASUREMENT	TIME OF ACQUISITION	
- TRADITIONAL ANTHROPOMETRY	LINEAR MEASUREMENT	60 TO 120 MEASUREMENTS BY SUBJECT PER HOUR	MANUAL HANDLING WITHOUT REFERENCE TO A 3-D SPACE.
- ANTHROPOSTEREOMETRY : . DIRECT MEASUREMENT	3 - D	100 TO 300 POINTS BY SUBJECT PER HOUR	WITH REFERENCE TO A 3-D SPACE. MANUAL HANDLING DETERMINATION OF VOLUMES OF ACTIVITY.
. AUTOMATISED MEASUREMENT .	3 - D	100 TO 1000 POINTS BY SUBJECT PER HOUR	AUTOMATICAL DATA PROCESSING.
- PHOTOGRAMMETRY :	3 - D	PHOTOGRAPHIES 1 TO 2 MN. BY SUBJECT ∞ OF POINTS.	DETERMINATION OF SURFACES, VOLUMES DATA PROCESSING THROUGH AN OPERATOR.
- OPTO-ELECTRONICAL TECHNIQUES . LASER	3 - D	30000 POINTS IN 5 SEC. BY SUBJECT.	AUTOMATICAL DATA PROCESSING

EVOLUTION OF THE MEASUREMENT TECHNIQUES IN BIOMETRY

Relationships with morphological parameters

3   SPATIO-TEMPORAL STUDY -

Now, the biostereometry which is defined as "the spatial and spatio-temporal analysis of the biological form and function based on the principals of analytic geometry" (HERRON, 1972) has realized a certain development because of finalized stereophotogrammetry.

3.1 Modification of body volumes linked with different biological functions -

In the 19th century, the works of physiologists enabled us to show the narrow relations between the body surface and different biological processes : respiration, thermotaxis, metabolism. SARRUS and RAMEAUX have noticed that the phenomens of metabolism and consumption of oxygen were directly related to the surface of human body. It is the same for residual volume of lungs. The gravity of prognosis of burns are always estimated according to percentage of the surface of the skin which has been destroyed.

In the field of biomechanics, as we have already mentioned, B. SHELDON used a stereophotogrammetric system for the detection of the prosthesis loosening in total hip arthroplasty (8). In the same way stereophotogrammetry can be used for the measuring of the body surface by a projected grid (W. FROBIN, H. HIERHELZER) (9).

The different research in fundamental or applied character, and in human biology are being confronted with the problem in the lack of knowledge in the narrow and permanent relations which are set up during a life time between the acquisition and the variation or morphological characteristics : dimensions, masses, surfaces, inertial properties and the conditions of the environment. The relationships that have been established in the course of existance play an essen-

tial role on the conditions in development of the body growth :
aging, senescence, biological rhythms, pathological conditions or
nutrition conditions.

3.2 Growth and development -

Studies on the somatic growth of young children have traditionally
been made using conventional anthropometry techniques. As a result,
while the conditions of growth of morphological variables such as
weight or segmental dimensions are well known, the same cannot be
said of the more general aspect of the development of the body in
a three dimensional reference space.

Up to today, in literature, we were measuring height, length,
breadth, perimeters, weight, unit of dimensional characters among
which we could only establish relationships of static type : correlations, regressions, curve of allometry, curve of growth.

Such an approach does not really take into account the relative
evolution in three dimensional space and as well the accordance
with time of all the anatomical elements in reference with a common three dimensional system. In fact, the acquisition of a specific
morphology, linked to a certain bodily posture, is being done
according to general diagram of development depending on constraint
of environment (earthly gravity).

The global or segmentary body volumes and surfaces, compose
morphological somatic characteristics which begin to explain the
physiological phenomenon - thermoregulation, energetic assessment,
thermic exchanges - more than the usual linear data.

Among the possible methods of study, the stereophotogrammetry
and the opto-electronic techniques appear to us as the most rewarding. They enable us to draw up the curves of growth on segmentary
surfaces of corresponding volumes (10). Further, it will be possible for us to verify the various relationships that exist with
masses, dimensions and the other morphological parameters (Figure
n°7).

3.3 Variations in the space of different segmentary elements -

The importance of such biostereometrical techniques lies at the
level of specific displacement of certain anatomical points in the
process of growth in relation to units of reference (axis, planes,
points) defined beforehand.

For example, if we consider the position of the center of gravity
(C.G.) of the human body, the latter has a functional evolutionary
significance in relation to the acquisition of the erected posture
which is characteristic of the human race. With the aid of this
center of gravity and two other anatomical vertex and acromial
points, we can define a reference plane considered as invariant in
the course of growth time.

12

Thus, we can progressively, in relation to this reference of mode, organize other anatomical elements of the body until they realize a definitive structure (Figure n°8).

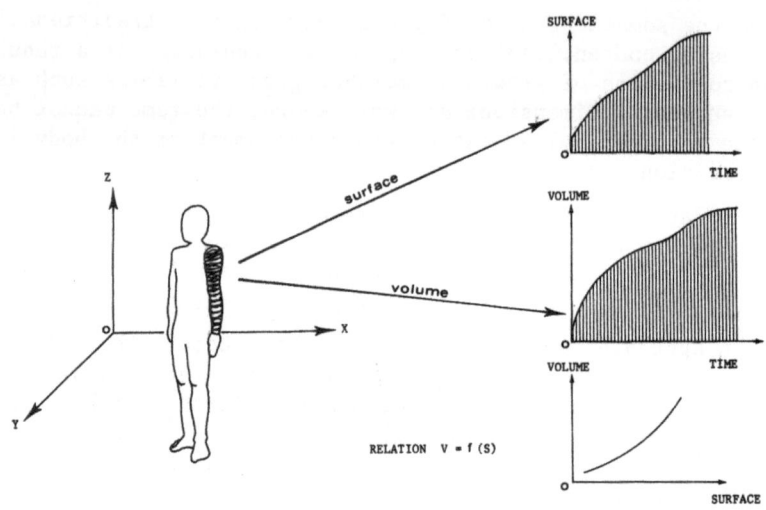

Figure n°7 - Biostereometry and measurement of the evolution of parameters surface volume in the course of time.

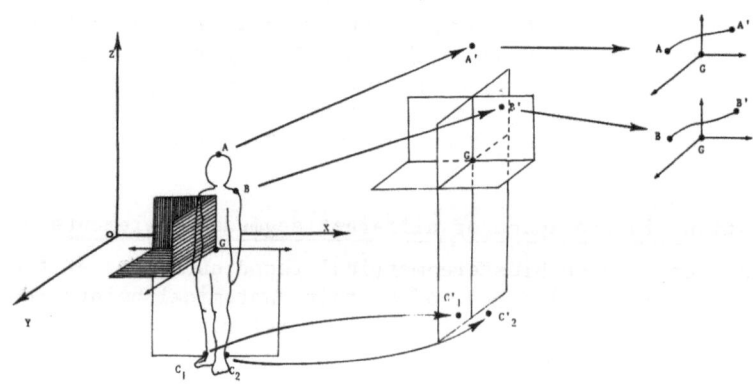

Figure n°8 - Biostereometry and measurements of the displacement of anatomical elements in space.
    - Modification of posture
    - Isotropy and anisotropy

Such approaches will provide new elements for the progress of phenomena not yet well known. Especially in the study of the acquisition of a real erected posture of a young child, the creation of a functionally and anatomically adapted morphology to bipedal locomotion, the advanced detection of troubles and malfunction in the attitudes, show paths for desirable research.

It is the same in the study of fundamental aspects of the body growth and the diversification in morphological types, the biostereometrical approach will allow clarification of the importance and the variability of the development according to the important directions of growth (concept of isotropy and anisotrophy).

4 MODELIZATION AND THREE DIMENSIONAL GRAPHIC REPRESENTATIONS OF THE HUMAN BODY -

Among the various applications of biostereometrics, the graphic representation of the human body by simulation on computer, composes the most sought after application in a number of disciplines, such as ergonomy, and biomechanics, etc.

In this case, the biostereometrics is a primary data base from which applications requiring a variety of levels of detail may be prepared.

4.1 Importance of stereometric techniques -

In an era where the development of data processing takes a considerable scope, it is quite evident that the different stereometric techniques (anthropostereometry, photogrammetry) provide a source of essential information for the knowledge of form and function of the human body.

Beyond the conventional anthropometric data, where either not very precise or very specific means of acquisition provided only one partial information, now the stereometry opens up a great deal of possibilities on the plane of fundamental and applied research.

Its principal, whatever may be the used technique is the determination of three dimensional coordinates in relation to a trirectangular system of reference.

Thus, the stereometric data shows a considerable enrichment since they provide the possibilities:

- to determine linear distances between the anatomical points taken two by two and then to find again the conventional anthropometric measurements with the aid of independent technique from the observer
- to have the access to new information such as :
  . exact position and the orientation of a segment in the space,
  . distances between anatomical points and planes of reference,
  . angles between segments,
- to define in a precise manner : forms, volumes and surfaces.

Further, the biostereometry enables one to integrate the fourth dimension : "time". This aspect leads to new perspectives mainly in the direct study of the growth phenomenon (cf. § 3.2).

Eventually, we think that the use of this stereometric data stock, derived from many surveys, then from many populations, will be extremely profitable.

4.2 Importance of the use of data bank and graphic software -

The necessity of making automatic the measurements of stereometric data is on the way to totally modifying the quality and the quantity of the formed measurements. The use of stereometric characteristics for the static and dynamic representation of the human body usually comes up against a considerable heaviness of means in expression and reproduction of advanced propositions. It is because of this reason the use of the Bank of International Data of Human Biometry and Ergonomy : ERGODATA, installed in the Laboratory of Anthropology and Human Ecology (L.A.E.H.), enables us to manage the stereometric data collected from the previously mentioned techniques.

All this data is directly applicable at the level of ERGODATA for the more or less complex calculations. The three dimensional data are further integrated at the level of graphic processing system at the Laboratory (L.A.E.H.) which uses the interactive software of three dimensional representation (EUCLID).

EUCLID is a data processing system of three dimensional form description, fulfilling complete simulation of the language and operators in conventional geometry. It appears to be an excellent core for the creation of a specific system of computer aid design.

The specific possibilities for EUCLID are not limited at a simple graphic extension and they provide a complete coherent unit allowing :
- creation of basic geometric forms,
- creation of complex forms by assembly,
- displacement and distortion of existing forms or the creation of new forms through transformation,
- creation by constraints of positioning and redimensioning,
- creation by rules of generations (surfaces of revolution),
- création by conjunction, fusion or substraction of existing forms.

The graphic software that is generated allows us to "see" the forms on which we work. The hidden parts can be carried out according to two modes of operation : the processing by sets or "batch" and the interactive processing.

To represent a human being with the help of EUCLID software, it is necessary to define a certain number of relative hypotheses in the form of biomechanical functions of such a silhouette representation.

In the first place it is not a question of elaborating a very much more complex human silhouette and it is necessary to define first of all the different modules which once gathered, compose this silhouette. The module are composed of : upper limbs, lower limbs, truck, and the head to which will be graphed the sub-modules corresponding to the inner articular mobilities, which are essential in a biomechanical point of view to the design of the living being. Thus, an analogous way for ŞAMMIE Research Group (11), we are capable of elaborating models holding in account of the variability of anthropometrical measurements and at the same time indexes of proportionality (Figure n°9). The graphic software using the stereometric data will allow us to displace the modules the one in relation to the other in a real situation.

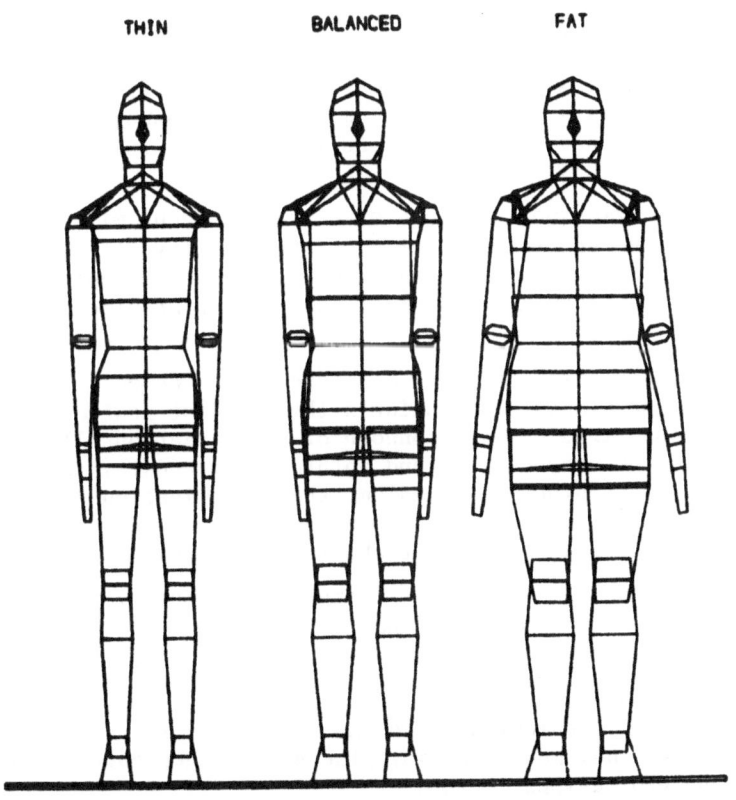

THIN   BALANCED   FAT

Figure n°9 - Examples of modelization of the human body from principal types morphologies that exist according to a population.

In this way, the elaboration of human silhouettes can be accomplished from the parametrage of certain anthropometric measurements (length, height, breadth, perimeters) and articular possibilities will be priminarily determinated by the stereometric techniques (intersegmentary angles).

4.3 Importance of the C.A.O. in the prediction of necessary volumes for the execution of one or more gestures -

The analytical study of man-machine relationships in design point of view and workplace installation led us to envisage an analysis of the dynamics of the complex and efficient gesture which include :

- the knowledge and the analysis of the space of activity as well as the volume of sitting or standing operator,
- the knowledge, by modules more or less representative of the population, of the biometry and the basic biomechancis of the users
- the systematization and the hierarchial organization in the spaces of efficient professional gestures necessary for the optimal accomplishment of the task.

From these elements, it is possible to identify the optimal conditions of designing the elements of the machine in saving the population from useless efforts and risks in the fulfillment of the task.

Thus the principe knowledge of a space made up with extreme reachable zone and preferential zones of activity allows us to arrive at best a compromise between optimal zones of functional limits associated with man and the load that the machine imposes on him.

The computer aid design is composed by the essential complement of methods and biometric techniques that we just mentioned. The method of modelization on a console of visualization allows us, with the aid of stereometric and anthropometric data, to create, through the data processing medium, the visualization on the module screen of an operator the necessary gestures for the accomplishment of a series of tasks (figure n°10).

Such a method considerably widens the perspective ot the use of equipment so far as this method :

- provides the evaluation of the workload according to the âge, sex and personal aptitudes,
- supplies biomechanical data to the manufacturers enabling them to elaborate new models of workplaces which decrease physical load and professional risks,
- allows the engineer of research departments to plan out useful new equipments, for the design of future machines, what ever be the morphology, age, sex, ethnic origin or socioprofessionals of the users.

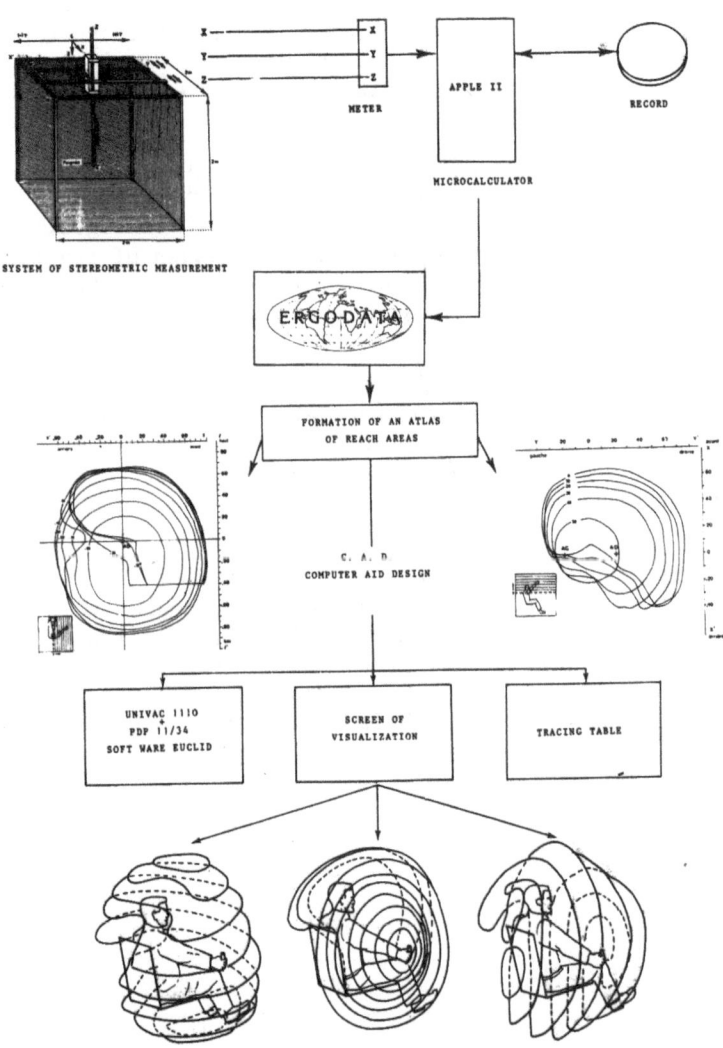

Figure n°10 - Computer Aid Design

5   CONCLUSIONS –

After ten years, the biostereometry still remains as a well expanding discipline full of rewarding data as much at the level of fundamental research as at the level of applied research.

What ever may be the technique, its principal stands on the determination of three dimensional coordinates in relation to a trirectangular reference. The photogrammetry, the stereophotogrammetry and the tomodensitometry supply a rigorous description of human shapes and once complete, this precise data gives us, the qualitative picture of what we observe.

The knowledge of volumes and that of the surface of the body, supply essential data for understanding many physiological phenomenons : the growth, the thermoregulation, the energetic assessments, the thermic exchanges, etc. In the domain of functional anatomy that of biometry or ergonomy, the biostereometry supplies quantitative data that the conventional anthropometry has never been able to obtain.

The stereometric input data at the Bank of International Data of Biometry and Ergonomy at the Laboratory of Anthropology and Human Ecology and their integration at the level of the graphic processing system (software EUCLID), composes a stock of essential data for the elaboration of the human body's model and its development.

The computer aid design represents the logical extension of previously mentioned methods and techniques. Particularly, it enables us to analyze the design and the installation of workplaces, the prediction of the necessary volumes for the execution of a particular task and the reconstitution of professional or athletic gestures in point of view of their optimization. We can well assert that biostereometry opens a way to many new possibilities in human biology.

REFERENCES

1. Whittle (M.W.); Herron (R.E.); Cuzzi (J.R.); Hugg (J.E.).-
*Effects of extented space flight on body form of Skylab astronauts
using biostereometric methods.-* in Biostereometrics 74. Washington
D.C. Septembre 10-13 1974.- Falls Church (U.S.A.) : American Society of Photogrammetry, 1974.- pp.588-589.

2. Crété (N.); Deloison (Y.); Mollard (R.).- *A study of facial
asymetries by the stereometric method.-* In Proceedings of the NATO
Symposium on Applications on Applications of Human Biostereometrics.
Paris. July 9-13 1978.- Washington : S.P.I.E., 1980.- pp.311-319.

3. Sheldon (B.); Harry (K.G.).- *A stereophotogrammetric system
for the detection of prothesis loosening in total hip arthoplasty.-*
in Proceedings of the NATO Symposium on Applications of Human Biostereometrics. Paris. July 9-13, 1978.- Washington : S.P.I.E., 1980.-
pp.112-123.

4. Selvik (G.).- *Roentgen stereophotogrammetry in Lund.-* in Proceedings of the NATO Symposium on Applications of Human Biostereometrics. Paris. July 9-13, 1978.- Washington : S.P.I.E., 1980.-
pp.184-189.

5. Frobin (W.); Hierholzer (E.).- *A stereophotogrammetric method
for the measurement of body surfaces using a projected grid.-* in
Proceedings of the NATO Symposium on Applications of Human Biostereometrics. Paris. July 9-13, 1978.- Washington : S.P.I.E., 1980.-
pp.39-44.

6. Tereda (H.); Ikeda (T.).- *Biostereometrical application of moi-
ré fringe method with special reference to our optical device in aid
of parallel light.-* in Proceedings of the NATO Symposium on Applications of Human Biostereometrics. Paris. July 9-13, 1978.- Washington : S.P.I.E., 1980.- pp.24-30.

7. Shapiro (J.M.).- *Topographic mapping of the ocular fundus by
laser contour angiography : the man-machine interaction.-* in Proceedings of the NATO Symposium on Applications of Human Biostereometrics.
Paris, July 9-13, 1978.- Washington : S.P.I.E., 1980.- pp.24-30.

8. See 3.

9. See 5.

10. Coblentz (A.); Ignazi (G.).- *A biostereometric approach to the study of infant's and children's body growth.*- in Proceedings of the NATO Symposium on Applications of Human Biostereometrics. Paris. July 9-13, 1978.- Washington : S.P.I.E.- pp.270-273.

11. Sammie Research Group.- *System for aiding man-machine interaction evaluation (SAMMIE).- Nottingham : University of Nottingham, 1980.*

SIGNAL DETECTION THEORY: LIMITATIONS AND APPLICATIONS

David J. Goodenough, Ph.D.

The George Washington University Medical Center
Department of Radiology
Division of Radiation Physics
2300 K Street, N.W.
Washington, D.C. 20037

ABSTRACT

The evaluation of system performance in diagnostic imaging has raised substantial questions concerning the importance and interplay of many physical and psychophysical parameters. It has become clear that many diagnostic decisions are related to complex processes of human pattern recognition and decision-making, as well as the more classical parameters of signal detection theory such as: contrast, noise, resolution, and dynamic range.

In this paper, attention will be given to some of the limitations and applications of the use of signal detection theory for the evaluation of medical imaging systems. Basic concepts of signal detection theory will be reviewed. Emphasis will be placed on the differences between relatively straightforward application to physical systems with known physical parameters and decision criteria versus the application to the human sensory system wherein the actual signals, noise and decision criteria may not be known.

In the physical domain, signal-to-noise ratios will be developed and examined for CT, radiography and nuclear medicine. In the sensory domain, examples of ROC experiments for each of these modalities will be studied for what might be considered relatively simple detection tasks, as well as more complex diagnostic decision tasks.

In the physical domain, it will be shown that important conclusions regarding the need for signal contrast and adequate dynamic range can be drawn. In the sensory domain, the importance of history, localization and differential diagnosis of abnormality will be discussed.

INTRODUCTION

In the beginning of the evaluation of medical imaging systems was the declarative statement, e.g.: "It's better," "It's worse," "It's about the same." The problem was that not only did two different people sometimes give different answers, but an individual might even seem to disagree with his own interpretation if tested in a "blind" fashion at a different time. One major problem of evaluation was in analyzing judgments based on an unknown or unspecified value scale. A second major problem was in learning to understand legitimate differences in inter- and intra-observer responses.

To begin to understand the background to these two problems, it is important to take note of the fact that any decision regarding the existence of a signal in the presence of noise can be associated with two kinds of errors: (1) false-positive, i.e., an incorrect decision that a signal (or abnormality) is present; and (2) false-negative, i.e., an incorrect decision that a signal is absent.

The true-positive fraction $P(S|s)$, or the "sensitivity" of a detecting system, represents the probability of responding correctly to the presence of a signal (disease) when the signal is actually present. Likewise, the true-negative fraction $P(N|n)$, which is just one minus the false positive fraction (frequently called the "specificity" of the detecting system), represents the probability of responding correctly to the absence of the signal when the signal is not present. Another term often encountered in error analysis is "accuracy". The accuracy rate is related to both sensitivity and specificity in that it may be defined as a number of correct decisions divided by the total number of decisions made (1). Thus, if $P(s)$ is the prior probability of a signal, then accuracy (A) can be calculated by the formula:

$$A = P(S|s) \ P(s) + P(N|n) \ (1-P(s)) \tag{1}$$

It should be noted that $P(S|s)$ and $P(N|n)$ are functions of the decision criterion and reflects the degree of conservatism of the reader and/or his estimates of the relative consequences of false-positive versus false-negative errors. Thus sensitivity, specificity and accuracy are not unique single values of a given imaging device or detecting system; rather, they depend on the threshold setting or criterion level of the detecting system or human observer!

A salient point of Receiver Operating Curve (ROC) analysis is explicit documentation of possible trade-offs between sensitivity and specificity as the decision criterion is varied from extreme conservatism to extreme liberalism.

ROC curve analysis was first developed for the evaluation of radar signal detectability and was later used to evaluate human detection performance in psychophysics (2,3). Several introductory discussions of the principles of ROC analysis have been published (4,5,6).

ROC analysis was introduced in Radiology in 1968 by Lusted (4), who reanalysed two classical studies of radiological performance (Garland, 1949 (7); Yerushalmy, Harkness, Cope, and Kennedy, 1950 (8)). One study examined the accuracy of a team of two readers and counted either positive responses from both readers or a positive response from one reader as a positive team response. The other study examined the effect of repeated readings by a single reader -- first with a conservative, then with a liberal, criterion for a positive response. Analysis in terms of the probability of a correct decision (of both kinds) led to values ranging from the 0.70 to the 0.90, suggesting different degrees of discrimination. The ROC analysis, on the other hand, showed that all the data fell along one curve, representing a single performance capacity but differences in decision criteria. The ROC provides a measure of the accuracy afforded by a system or that is independent of the reader's decision criterion, or his tendency to "underread" or "overread".

ROC has also been used in cost-benefit analyses of diagnostic techniques (e.g., McNeil, Varady, Burrows, and Adelstein, 1975 (9)).

Applications of ROC analyses have been made to remote viewing of images, including television display of chest X-ray films (Kundel, 1972 (10); Andrus, Dreyfuss, Jaffer, and Bird, 1975 (11)), and picturephone transmission of radionuclide scans (Anderson, Mintzer, Hoffer, Lusted, Smith, and Pokorny, 1973 (12)). ROC analysis has been applied to training of paramedics to read film -- at the professionals' level of performance for mammography (Alcorn and O'Donnell, 1969 (13)) and chest X-rays (Sheft, Jones, Brown, and Ross, 1970 (14)). Recent reviews describe use of the ROC in more than 20 medical studies (15).

Consider the simplified situation of estimating the presence or absence of a signal from a single outcome of known probability distribution describing probability of various outcomes. Let $f(x|n)$ be the normalized probability distribution describing the outcome, x of some random variable $\underset{\sim}{x}$ when noise alone is present, and $f(x|s)$ be the corresponding normalized probability distribution when a signal is present as well. Let each outcome of $\underset{\sim}{x}$ become

24

the input to a detecting system which must decide whether the input is due to noise or to a combination of signal plus noise.

Suppose the system is designed to respond with "Signal" ("S") for each outcome of $x \geq x_c$ and "Noise" ("N") for each outcome of $x \leq x_c$ (Figure 1). The specified value x_c (called the criterion level) of the random variable x (called the decision variable) defines two areas of each of the two probability distributions $f(x|n)$ and $f(x|s)$ such that x_c forms the lower boundary of one area (the right-hand tail) of each distribution. The probability that a given outcome of x arising from the signal-plus noise distribution will evoke the response "S", denoted by $P(S|s,x_c)$, is then given by the area under the signal-plus-noise distribution to the right of x_c.

$$P(S|s,x_c) = \int_{x_c}^{\infty} f(x|s)dx \qquad (2)$$

Similarly, the probability that a given outcome of x arising from the noise distribution alone will evoke the response "S", denoted by $P(S\,n,x_c)$, is given by the area under the noise distribution to the right of x_c.

$$P(S|n,x_c) = \int_{x_c}^{\infty} f(x|n)dx \qquad (3)$$

Because $f(x|s)$ and $f(x|n)$ are normalized to the unit area, the probability that an outcome of x arising from the signal-plus-noise distribution will evoke the response "N" is $P(N|s,x_c)$ or $1 - P(S|s,x_c)$, while the probability that an outcome of x arising

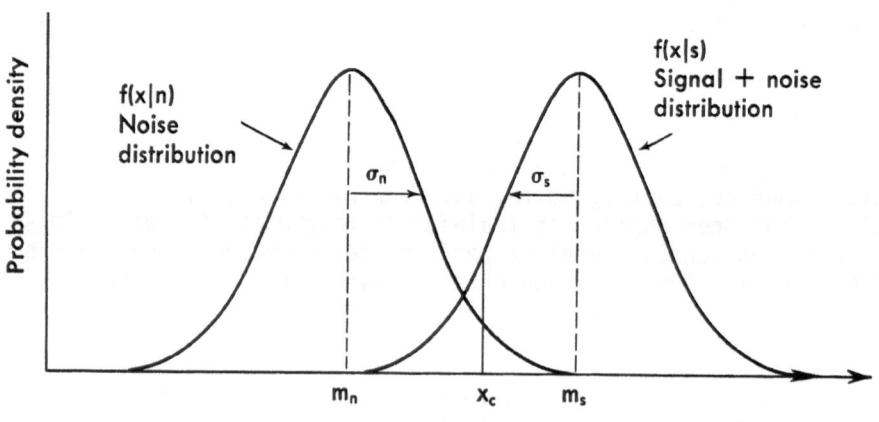

X — axis

Figure 1: Normalized probability distributions for noise $f(x|n)$ and signal-plus-noise $f(x|s)$, where m_n and m_s are the means and σ_n, σ_s are the standard deviations of the respective distributions.

from the noise distribution will evoke the response "N" is
$P(N|s,x_c)$ or $1 - P(S|n,x_c)$. These probabilities are shown in
matrix form in Figure 2 as the right-and-left-hand tails of the
corresponding distributions. This form is often called the stimulus-
response matrix. As suggested above, it is only necessary to specify
one of the conditional probabilities of the signal-plus-noise distribution, since the other probability can then be determined from
the equation

$$P(S|s,x_c) + P(N|s,x_c) = 1 \qquad (4)$$

Likewise, only one conditional probability of the noise distribution
is necessary, since

$$P(S|n,x_c) + P(N|n,x_c) = 1 \qquad (5)$$

The stimulus-response matrix, and the accompanying conditional
probabilities of signal and noise outcomes, may be used to describe
various terms often used to characterize the efficacy of medical
x-ray imaging systems. For example, $P(S|s)$ is often called the
"hit" or true positive rate (fraction); $P(S|n)$ is often called the
false positive or false-alarm-rate (fraction); $P(N|n)$ is often
called the true negative rate (fraction); and $P(N|s)$ is the miss or
false negative rate (fraction).

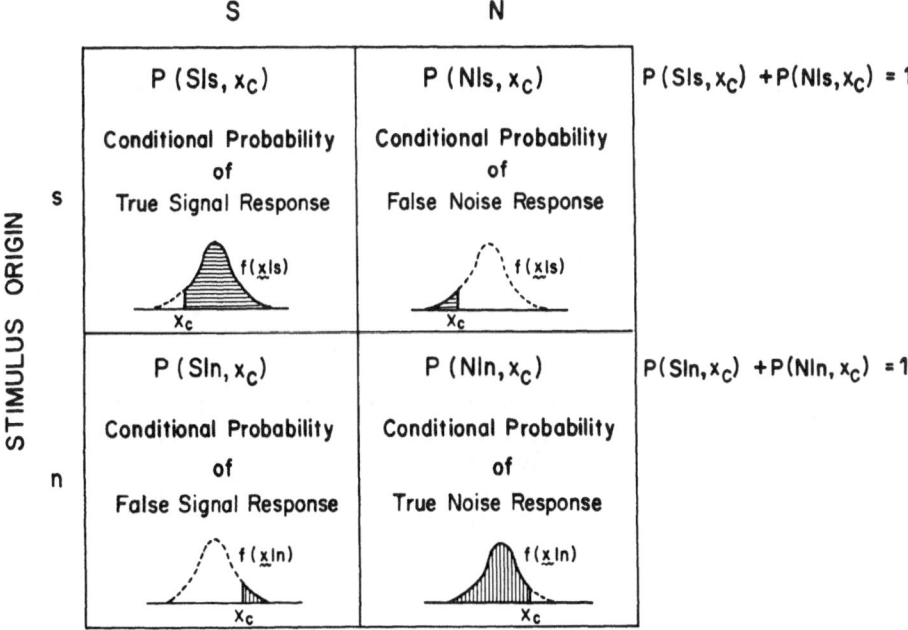

Figure 2: Stimulus-response matrix.

ROC CURVES - INTERPRETATION, MEASUREMENT

The information in the stimulus-response matrix characterizing the sensitivity and specificity of an imaging system operating at a given threshold level can be represented as a point on a two-dimensional graph. As the threshold is varied and x_c takes on each possible value of $\tilde{x}$, the set of points generated will determine the so-called receiver operating characteristic (ROC) curve which is

$$P(S|s,x_c) \text{ vs } P(S|n,x_c). \tag{6}$$

The ratio of the conditional probability of a true "Signal" response (based on criterion level x_c) to the conditional probability of a false "Signal" response (based on criterion level x_c) is given by:

$$\frac{P(S|s,x_c)}{P(S|n,x_c)} = \frac{\int_{x_c} f(x|s)dx}{\int_{x_c} f(x|n)dx} \quad \frac{\text{the area under the right-hand tail of the signal-plus-noise distribution}}{\text{the area under the right-hand tail of the noise distribution}} \tag{7}$$

Figure 3 illustrates the way in which the noise distribution as well as the signal-plus-noise distribution are partitioned into various areas by the indicated decision criterion levels, $x_c(1)$ to $x_c(5)$. Each of these criterion levels then defines an appropriate $P(S|s)$ and $P(S|n)$ as can be seen from equation 7. As one adopts an increasingly conservative criterion level moving from $x_c(1)$ to $x_c(5)$, one can reduce the false positive decision rate at the cost of a decreased true positive decision rate, i.e., one is essentially trading sensitivity for specificity.

Thus, criterion level $x_c(5)$ used to define category 5, in which the decision-maker feels that an outcome of $x > x_c(5)$, is much more likely to have come from the signal-plus-noise distribution than noise distribution, i.e., the signal is "almost definitely present." Decision criterion levels $x_c(4)$ and $x_c(5)$ define category 4, in which the decision-maker feels that outcomes of x_c $x_c(4)$ but less than $x_c(5)$ are more likely to have come from the signal-plus-noise distribution than the noise distribution, but not as likely as outcomes of x_c $x_c(5)$, i.e., the signal is "probably present". In general, decision criterion levels $x_c(n-1)$ and $x_c(n)$ came from the signal-plus-noise distribution rather than the noise distribution. The categories may thus be given qualitative description such as:

(5) = "almost definitely present"

(4) = "probably present"

(3) = "unsure"

(2) = "probably not present"

(1) = "almost definitely not present"

h categories can be used to develop an ROC curve by the use of a
ing procedure wherein the decision-maker rates his degree of
fidence regarding the presence of a signal. For example, in a
ing procedure an observer might be asked to respond on a scale
1-5, corresponding to his degree of confidence that a signal is
sent in a given trial (image). These five confidence levels
ht, for example, correspond to $x_c(1)$ through $x_c(5)$ in Figure 3.
 total data obtained in such a rating experiment may then be
lyzed in Figure 4 which shows how the category scores may be
ratively combined moving from category 5 back to 1, indicating
 total number of outcomes that would have exceeded each category
eshold. This hypothetical data results in the ROC curve shown
Figure 5. It is not important that all observers adopt the same
terion levels or thresholds; rather, that the various categories
vide a discrete sampling of the decision thresholds available to
h observer.

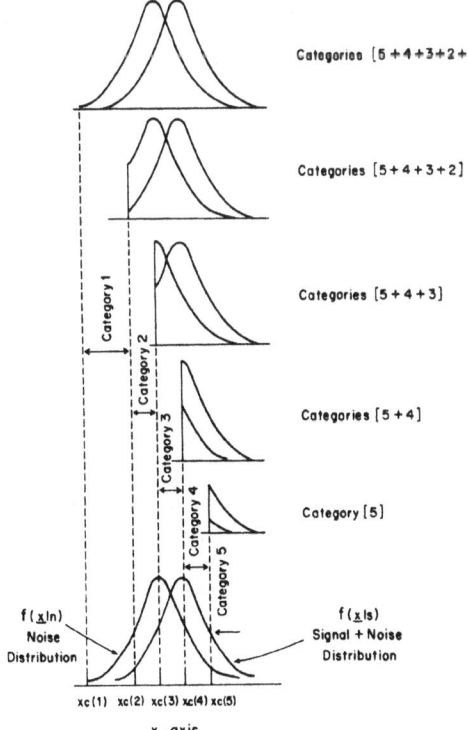

Figure 3: Decision
criterion levels.

CATEGORY

	1	2	3	4	5	
	Almost definitely not present	Probably not present	Unsure	Probably present	Almost definitely present	
No. of signal outcomes placed in category:	2	14	34	34	16	TOTAL = 100 SIGNAL OUTCOMES
No. of noise outcomes placed in category:	16	34	34	14	2	TOTAL = 100 NOISE OUTCOMES

A

CATEGORIES:

	(1+2+3+4+5)	(2+3+4+5)	(3+4+5)	(4+5)	(5)	
No. of signal outcomes placed in categories:	100	98	84	50	16	
No. of noise outcomes placed in categories:	100	84	50	16	2	B

CATEGORIES:

	(1+2+3+4+5)	(2+3+4+5)	(3+4+5)	(4+5)	(5)	
% of signal outcomes placed in categories:	100	98	84	50	16	
% of noise outcomes placed in categories:	100	84	50	16	2	C

CATEGORIES:

	(1+2+3+4+5)	(2+3+4+5)	(3+4+5)	(4+5)	(5)	D
Probability of a signal outcome placed in	1.0	.98	.84	.50	.16	= P (S|s)
Probability of a noise outcome placed in	1.0	.84	.50	.16	.02	= P (S|n)

Figure 4: Hypothetical example illustrating the method in which ROC curves are developed from the data collected in a rating procedure experiment.

A. Responses of a decision-maker to 100 trials containing both signal and noise (i.e., 100 signal outcomes) and 100 trials involving noise (i.e., 100 noise outcomes).

B. Category scores from Figure 4, A, cumulated successively from right to left.

C. Cumulated category scores from Figure 4, B, expressed as percentages of the total number of signal outcomes and noise outcomes, respectively, showing the relative areas under the respective right-hand tails of the signal-plus-noise and noise distributions defined by each criterion level (Fig. 3).

D. Results from Figure 4, C, expressed as conditional probabilities of correctly identifying the stimulus origin.

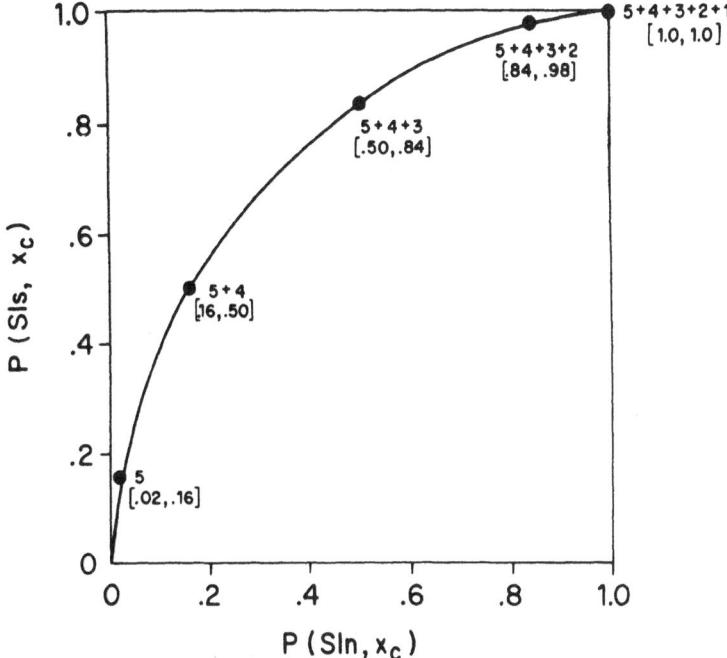

Figure 5: ROC curve resulting from the data shown in Figure 4, D. The ordinate represents the conditional probability of a correct signal response, while the abscissa represents the conditional probability of a false signal response.

The ability of a detecting system to distinguish between outcomes of the signal-plus-noise and noise distributions will increase as the amount of overlap between the two distributions decreases. The amount of overlap of gaussian distributions of equal variance $(\sigma_s^2 = \sigma_n^2)$ may be characterized by the parameter $d' = (m_s - m_n)/\sigma_n$, where d' increases as the amount of overlap of the two gaussian distributions decreases. Hence, the amount of overlap of the two distributions will decrease and d' will increase as the separation between the means of the two distributions $(m_s - m_n)$ increases and/or the standard deviation $(\sigma_s = \sigma_n)$ of the distributions decreases. The parameter d' is an index of detectability and may be considered to be a measure of the signal-to-noise ratio. ROC curves as a function of increasing signal detectability, i.e., increasing d', are shown in Figure 6. It may be said that for these types of ROC curves, detectability increases as the entire ROC curve moves upwards; and that in moving along a given ROC curve from bottom to top, an observer is generally trading increased sensitivity for decreased specificity.

One problem of relating ROC curves to the signal and noise parameters of the image is that the actual decision variable of the

30

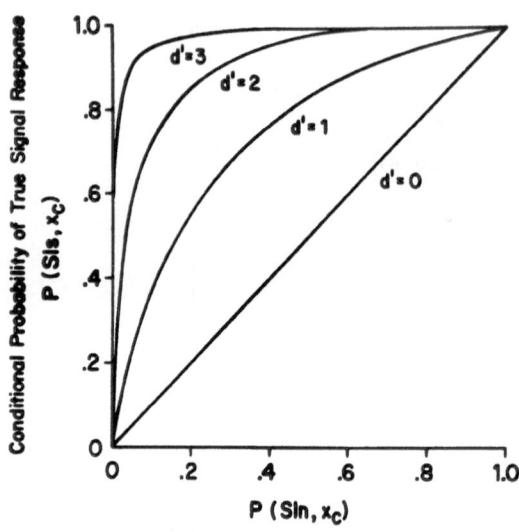

Figure 6: ROC curves for d' = 0, d' = 1, d' = 2, and d' = 3. The
d' = 0 curve generated by the values of $P(S|s,x_c)$ and $P(S|s,x_c)$ as
x_c takes on each possible value of x, when $f(x|s)$ and $f(x|n)$ are
completely overlapping gaussian distributions of equal variance
$(\sigma_s^2 = \sigma_s^2)$, is the positive diagonal of the ROC graph. This ROC
curve will result from any completely overlapping distributions,
because $p(S|s,x_c) = P(S|n,x_c)$ for all values of x_c.

human observer is not known. If one considers the situation presented in Figure 7, one sees that outcomes of some random variable
x describing some physical stimulus are now the input to the eye-
brain system of an observer rather than the input to an ideal
detecting system.

The external random variable x is now processed by the eye-
brain system of the observer. The external variable x may be transformed to some new random variable $y = g(x)$ at the sensory level
(for example, changes in the light photons per given area per given
time may yield logarithmic changes in spike (action potential
firing) frequency of the optic nerve). The transformation process
may be accompanied by incomplete transmission of information as
represented by the non-perfect transfer function of Figure 8 (16).
Additional noise may be added by the processing system itself, and
thus at the sensory level one may find the probability distribution
due to the noise, and due to the signal plus noise to be $f_1(y|n)$
and $f_1(y|s)$ respectively.

It is necessary to discuss an often overlooked factor in a
signal-detection task; namely, the process of visual search wherein
many different areas must be tested for the possible presence of

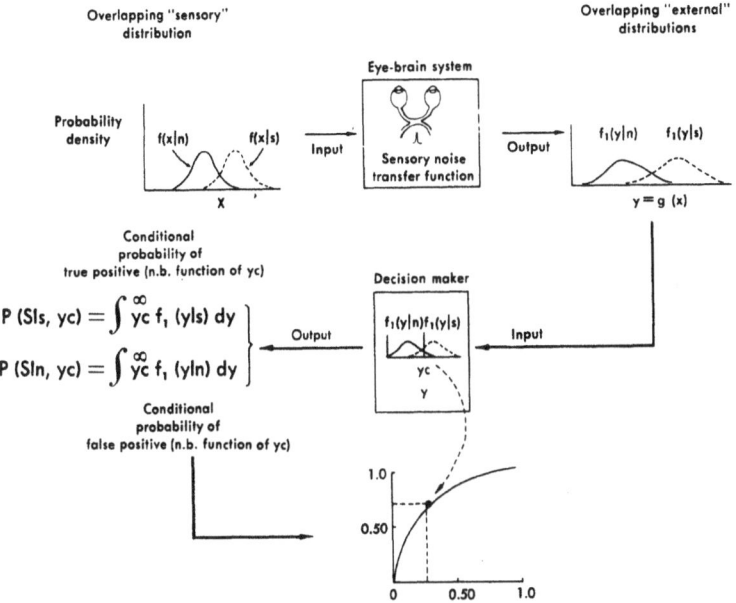

Figure 7: Schematic illustration of transformation of physical variable to sensory variable.

the signal (17). Figure 9 illustrates the expected change in a typical ROC curve as the number of M, of possible independent test areas in which a single signal may occur once or not at all, is increased. In this case, the predictive equations are:

$$P(N|n,y_c,M) = (N|n,y_c)^M \tag{8}$$

and

$$P(S|s,y_c,M) = \{1-P (N|s,y_c)\} P(N|n,y_c)^{M-1} \tag{9}$$

It should be noted that this model does not require the decision-maker to identify correctly the one signal outcome from the (M-1) noise outcomes, in order for response "S" to be considered correct. Excellent agreement has been found between the theoretical predictions of this model and the experimental results of increasing the background area of a radiograph being searched for the possible presence of a signal (17).

The use of this search model results in a possible explanation of the differing reported values of the signal-to-noise ratio necessary for threshold detection. Figure 10 shows how the threshold signal-to-noise ratio will vary as a function of the number independent areas that must be tested. In this case, one must also choose a value of the false positive rate that will accompany the

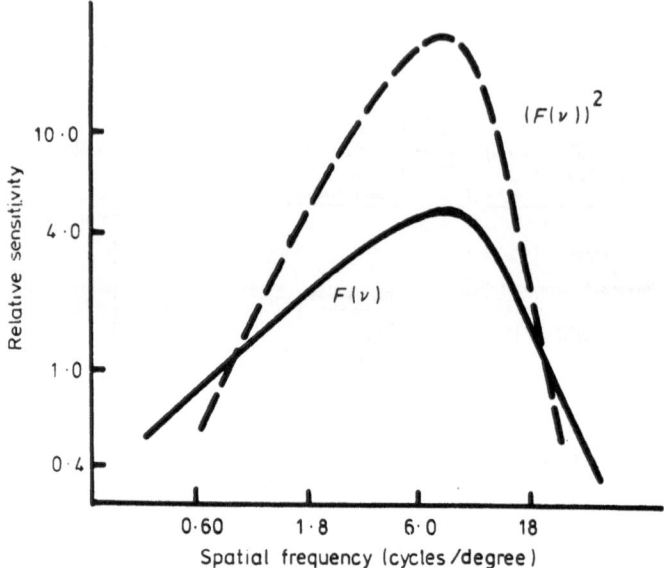

Figure 8: A describing function for the human visual system.

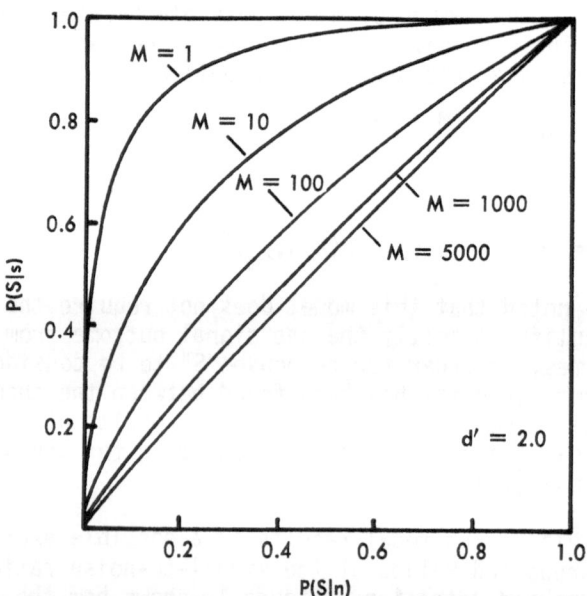

Figure 9: ROC curves as a function of the number (M) of independent test areas in which the signal may occur.

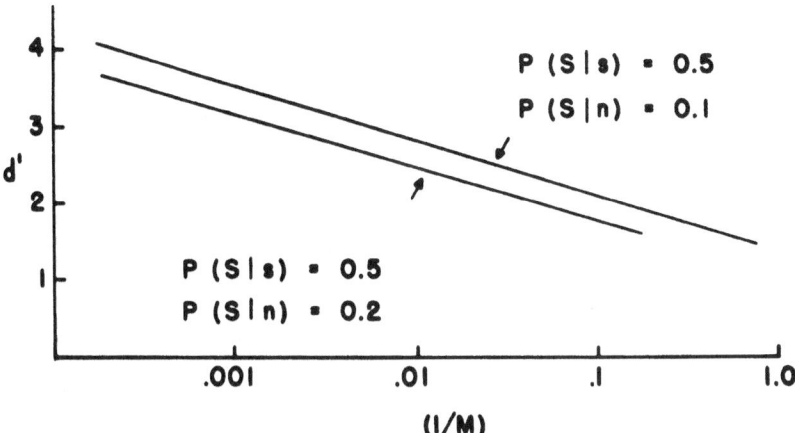

Figure 10: Signal-to-noise ratio needed for specified detection rates as a function of 1/M.

50% true positive rate usually required. One can see that for realistic values of M, the threshold value of d' will range from about 1 to 5, in agreement with several published studies (18,19).

Modification of the above arguments and recent experiments have confirmed that signal-detection theory can be extended to observational tasks where the observer is required to identify the correct localization L, (up to some predetermined limits) of a visual signal in order to receive credit for a true-positive response.

The extremely grave errors that can result from failing to take localization requirements into account, was first documented by Metz and Goodenough (13), who reanalysed data on noise smoothing in Nuclear Medicine images.

Kuhl et al. (21) had studied observer performance as a function of the amount of scan smoothing in nuclear medicine images. Resulting values of d' characterizing observer performance were compared and shown to range from -0.5 to +0.5 with no apparent trend in increase performance due to increased smoothing. This data was reinterpreted by Metz and Goodenough (20). To extract a meaningful measure of d', the data must first be corrected for the fact that the signal could occur in any one of four (independent) test areas. A model was applied that corrected the data for the "quadrant" identification detection task, and new d' values that result are shown to the right of Figure 11. The data points shown in the figure correspond to the unprocessed data (Case 1) and three degrees of increasing smoothing (2 to 4).(21)

34

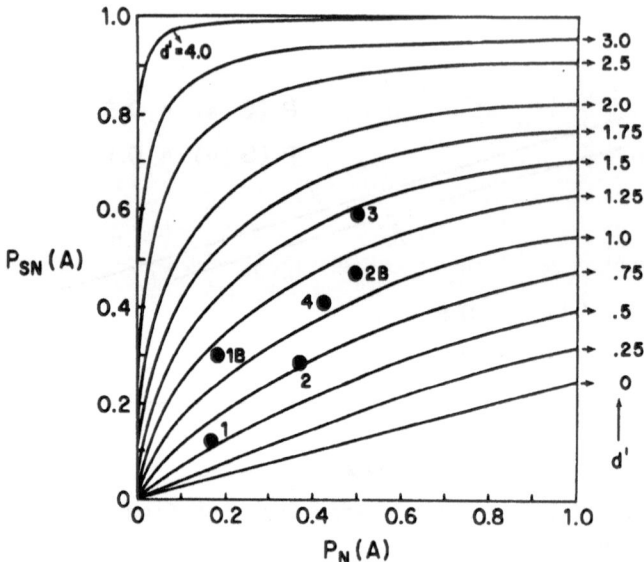

Figure 11: ROC curves for localization experiment with four data points indicating increased amounts of smoothing. (20)

After correction for search, the experimental data shows increased observer performance (i.e., the sensory value of d' is increased) by all three degrees of smoothing. It is of interest that process 3 yields a "corrected" sensory signal-to-noise ratio d' of about 1.5, which in the uncorrected value of d', is not much greater than zero or "guessing". This corrected sensory value is close to the stated physical signal-to-noise ratio of 1.8 ± 0.3, which is the largest sensory value of d' theoretically attainable by the observer performing a matched filtering operation on the input data (22).

Additional experiments were later reported confirming the general validity of the localization modification to conventional ROC curves (23). The resulting ROC curves were called LROC curves. It is important to note that LROC curves can be predicted and related to conventional ROC curves, which are usually easier to develop and record experimentally.

Success has been reported in extending signal-detection theory to the case where the observer may be required to determine the number of signals or lesions present in the field (24). Experimental data has been shown which supports a theory describing the relationship between the ROC curve describing detection of a single signal and the ROC curve(s) describing the detection of multiple signals in the field. The observer is required to state, in effect, how many signals he decides to be present. It has been shown how signal detection theory can be used to predict observer performance in this complex task from knowledge of the conventional ROC curves measured for the simple detection task. These predictions were tested for the case in which zero, one, or two visual signals were known to be present. For this case, the generalized ROC curve is a curve in six-dimensional space, which can be represented by a set of five two-dimensional graphs (24).

Indices of ROC Performance

A recent comprehensive review of indices of complete ROC curves or points thereon, has been given by Swets (25). One major approach is the empirical observation that empirical ROC curves tend to plot as straight lines on double probability (normal deviate) graph paper. The curve (line) then can be characterized by its slope and intercept. The previously discussed measure d' applies rigorously only to ROC curves having unit slope.

The area under the conventional ROC curve can be shown to equal the fraction of correct responses that would result from an experiment in which the observer considers two images (or sets of data) simultaneously, one of which contains a signal (or is due to a disease state), and must choose the image containing the signal (or the data set associated with the disease state). Thus the area under an ROC curve provides a measure of discrimination ability (2).

Several caveats must be kept in mind in estimating ROC curves from single points on the curve. Conventional ROC curves are such that the estimate of d' based on one point will be lower as that point is more to the right.

In comparing two points, the value of d' associated with P_1 may be higher than the value of d' for P_2, even though P_1 may be on a curve consistently lower than the curve on which P_2 falls (26).

A reasonably good estimate of accuracy could be obtained from a single point if accuracy were indexed by the amount of information (in bits) obtained from each observation (27).

Isoinformation curves (on probability coordinates) are concave toward the upper left corner; their slope is generally less than unity for prior probabilities of signal greater than 0.5, and their slope is generally greater than unity for prior probabilities of signal less than 0.5. Considering a prior probability of 0.5, the concavity is pronounced enough so that data points lying along an ROC of unit slope could vary considerably in information transmitted for constant accuracy (25).

A recent modification of ROC theory is the development of the Free Response Operating Characteristic (FROC) curve (28). This

modification offers theoretical justification for a practically
simpler methodology of developing "ROC-type" data in a two dimensional format that includes aspects of both localization and multiple
signal occurrence (28). The basic assumption of this modification
is that the probability of a false positive follows a Poisson distribution and, therefore, that the mean number of false positives per
region is sufficient to fully describe their rate of occurrence.

The earlier work (24) on multiple-signal detection has stated
that, although not representable in two dimensions, the data can be
reasonable well predicted from the simpler single-signal experimental approach. The FROC study claims that rather than being
consistent with two-dimensional data, the multiple-signal results
actually are two-dimensional data. Furthermore, FROC multiple-
signal experiments with accurate location is basically simple. The
practical importance of this simplicity is that multiple-signal
experiments with accurate location can be quick and efficient.

In essence, the FROC approach involves a trained observer
inspecting an image with multiple signals and indicating on the
image possible signal locations with appropriate confidence levels.
The data is then plotted as $P(S|s)$ versus mean number of false posi-
tives per sample area (this latter quantity can be explicitly trans-
formed to $P(S|n)$ for the assume Poisson process).

Recent work by Hanley and McNeil (29) has shown that in the
"rating" method of ROC curves, the area under the ROC curve represents the probability that the image obtained on a randomly chosen
diseased subject is correctly rated with greater suspicion than an
image on a non-diseased subject. In addition, they show that this
probability can be described by the non-parametric Wilcoxon statis-
tic, thus providing expressions for sampling variability independent
of functional form of the underlying distributions (29).

EXPERIMENTAL RESULTS OF OBSERVER PERFORMANCE WITH MEDICAL IMAGES WITH PRESCRIBED SIGNALS

The available literature, although relatively sparse and non-
conclusive, indicates that in considering detection of low contrast
objects, the medical imaging modality must render a large signal-
contrast-to-noise amplitude ratio; that is, not only must there
exist enough contrast in the signal compared to the size and the
mean luminance level of the display, but also the signal contrast
must be sufficiently (different) large compared to the noise, in
order to avoid confusion between the signal and the statistical ex-
cursions of the noise. The signal-to-noise ratio, d', however, is
not a generally reliable figure of merit for evaluating "diagnostic"
importance of contrast and noise in a medical image. One must consider not only the amplitude of the statistical fluctuations, but

also the characteristic appearance or pattern of the noise. This character or pattern of the noise can become very important and is experienced in CT and radiography as quantum mottle or in nuclear medicine as a "blobby" pattern following certain noise smoothing operations. The appearance of the noise is important in that certain types of noise may look more or less like the signal or object of interest, and thus may be more or less easily confused with the object. In addition, certain types of noise may effectively "mask" a given signal. In a related sense a general perceptual problem which may arise in viewing a noisy image, is that not only may the particular object of interest be obscured by the noise, but the overall image can in a more global sense be "disturbing". This latter type of perceptual problem -- involving questions of pattern recognition -- is one of the more fundamental problems in the medical imaging field. Let us examine two fairly straightforward applications of ROC theory for radiography and nuclear medicine.

Radiography

A signal detection experiment was conducted on the detection of a simulated radiographic signal in a situation where contrast and noise could be controlled separately (17, 30). In this experiment a low contrast 2 mm diameter light signal could be projected onto random locations of uniformity exposed radiographic samples of the types mentioned above, with each type exhibiting the coarse fluctuations in density, called radiographic mottle, which results from the interaction of the optically degrading point spread function characteristics of an intensifying screen with the Poisson fluctuations of the number of x-ray quanta absorbed in the screen.

Figure 12 shows the experimental ROC curves which resulted from using three different contrast levels of the signal added to the noise background resulting from the RPR/PS intensifying screen/film combination. The designation B, 1.25B and 1.56B indicates two successive 25% increases in signal contrast $(m_s - m_n)/m_n$, relative to the signal contrast B which is approximately 1%, where m_s and m_n represent the respective signal and noise luminance levels (31).

Figure 13 can be used to examine the signal detectability of the same small light spot signal projected onto the two different types of noise background. It is interesting to note that these experiments indicated that increases in contrast or decreases in noise amplitude both produced increases in sensory signal-to-noise ratio (d'). In fact, for this particular experiment a slight advantage was observed for increased contrast rather than nominally equivalent decreases in noise.

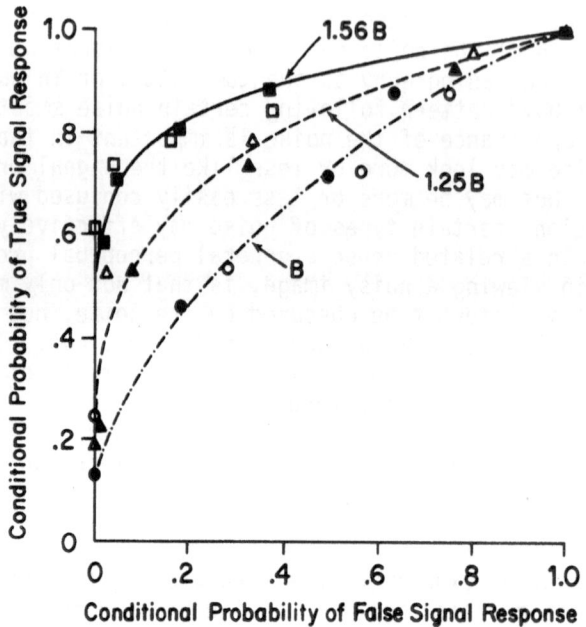

Figure 12: ROC curves resulting from changes in signal contrast.

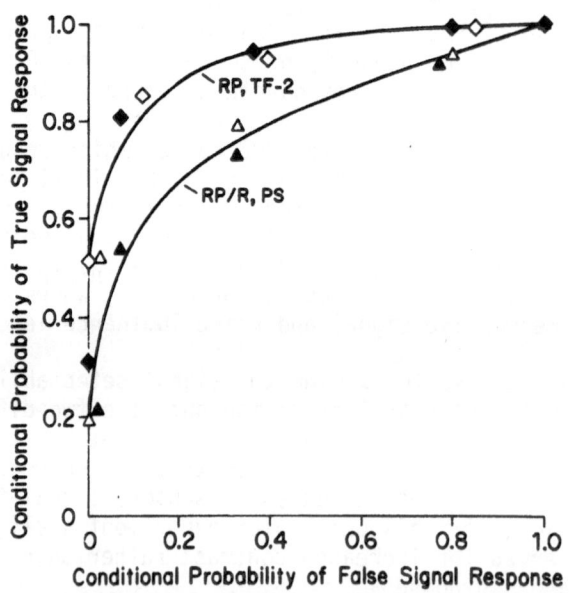

Figure 13: ROC curves resulting from two different types of radiographic mottle backgrounds, onto which is projected a 2 mm diameter signal of 1% contrast level.

Nuclear Medicine

It is well known that certain filter functions may be used in image manipulation of medical images, in order to achieve resolution enhancement or noise smoothing. As mentioned previously, the data by Kuhl et al. (21) after correction for search, show that the sensory value of d' is increased by all three cases of smoothing. It is interesting to note that process 3 yields a sensory signal-to-noise ratio of 1.8 ± 0.3, which would be the largest sensory value for d' attainable theoretically by the observer performing a matched filtering operation on the input data (22).

Models of Observer Performance

It should be pointed out that the noise (σ_D) introduced by decision-making need not necessarily be noise associated with the eye's acquisition of the physical data (e.g., additive random bio-logical fluctuations down the optic nerve), but rather, this noise could also be introduced by the relative inability of a decision-maker to correctly store and reproduce his decision-criterion level. As his ability to store the exact position of this criterion level varies, then it can be shown that his effective signal and noise distribution will be a convolution of the processed physical distributions with the probability distribution describing his ability accurately to reproduce his criterion level (32, 33).

If one assumes that in certain cases the human observer can adopt a 'matched filter' appraoch to detection of noise-limited signals -- that is to 'tune' his eye for a specific signal type -- then, for certain simple cases (e.g., detection of disc-shaped signals in white; Poisson, stationary noise), one would expect d', the signal-to-noise ratio, to be given by:

$$d' = C/\sigma_T \tag{10}$$

where C is the signal contrast, and σ_T is the total relative standard deviation of the noise at the decision-making level, which in the simplest case (independent, additive noise) would be given by

$$\sigma_T{}^2 = \sigma_P{}^2 + \sigma_D{}^2 \tag{11}$$

where σ_P is tha standard deviation of the physical noise and σ_D is the standard deviation of the decision-making noise.

Moreover, one can use the data shown in Figure 10 and the rela-tionships between d', C and σ to predict that

$$C_{req} \propto (K_1 \log (\frac{1}{M}) + K_2) \ (\sigma_P{}^2 + \sigma_D{}^2)^{\frac{1}{2}} \tag{12}$$

This equation predicts that the required contrast will have logarithmic dependence on M -- the number of "independent" test areas in which the signal may occur -- (which will be affected by the total field size A and the signal area a {disc signals}), K_1 and K_2 being constants derived from Figure 10.

Thus, for $P(S|s) = 0.50$, $P(S|n) = 0.20$, values can be estimated for $K_1 = 0.75$ and $K_2 = d'$ (at $M = 1$) $= 1$. This relationship seems reasonable in the sense that for $M = 1$, the required contrast C_{req} will be given by:

$$C_{req} \propto (\sigma_p + \sigma_D)^{\frac{1}{2}} \tag{13}$$

$$\propto (\frac{1}{na} + \sigma_D^2)^{\frac{1}{2}}$$

Where n is the mean count density of a white, Poisson noise distribution and a is the area of the signal.

This relationship can be fitted quite well to the data of Kohlenstein (34) shown in Figure 14 describing observer performance in detecting lesions in simulated radionuclide scans, in which similar results were obtained from about 10,000 observations.

In these simulation experiments, signal and noise parameters were independently controlled.

The principal conclusion from the radiographic signal-detection experiment and the radionuclide scan experiments is that, in both studies, changes in relative signal amplitude (contrast) were slightly more effective in a signal-detection sense than corresponding changes in $(\sigma_p)^{-1}$, a conclusion that is in good agreement with the theoretical predictions of an internal noise source, or similar uncertainty in maintaining a decision criterion.

The implications of an internal noise source should be very important in the design of imaging systems and data processing techniques. Techniques such as certain types of resolution enhancement, which tend to increase contrast and noise σ_p at the same rate, should actually increase human detection performance, especially at fairly high count rates ($\sigma_p \leq \sigma_D$). Equivalently, techniques which tend to decrease contrast and noise at the same rate, such as certain types of smoothing, should tend to decrease human detection performance.

Caution, however, must be advised in interpreting these statements without carefully weighing the effect of processing techniques on signals and noise of very different spatial frequency composition, for example, coarsely digitized images. In this case contrast and

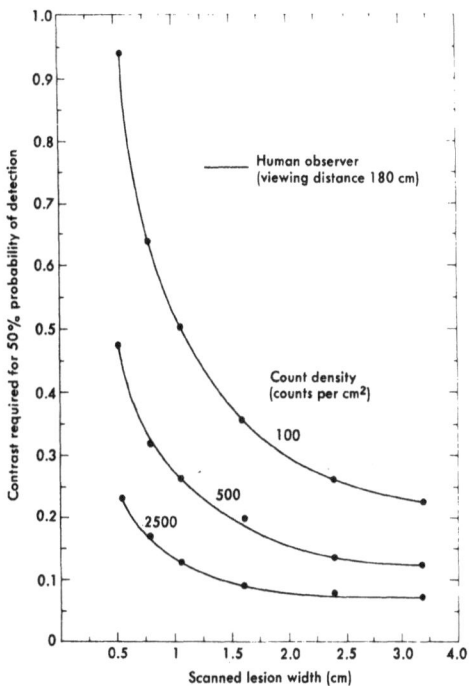

Figure 14: Contrasts required for the human observer to have a
50% probability of detection.

noise might not be changed at the same rate, as for example in the
Kuhl (21) studies; moreover, certain noise patterns may be psycho-
logically objectionable to the human observer as mentioned earlier.

This latter point concerning the importance of the character
of the noise resulting from image processing techniques has been
investigated by Pizer and Todd-Pokropek (35) in an ROC experiment
in which the observer would try to locate lesions in smoothed scintigrams with fixed resolution and fixed signal to noise ratio but
varying noise character. Figure 15 shows observer performance data
for detection of varying sized signals (holes) and varying types of
noise sizes (or, character). In particular, the detection data
shown in Figure 15 reveals that if smoothing is to be done, then
with regard to noise character alone, the following holds: for
small lesions, much smoothing is most desirable, and a medium amount
of smoothing (producing many medium-sized noise blobs) is least
desirable; and for large lesions, little smoothing is most desirable
and much smoothing (producing many large noise blobs) is least
desirable.

This conclusion might be loosely summarized as saying that the
character of the noise causing the most "signal-like" undulations

42

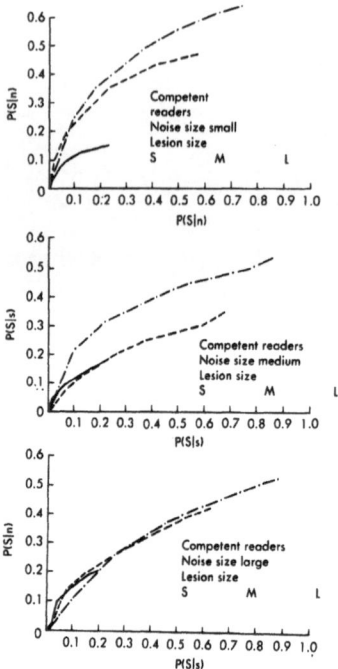

Figure 15: ROC curves for three different lesion sizes and three different noise sizes. (35)

(blobs) is most deleterious to signal detection performance.

Extension of Detection Theory to Complex Radiologic Diagnoses

It was pointed out in the introduction that signal detection theory has been applied to the evaluation of complex radiologic diagnostic procedures. These studies have generally used ROC techniques only as an empirical measurement of relative error rates (true- and false-positive response frequencies) associated with different diagnostic systems or diagnostic procedures. It is important to establish a data base for describing decision-making at the output end of the diagnostic process. Moreover, there is much recent progress in establishing the relationship between ROC analysis and determination of diagnostic benefit (1, 24). However, relatively little success has been reached in establishing the relationship between diagnostic error rates and the physical parameters of the image. This relationship seems fundamental in the sense that improvements in the physical parameters of the image may be relatively insignificant at the diagnostic level if uncertainties in the decision-making factors should turn out to be the limiting factor in accurate diagnosis.

One might then ask what factors might enter into the overall diagnostic process in such a way as to perturb the extension of the results of simple signal-detection experiments to complex diagnoses. One such factor which must certainly enter into the process is the formidable task of pattern recognition in an image which is basically a 2-d display of 3-d data. The structures within the image are obtained from differing angles of projection and differing magnifications. Images of structures overlapping the signal may be enhanced or diminished causing various levels of complexity in detecting the signal. A signal found in one location may have a detectability and implication different from a signal found in another location. The pattern of the signal is often noncontinuous and must be integrated across breaks in the pattern due to structural or stochastic sources of variation. Thus, one must determine the effect of the image parameters on the ability of the radiologists to perform such perceptual tasks as gestalt completion (or 'closure' of broken figures) and 'hidden' figure identification.

It may not be surprising that recent studies utilizing pattern recognition principles for computer diagnosis of pneumoconiosis have shown that the 'trained' computer could rather readily obtain a normal-abnormal classification rate comparable to the average physician error rate when reading the same representative sample of pneumoconiosis films (36,37). Moreover, on this latter point on the nature of the perceptual task, important articles (38,39) have pointed out the importance of peripheral (global) vision in interpreting chest radiographs in even short flashes of a radiograph. Thus, results based on scanning an image for an isolated abnormality on a region-by-region basis with an aperture type (fovealvision) detector should be carefully weighed before assuming application to a more complex diagnostic task.

It seems clear that signal detection theory and ROC curves appear to offer strong theoretical appeal to assessment of medical imaging systems when the signal (or signals) can be appropriately defined and adequate task definition (e.g., localization) provided. The major limitation at this time, to the extension of this methodology to complex medical images (such as chest radiographs), appears to be in the ability to define an unambiguous signal or disease state, for which a truly representative sampling set can be provided under controlled conditions. An elegant example of a well constructed ROC protocol (40) for rigorous evaluation of diagnostic systems in medicine was recently applied to a comparative study of two radiologic techniques. Accuracies of computed tomography and radionuclide scanning in detecting, localizing, and diagnosing brain lesions were assessed in an ROC methodology with a sample of patients in whom tumor had been suspected. Computed tomography was found to be substantially more accurate than radionuclide scanning. Moreover, significant impace could be seen from localization, history and differential diagnostic requirements (40).

To explain further the problems of the "ambiguous" signal, consider a study which amy appear at first to run counter to the ROC approach, but which rather is intended to begin to investigate the complexities of identifying physical and anatomical signal)s) and noise in chest radiographs (41).

The selection of a screen/film system for portable chest x-ray procedures if often a difficult choice. In particular, the advent of fast screen/film systems, many of them using rare-earth phosphors, has compounded the task facing the physician who must make a decision based on the diagnostic trade-offs between motion unsharpness, spatial resolution (including geometric unsharpness), contrast, noise (graininess of quantum mottle), patient exposure and practial utility Whereas the faster systems may offer advantages for reduced motion unsharpness (particularly for the limited radiation output of certain portable chest units), they may also be accompanied by decreased spatial resolution and increased noise.

A panel of radiologists were asked to choose on the basis of their clinical experience, anatomic landmarks appearing in posterior/ anterior (P/A) chest radiographs whose visualization is related to the visualization of significant findings. These anatomic landmarks were then assigned weights and integrated into an evaluation form shown in the accompanying Table I. In addition, physical factors, as defined and interpreted by radiologists, were assembled into a second evaluation form as shown in Table II. Phantom and patient radiographs were then prepared for evaluation.

In this preliminary experiment, the data for total anatomical and physical parameters agreed closely for both patient and phantom radiographs. The data for the detail parameter showed that slow speed systems score highest when used with phantoms, while fast systems score best when used with patients. The phantom data show perceived system quantum mottle increasing with system speed as is usually observed. However, one fast System (D) was an important exception in that the phantom graininess curve was ranked highest (best). In addition, System (D) seemed to show a clear preference for contrast in the phantom radiograph as opposed to the patient radiographs. The performance of System (D) appears to be the result of optimizing the combination of motion unsharpness, intrinsic resolution, and noise.

A major weakness of the study is the somewhat arbitrary assignment of initial weighting factors. On the other hand, the value of such studies is that they might eventually help yield the actual weighting factors.

A statistical analysis was performed using one-way analysis of variance with unequal cell sizes followed by the Student-Newman-Keuls Test to compare the statistical significance of mean score

TABLE I

SUBJECTIVE ASSESSMENT OF ANATOMICAL PARAMETERS

Total Score = 100

BONY THORAX (ribs & clavicles) (10)   RETROCARDIAC AREA (30)   TRACHEA (15)

Cortical Margins (5)   Left Diaphragm (15)   Visible To: (15)

( ) optimally visualized (5)   ( ) totally visualized (15)   ( ) left main stem bronchus (15)
( ) adequately visualized (4)   ( ) partially visualized (7)   ( ) carina (10)
( ) poorly visualized (2)   ( ) not visualized (0)   ( ) neck and upper mediastinum (5)
( ) not visualized (0)   ( ) disease precludes   ( ) not visible (0)
( ) disease precludes   evaluation (N)   ( ) disease precludes
  evaluation (N)   evaluation (N)

Trabeculae (5)   Spine (15)

( ) optimal detail (5)   ( ) too well visualized (7)
( ) adequate detail (4)   ( ) optimally visualized (15)
( ) poor detail (2)   ( ) acceptably visualized (7)
( ) not visualized (0)   ( ) poorly visualized (3)
( ) disease precludes   ( ) not visualized (0)
  evaluation (N)   ( ) disease precludes evaluation (N)

DIAPHRAGM (15)   PULMONARY VASCULATURE (30)

Diaphragm Outline (15)   Maximum Measurable To: (30)

( ) both visualized (15)   ( ) right costophrenic angle (30)
( ) right only (7)   ( ) right mid-lung (20)
( ) left only (7)   ( ) right descending pulmonary artery (10)
( ) not visualized (0)   ( ) none (0)
( ) disease precludes   ( ) disease precludes evaluation (N)
  evaluation (N)

TABLE II

SUBJECTIVE ASSESSMENT OF PHYSICAL PARAMETERS

OVERALL FILM QUALITY (100)

( ) optimal (100)
( ) good (67)
( ) poor, but diagnostic (33)
( ) unacceptable (0)

PHYSICAL FACTORS (100)

Contrast (35)   Density (15)

( ) optimal (35)   ( ) optimal (15)
( ) good (23)   ( ) good (10)
poor, but diagnostic   poor, but diagnostic
  ( ) too gray (11)   ( ) too dark (5)
  ( ) too black/white (11)   ( ) too light (5)
unacceptable, not diagnostic   ( ) unacceptable (0)
  ( ) too gray (0)
  ( ) too black/white (0)

Graininess (20)   Detail (30)

( ) no grain visible (20)   ( ) optimal (30)
( ) minimal grain (13)   ( ) good (20)
( ) grainy, but does not   ( ) poor detail, but does not
  interfere with diagnosis (6)   interfere with diagnosis (10)
( ) grain interferes with diagnosis (0)   ( ) lack of detail, interferes
      with diagnosis (0)

data. More significant differences were observed for phantom radiographs than for patient radiographs. This result may have been due to the inherent differences between a phantom and a patient (e.g., patient motion and overlying structure), or variations between patients. The difference in the data between patient and phantom data is most noticeable for the "detail" parameter. For "detail", the only significant difference for patient radiographs was seen between the highest speed systems, consistent with, but not proving, the hypothesis that the extent of patient motion is probably an important aspect of perceived detail.

One of the more interesting results of the preliminary work is the fact that one finds a statistically significant reversal preference on the total physical score when comparing phantom radiographs versus patient radiographs for System B (the conventional system) and System D (over twice as fast). It is concluded that motion and/or other yet unidentified sources of difference between static phantoms and patients should be carefully kept in mind in attempted evaluation schemes.

It is hoped that more sophisticated ROC observer performance tests can be developed which will allow the "unfolding" of one disease state from another, and that multidimensional analysis will allow meaningful assessment of diagnostic weighting factors.

This paper examines relative image parameters of screen/film radiography and Computed Tomography. The examination concentrates primarily on large area contrast, noise, and signal-to-noise parameters that might be used to describe the limitations on the detection of an isolated tumor-type signal embedded in a homogeneous surround. It is recognized that this model is useful primarily to determine basic physical limitations of the two types of diagnostic imaging systems. (Figure 16)

PHYSICS AND PSYCHOPHYSICS OF COMPUTED TOMOGRAPHY & RADIOGRAPHY

Certain parameters are known classically to affect the human ability to perceive visually the existence or absence of some abnormality or "signal" in a diagnostic image. These parameters include contrast, noise and sharpness (42).

At normal viewing levels of about 100 foot-lamberts, one is limited to perceiving signals of about .01 contrast (1%) even under optimal circumstances of a large signal and noiseless background (43).

The noise in a diagnostic x-ray image is ultimately limited by the finite number of x-ray photons that may be used in making up the image. This finite number of x-ray photons is related to the sensitivity of the diagnostic system used to obtain the image. The amplitude and appearance (character) of the noise fluctuations can diminish the ability to perceive a radiologic signal (44).

The sharpness of the signal boundary is determined by the intrinsic resolution properties of the diagnostic imaging system, as well as by motion unsharpness arising from the inherent movement of the anatomical part of interest and the particular exposure time required to record the image (45).

The overall assessment of diagnostic image quality reflects a complicated interrelationship of many physical and psychophysical parameters, as may be seen in the accompanying Table 3. In addition, the important questions of pattern recognition and structure noise further complicate the evaluation of diagnostic image quality (42).

CONTRAST IN RADIOGRAPHY AND COMPUTED TOMOGRAPHY

Contrast in Radiography

The relationship between density and the transmitted light, T, coming through the radiograph (when placed on the viewbox) is given by:

$$D = -\log_{10} T \qquad (14)$$

If T_S and T_B represent the respective transmission through the signal and background, then it can be shown that the radiographic contrast, (C_R) is approximately equal to:

TABLE 3

Experimental parameters to be controlled and specified in evaluation of human observer detection performance.

(1) Image parameters

  a. Signal to be detected: size, shape, inherent contrast

  b. Number of possible signals

  c. Image system: spatial resolution (MTF), sensitivity,
      linearity, noise (amplitude and character), speed
      (dose)

  d. Non-signal structure: grid lines, anatomy

(2) Observational parameters

  a. Display system

      Brightness scale
      Gain
      Offset
      Any nonlinearity
      Magnification/minification

  b. Viewing condition

      Viewing distance
      Ambient room brightness

  c. Detection task

  d. Number of observations

(3) Psychological parameters

  a. a priori information given observer

  b. Feedback given observer (if any)

  c. Observer experience for other given parameters:

      Clinical versus non-clinical familiarity with signal,
      display, and especially with type of noise artifacts
      to be expected.

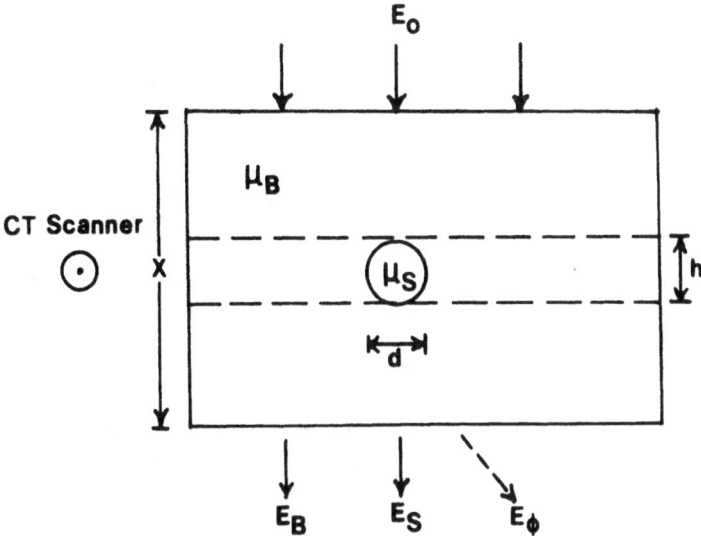

Figure 16: Schematic illustration of model used to compare radiography and Computed Tomography. Spherical signal of diameter d and
absorption coefficient μ_S embedded in homogenous media μ_B. E_0 is
the incident exposure, E_B the exit exposure from the surround, E_S
the exit exposure under the signal region, and E_ϕ the exposure from
scattered radiation. The CT slice width is given by h.

$$C_R = \frac{T_S - T_B}{T_B} \tag{15a}$$

$$C_R = G(\mu_S - \mu_B) \, d \, \frac{E_B}{E_B + E_\phi} \tag{15b}$$

where d is the diameter of the signal, E_ϕ is the exposure due to
scattered radiation, and E_B is the exposure due to primary radiation.
Equation 15b indicates that increased radiographic contrast can be
obtained from increasing the film gradient G, or from increasing
difference between the x-ray linear attenuation coefficient of the.
signal μ_S and background, μ_B, (i.e., subject contrast), or by
increasing the diameter d of the signal, or by reducing scattered
radiation.

Contrast in Computed Tomography

In the case of homogeneously composed volume elements, the
CT output has been reported to be related linearly to the "effective" linear attenuation coefficient (μ), characterizing the volume
element under investigation. In fact, it has been reported that
the CT number, ξ, is given by:

$$= K_1 \ \frac{(\mu - \mu_W)}{\mu_W} \tag{16}$$

where μ_W is the linear attenuation coefficient of water and K_1 is a constant (46). This relationship states that for homogenous substances, differences in μ from μ_W (the approximate linear attenuation coefficient of water at E = 73 kev, is 0.190 cm^{-1}) are linearly amplified by a factor of K_1 in order to establish the CT number, which can then be displayed as some relative light intensity on a CRT screen. In the original Hounsfield numbering scale, (Air = -500, Water = 0, and Bone = +1000), K_1 is approximately 1000 and k_1/μ_W is approximately 5260. The exact relationship between the CT number and the linear attenuation coefficient is complicated by the fact that the CT system uses a polychromatic spectrum of x-ray energies (for example, an x-ray tube operating at 100 kVp, 120 kvP, or 140 kVp)(47).

Another question of the applicability of this linear relationship is that the x-ray intensity contribution may vary over the object volume. Therefore, the relative x-ray intensity distribution at each point within the object volume must be determined to predict the (weighted average) attenuation coefficient that will be assigned to the particular volume element. An example of this position dependent effect can be seen by the differences in the images of the same nominal beads, which differ only in their depth within their own relative volume elements (48).

To estimate the contrast between the signal region and the background region in CT, one can assume that the luminance display function is linear over some local range of interest.

In viewing a CT image, a "window" is selected for viewing a given subset of the total range of CT numbers available from the reconstruction. This window has a lower value, a central value and an upper value. The difference between the upper and lower value constitutes the "window width". The width of the window describes the total range of CT values selected for viewing. In the sense that the CT number is essentially a scaled version of an effective linear attenuation coefficient, the selection of the window width can then be considered as selection of two effective linear attenuation coefficients, namely: the lower window width is the particular CT value, ξ_L (or corresponding linear attenuation coefficient - μ_L), below which all CT values appear at the same darkest shade of grey available on the display; the upper window width is the particular CT value (ξ_U) (or effective linear attenuation coefficient μ_U, above which all CT values appear at the lightest shade of grey available on the display. The window is usually centered on the value of the average background CT value (ξ_B) or attenuation value

(μ_B) of interest (e.g., tissue on water-like value).

For example, typical window settings might be: central value of 0 Hounsfield units and window width of 100 Hounsfield units. Such window settings might correspond to linear attenuation values of:

$$\mu_B = \mu_w \simeq .190 \text{ cm}^{-1}$$

$$\mu_L = .180 \text{ cm}^{-1}$$

$$\mu_U = .200 \text{ cm}^{-1}$$

$$\mu_L = \mu_B = -.010 \text{ cm}^{-1}$$

Then let

$$= CT\# = K_1 \frac{(\mu - \mu_w)}{\mu_w} \tag{17}$$

$$T = \text{luminance function} = K_3 (\xi - \xi_L) = K_4 (\mu - \mu_L) \tag{18}$$

$$\xi_L = CT\# \text{ of lower window settings } (\mu_L) \tag{19}$$

Then

$$C_{CT} = \frac{T_S - T_B}{T_B} = \frac{\mu_S - \mu_B}{\mu_B - \mu_L} \tag{20}$$

Where

μ_B = linear attenuation coefficient of background

μ_S = linear attenuation coefficient of signal

μ_L = linear attenuation coefficient corresponding to lower window setting

μ_w = linear attenuation coefficient of water

K_1, K_3, K_4 = Constants

The term in the denominator of the CT equation (μ_B minus μ_L) is an extremely important parameter in CT imaging. The normal contrast-latitude loop of a radiographic screen film is usually invariable after photographic development, but within a CT system, the contrast-latitude loop is left variable and subject to operator selection. Thus, in choosing to examine some given subregion of the continuum of attenuation values found between air and bone, one is basically selecting a "window" or subset of values to view at a given time (for example, a high contrast and low latitude; or a low contrast and a wide latitude view of the same object). Freeing the viewer from a given contrast-latitude range is an important attribute of CT systems.

Comparison of Contrast in Computed Tomography and Radiography

Using the relationships between the visual contrast given by radiography, and that of CT, then;

$$C_{CT} = C_R / \{ G(\mu_B - \mu_L) \ d \} \tag{21}$$

This relationship predicts that contrast in CT is greater than that in radiography whenever the product of G, $(\mu_B - \mu_L)$, and d is less than unity. Then, in the sense that a typical window setting, $\mu_B - \mu_L$ is approximately .02 cm^{-1}, this equation shows that in terms of visual contrast, radiographic signals will have to have extremely large diameters (several centimeters or larger), and/or have high differential attenuation coefficients to present contrast level competitive with CT. Note, however, the parameter $(\mu_B - \mu_L)$ involved in the so-called window settings (choice of contrast and latitude in the CT system) is a key factor enhancing the relative performance of CT versus radiography. Using other means of expanding the contrast scale in radiography, such as certain kinds of television contrast stretching techniques, might decrease the contrast advantage of CT.

What limits the ability to do this?

Any image processing technique, including those used in CT and those that one might seek to apply to radiography, will be limited by the signal-to-noise ratio levels that are an intrinsic property of the acquired information. Thus, if the noise level is very large, it makes little sense to augment or stretch the contrast of objects within the image, because this will increase or blow up the noise fluctuations as well as the signal contrast.

Does CT have inherent advantages over radiography in terms of signal-to-noise ratio?

NOISE IN RADIOGRAPHY AND COMPUTED TOMOGRAPHY

Noise in Radiography

Certain fundamental limitations are imposed upon image quality

by the necessity for use of a finite radiation dose in most radiographic procedures. A finite radiation dose implies an upper limit
to the number of x-ray photons that will be stopped by the recording
system (the image receptor). In most photon-limited imaging systems,
a basic uncertainty in information level results from the Poisson
statistics characterizing the x-ray beam.

The blurring or unsharpness which accompanies the transducing
operation of a radiographic screen/film combination, also introduces changes in the appearance and amplitude of the statistical
x-ray fluctuations which constitute the primary source of "noise" in
the radiographic x-ray beam (35). In a sense, these fluctuations
are also "imaged" by the screen. Sharply varying (uncorrelated from
point to point) noise fluctuations in the image are not found;
rather, the noise (or density fluctuations) take on a characteristic
mottled (or correlated) appearance. Instead of "salt and pepper"
sharply varying density values across a uniformly exposed film,
relatively larger areas of "Quantum mottle", high and low density
patches are found (34). In many ways the blurring operation can be
considered as a "noise smoothing" effect.

In terms of the light (T) transmitted through the illuminated
radiograph, the relative (noise) fluctuations around the mean transmission value ($\sigma(T)/T$) are given by the following equation (42):

$$\frac{\sigma(T)}{T} = \frac{G}{\bar{n}_x^{\frac{1}{2}} a^{\frac{1}{2}}} F \qquad\qquad (22)$$

As noted earlier in the equation describing radiographic contrast, the parameter G and a parameter related to the size of the
signal (in this case the area of the signal being searched "a") are
found. In addition, one now finds the expected number of absorbed
photons per unit area $\bar{n}_x$, as well as an important parameter "F"
which is related to the inherent resolution properties or Modulation
Transfer Function of the recording system (34,42).

In particular, note that the relative noise fluctuations for
1 cm diameter signals for present medium speed film/medium speed
screen combinations are less than one part in a thousand (this
results from stopping about 10^7 x-ray photons per cm^2 of screen)
(41). However, the other problem with noise is that the human
observer responds to borders or edges (high spatial frequencies) and
even a large signal with a low contrast unsharp edge may have important edge information obscured by noise fluctuations (42,49).

Noise in Computed Tomography Systems

An equation often used to describe the relationship between the standard deviation of the attenuation values per unit pixel element, $\sigma(\mu)$, in a CT scanner with pixel element dimension (w), slice thickness (h), and the patient dose (D), is given by

$$\sigma(\mu) \sim \frac{1}{D^{1/2} w^{3/2} h^{1/2}} \tag{23}$$

This relationship, however, is simplistic in that it ignores the important question of the character of the noise that results from the combination of photon statistics and the choice of a filter function. A rigorous treatment of the noise in a CT scan requires consideration of the auto-covariance properties of the noise (51).

Signal-to-Noise Ratios

Let the signal-to-noise ratio, d', be defined as signal contras to noise amplitude; then, it can be shown that for signals considerably larger than resolution blur sizes, that for CT:

$$d'_{CT} \doteq \frac{10^4}{2} (\mu_S - \mu_B) a^{\frac{1}{2}} (whD)^{\frac{1}{2}} \tag{24}$$

and for Radiography

$$d'_R \doteq (\mu_S - \mu_B) d \bar{n}_x^{\frac{1}{2}} a^{\frac{1}{2}} \tag{25}$$

Then, for the same x-ray spectrum, if we assume, $\bar{n}_x^{\frac{1}{2}} = 3 \times 10^3 cm^{-1}$, w = .15cm, h = 1.3cm, D = 2 rad, and in the absence of a significant scatter fraction:

$$\frac{d'_{CT}}{d'_R} = \frac{10^4 (whD)^{\frac{1}{2}}}{2d \bar{n}_x^{-\frac{1}{2}}} \simeq \frac{3}{2d} (whD)^{\frac{1}{2}} \sim \frac{1}{d} \tag{26}$$

where d, the diameter of the circular target is expressed in centimeters.

In the presence of scatter, this relationship must be modified to:

$$\frac{d'_{CT}}{d'_R} = \frac{1}{d} \frac{(E_B + E_\phi)}{E_B} \tag{27}$$

The exact relationship between the signal-to-noise ratios is obviously dependent on the degree of scattered radiation, and the choice of values for K_2, w, h, D, and $\bar{n}_x$. The inverse relationship of this ratio on the signal size seems clear. Thus, at some signal size (on the order of a few centimeters) the signal-to-noise ratio of CT should become less than that of radiography. The principal signal-to-noise ratio advantage of CT over radiography appears to be in detection of a signal with a diameter of a few centimeters or less.

Several caveats must be kept in mind in this analysis: (1) even if signal-to-noise ratios were equal for CT and radiography, contrast enhancing techniques may still be necessary in radiography to make the signal contrast perceptible -- however, the basic signal-to-noise ratio would be adequate to do so; (2) the degrading effect of the scatter contribution is important in radiography, and its magnitude could require signals to be an order of magnitude larger than previously suggested before radiography could compete (for example, in dense regions of the abdomen) with CT; (3) the analysis so far has ignored potential differences in spatial resolution and motion unsharpness; (4) the simple model does not present differences in the perceptual tasks of "projection" radiography versus "tomographic" imaging, nor does it include effects of peripheral vision (52).

RESOLUTION FACTORS IN RADIOGRAPHY AND COMPUTED TOMOGRAPHY

Resolution in Radiography

There are three basic sources of resolution degradation or unsharpness in screen/film radiography: (1) motion unsharpness -- the blurring of a point due to the motion of the patient during the exposure time of the procedure; (2) receptor unsharpness -- the inherent blurring operation caused by the transducing or conversion of x-rays into light within the intensifying screen; and (3) geometric unsharpness (focal spot unsharpness) -- the blurring due to the finite size and x-ray intensity distribution of the x-ray focal spot. Combinations of these sources generally lead to an overall blurring or defocusing effect.

This blurring or unsharpness may be characterized by its spatial extent, which is generally the blur size or "point spread function", or by the Modulation Transfer Function (MTF), which describes how the spatial frequencies that make up an object are transferred by the image recording system.

The overall system point spread function might be considered a Gaussian-shaped function. This approximation is convenient in that a rotationally symmetric Gaussian distribution may be fully described by a single parameter, namely its standard deviation ($_T$) which is a measure of the width of the distribution and the extent of the blurring. A specification of u for each of the three blurring sources mentioned previously, may be used to describe the relative blurring effect of each source of unsharpness; motion unsharpness (u_m), receptor unsharpness (u_r) and geometric unsharpness (u_g). In addition, by assuming that the individual blur functions are Gaussian, the overall unsharpness or blurring function is given by the root mean square (rms) of the individual blur contributions.

$$u_T = \sqrt{u_m^2 + u_r^2 + u_g^2} \tag{28}$$

This equation and Table 4 indicate how the various blur sources combine into an overall general blur or degradation function for radiography where, M is the magnification and "t" the exposure time (41). A good estimate of the total overall blur width is given by 4u or 95% of the area under the Gaussian distribution.

$$u_T = (\frac{u_r^2}{M^2} + u_m^2 t^2 + u_g^2 \{\frac{M-1}{M}\}^2)^{\frac{1}{2}} \tag{29}$$

In particular, a motion unsharpness value of $4u_m$ = 5 mm/sec is used. Certain advantages can be obtained from magnification studies, in that the focal spot, image receptor and patient motion blur factors may be carefully selected so as to produce some reduced overall unsharpness. Scatter is generally considered independently of MTF and is considered a contrast reducing factor. Moreover, magnification is often used with an airgap technique which reduces the scatter contribution without the need for grids. Of course, it can be noted from Table 4 that the x-ray generator output and the focal spot size (both the nominal and actual size) will be important in determining the limits of magnification (41,53).

Resolution in Computed Tomography

Some of the same resolution factors encountered in Radiography enter into the overall consideration of resolution in CT; e.g., u_r and u_g. Motion, however, is not a tractable and may manifest itself differently as artifact(s) rather than blurring, depending on the sampling scheme and type of motion encountered.

One may consider u_r to be related to the detector aperture width and u_g to be related to the focal spot width. Both unsharpness values must, of course, be related to a given image plane and will therefore be influenced by the geometric design, particularly M. M is the focal spot-to-detector distance divided by the focal

TABLE 4

Magnifi-cation M	Relative Exposure Time t	Focal Spot Unsharpness 4_{u_g}	Screen/Film Unsharpness 4_{u_r}	Motion Unsharpness 4_{u_m}	Total Unsharpness 4_{u_T}
1.0	0.2 secs	1 mm	0.33 mm	5 mm/sec	1.05 mm
1.5	0.3	1	0.33	5	1.55
2.0	0.4	1	0.33	5	2.07
1.0	0.2	2	0.33	5	1.05
1.5	0.3	2	0.33	5	1.66
2.0	0.4	2	0.33	5	2.24
1.0	0.1	1	0.66	5	0.83
1.5	0.15	1	0.66	5	0.93
2.0	0.2	1	0.66	5	1.17
1.0	0.1	2	0.66	5	0.83
1.5	0.15	2	0.66	5	1.10
2.0	0.2	2	0.66	5	1.45

spot-to-pivot distance, and is on the order of 1.4 to 2 for conventional systems and up to the order of 2.5 for CT systems offering geometric enlargement. Even first-order consideration of these blurring functions, with u_g and u_r on the order of 1 mm or so, will rapidly reveal that CT systems will be challenged to achieve spatial resolution levels much beyond 1 cycle/mm, particularly if one requires a full body section (or head) scan to be obtained within a few seconds. Small focal spot size required for increased resolution will be challenged to produce adequate x-ray intensity (and thus "contrast resolution" as dictated by low noise levels) within short scan times.

Then, too, for CT one must consider an important factor which is not usually encountered in radiography; namely, sampling rate and sampling pattern. Moreover, the sampling rate and sampling pattern are dependent on the type of geometry (generation) utilized in the CT scanner. First, second and fourth generation designs tend to offer a redundancy of spatial sampling becuase of the ability to interrogate (sample) the detector at an almost unlimited number of times (or spatial positions) for a given "view" or angular position of the scan. Of course, a certain penalty may be paid by total scan time, but artifacts due to undersampling (aliasing) may be essentially removed. Current third generation designs, with fixed focal spot source location, on the other hand, may be ultimately limited by the fact that the fixed source-detector configuration enables a redundancy of "views" (sampling at different angular positions), but a limited number of rays or spatial sampling for a given view.

The question of the practical limitation of this technique transcends commercial exploitation and depends ultimately on the degree of spatial resolution required by the diagnostician, and the limit to which he is able to tolerate aliasing (undersampling) artifacts.

In addition, in a 3-D resolution sense, there is a limit to how small a signal CT systems might detect because of the volume averaging effect (the influence of slice width as well as the pixel) and the inferior spatial resolution of CT systems compared to that of radiography. For small objects where the contrast (in particular the edge perception) is strongly influenced by MTF, (i.e., related approximately to the integral of the square of the MTF), the contrast in CT and radiography will be weighted by the spatial resolution properties of the radiographic system compared to the spatial resolution properties of the CT system in a quadratic or square nature (54).

ANALYSIS OF UPTAKE RATIO FOR NUCLEAR MEDICINE

One may wish to know the minimum uptake ratio for a given size lesion at a given depth which makes a lesion just perceptible in a nuclear medicine study (55). One can solve for the uptake ratio in terms of the physical parameters, by assuming that the uptake is greater than the background. The minimum uptake radio (u), is then given by (55):

$$U = 1 + \frac{SNR \cdot (1 - \exp(-\mu t)) \cdot (1 + \alpha/\mu)}{\mu \sqrt{n_B/A} \cdot V \cdot \exp(-\mu d)} \qquad (30)$$

From this formulation one can solve for the value of U necessary to image various effective lesion areas (A), and volume V, at various depths (d). n_B is the areal count density, μ is the attenuation of the background of thickness t, and α is scatter correction function depending on window settings, etc. It is uncertain as to the value of signal-to-noise ratio (SNR) to use, but a conservative estimate of 5 may be necessary for the complex tasks involved in clinical imaging. Note that because of the definition of SNR used in this test, this actually reflects a value of about 3.5 by most definitions (55,56).

To illustrate the results, assume the values listed in Table 5. Using these parameters, the uptake ratio needed to achieve this level of the SNR has been calculated as a function of lesion diameter, lesion depth, and background count density. It can be seen in Figure 17 that small lesions at depths >5cm become exceedingly difficult to detect.

TABLE 5

PARAMETERS USED IN LESION DETECTABILITY MODEL

Signal-to-noise ratio, SNR   5.0

Linear attenuation coefficient, μ .15 cm^{-1}

Intrinsic detector resolution, σ_i .2 cm

Collimator resolution, $\sigma_G(0)$ .1 cm

Collimator thickness, ℓ 2.54 cm

Medium thickness, t   30.0 cm

At a depth of about 5 cm using what might be considered a high resolution collimator (FWHM = .8 cm at this depth), these considerations require an uptake ratio of about 14 to detect a 1 cm diameter lesion with a background count density of 1000 counts/cm^2. As the lesion size becomes small compared to the system resolution, the image size and the effective area approach a constant value determined by the spread function of the imaging system. The net number of counts within this area is dictated by the total activity within the lesion, which in turn is a function of the volume of the lesion. This quantity which depends on the 3rd power of the lesion diameter accounts for the rapid increase in the minimum uptake ratio necessary for detection as the lesions become smaller. This relationship is demonstrated in more detail in Figure 18, which shows the uptake ratio as a function of lesion diameter for several depths.

The effect of the background count density is important. For the case where the uptake ratio is large compared to the value 1, the second term in this equation dominates, and the uptake varies inversely with the square root of the background. For example, if an uptake ratio of 10 is necessary when the background is 1000 counts/cm^2, then an uptake of about 5 would be required if the background were increased to 4000 counts/cm^2 with all other parameters being the same.

While the results have been applied to the situation of "hot" lesions, the formalism is valid for "cold" lesions as well. The quantity (U-1) can be replaced with its absolute value in order to handle both cases. A lesion which contains no activity gives a factor which is equivalent to an uptake ratio of 2, which is the maximum that a "cold" lesion can present. It can be seen from

60

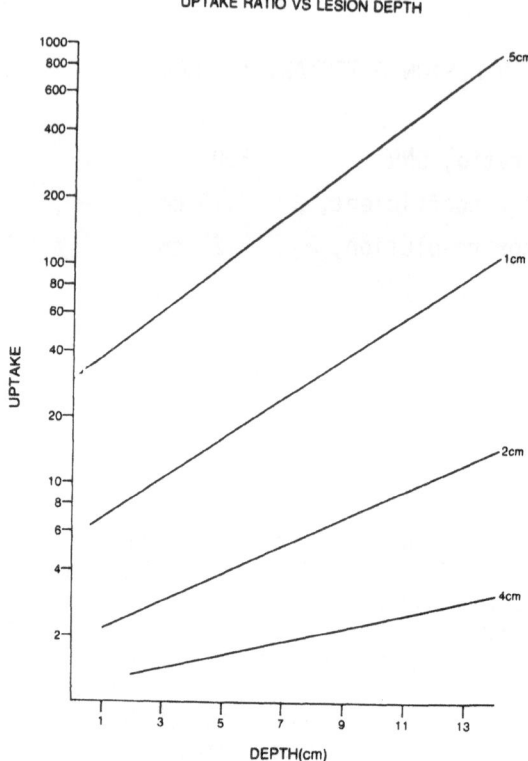

UPTAKE RATIO VS LESION DEPTH

<u>Figure 17</u>: Uptake ratio versus lesion depth for four different signal diameters.

Figures 17 and 18 that there are very few conditions in which the uptake ratio necessary for detection is less than or equal to a value of 2. A 4 cm diameter "cold" lesion satisfies this for all depths up to the midline of a 30 cm medium, and hence should always be detectable if multiple projections are obtained. Likewise, a 3 cm "cold" lesion would be detectable at most depths. However, a 2 cm diameter "cold" lesion could be visualized only when it is near the surface (<3cm). The task of detecting sub 1 cm lesions is clearly formidable within the current state-of-the-art camera imaging as reflected by this model. To detect this lesion at greater depths would require some combination of higher spatial resolution and count densities. It may, in fact, turn out that emission computerized tomography may provide the only approach to imaging small "cold" lesions in the range of 1 cm diameter at depth.

Finally, it should be mentioned that the display system or image recording medium will affect the contrast and noise presented to the observer and has not been addressed in this first order

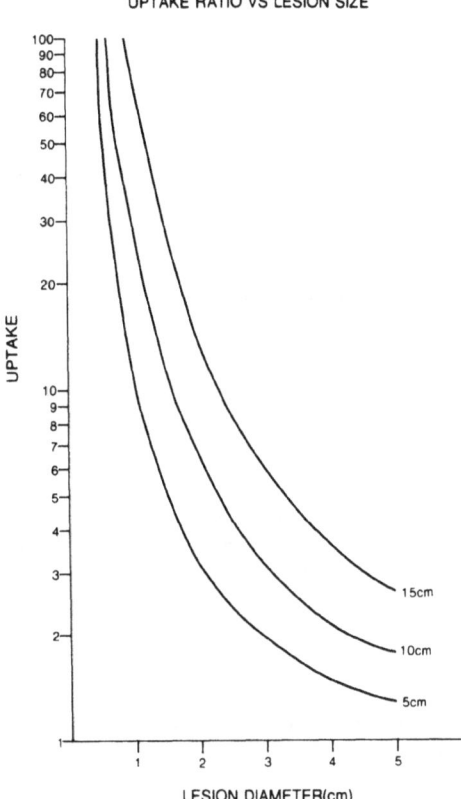

Figure 18: Uptake ratio versus lesion size for three different depths.

model, although other authors have considered this effect. In addition, image processing techniques might also prove to be useful in the future in enhancing the detectability of low contrast lesions which would reduce the minimum uptake ratio further.

REFERENCES

1. Metz, C.E. "Basic Principles of ROC analysis." Seminars in Nuclear Medicine 8:283, 1978.

2. Green, D.M. and J.A. Swets. "Signal Detection Theory and Psychophysics." (New York, John Wiley & Sons, 1966) Reprinted: Huntington, New York, Robert E. Krieger Publishing Co., 1974.

3. Peterson, W.W., Birdsall, T.G., Fox, W.C. "The theory of signal detectability." Transactions IRE Professional Group on Information Theory PGIT 4:171, 1954.

4. Lusted, L.B. "Observer error, signal detectability and medical decision making." Computer Diagnosis and Diagnostic Methods. (Springfield, Charles C. Thomas, 1972)

5. Egan, J.P. and F.R. Clarke. "Psychophysics and signal detection." Experimental Methods and Instrumentation in Psychology (J.B. Sidowsky: McGraw-Hill, 1966, p. 211).

6. Swets, J.A. "The relative operating characteristic in psychology." Science 182:990, 1949.

7. Garland, L.H. "Scientific evaluation of diagnostic procedures." Radiology 52:309, 1949.

8. Yerushalmy, J., Harkness, J.T., Cope, J.H., et al. "Role of dual reading in mass radiography." American Review of Tuberculosis 61:443, 1950.

9. McNeil, B.J., Varady, M.S., Burrows, B.A., et al. "Cost effectiveness in hypertensive renovascular disease." New England Journal of Medicine 293:216, 1975.

10. Kundel, H.L. "Factors limiting roentgen interpretation -- physical and psychologic." Current Concepts in Radiology (E.J. Potchen: C.V. Mosby, St. Louis, 1972, p. 1)

11. Andrus, W.S., Dreyfuss, J.R., Jaffer, F., et al. "Interpretation of roentgenograms via interactive television." Radiology 116:25, 1975.

12. Anderson, Jr., T.M., Mintzer, R.A., Hoffer, P.B., et al. "Nuclear image transmission by picturephone." Investigative Radiology 8:244, 1973.

13. Alcorn, F.S., E. O'Donnell. "The training of nonphysician personnel for use in a mammography program." Cancer 23:879, 1969.

14. Sheft, D.J., Jones, M.D., Brown, R.F., S.E. Ross. "Screening of chest roentgenograms by advanced roentgen technologists." Radiology 94:427, 1970.

15. Swets, J. and D. Green. "Applications of signal detection theory." Psychology: From Research to Practice (H.L. Pick, Jr.: Plenum Press, 1978).

16. Cornsweet, T.N. Visual Perception, Academic Press, New York.

17. Goodenough, D.J., Rossmann, K., Lusted, L.B. "Radiographic applications of signal detection theory." Radiology 105:199, 1972.

18. Coltman, J.W. and A.E. Anderson. 1960 Proc. IRE 48:858.

19. Rose, A. Vision - Human and Electronic, New York, London, Plenum Press, 1974.

20. Metz, C.E. and D.J. Goodenough. "On failure to improve observer performance with scan smoothing: a rebuttal." Journal of Nuclear Medicine 14:873, 1973.

21. Kuhl, D.E., Sanders, T.D., Edwards, R.P., et al. Journal of Nuclear Medicine 13:752, 1972.

22. Metz, C.E. A Mathematical Investigation of Radioisotope Scan Image Processing. Ph.D. Thesis, University of Pennsylvania, 1969.

23. Starr, S.J., Metz, C.E., Lusted, L.B., Goodenough, D.J. "Visual detection and localization of radiographic images." Radiology 116:533, 1975.

24. Metz, C.E., Starr, S.J., Lusted, L.B., Rossmann, K. "Progress in evaluation of human observer visual detection performance using the ROC approach." Information Processing in Scintigraphy (Raynaud, G, Todd-Pokropek, A.E., eds., Commissariat a l'Energie Atomique, Department de Biologie, Service Hospitalier Frederic Joliot, Orsay, France (1975) 420.

25. Swets, J. "ROC analysis applied to the evaluation of medical imaging techniques." Investigative Radiology 14:109, 1979.

26. Goodenough, D.J., Metz, C.E., Lusted, L.B. "Caveat on use of the parameter d' for evaluation of observer performance." Radiology 106:565, 1973.

27. Metz, C.E., Goodenough, D.J., Rossmann, K. "Evaluation of receiver operating characteristic curve data in terms of information theory, with applications in radiography." Radiology 109:297, 1973.

28. Bunch, P.C., Hamilton, J.F., Sanderson, G.K., Simmons, A.H. "A free response approach to the measurement and characterization of radiographic observer performance." S.P.I.E. Optical Instrumentation in Medicine. 127:124, 1977.

29. Hanley, J.A. and B.J. McNeil. "The meaning and radiologic use of the area under an ROC curve." Radiology. (In Press)

30. Goodenough, D.J., Rossmann, K., Lusted, L.B. "Radiographic applications of receiver operating characteristic (ROC) curves." Radiology 110:89, 1974.

31. Goodenough, D.J., Rossmann, K., Lusted, L.B. "Factors affecting the detectability of a simulated radiographic signal." Investigative Radiology 8:339, 1973.

32. Wickelgren, W.A. Journal of Math. Psychology 5:102, 1968

33. Goodenough, D.J. and C.E. Metz. 1976 Information Processing in Scintigraphy (Raynaud C., Todd-Pokropek, A., Orsay, France: Commisariat a l'Energie Atomique, Departmente de Biologie, Service Hospitalier Frederic Joliot) p. 400.

34. Kohlenstein, L.C. The Johns Hopkins Applied Physics Laboratory Report, CP 028, 1973.

35. Pizer, S.M., Todd-Pokropek, A.E. "Noise Character in processed scintigrams." 1976 Information Processing in Scintigraphy (Raynaud, C., Todd-Pokropek, A.E., Orsay, France: Commissariat a l'Energie Atomique, Departmente de Biologie, Service Hospitalier Frederic Joliot).

36. Kruger, R.P., Thompson, W.B., Turner, A.F. 1974 IEEE Transactions on Systems, Man., and Cybernetics (January) p. 1, 1974.

37. Goodenough, D.J., Weaver, K.E., Davis, D.O. "Development of a Phantom for Evaluation and Assurance of Image Quality in CT Scanning." 1976 Proceedings of The Society of Photo-Optical Instrumentation Engineers Symposium 56:64.

38. Kundel, H.L. "Peripheral Vision: Structured noise and film reader error." Radiology 114:269-273, 1975.

39. Kundel, H.L. and C.F. Nodine. "Interpreting chest radiographs without visual search." Radiology 116:527, 1975.

40. Swets, J.A., Pickett, R.M., Whitehead, S.F., et al: "Assessment of diagnostic technologies." Science 205:753, 1979.

41. Goodenough, D.J. and K.E. Weaver. "Physical Aspects of the Portable Radiograph," in Goodman, L.R. and Putnam, C.E., eds. Intensive Care Radiology: Imaging of the Critically Ill. St. Louis, C.V. Mosby, 1978:315-341.

42. Goodenough, D.J. "Assessment of Image Quality of Diagnostic Imaging Systems," in G.A. Gray, ed., Medical Images: Formation, Perception and Measurements. Proceedings of the 7th L.H. Gray Conference. New York, John Wiley and Sons, 1976:263-277.

43. Blackwell, H.R. "Contrast Thresholds of the Human Eye." Journal of the Optical Society of America 36:624-643, 1946.

44. Rossmann, K "Spatial Fluctuations of X-ray Quanta and the Recording of Radiographic Mottle." American Journal of Roentgenology 90:863-869, 1963.

45. Rossmann, K. "Point Spread Function, Line Spread Function and Modulation Transfer Function: Tools for the Study of Imaging Systems." Radiology 93:257-272, 1969.

46. McCullough, E.C., Baker, H.I., Hauser, O.W., Reese, D.F. "An evaluation of the quantitative and radiation features of a scanning x-ray transverse axial tomograph: the EMI scanner." Radiology 111:709-716, 1974.

47. Weaver, K.E., Goodenough, D.J., Briefel, E. "Sensitometry in computerized tomography." Proceedings of S.P.I.E., Medicine VI, 1977, 127:87-94.

48. Goodenough, D.J., Weaver, K.E., Davis, D.O. "Potential artifacts associated with the scanning pattern of the EMI scanner." Radiology 117:615-619, 1975.

49. Goodenough, D.J., Rossmann, K., Lusted, L.B. "Factors affecting the detectability of a simulated radiographic signal." Investigative Radiology 8:339-344, 1973.

50. Goodenough, D.J. "Psychophysical perception of computed tomography images," in Newton and Potts, eds., Radiology of the Skull and Brain: Technical Aspects of Computed Tomography. C.V. Mosby, St. Louis, 1981.

51. Tanaka, E., Iinuma, T.A. "Correction functions for optimizing the reconstruction image in transverse section scan." Physics in Medicine and Biology 20:789-798, 1975.

52. Kundel, H.L. "Peripheral Vision: Structured noise and film reader error." Radiology 114:269-273, 1975.

53. Weaver, K.E., Wagner, R.F., Goodenough, D.J. "Performance considerations of x-ray tube focal spots." Proceedings of the 1974 BRH/SPIE Symposium on Medical X-ray Photo-Optical Systems Evaluation 56:150-158, 1975.

54. Goodenough, D.J., Weaver, K.E., Davis, D.O. "Physical measurement of the EMI imaging system," in Ter-Pogossian, M.M., Phelps, M.E., Brownell, G.L., Cox, J.R., Jr., Davis, D.O., Evens, R.G., eds. Reconstruction Tomography in Diagnostic Radiology and Nuclear Medicine. Baltimore, University Park Press, 1977:225-243.

55. Atkins, F.B., Goodenough, D.J. "Simulated Uptake Ratio Requirements for Spherical Lesions Imaged with a Conventional Scintillation Camera," in W.C. Eckelman, ed., Receptor-Binding Radiotracers, CRC Press, Inc. (In Press).

56. Tsui, B.M.W., Metz, C.E., Atkins, F.B., Starr, S.J., and Beck, R.N. "A comparison of optimum detector spatial resolution in nuclear imaging based on statistical theory and on observer performance." Physics in Medicine and Biology 23:654-676, 1978.

Part II: Advances in Source and Detector Technology

METHODS OF MICROWAVE
IMAGERY FOR DIAGNOSTIC APPLICATIONS

Lawrence E. Larsen, M.D. and John H. Jacobi, M.S.

Department of Microwave Research
Walter Reed Army Institute of Research
Walter Reed Army Medical Center
Washington, D.C. 20012

INTRODUCTION

The spatial distribution of microwave energy transmitted
from an incident field through a biosystem to a receiving
antenna depends upon features of both the biosystem and the
incident energy. With respect to the incident field, features
such as frequency, polarization, and mode are important
parameters of such a radiative transfer. With respect to the
biosystem, the spatial distribution of dielectric properties and
their time as well as frequency dependencies are the important
parameters. Further, to the extent that the incident flux
density is sufficient to heat the biosystem, power density may
itself effect the spatial distribution of absorbed microwave
energy. This is a consequence of two facts: first the
microwave constitutive parameters of biological dielectrics are
temperature dependent per se; secondly, in situ
thermoregulatory mechanisms may substantially alter the spatial
distribution of complex permittivity as a result of vasomotor
activity.

The basic motivation for diagnostic applications of
microwave imagery is improved physiologic and pathophysiologic
correlation, especially in soft tissue. This expectation is
based on the molecular (dielectric) rather than atomic (density)
based interactions of the radiation with the target when
compared with x-ray imagery. Furthermore, the more than order
of magnitude range of microwave constitutive parameters in soft

tissue compared to the few percent range of densities in soft tissue, suggests improved contrast and better tissue characterization.

The tutorial sections of this paper deal with characteristics of the incident radiation and properties of biosystems as media which are important for the propagation of microwave energy. After a discussion of dielectric properties and various biological considerations, electromagnetic wave descriptors and system design criteria will be considered. This will be followed by a description of actual data collection systems, subsequent image processing and finally image interpretation keyed to known regional specialization in the canine kidney.

The Nature of Dielectrics

Since microwave images are formed on the basis of the spatial distribution of complex permittivity, the nature of biological dielectrics and their role as media for propagation of microwave energy are items of necessary background (1, 2, 3). Electromagnetic waves in the microwave region of the spectrum (typically defined as 300 MHz to 300 GHz in frequency, although a much smaller range of ca. 1 to 10 GHz is suitable for diagnostic imagery) propagate in uniform dielectrics according to

$$E = E_o \exp(-\gamma z)$$

where E_o is the electric field at the origin, E is the scalar instantaneous electric field in the dielectric at a distance z from the origin and γ is the complex propagation coefficient. The complex propagation coefficient is defined as

$$\gamma = \alpha + j\beta = j\omega \sqrt{\epsilon^* \mu^*}$$

where α is the attenuation factor, β is the phase factor, ϵ^* is the complex permittivity, μ^* is the complex permiability and j has its usual significance. The factors α and β are related to the microwave constituative properties of the medium as follows:

$$\alpha = \lambda \omega^2 / 4\pi \, (\epsilon'\mu'' + \epsilon''\mu')$$

and

$$\beta = \frac{2\pi}{\lambda} = \omega \left[\frac{\varepsilon'\mu' - \varepsilon'\mu''}{2} \cdot \sqrt{1 + \frac{\varepsilon'\mu'' + \varepsilon''\mu'}{\varepsilon'\mu' - \varepsilon''\mu''} + 1} \right]^{1/2}$$

where λ is the wavelength, ω is the angular frequency, ie.
$\omega = 2\pi f$, and f is the frequency in Hertz of the electromagnetic
wave. The constituative parameters of μ^* and ε^* refer to the
magnetic (complex permiability) and dielectric (complex
permittivity) properties of the medium. The magnetic properties
are assumed to be those of free space, i.e. purely real with no
attenuation or phase shift. The dielectric properties are
complex as the result of the fact that biological dielectrics
(other than air) contain both conduction and displacement
currents when polarized by an electric field or when immersed in
a time harmonic electric field. The conduction currents
represent current flow that is in phase with the applied voltage
whereas displacement currents are in phase quadrature with the
applied voltage. The complex nomenclature is applied as
follows:

$$\varepsilon^* = \varepsilon' - j\varepsilon''$$

where ε' is the real part of the complex permittivity, known as
the dielectric constant, and ε'' is the imaginary part known as
the dielectric loss factor. It is important to understand that
the loss in question is dielectric, that is, such loss exists in
the absence of D.C. conductivity. The real and imaginary parts
of the complex permittivity represent the complementary
processes of energy storage and energy dissipation,
respectively. Since heat production is related to the product
of frequency and the dielectric loss factor, these are often
combined in the quantity known as dielectric conductivity, σ

$$\sigma = \omega\varepsilon''$$

As a matter of convenience, the complex permittivity is often
normalized to that of free space. That is,

$$\varepsilon^*_r = \varepsilon^*/\varepsilon_o$$

where ε_o is the permittivity of free space and ε^*_r is the relative complex permittivity. Likewise, the real and imaginary part are normalized as follows

$$\varepsilon^*_r = \varepsilon'_r - j\varepsilon''_r = \varepsilon'/\varepsilon_o - j\varepsilon''/\varepsilon_o$$

where ε'_r is the relative dielectric constant and ε''_r is the relative loss factor.

Both ε'_r and ε''_r are important for diagnostic imagery of biological targets in the decimeter wavelengths where the experiments to be later described were conducted. Most biological dielectrics are water dominated. Water has a rather high relative dielectric constant of about 80 at middle microwave frequencies. This accomplishes a significant reduction in wavelength as compared to air since the phase velocity in lossless dielectrics is

$$dz/dt = v = \omega/\beta \text{ and } \lambda_{air}/\lambda_{diel} = c/v \simeq 1/\sqrt{\varepsilon'_r}$$

where β is approximately $c\sqrt{\varepsilon'_r}$ and c is the velocity of light in a vacuum. Thus, the retarded phase velocity results in wavelength contraction to about 1/9 of its value in air. This property is very useful in microwave imaging systems when water serves as a coupling and loading medium for waveguide antennas to probe the fields scattered by organs under study. Water is also rather lossy. At a frequency of 3 GHz, pure water attenuates at a rate of about 3.82 dB/cm. This provides for effective attenuation of wave propagation along the first dielectric interface which suppresses a major component of multipath in forward scatter system geometries. With respect to biologic dielectrics in situ, the measured insertion loss for thorax and abdomen at 2 GHz agree rather well for that predicted on the basis of bulk equivalent muscle at about 50 Nepers/meter or about 85 dB loss for a 20 cm path length (4). At 3 GHz, attenuation is about 60 Np/m or about 104 dB for the same path length. At 4 GHz the loss would be about 134 dB. Because of additional "loss" due to the phase factor, 4 GHz is about the highest practical frequency in abdomen and thorax when using state of the art receivers (noise floor at ca. -140 dBm) and modest amplification prior to the transmitting antenna. In the case of breast scanners, however, appreciably higher frequencies (ca. 10 GHz) may be employed and in the case of head scanners

intermediate frequencies (ca. 6 GHz) may be useful in
transmission systems as a result of the appreciably lower
attenuations of these tissues and the shorter path lengths
involved.

Dielectric properties at microwave frequencies represent
the electrical behaviour of biological materials at wavelengths
short enough that useful spatial resolution may be obtained and
images can be produced. Dielectric properties are relatable to
molecular structure by way of charge asymmetries and rotational
mobilities. These factors are expressed in large part by the
dipole moment. Net charge imbalance along one axis may be
reduced to an equivalent dipole whereupon two charges equal to
plus and minus one electron charge when separated by one
nanometer represent about one half Debye. In these terms, water
has a dipole moment of about 2 Debyes. This may be deduced from
a knowledge of the static (low frequency) dielectric constant of
water. Large molecules may have charge asymmetries that cannot
be resolved along a single axis. Under these conditions, higher
order moments may result such as quadrapole and octapole
moments. Also, a number of dispersion mechanisms exist which
involve various irrotational states of water, side groups and
end groups of large molecules. Alterations in conformational
state also effect dielectric properties in large molecules.
Numerous small molecules such as amino-acids, oligopeptides,
etc. also contribute to dielectric properties in the microwave
region.

Dielectric properties at microwave frequencies of various
tissues in situ are a relatively new area of study with respect
to physiologic and pathophysiologic correlations (5). However,
it may be stated with certainty that various regional
specializations in brain (e.g. white matter as opposed to grey
matter) and kidney (medulla as opposed to cortex) are
represented in both ε_r and σ. Furthermore,
antemortem/postmortem comparisons in brain and changes in renal
permittivity with blood flow do not limit interpretation to
simple changes in blood volume. Certainly, the images to be
presented later in this paper attest to the fact that spatial
variations in complex permittivity are relatable to known
regional specialization in the canine kidney.

A brief comparison of microwave interactions in distinction
with x-ray interactions in biosystems may be useful at this
point. The chief difference between x-ray photons and microwave

photons is their difference in energy. This is a consequence of the ca. 10^9 times higher frequency of photons in the x-ray region of the electromagnetic spectrum. That is

$$e = hf$$

where h is Planck's constant and e the photon energy. Diagnostic x-rays typically have photon energies in the 100 KeV (Kilo-electron-volt) range where as microwave photons at decimeter wavelengths have photon energies in the 10^{-4}eV range. X-ray absorption mechanisms in this range are chiefly K-capture and Compton scattering, both of which may be modeled by exponential functions of the atomic number (s) of the constituent atoms (6). Microwave absorption is based on rotation of molecules or component side chains, end groups, etc. The central notion is that the photon energy of the incident radiation determines which work functions in the target will be addressed. K-capture requires the incident photon to supply the correct energy to dislocate a K-band electron. This is a vastly more energetic process than overcoming the weak inter- and intra-molecular forces in rotatable dipoles. Inasmuch as atomic composition is not uniquely associated with biological function, the biological relevance of x-ray interrogation may be expected to be chiefly structural. This is evidenced by the popularity and often necessity of contrast enhancement procedures in diagnostic radiology. On the other hand, there is reason to believe that the molecular level (especially with respect to secondary and tertiary structure) offers greater promise for biological relevance to health and disease. Examples of this assertion include the importance of secondary, and tertiary structure for enzyme substrate interactions, ligand-receptor interactions and the role of water in the structural stability of biopolymers. It is these hopeful expectations that motivate attempts to form images on the basis of dielectric properties. Since the information addressed by x-ray and microwave interrogation are not redundant, the combination of properties will provide a more complete description of the target than either one alone. Furthermore, the low photon energies of microwave radiation are of little added risk when compared to the ionization produced by x-ray photons (7).

At this juncture, the next item of necessary background is the choice of the target organ for microwave imagery demonstration and its relationship to dielectric properties. After this, methods of description for electromagnetic waves will continue. Of course, this has begun in the present section, but the item remaining - polarization - deserves special treatment after the biological and dielectric preliminaries are concluded.

Choice of Target Organ

The choice of a target for demonstrations of microwave imagery in biosystems is an important topic. Since water is an important constituent molecule in biological dielectrics, an organ with specialization for water transport would be a good choice. Further, since tomographic reconstruction of organ images has not yet been achieved, an organ with symmetry in a plane perpendicular to the direction of propagation would be desirable. Finally, an organ with regional specialization and a fibrous capsule to maintain its shape in vitro would be helpful. All of these considerations suggest that the kidney is a good choice for imagery demonstration.

Another set of considerations apply to the choice of in vitro rather than in situ imagery. Obviously, in situ imagery is the desired goal, but imagery demonstrations in vitro limit the number of problems which require simultaneous solution. Imagery in vivo is complicated by several important but temporarily subsidiary problems. Among these, three are of prime importance: In vivo imagery will be contaminated by significant movement artifact even in abdominal organs due to diaphragm contraction during respiration. Since data collection times are so long (ca 4.5 hr), this movement would seriously degrade the image and make it difficult to assess the fundamental problem of biological relevance/interpretation of microwave imagery in biosystems. Secondly, the images would be contaminated by greater refractive error when intervening heterogeneous dielectrics are interposed between the antennas and organ of interest. This problem requires solution, but only after the questions of biological relevance and pathophysiological correlation confirm the motivation for use of microwave energy as the interrogating radiation. Thirdly, the present receiver could not accommodate the insertion loss commensurate with the long path lengths in canine kidneys in situ. The solution to this problem requires no new technologies for S band receivers; rather, it is a statement of the relative insensitivity of the existing receiver (noise floor of ca. -80 dBm) compared to of-the-art S band receivers (ca. -140 dBm).

Polarization Concepts

Microwave energy in free space is often described as a transverse electric and magnetic wave which is characterized by its amplitude, frequency and initial phase. This description is incomplete at least to the extent that the direction of the electric and magnetic components are only required to be mutually perpendicular and perpendicular to the direction of propagation. That is to say, polarization is not described and the vector nature of the radiation is not fully specified.

A reference co-ordinate system for polarization description is needed. Such a reference is established by projection of the electric field component onto a plane which contains all possible directions of the electric field vector within the constraint that the electric field must be perpendicular to the direction of propagation. The electric field projection plane may be resolved into two orthogonal directions. In general, the electric field may occupy any position on that plane. This condition represents random polarization. However, random polarization is rarely encountered in radar or communication systems insofar as propagation and power transfer is substantially affected by polarization. This is especially true when heterogeneous conductors and/or dielectrics are interposed in the propagation path (8).

The conventional definitions of polarization are referenced to the locus of the electric field vector as projected onto the plane viewed from the direction of propagation as illustrated by Figure #1. A co-ordinate system is then applied to the two components of the projection plane. The IEEE standard provides a basis for this co-ordinate system which is an orthogonal pair parallel and perdendicular to the horizon. The simplest locus of polarization is linear wherein the oscillations of the electric field are confined to a single line when viewed from the direction of propagation. When the electric field component of the electromagnetic wave is colinear with either basis, the plane of oscillation is either perpendicular to the horizon (linear, vertical) or parallel to the horizon (linear, horizontal). On the projection plane, these are vertical and horizontal lines, respectively. Slant linear polarizations result from rotation of the plane of polarization. Another common condition is circular polarization wherein the electric field rotates in space such that on the projection plane a circle is traced by the tip of the electric vector for each cycle. As a matter of convention, the time harmonics are supressed in the projection. Circular polarization of the

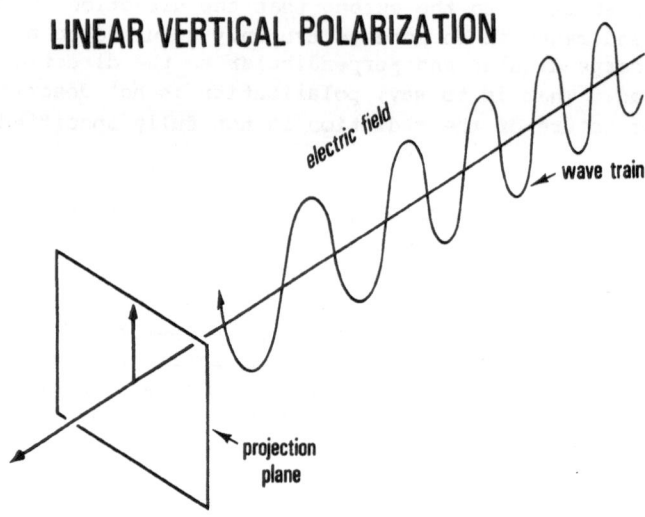

Figure #1. Linear Polarization of an Electromagnetic Wave.

electromagnetic wave train is then often described as a cork-screw where the direction of propagation is along the axis of the cylinder and the sense of polarization may be either clockwise when viewed from the direction of propagation (left hand circular) or counter-clockwise (right hand circular). Note that the sense of rotation is switched on the projection plane from that in the wavetrain, as shown in the Figure #2. Circular polarization is especially attractive in that the waveguide aperture is symmetric i.e. either round or square. This may provide some advantage as will be apparent later in this paper.

Since all positions on the projection plane of the electric field may be described by an orthogonal bivariate quantity, the most general polarization is elliptical whereby the tip of the electric field vector traces an ellipse on the projection

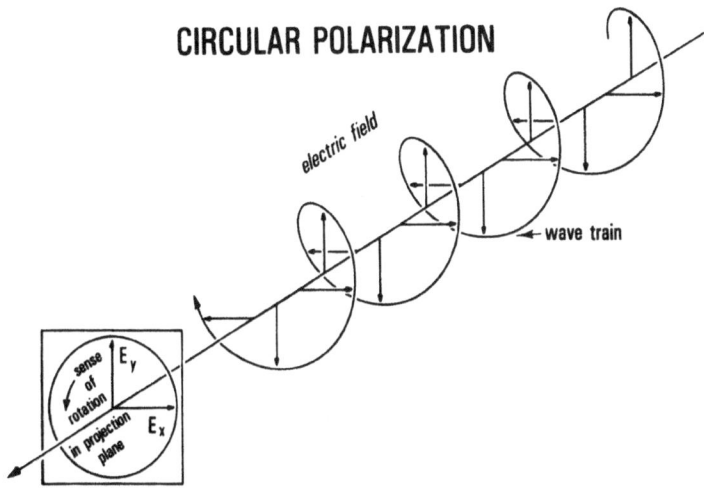

Figure #2. Circular Polarization of an Electromagnetic Wave.

plane. In this way, linear and circular polarization represent specializations of elliptical polarization: namely, when the two orthogonal components are equal, circular polarization results; and when one or the other orthogonal component is zero, linear polarization results. Slant linear polarization may result from mixtures of left and right-hand circular polarization with differences in initial phase.

Power transfer between two dipole antennas nicely illustrates the importance of polarization. In this case, linearly polarized fields produced by the transmitting antenna couple energy into the receiving antenna according to a cosine law. That is, when the plane of the transmitted electric field is parallel to the plane of the receiving dipole (i.e. the transmitter dipole and receiver dipole are co-planar and parallel), the polarizations are matched and power transfer is maximized. In other words, the angle between them is zero and the cosine is unity. As the angle approaches 90°, the power transfer approaches zero.

With respect to the general elliptic polarization, several parameters of description are pertinent. The orthogonal field components are

$$E_x = |E_x| \exp (i \theta_x)$$

and

$$E_y = |E_y| \exp (i \theta_y)$$

where the magnitudes are for any orthogonal pair with phases of θ_x and θ_y. The time harmonics are suppressed. The amplitude of an elliptically polarized wave is

$$E^2 = |E_x|^2 + |E_y|^2$$

The axial ratio, r, is the ratio of the minor to the major axes of the polarization ellipse as viewed on the projection plane. The angle the major axis of the ellipse makes to the reference coordinate frame is known as the orientation angle, β. The ellipticity angle, α is related to the axial ratio as follows:

$$\alpha = \pm \arctan r$$

where the sign represents the sense of rotation. These definitions are illustrated in Figure #3. The complex polarization ratio is defined as,

$$P = |E_x|/|E_x| \angle \underline{\theta_y - \theta_x}$$

That is, the complex polarization ratio magnitude is the ratio of the magnitudes of the orthogonal component magnitudes and its phase is the difference of phases of the orthogonal components.

POLARIZATION ELLIPSE

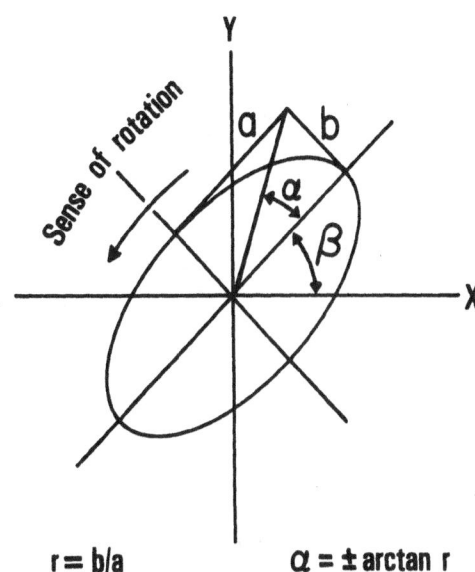

$$r = b/a \qquad \alpha = \pm \arctan r$$

Figure #3. Parameters of Elliptical Polarization.

In more general terms, the polarization state may be represented as a point on the surface of a sphere as shown in Figure #4. The point is located by a longitude of 2β and a latitude of 2α. One half of the sphere represents right sensed polarization (positive α) and the other half represents left sensed polarization (negative α). The poles represent circular polarization and the equator represents linear polarization states. This representation of polarization on the surface of a unit sphere was first described for optical radiation by Poincare. The sphere is known as the Poincare sphere (9).

Polarization is more conveniently shown with a projection of the pertinent hemisphere onto a plane which is shown in figure #5. Note that horizontal linear polarization is at the

POLARIZATION SPHERE

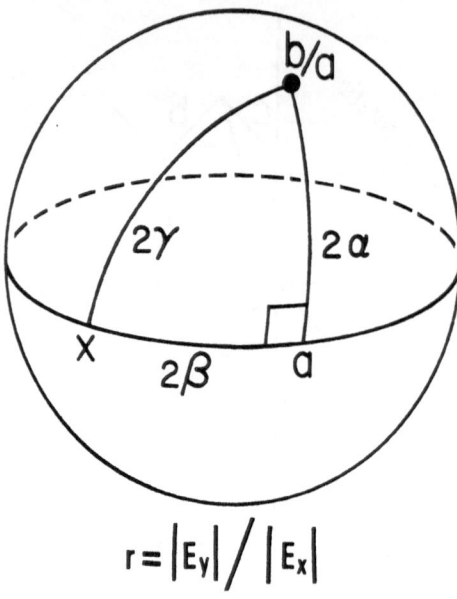

$$r = |E_y| \,/\, |E_x|$$

Figure #4. Polarization State on the Poincare Sphere

right hand perimeter whereas vertical polarization is at the
left hand perimeter. Further, the radial distance to a
polarization state on the chart is 2 α. This polarization
representation is very useful for the concept of power
transfer. If the polarization of each antenna is defined as the
polarization of the wave it would produce in the far field of
its radiation pattern when energized, and each polarization is
represented as a point on the Poincare sphere, then the
efficiency of power transfer is proportional to the cosine of
the polar angle, Δ, between the two points as shown in Figure
#6. This polar angle, Δ, is twice the difference between the
orientation angles of the major axis of the two elliptical
polarizations.

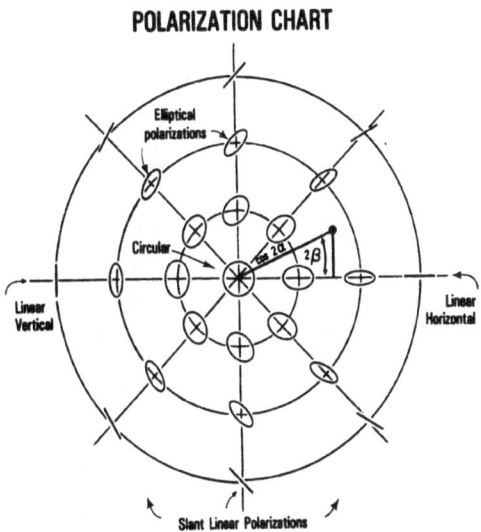

Figure #5.   Polarization Hemisphere Projected Onto a Plane.

$$\Delta = 2|\beta_1 - \beta_2|$$

The functional form of the power transfer efficiency, Γ , depends upon the polarization states involved. In the case of linear polarization,

$$\Gamma = 1 + \frac{\cos \Delta}{2}$$

In terms of axial ratios, the power transfer efficiency is

$$\Gamma = \frac{(1 \pm r_1 r_2)^2 + (r_1 \pm r_2)^2 + (1 - r_1{}^2)(1 - r_2{}^2) \cos \Delta}{(1 + r_1{}^2) \qquad (1 + r_2{}^2)}$$

POWER TRANSFER

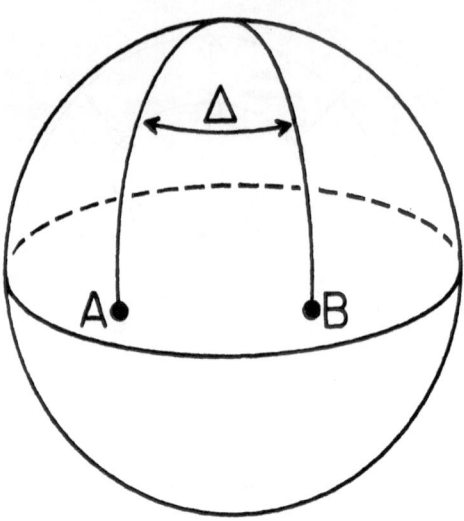

Figure #6.   Power Transfer Between Two Polarizations.

where the sign indicates sense of rotation and Δ is the polar
angle previously defined.   Power transfer is maximized when
the axial ratios and direction of rotation are matched.

Polarization Transformation

The polarization of the electromagnetic wave launched by
a transmitting antenna may be modified by the spatial distribution propagation constants present in the media of propagation.
To the extent that the polarization of the wave is different at
the receiving antenna than that which was transmitted, the target
has effected a polarization transformation upon the incident radiation.   Such a polarization transformation may provide a useful
description of the target.

Considerable theory exists for the case of backscattered microwave energy for a fixed aspect between the transceiver and target. The work of Kennaugh, Sinclair, Copeland, and Huynen are pertinent examples (10, 11, 12, 13). Less work exists in the forward scatter case, but it is certainly well known that polarization transformation is possible. In the case of linearly polarized radiation, the transformation is depolarization since linear transmit is converted to elliptical receive. Some examples of polarization transformation are shown in Figure #7. By analogy with the monostatic case, some physically reasonable assertions may be made for forward scatter, but in the case of imagery it is important to

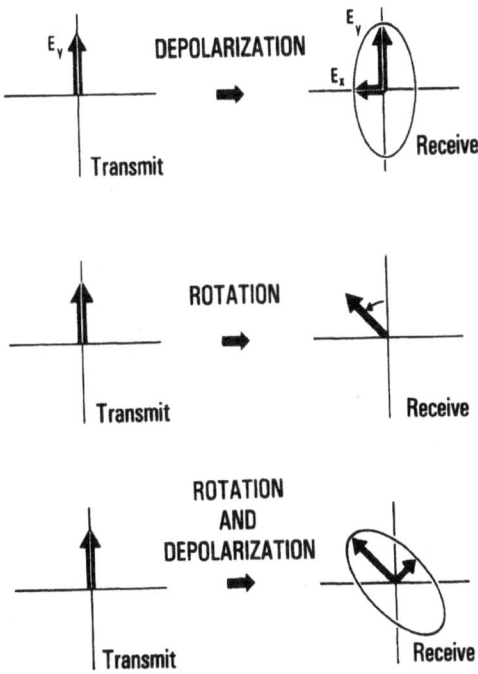

Figure #7. Various Examples of Polarization Transformation.

distinguish the additional factors of near field operation
(whereby the fields have axial as well as transverse components)
and the variable aspect of illumination. Also the effects of
charges and magnetic fields (Faraday rotation) are ignored.

By analogy with the monostatic case, the polarization
properties of the target may be described for various bases.
One convenient basis is linear polarization where the orthogonal
pair is horizontal and vertical polarization. One useful
representation is to define a target's polarization scattering
matrix, T_π, for the bistatic angle of π (i.e. forward scatter),

$$\begin{bmatrix} E_{s_x} \\ E_{s_y} \end{bmatrix} = \begin{bmatrix} E_{i_x} \\ E_{i_y} \end{bmatrix} \begin{bmatrix} T_\pi \end{bmatrix}$$

where T_π is a two by two symetric matrix of complex numbers
which relate the incident electric field components, E_{i_x} and
E_{i_x}, to the scattered electric field components, E_{s_x} and E_{s_y}.

The scattering matrix for the far field is:

$$\begin{bmatrix} T_\pi \end{bmatrix} = \begin{bmatrix} |t_{11}|\exp(i\phi_{11}) & |t_{12}|\exp(i\phi_{12}) \\ |t_{21}|\exp(i\phi_{21}) & |t_{22}|\exp(i\phi_{22}) \end{bmatrix}$$

The elements of the matrix (T_π) are magnitudes of the
forward scattered fields, $|t_{m,n}|$, and their associated phase
angles, $\phi_{m,n}$, for each combination of the two basis vectors, m
and n, indicated as subscripts.

In the near field, the axial component requires an
additional element to make a 3 by 3 matrix

$$
\begin{bmatrix} E_{s_x} \\ E_{s_y} \\ E_{s_z} \end{bmatrix} = \begin{bmatrix} E_{i_x} \\ E_{i_y} \\ E_{i_z} \end{bmatrix} \quad \begin{bmatrix} T_\pi \end{bmatrix}
$$

where

$$
\begin{bmatrix} T_\pi \end{bmatrix} = \begin{bmatrix} |t_{11}|\exp(i\phi_{11}) & |t_{12}|\exp(i\phi_{12}) & |t_{13}|\exp(i\phi_{13}) \\ |t_{21}|\exp(i\phi_{21}) & |t_{22}|\exp(i\phi_{22}) & |t_{23}|\exp(i\phi_{23}) \\ |t_{13}|\exp(i\phi_{31}) & |t_{23}|\exp(i\phi_{23}) & |t_{33}|\exp(i\phi_{33}) \end{bmatrix}
$$

In either case, the time harmonic notation is surpressed. The quantities actually measured are the magnitudes and phase angles at a single aspect for the Kurokawa scattering parameter S_{21} (i.e. coherant transmission or insertion loss) under all possible combinations of the basis polarizations (14). In the far field case, the two polarizations may be vertical and horizontal. In the near field case, the three polarizations may be vertical, horizontal and axial. That is, for example, in the far field case with vertical and horizontal bases, the polarization transformation matrix may be written in shorthand notation as

$$
\begin{bmatrix} T_\pi \end{bmatrix} = \begin{bmatrix} HH & HV \\ VH & VV \end{bmatrix}
$$

where the first letter (or subscript) in the previous notation applies to the polarization of the transmitting antenna and the second applies to the receiving antenna. It is understood that the matrix elements are complex quantities as shown in complete form above. The physical interpretation to be applied is, for the case of element HH, that the complex scattering parameter S_{21} is measured for one aspect of illumination and bistatic reception with both the transmitting and receiving antennas linearly polarized in the horizontal direction. In the case of element VV, both are vertically polarized. The off-diagonal elements are cross polarization states. For example, element HV is horizontal transmit and vertical receive.

In the case of an image, each element of the polarization transformation matrix becomes a two dimensional spatial series of complex numbers. Thus

$$\left[T_{\pi_i} \right] = \begin{bmatrix} HH_{mn} & HV_{mn} \\ VH_{mn} & VV_{mn} \end{bmatrix}$$

where the indices m and n are bistatic measurements at various positions azimuth and elevation.

In imagery systems, the magnitude and phase angles are represented by two real valued spatial series. In the case of the first copolarized images, t_{11} becomes indexed over azimuth and elevation to create the images; one is for phase, one is for magnitude. The magnitude image is known as the vertical-vertical or co-polarized (VV) image. The t_{12} component is similarly indexed over azimuth and elevation to create the t_{12} magnitude image. This image is known as the vertical-horizontal or cross polarized (VH) image. Similar procedures create the other possibilities in the 2 x 2 matrix T_π. Thusfar, axial field components have not been measured and none of these elements (third row and/or third column) in the near field polarization transformation matrix have been used for imagery. Similarly, cross polarized phase images have not yet been utilized.

The various magnitudes in T_{π_i} may be combined to create a composite image. One of the possibilities in the so-called polarization invariant quantity Q (15), which for a pixel is

$$Q_{mn} = \left| t_{11} \right|^2_{mn} + \left| t_{12} \right|^2_{mn} + \left| t_{21} \right|^2_{mn} + \left| t_{22} \right|^2_{mn}$$

Another possibility is linear combinations of cannonical representations of the matrix T_π. Clearly, many fruitful avenues for research exist in this area; but in the present case only two magnitude images will be presented and these are from different kidneys. The reason for this slow start is the fact that data collection takes so long (ca. 4.5 hr). As a result, multiple images of a single target are not feasible with the existing scanner. The electronically scanned array under development should improve the data acquisition time to the order of minutes rather than hours. The shorter data acquisition time will permit many polarization transformation studies (among them, pathophysiological correlations) which are not presently possible.

SYSTEM DESIGN CONSIDERATIONS

The advantages of the microwave region of the spectrum as a means for interrogation of biosystems have previously been frustrated by the problem of how to reconcile two contradictory requirements: adequate spatial resolution and managable propagation loss. These requirements are contradictory since shorter wavelengths improve spatial resolution, but simultaneously increase propagation loss. This dilema may be mitigated by the use of high dielectric constant materials to fill waveguide based antennas as well as to provide a coupling medium between the antennas and the target. This technique has been presented elsewhere (16), hence, only a summary will be provided here. The coupling/loading medium of choice is water. It provides high dielectric constant sufficient to contract the wavelength by a factor of approximately 9 (relative to air); it is sufficiently lossy as a coupling medium to attenuate multipath (chiefly at the first inerface of the target); it provides an easily implemented anechoic environment to prevent interference; and it provides a reasonably good, yet broad band, match to water dominated biological dielectrics.

The use of water as a loading/coupling medium, therefore, accomplishes wavelength contraction without the propagation loss penalty associated with increased frequency. Operation in the S band leaves the propagation losses managable at those of 2-4 GHz in water, but accomplishes resolution comparable to 18-36 GHz in air.

This technique has been used in the near field environment (i.e. when the target is in the near field of the antenna, or about one penetration depth away) where resolution is determined largely by aperture dimensions of the antenna. It is presently being generalized to far field operation by means of a water coupled, phased array antenna. The array will offer several significant advantages: electronic beam steering will reduce data collection time; the low f number of the array should provide resolution in elevation and azimuth comparable to that achieved in the near field of a simple unfocused element; and electronic focusing will vastly improve beam width in range when compared to the single element previously employed.

Scattering Geometry

The system configuration as a forward scatter imager deserves some discussion. Foreward scatter is, of course, uncommon in radar applications. This is largely because a simple foreward scatter radar system can only provide information concerning detection of targets with no information concerning location or Doppler. In medical applications, location can be resolved in elevation and azimuth by scanning, but recovery of the range coordinate requires tomographic reconstruction. Range is easily obtained with a back scatter system, but the scattering cross section is often orders of magnitude smaller than in the case of forward scatter (17). This is less true for small scatters (i.e., small relative to the wavelength in the medium), e.g., in the Rayleigh region. Resonances are a special case, but these are generally dampened in dissipative dielectrics. The behavior of foreward scatter cross section as a function of the size of the scattering object relative to a wavelength in the medium (or, alteratively a fixed target object illuminated with increasing frequency) is a smoother function than in the case of backscatter. In the case of simple scatters such as spheres, the forward scatter cross section is a smooth, monotonic function of frequency/size; whereas for back scatter, the cross section is oscillatory and not monotonically related to frequency (size) as shown in Figire #8. Polarization does not affect the scattering cross-section in the case of spherical objects. In the case of double layered dielectric cylinders (see Figure #9) it is apparent that the foreward scatter cross-section exceeds the back-scatter cross-section. Further, the object size with respect to wavelength bears a nearly montonic relationship to the cross-section in the case of forward scatter whereas this is conspicuously not true with back-scatter. Note also the effect of polarization. Furthermore, spectroscopic methods for characterization of the medium in the propagation path are often more easily applied to forward scatter than to back scatter. These arguments were illustrated by improved sensitivity to small, concentric dielectrics with foreward scatter rather than back scatter configurations as shown in Figure #10.

The chief disadvantages to foreward scatter are both consequences of the longer path length. These are the need for greater sensitivity of the receiver and more serious degradation of the image by refractive effects.

On balance, these considerations appear to favor forward scatter systems although solution of refractive effects may delay _in situ_ operation. This is especially troublesome with

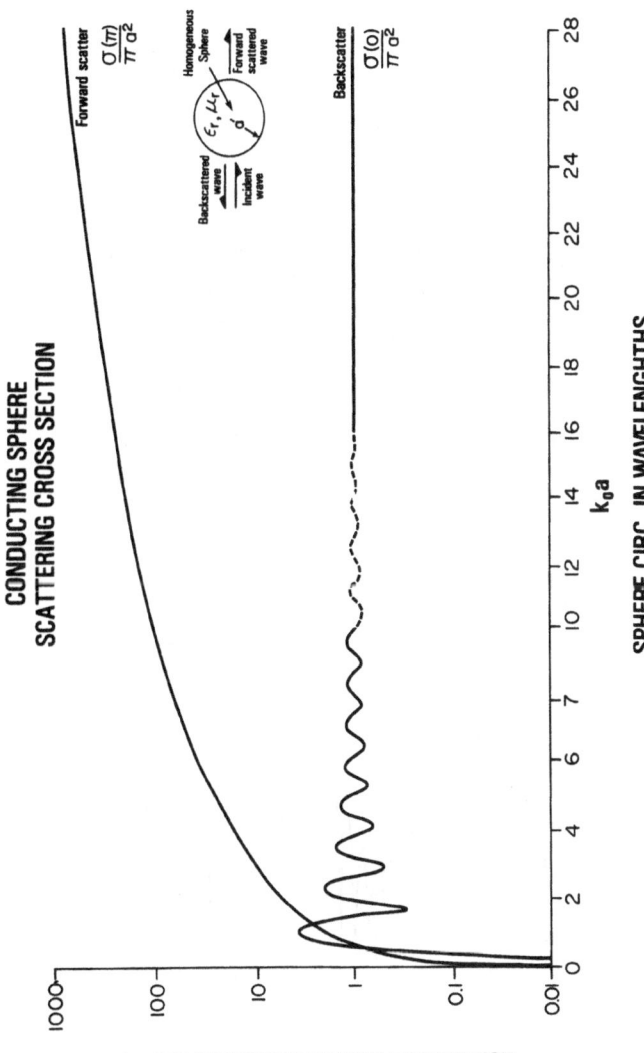

Figure #8.   Scattering Cross-Section for Conducting Sphere (from Ruch, et. al.).

90

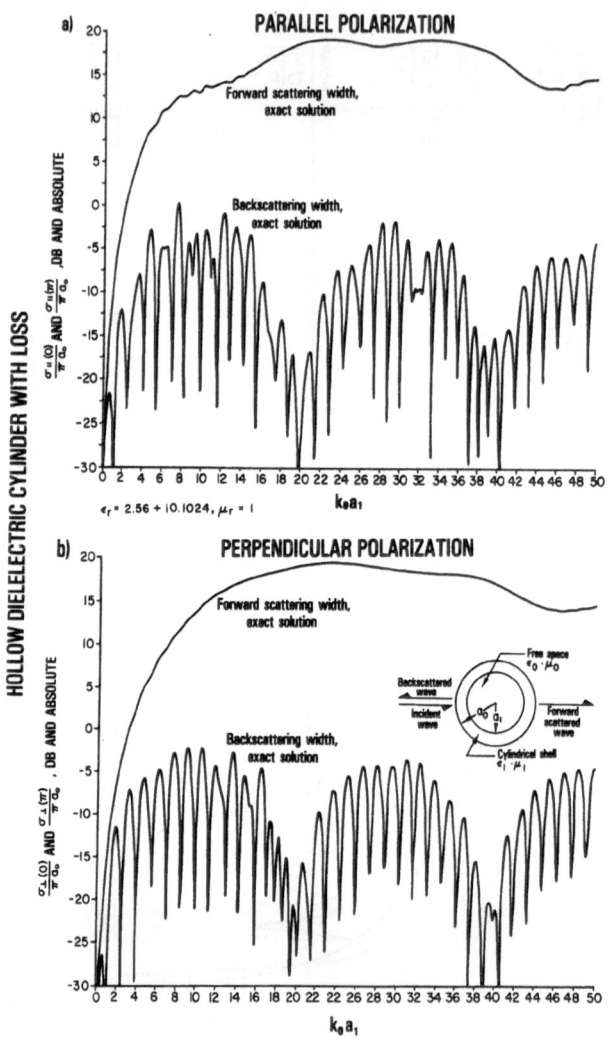

Figure #9. Scattering Cross-Section for Heterogeneous
Dielectric Cylinders with Lossy Walls (from
Ruch et. al.).

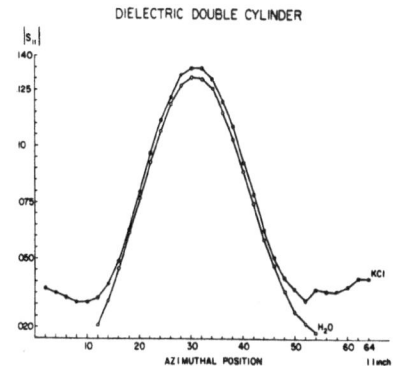

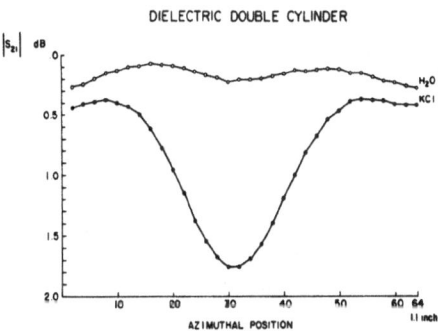

Figure #10 a, b. Glass Tubing 6 mm OD and 3 mm ID Filled with Water and Kcl Solution, $|s_{11}|$ and $|s_{21}|$, Respectively.

tomographic systems, although reconstruction is certainly possible by conventional linear methods which ignore the difficulties of refraction, reflection and diffraction (18). One special case does argue for back scatter systems. That is when the target of interest is superficial (e.g. a blood vessel) and much higher frequencies (e.g. 10 GHz) are needed for resolution.

IMPLEMENTATION

The basic system configuration is a forward scatter (bistatic at 180°) design with one transmitting antenna and one receiving antenna. The antennas are water loaded and water coupled to the target which is interposed between the two antennas as shown in Figure 11. The two antennas are rigidly interconnected and scanned as a pair in a raster pattern over the isolated canine kidney. The basic datum is the complex Kurokawa scattering parameter S_{21} for each of two combinations of linear polorization (19, 20). One case is copolarized (VV), the other is cross polarized (VH). The transmitting antenna is always vertically polarized whereas the receiving antenna is polarized alternately in the vertical and horizonital directions (21). The data are converted into images by intensity modulation of a raster scanned display. Various image processing steps are applied in the amplitude and spatial frequency domain. Image interpretation is made on the basis of known regional specialization in the kidney.

Data Acquisition

The data presented later in this paper are two dimensional arrays of microwave transmission coefficients (magnitude and phase of S_{21}) which describe the relative insertion loss and relative phase shift of a 3.9 GHz signal as it propagates through the target of interest. This insertion loss and phase shift is affected by the path length, complex permittivity and geometry of the biological material, and the degree to which polarization transformation occurs as a signal is propagated through the target. The image was collected as a square 64x64 array at 1.4mm sampling increments. The basic data are scattering parameters S_{21}, i.e. insertion loss and phase shift at each location on the raster. The block diagram of the data collection system is shown in Figure #12. This diagram has been divided into three functional subsystems, control and recording, microwave stimulus/response, and the electromechanical scanner.

The electromechanical scanner consists of a water tank (.914 meters cubical tank), vertical and horizontal translation axes, independant drive motors for the axes, independant position transducers for the axes, and mounting frames upon which to connect the antennas and the specimen. The linear position transducers were of the electro-optical type (Heidenhain Pos-Econ 1) with a total range of approximately 200 mm and an accuracy of ± 0.002 mm (this accuracy is slightly degraded by the stepping motors). The position transducer readouts have + 8421 BCD out puts which are interfaced to the Hewlett Packard (HP) 2100 mini computer using two HP 12604B Data Source Interface Cards. This interface required construction of an intermediate buffer that provided special signals such as flag and control logic required by the HP12604B.

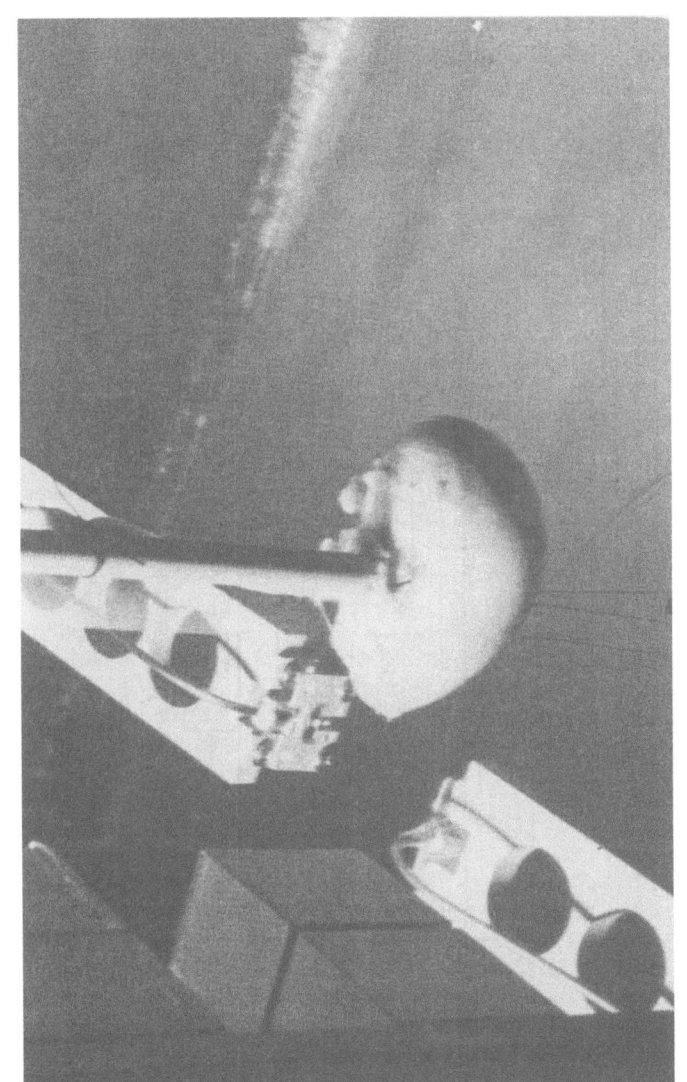

Figure #11. Canine Kidney in Microwave Scanner with Water Coupled Antennas.

94

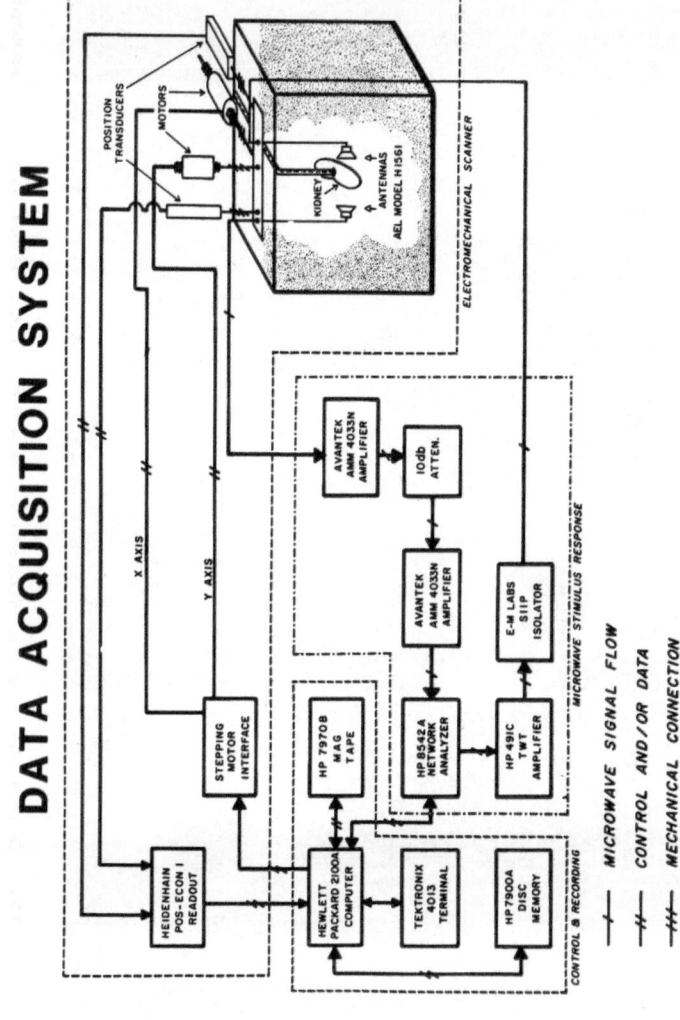

Figure #12. Scattering Parameter Imaging System Block Diagram.

The X and Y axes were driven by a Superior Electric M112-FJ25 synch-ronous stepper motor through a gear reduction box and worm gear. The motors were interfaced to the HP2100A computer through a SloSyn Translator Model BTR103RT and HP sixteen bit duplex register in the computer. The computer controlled the X and Y coordinates of the positioner by sending pulses to the stepper motors under software control. This arrangement, in which the computer read the X and Y positions and controlled the motors, allowed closed loop control of the scanner position under softward control. In this manner, the accuracy between image elements (pixels) was set to ±0.01 mm. Although higher accuracy was possible (±0.003 mm) it was not used because it considerably dilated the data acquisition time.

The cubical tank contained the water into which the antennas and specimen were immersed. The water was continuously filtered through ion-exchange columns and iodinated as a bacteriocidal measure.

The 3.9 GHz microwave interrogation signal was generated by a phase-locked HP8542 A Automatic Network Analyzer. This signal was amplified to the level of approximately 1 watt in an HP491C Traveling Wave Tube amplifier, passed through an isolator to protect the TWT and sent to the transmitting antenna (American Electronics Laboratories Model H1561). The signal was received on an identical antenna; amplified by two Avantek low noise amplifiers in a series and passed to the receiver of the HP8542A. The uncorrected transmission coefficient (S_{21}) is generated in the HP8542A receiver, digitized, and stored in the HP2100A computer. This data is corrected for errors such as source mismatch, tracking errors, etc. by techniques described in the literature (22).

The corrected data was recorded on a disc file and later transferred to magnetic tape in a format compatible with the image processing system.

Methods for Suppression of Multipath

Multipath describes the fact that microwave energy reaches the receiving antenna through a variety of paths. This is the result of diffraction, refraction, reflection, and beam spreading as the radiation propagates through the target organ and coupling media. Since this problem and its amelioration have been discussed in detail elsewhere (23, 24), we shall only summarize the method here.

The basic method is related to the chirp or linear FM radar whereby time and frequency are associated in a swept signal. The linear FM signal is passed through a power divider (as shown in the system block diagram of Figure #13) after which two paths exist. One path is the reference channel which suffers a known propagation delay through a section of coaxial cable. The other path goes through the organ under study by means of two antennas which move in a raster pattern over the organ. The two signals are recombined in a mixer and low pass filtered. The output frequency is proportional to the instantaneous frequency difference at the two input ports. As a result of the time-encoded-by-frequency input signals, the difference frequency at the mixer output port is proportional to the differential time delay between the two paths. A small frequency window (corresponding to a range of arrival times) is placed on the mixer output and the maximum signal amplitude within that window becomes the basic datum at each position of the transmit/receive pair. Thusfar, only co-polarized magnitude images have been produced over a ca. 3-4 GHz sweep in 16 msec.

Image Processing

Two types of digital image processing were performed: amplitude domain and spatial frequency domain. The processing sequence began in the amplitude domain. The first step was interpolation from the 64x64 data collection raster to a 256x256 raster. The data begins as 15 bits plus sign, but it is truncated to 7 bits plus sign. The interpolation function used was the cubic spline (25). Interpolation properly consists of an ideal low pass filter applied to the data acquired on the scanner grid to regenerate the continuous, band limited (i.e. in spatial frequencies), two dimensional image of signal amplitudes. The reconstituted image is then in principle resampled at new grid positions. The interpolation kernal is convolved with the available data such that existing data values are not modified. The ideal kernal is the sin (x)/x function. This kernal is approximated by a cubic spline (26).

The cubic spline function has three ranges of values as shown below:

$$
f(x) = \begin{cases}
f_1(x) = a_1|x|^3 + b_1|x|^2 + c_1|x| + d_1; & 0 \le |x| \le 1 \\
f_2(x) = a_2|x|^3 + b_2|x|^2 + c_2|x| + d_2; & 1 \le |x| \le 2 \\
f_3(x) = 0 ; & |x| \ge 2
\end{cases}
$$

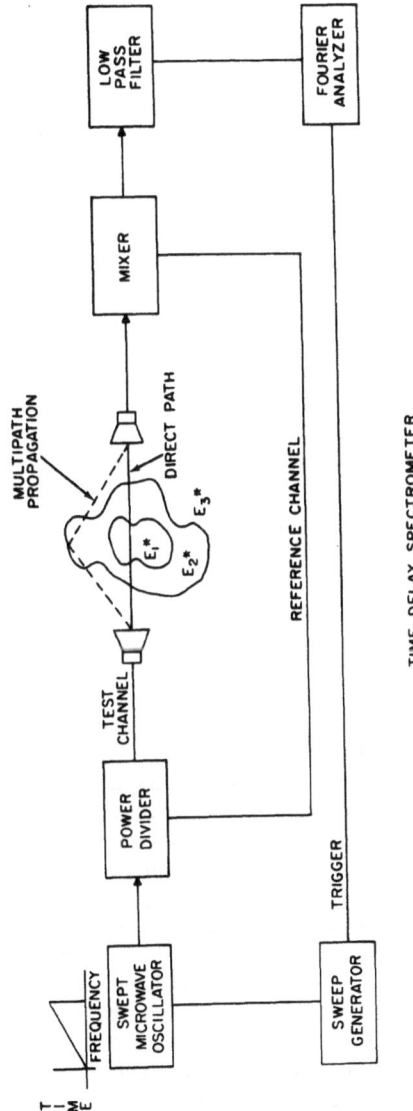

Figure #13. Microwave Time Delay Spectrometer Imaging System Block Diagram.

The function is evaluated for a range of ±4 pixels in azimuth and elevation to result in a 16 point kernal. The function approximates a sin (x)/x function in two dimensions and it is normalized to unity in magnitude. When the main lobe is coincident with existing data, the nulls are at 16 existing grid points. Thus, the function simply multiplies the value at the main lobe by one and adds zeros. At new locations, the interpolation error has a peak value of ca. 5% and a average error of ca. 2% (27).

The cubic spline is preferable to the two more common interpolation operators which are simple pixel replication and bilinear (two dimensional linear) interpolation. The former suffers from image blocking (checkering) and the latter substantially departs from the ideal low pass filtering. That is, spatial frequencies near but below the folding frequency are attenuated. Cubic spline interpolation also provides continuity in the first and second derivitives of the pixel values whereas bilinear interpolation provides continuity only in the displayed values. Pixel replication operates without regard to continuity of the displayed values. Of course, interpolation does not increase the number of "independant" pixels, neither does it compensate for any possible aliasing from the ca 1.4 mm sampling increment in azimuth and elevation. The objective is entirely to enhance the perceived image "quality" by simulating a continuous rather than a discrete representation of the data.

The next processing stage was also in the amplitude domain, but the objective was to adapt the dynamic range of the data to the dynamic range of the video display. The operation is known as grey scale mapping whereby the original scale of intensity values are mapped onto a different scale. The archetype of the operation is the ramp-intersect map which stretches some subset of the original range onto the full range of the new scale. This contrast stretcher is useful for part-range expansion, but it has the disadvantage that the lower and upper interecept points map all values at or above the upper intercept into one value at the new scale maximum and all values at or below the lower intercept onto the scale minimum. This, of course, is often an undesirable data compression. The map used in this study is different in that all values from the original scale are mapped into unique values on the new scale. The map actually used is a two-piece linear function with an interactively alterable hinge point. Since a null operator would be a 45° line through the origin, the expansion is proportional to the slope of the mapping function. Thus, the map expands the scale for values below the hinge and compresses those above the hinge when the hinge point is above the 45°

line. The situation is reversed for hinge points below the 45°
line. These grey scale operators are illustrated in the Figure
#14.

The last amplitude domain step is pseudocolor processing.
This processing is often referred to as density slicing. This
nomenclature is an atavism from digital processing of
photographic images where by the optical density was assigned a
color in a color map corresponding to the range of measured
light transmssion via a scanning desitometer. In the present
context, the color map is applied to the scale of magnitudes of
scattering parameter S_{21} as shown in Figure #15. The color maps
used in the present work are those from the NASA LANDSAT series.

Spatial frequency domain processing is accomplished by
two-dimensional digital filters (28). These are specified with
radially symmetric transfer function magnitudes. The transfer

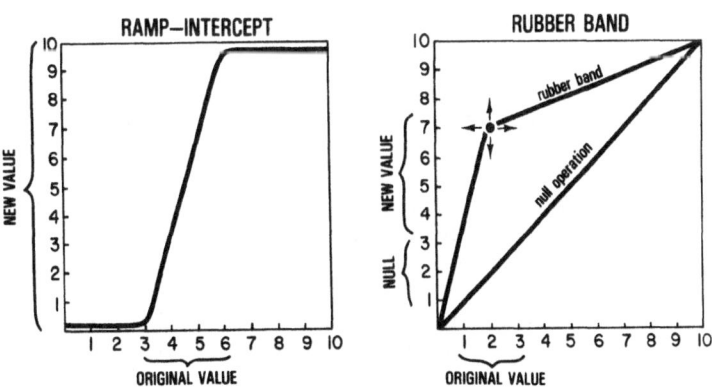

Figure #14. Grey Scale Mapping Operators.

PSEUDOCOLOR DENSITY SLICING

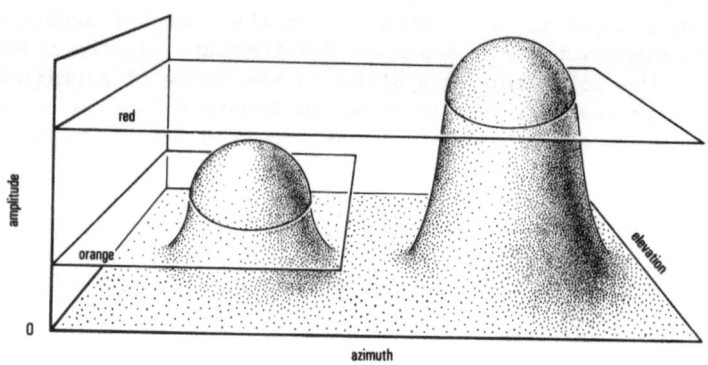

Figure #15. Pseudocolor Processing by Density Slicing

functions are comprised of only even terms (cosines); thus,
there is no detectable phase shift. The images are first
Fourier transformed in one-dimension, transposed and Fourier
transformed again in the same direction. Since the
two-dimensional Fourier transform has a seperable kernal, two
one-dimensional transforms may be used to implement the
two-dimensional transform. The Fourier processed image is then
multiplied by the specified transfer function and the product is
inverse transformed back to the spatial domain.

The form of the transfer function is a radially symmetric
band-pass-filter. Such a transfer function is shown in
perspective in Figure #16. This class of filter is designed to
reject spatial frequencies (i.e. spatial frequencies are the

TWO DIMENSIONAL BAND PASS FILTER

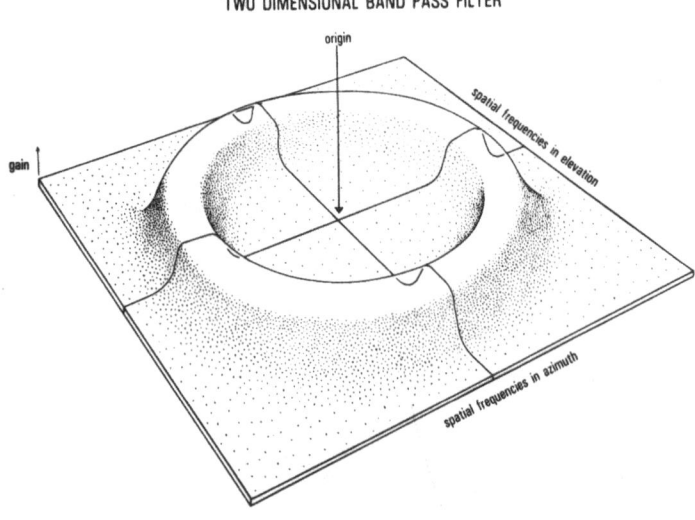

Figure #16.   Perspective View of the 2D Band Pass Filter.

reciprocal of length in the same sense that ordinary frequency
is the reciprocal of time) that are either above an upper "cut
off" or below a lower "cut off". The cut-off frequencies are
half power points. The operation of the filter may be viewed as
a cascade of a high pass filter set at a low cut-off frequency
and a low pass filter set at a high cut-off frequency. The
dampening factor is $\sqrt{2}$, and the asympotic rate of attenuation
is 12 dB/octave. These 2nd order filters were selected on the
basis that higher order filters tend to introduce ringing in
image in the same way that the step function responce of
ordinary filters exhibit greater time domain overshoot as the
order is raised. The dampening factor of $\sqrt{2}$ was selected to
minimize pass-band ripple.

The lower spatial frequency cut-off was selected with the aid of the two dimensional power spectrum of image as shown in Figure #17. Low spatial frequencies were rejected to remove effects of global changes in organ thickness and to ameliorate refractive effects in the image. High spatial frequencies were rejected to remove noise introduced by the cubic spline interpolation.

The convolution operator was used to enhance gradients within the image. This operation was implemented with a 3x3 kernal configured as a local high-pass-filter. It acts in a manner analogous to an isotropic three point moving average filter (the archetype being a differentiator) in two

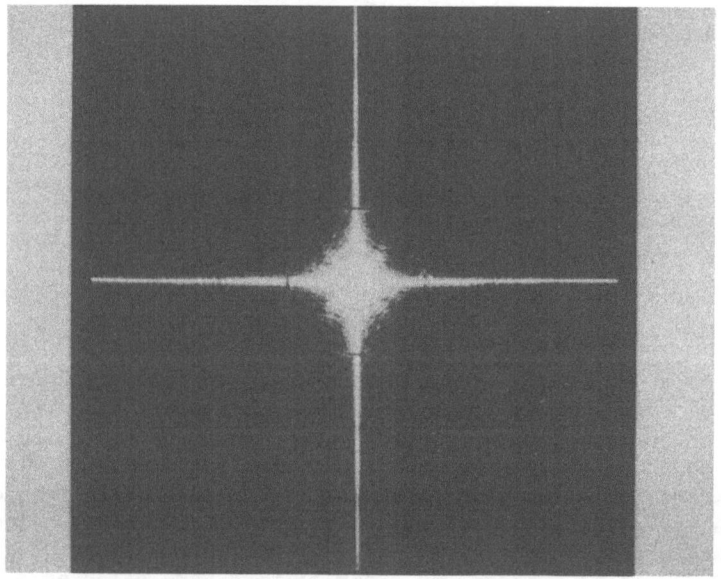

Figure #17. Band Pass Filter Overlaid on a Power Spectrum.

dimensions. The lack of directional sensitivity in such an isotropic filter requires symmetry in the kernal. That is, the generic form is

$$h(x,y) = \begin{bmatrix} A & B & A \\ B & 1 & B \\ A & B & A \end{bmatrix}$$

When both |A| and |B| are ≤1 and the coeficients are constrained to negative values for high pass filtering. Typically |A| > |B| in order to avoid undue emphasis of the asymmetries due the wave guide aperture. The operator is implemented by convolution of the kernal with the image as follows:

$$g(x,y) = f(x,y) * h(x,y)$$

where g(x,y) is the gradient enhanced image, f(x,y)is the original image and h(x,y) is the kernal. In all cases, only mild high pass filtering was employed in order to provide contrast for photographic recording of the image.

CANINE RENAL ANATOMY AND PHYSIOLOGY

A brief discussion of canine renal anatomy and physiology is a necessary background for plausible interpretation of the microwave images that will be presented later in this chapter. These topics will be treated largely in terms of generalization since many references exist with detailed discussion and extensive bibliographies (29, 30, 31).

In very broad terms, the kidney consists of five regions (see Figure #18). Of these, the central divisions are the cortex, medulla and pelvis. The other two regions are the outer margin, known as the capsule, and the medial structures of the hilus where blood vessels and the ureter have ingress and egress from the organ.

In similarly broad terms, the renal unit of function is the nephron (see Figure #19). Each kidney contains ca 10^5 nephrons. The individual nephron functions in a series of sequential processing steps. The first stage is ultra filtration of the blood at the glomerulus. Only blood cells and large protein molecules are retained; sugars, amino acids and electrolytes pass into the proximal nephron for further

104

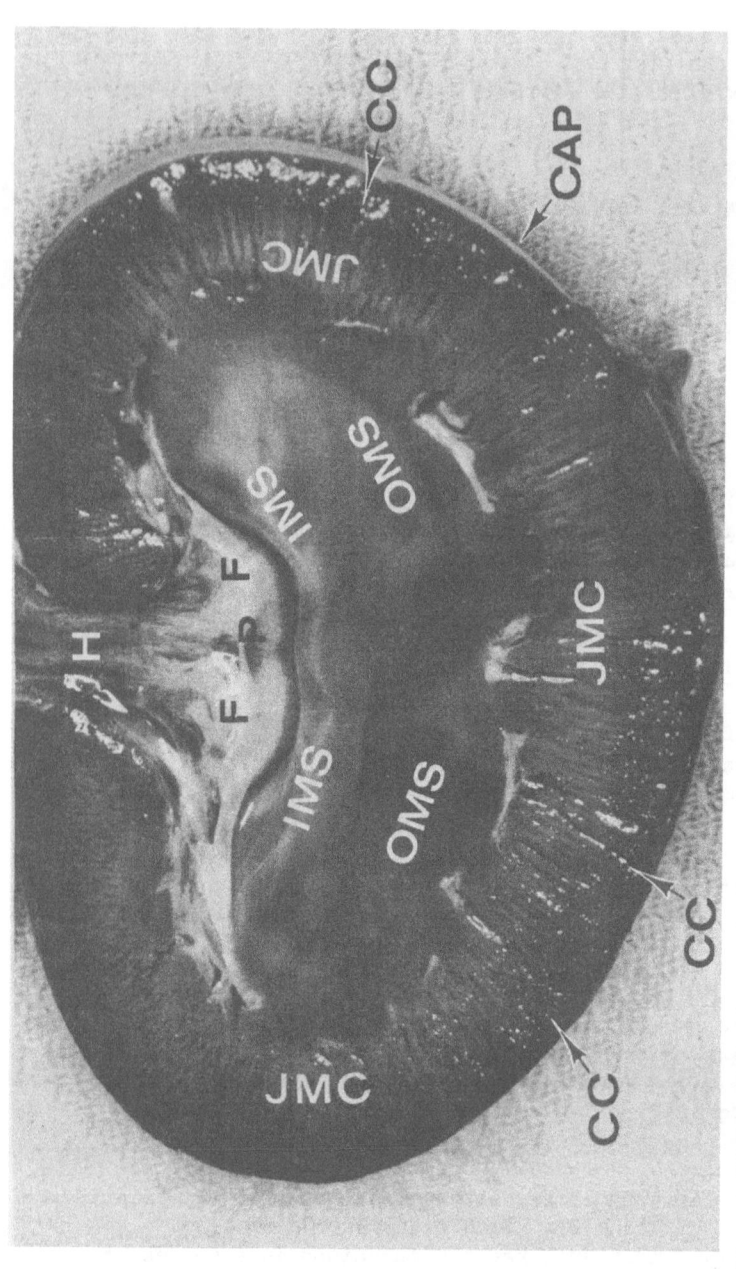

Figure #18. A Kidney Specimen with Dissection to Demonstrate Regional Anatomy. Code for Later Use: CC is Cortex Corticis, CAP is Capsule, JMC is Juxtamedullary Cortex, OMS is Outer Medullary Stripe, IMS is Inner Medullary Stripe, P is Pelvis, H is Hilus, F is Fat in Sinus, R is Support Rod, A is Artifact.

processing. The next processing step takes place in the proximal segment of the nephron where sugars, small protein molecules, amino acids and electrolytes are extracted from the ultrafiltrate and returned to the blood. The proximal segment also secretes p-aminohippurate into the partially processed ultrafiltrate. The next processing step is passive electrolyte and water movement out of the descending limb of the Loop of Henle. A counter current multiplier increases tonicity in the medulary interstitial spaces. Tonicity increases from a value of ca. 300 mosmols/l at the corticomedullary junction to a value of about 1200 mosmols/l at the tip of the medullary inner stripe. This is accomplished by sodium transport and the lack of water permiability in the ascending limb of the Loop of Henle. The vasa recta in combination with low medullary blood flow apparently reduces dissipation of the osmotic gradients produced by the Loop of Henle. The collecting ducts later serve as an osmotic exchanger in the medulla. The distal convoluted tubule further reabsorbs and secretes electrolytes.

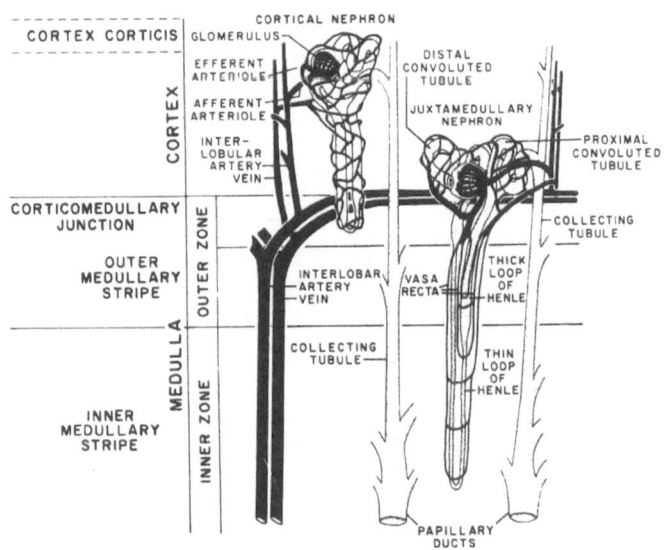

Figure #19. A Schematic View of the Nephron.

106

Finally, the product is transferred to the collecting tubules
where amonia secretion and water transport take place chiefly by
virtue of interstitial electrolyte concentrations produced via
the Loop of Henle. The urine thereby becomes concentrated on
route to the renal pelvis.

Canine renal anatomy differs from the more commonly known
human anatomy in that the canine organ is non-papillary. In
other words, the medullary pyramids that are prominant in
pylographic xray studies of humans are replaced by a single
central pyramid. This is evident on both the transverse and
longitudional sections shown in Figure #20. At the functional
unit level (i.e. the nephron) human and canine is quite similar.

The outer margin of canine kidney is a thin fiberous
capsule. Medial to the capsule is the cortex corticis. This is
a sub-region of the cortex that is characterized by a relative
pancity of glomeruli and high population density of proximal as
well as distal convoluted tubules.

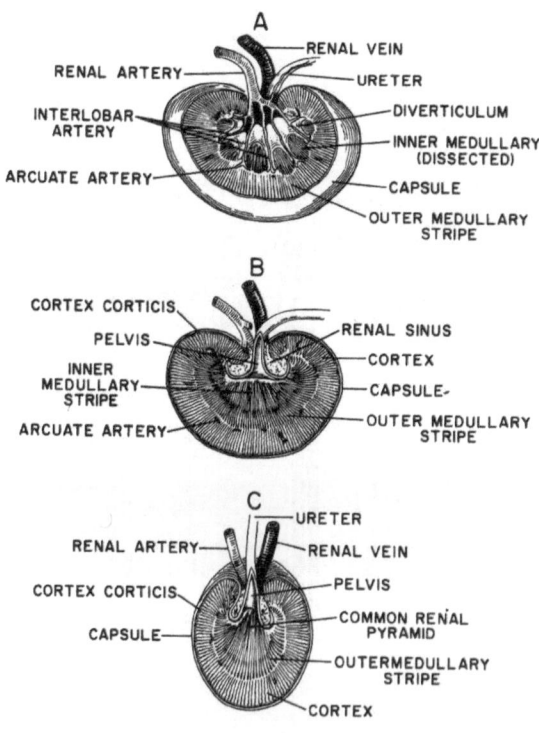

Figure #20. Graphic Illustrataion of Canine Renal Anatomy.

Medial to the corticis is the major portion of the cortex characterized by glomeruli, convuluted tubules and early urine collecting tubules. This region blends into the juxtamedullary cortex at corticomedulary junction. The cortex is lobulated by the interlobar arteries shown in Figure #20. These vascular patterns are further illustrated by angiography whereby x-ray contrast agent is injectd into the renal artery. A canine renal angiogram is shown in Figure #21.

The corticomedullary junction is formed by vascular patterns whereby the radially disposed lobar arteries produce a circumferential branch known as the arcuate artery. Small branches of the arcuate artery provide the lobular arteries, again in a radial pattern, from which the gromeruli are derived.

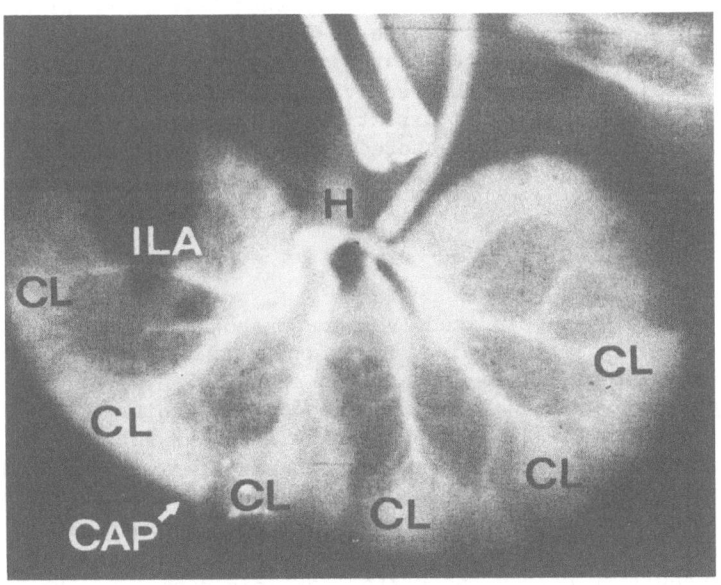

Figure #21. X-Ray Angiogram of Canine Kidney. Note the Cortical Lobulations, indicated by CL; and the Interlobar Arteries, indicated by ILA.

Medial to the corticomedullary junction is the first
subregion of the medulla, known as the outer medullary stripe.
This is a region characterized by the thick portion of the loop
of Henle and moderate size collecting tubules. The next
sub-region is the inner medullary stripe. This is a region
where the thin loops of Henle and the larger collecting ducts
exist.

Medial to medulla is the pelvis where the collecting ducts
empty the fully processed urine. The pelvis a muscular cistern
which is contiguous with the ureter in the hilar region of the
organ. The other hilar structures are the renal artery and
vein. Often a sinus or sinuses exists in the perihilar region
which is occupied by fat.

CANINE RENAL IMAGES

The presentation of imagery is grouped according to the
combination of polarization basis vectors used to generate the
image and the image processing steps that have taken place. The
first polarization basis is the co-polarized or VV pair. That
is, the transmitting antenna is linearly polarized in the
vertical direction and the receiving antenna is linearly
polarized in the vertical directions. The image, therefore,
represents the forward scattered radiation (i.e. insertion loss)
at 4096 positions in a raster scan of 1.4mm sampling increments
under the condition that the received polarization is the same
as transmitted polarization.

The first co-polarized (VV) image shown in monochrome (see
Figure 22a) is that obtained after only amplitude
processing steps. These processing steps began with
interpolation by a cubic spline from 64x64x15 bits deep to
256x256x7 bits deep.The interpolation step was followed by grey
scale mapping with the rubber band operator. This was followed
by the 3x3 convolution operator to enhance gradients. In the
image of Figure #22a, the pelvis and medullary inner strip are
certainly visible as is the corticomedullary junction with
juxtramedullary cortex and cortex corticis distal to the
junction. Some suggestion of cortical lobulations is also
visible.

The same sequence of image processing steps has been
applied to the cross-polorized (VH) image with the addition that
the grey scale is inverted. The image is formed by measurements
of the foreward scattered radiation under the condition that the

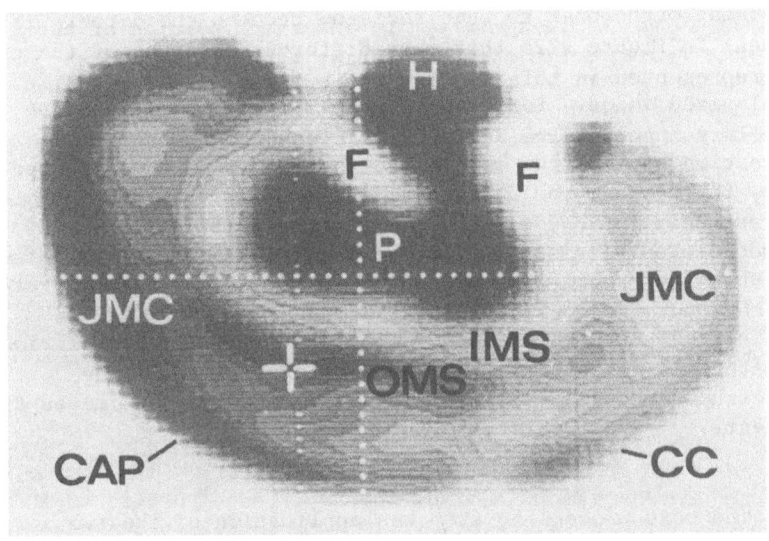

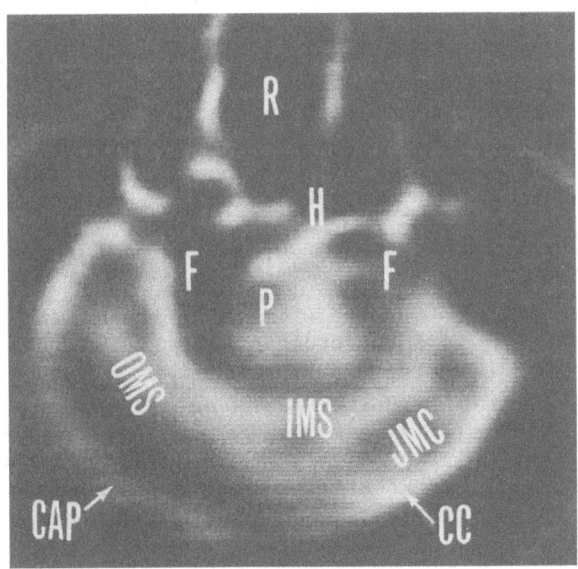

Figure 22a, b.   Copolarized (Upper) and Cross-Polarized (Lower)
                 Images

transmitted radiation is depolarized by the organ and the component orthogonal to that radiated becomes the datum. It is evident in Figure #22b that very different features of the organ are represented in this image when it is compared to the copolarized image. For example, the lamination between the medullary inner stripe and pelvis is enhanced as is the lamination between the cortex and the medullary outer stripe. Also, the support rod is clearly represented in the VH image whereas only the end of rod was evident in the VV image. Pseudocolored versions of the amplitude domain processed images are shown in Figure 23a, b. Of course, the same features are present; but the density slicing process enhances the distinctions between adjacent "grey" levels. The convolution operator was not used in the pseudocolored images. The differences between copolarized and cross polarized images are evident.

The next processing step was application of the two dimensional band pass filter followed by the rubber band and convolution operators. The copolarized magnitude image in Figure #24a is now much improved with respect to enhancing the cortical lobulations as well as the medullary inner and outer stripes. Similarly, the cortex corticis is enhanced. The co-polarized phase of S_{21} image after the same image processing sequence is shown in Figure #24b. The bright bars represent artifact. Once again, the cortex corticis, juxtamedullary cortex, medullary outer stripe, medullary inner stripe, pelvis, hilus and fat in the sinus are distinguishable. Note that the magnitude and phase co-polarized images are from the same kidney specimen.

The co-polarized magnitude image in pseudocolor is shown in Figure #25a, along with the cross-polarized magnitude image in Figure 25b. With regard to the cross-polarized magnitude image, the region between the two Pamina previously described is somewhat enhanced. It is also apparent in the band pass filtered cross-polarized image that the effects of the waveguide aperture assymetry are enhanced. This is an unfortunate consequence of the double ridged waneguide antenna in the cross-polarized configuration. Attempts to remove this effect by means of a horizontal notch filter were only partially successful. These factors argue for the use of a symmetrical aperture when band width is not a major concern.

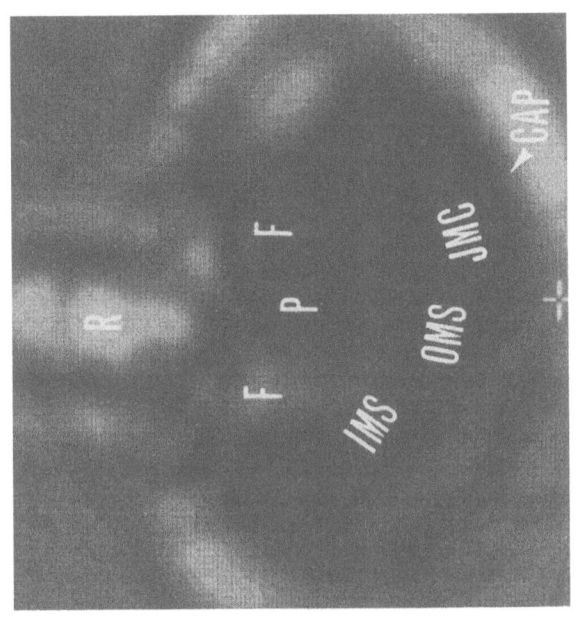

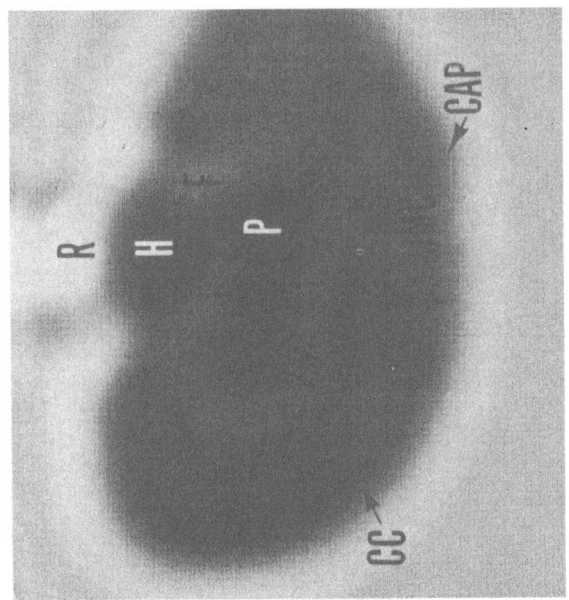

Figure #23a, b. Pseudocolored Image with Only Amplitude Domain Processing. Copolarized Image is at the Left, Cross-Polarized Image at the Right.

112

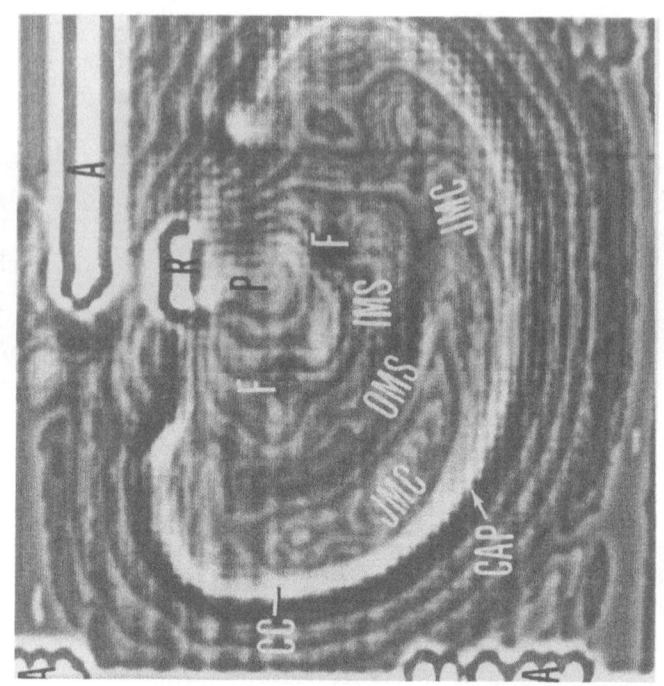

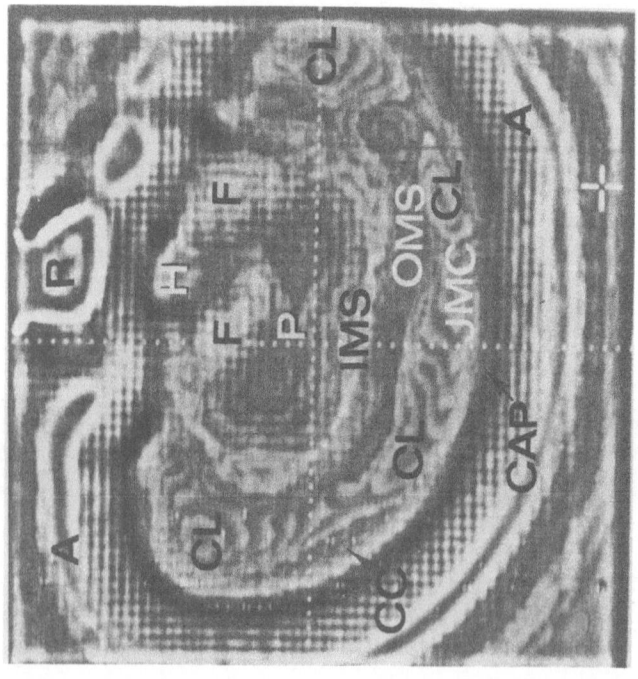

Figure 24a b. Fully Processed Images are Shown for the Magnitude and Phase of Scattering Parameter S_{21} on the Left and Right, Respectively.

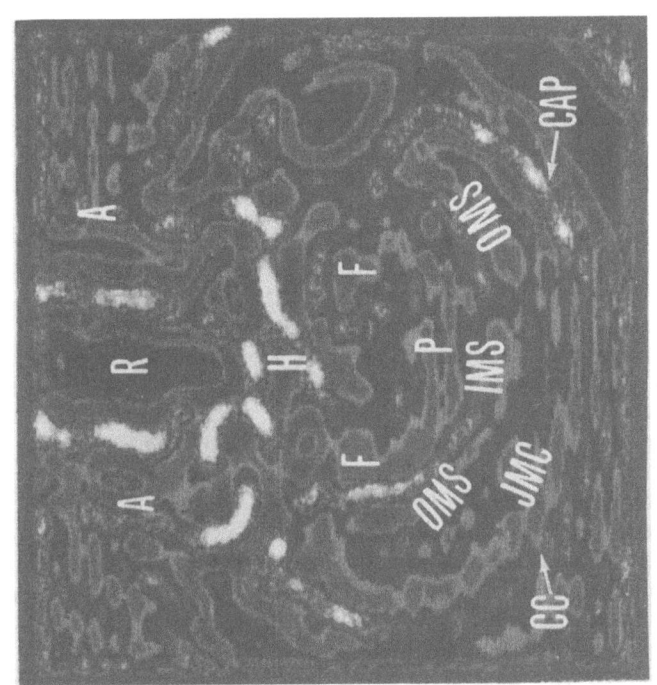

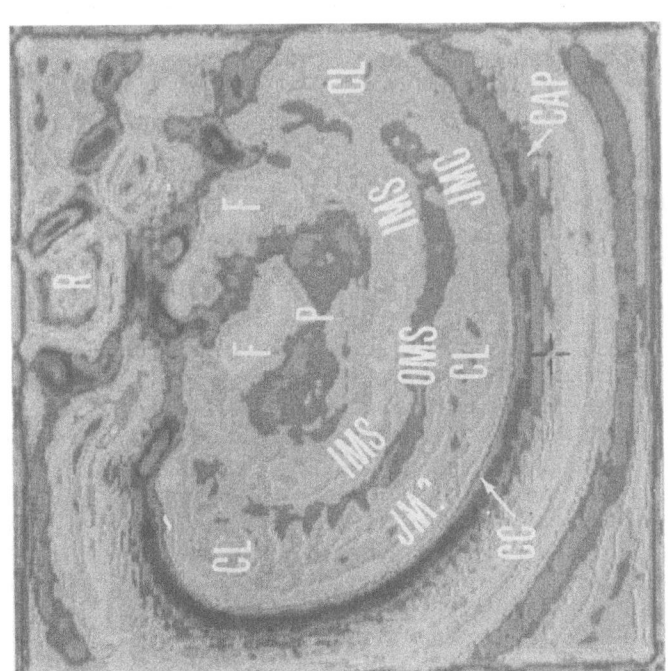

Figure #25a, b. Copolarized and Cross Polarized Magnitude Images are Shown After
Two Dimensional Band Pass Filtering and Pseudocolor Processing on
the Left and Right, Respectively.

The final presentations for both the copolorized (VV) and cross polarized (VH) scattering parameter images are in a contour format (see Figures 26a and 26b) to permit quantitive comparison. Note that the contour intervals are not identical for the two images due to the need to preserve relatability to the grey scale and pseudocolor presentations.

The images from the differential propagation delay or microwave time delay spectrometer (MTDS) are clearly interpretable in the same terms as were applied to the scattering parameter images. The most notable feature is the of artifact in the area outside of the capsule as shown in the monochrome image in Figure #27a. Signal processing steps have been limited to interpolation, grey level mapping and the convolution operator. Note that the cortex corticis and justamedullary cortex are distinguishable. Similarly, there is some suggestion of cortical lobulation, but these are better seen in the contour display which is shown in Figure 27b. The medullary outer stripe is distinguishable from both the inner stripe and the juxtamedullary cortex. Likewise, the inner stripe and pelvis are easily separable. Note also that the artifact, due to the support rod, is suppressed. The contour plot in Figure #27b better displays cortical lobulations and gradients within the pelvis. The enhanced dynamic range of the contour plot also reveals some slight artifact outside of the capsule.

DISCUSSION

The primary feature of the results is that both the copolarized and cross polarized images can be related to known regional specialization within the target organ. This reflects upon the choice of the kidney organ for microwave imagery demonstration wherein gross anatomy, in fact, corresponds rather closely to aggregate nephron morphology. Hence, aggregate physiology at the microscopic scale is correlated with regional specialization. The apparent corespondence between the microwave images and this regional specialization argues for the biological releveance of imagery based upon dielectric properties in the microwave region of the electromagnetic spectrum. We know of no other single form of radiation that offers comparable physiologic corelation in any soft tissue organ. The fact that four imagery methods yield self consistant

115

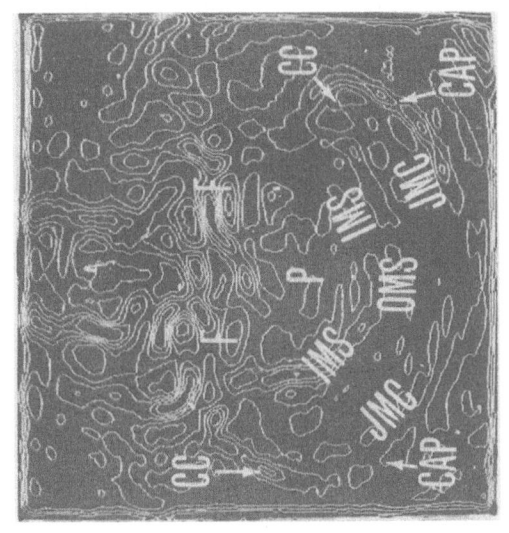

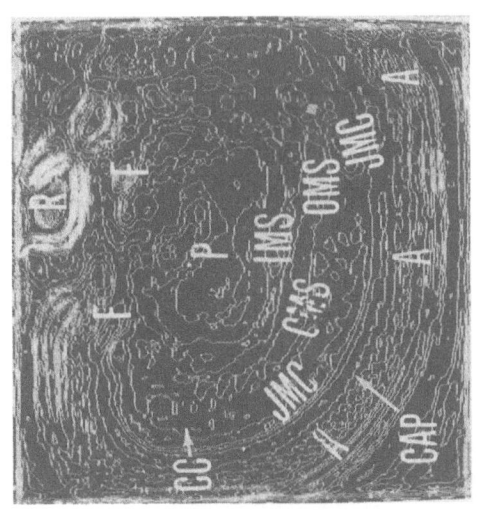

Figure #26a, b. The Fully Processed Data for the Co-Polarized and Cross-Polarized Images are Shown in Contour Format on the Left and Right, Respectively. The Contour Intervals are 10 and 50, Respectively.

116

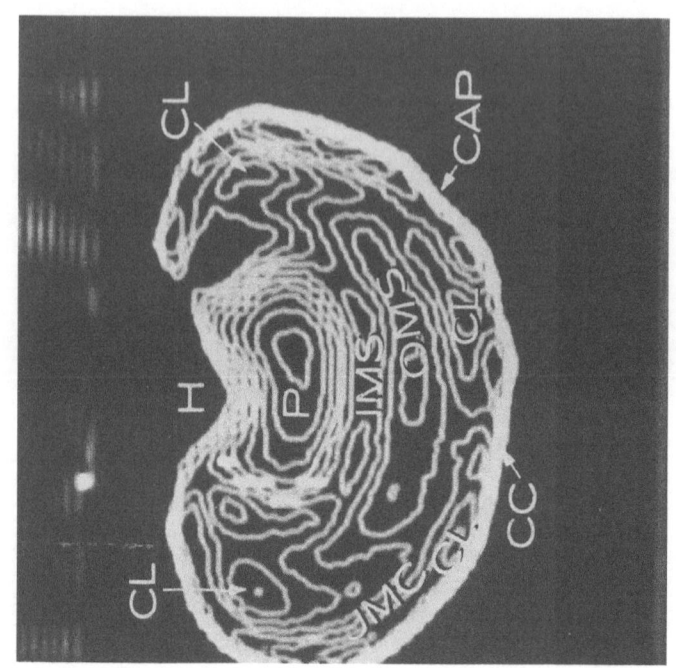

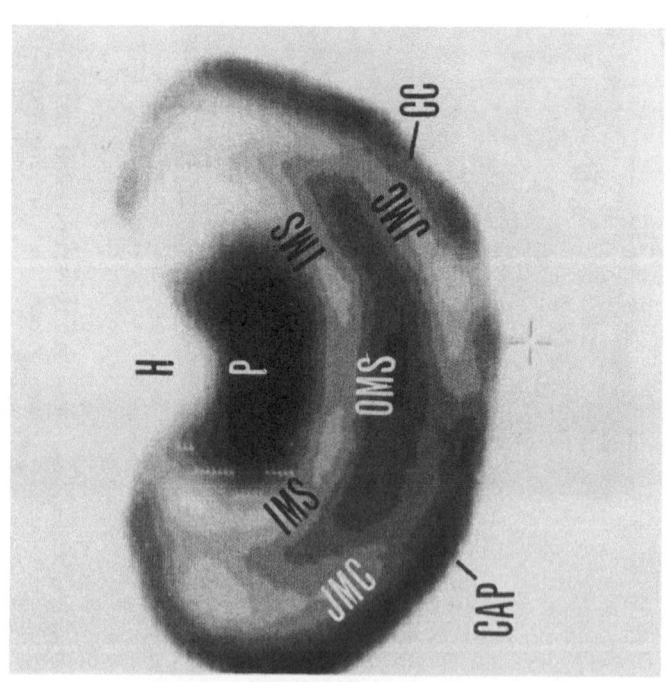

Figure 27a, b. The MTDS Image in Monochrome is Shown on the Left. The Same Image in
Contour Format is Shown on the Right with a Contour Interval of 50.

images and interpretations is further source for optimism. In addition to a high level of biological relevance, microwave radiation is clearly less hazardous than x-ray imagery and no artificial contrast enhancement need be used. These properties have the potential advantage that invasive procedures may be avoided and early diagnosis of disease may be improved.

Indeed, the contrast observed in all of the images presented here is less than that in situ because saline replaced urine in the pelvis. This step was taken to insure that no air was present although the ureter was cut between ligatures. Blood volume was retained at physiologic values since the renal artery and vein were cut between ligatures just prior to nephrectomy and commencement of the scan.

The non-invasive methods used herein do offer promise for providing spatial maps of the energy dissipation and energy storage in biologic dielectrics. Indeed, to the extent that insertion loss measurements can be made with resolution in three dimensions and the various scattering mechanisms can be discriminated, non-invasive dosimetry will become possible. The necessary intermediate step is to deduce the spatial distribution of the real and imaginary parts of the complex permittivity from scattering parameter measurements. For example, to the extent that higher insertion loss represents attenuation, the outer medullary stripe may be predicted to be subject to greater energy deposition than the adjacent juxtamedullary cortex and inner medullary stripe. This inference remains unproven at the present time.

The present work is encouraging, but several additional steps are required. The first of these is to decrease the data acquisition time by use of the phased array system. Present estimates suggest that spatial resolution comparable to that obtained in the near-field with a single element will be available to azimuth and elevation with data collection times in the order of minutes (or less) rather than hours. In addition to electronic beam steering, the array will provide off-line focusing in range, which may be expected to improve image quality. If these expectations are fullfilled, the isolated organ can be maintained on extracorporal circulation at 37°C. The use of physiologic temperature will decrease attenuation and pathophysiological correlations may be explored. Furthermore, the full use of polarization diversity may be explored without the inevitable specimen degradation that would otherwise take place.

In a speculative vein, it is also reasonable to inquire
about improvement in resolution and operation in situ.
Resolution is presently limited by dielectric constant of the
coupling loading medium and hence the size of aperture. Of
course, the frequency of operation could also be increased.
Since the later is of limited utility except in special cases,
the only other available avenue is reduction in aperture area by
the use of still higher relative dielectric constant (ϵ'_r)
material. However, decreasing the aperture area without
increasing the ϵ'_r of the loading medium adds loss to the
system. The important parameter of wavelength in the coupling
medium is ignored if only the aperture is arbitrarily reduced.
In the present system, the aperture is loaded by the same high
ϵ'_r material that provides coupling. These facts combine to
limit resolution to ca. one-half wavelength in the medium when
operated in the near field and forward scatter mode. This
interpretation is supported by the fact that two targets may be
easily resolved at spacings where the wavelength is the medium
surrounding the targets (as opposed to the wavelength in the
coupling medium) was clearly too long to resolve the targets
(16, 18). In simple terms, it would appear to be difficult to
state resolution limits more precisely than those already
demonstrated in the present system whereby the aperture
dimensions (i.e. one-half wavelength in the coupling/loading
medium for the broad and one-quarter wave length for the narrow
dimension, respectively) largely determine resolution.
Resolution in the cross-pol case is more difficult to describe
since it is clearly direction dependent and strongly influenced
by lamination.

The immediate future lies in the water coupled array
antenna (see Figure #28). It will be described here in only an
abbreviated form since a complete exposition exists elsewhere
(32). The system consists of a receive array of 128 double
ridged waveguide elements which measure the forward scattered
complex field amplitudes over a hexagonal lattice approximately
19 cm in diameter. Each element in the receive array is routed
through a series of electromechanical coaxial switches to a
harmonic down-converter and complex ratiometer. The complex
ratiometer provides a magnitude and phase for each element which
is digitized and stored on a magnetic disk. At the present

time, 9 seconds are required to poll the 128 receive array
elements. Focusing and beam steering take place off-line to
maximize flexibility as opposed to RF phase shifters or
dielectric lenses.

The transmit array consists of 153 double ridged wavequide
elements in a hexagonal lattice 15 cm in diameter. Two
illumination modes are possible: broad-side and a series of
pencil beams scanned over the target. Both modes are phase
matched.

At the present time, scan speed is largely determined by
the electromechanical switches, which require about 45 msec per
element. These switching times may be decreased to about 1% of
their present value by the use of PIN diode switches instead of
electromechanical switches. This implies that a high data rate
may be achieved, perhaps in the order of 10-100 msec per
frame. Even this is not fast by microwave standards. System
configurations for maximum speed would be rather different from
the one described here. It would appear to be technologically
feasible to achieve video frame rates if this objective was
included as a design goal.

Problems remain with respect to multipath, although these
may be ameliorated to a large extent with hybrid time/amplitude
measurements. Problems also remain with respect to diffractive,
reflective and refractive errors. The next area of technology
development to bear upon these problems and their solution is
the phased array antenna (32). Data collection time is
important not only for pathophysiological correlation in dynamic
studies, but it also impacts feasibility for various methods of
error correction prior to tomographic reconstruction. These
areas remain as topics of future research; but the motivation
for their solution must come from demonstration of the relevance
of microwave imagery to health and disease.

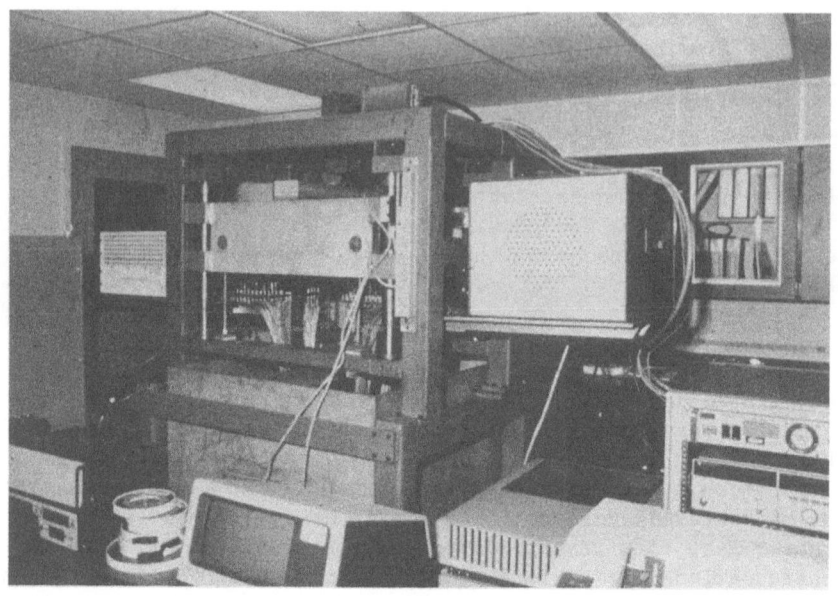

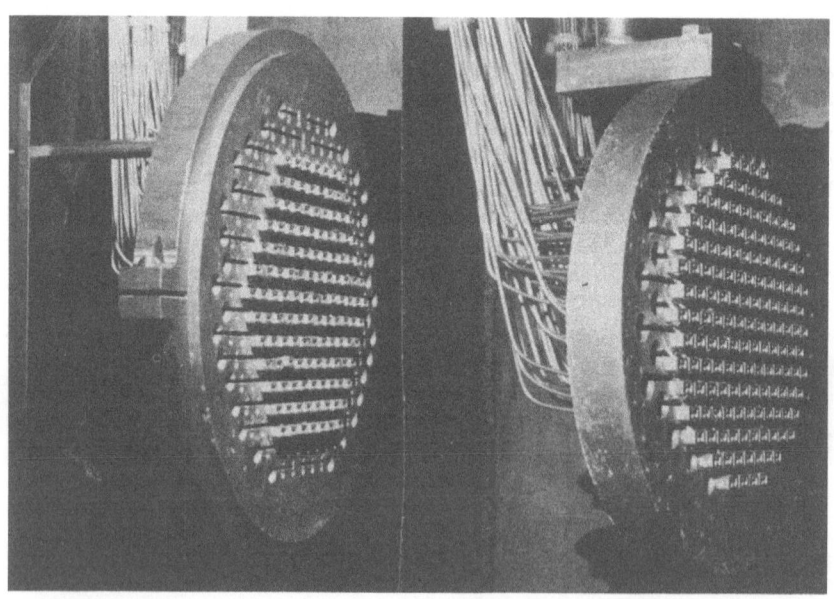

Figure #28a, b, c. Phased Array System;
Transmit Array, and Receive Array.

REFERENCES

1. Von Hippel, A.R. Dielectrics and Waves (MIT Press, 1954).

2. Hasted, J.B. Aqueous Dielectrics (Chapmand and Hall, 1973).

3. Grant, E.H., Sheppard, R.J. and South, G.P. Dielectric Behavior of Biological Molecules in Solution (Clarendon Press, 1978).

4. Yamaura, I. "Meausrements of 1.8 - 2.7 GHz microwave attenuation in the human torso." IEEE Trans. Microwave Theory and Techniques, MTT-25 (1977) 707-710.

5. Burdette, E.C., Cain, F.L. and Seals, J. "In vivo probe measurement techniques for determining dielectric properties at UHF through microwave frequencies." IEEE Trans. Microwave Theory and Techniques, MTT-28 (1980) 414-427.

6. Rutherford, R. A., Pullan, B.R. and Isherwood, I. "Measurement of effective atomic number and electron density using an EMI scanner." Neuroradiol., 11 (1976) 15-22.

7. Gregg, E.C. "Radiation risks with diagnostic x-rays." Radiology 123 (1977) 447-453.

8. Born, M. and Wolf, E. Principles of Optics (Pergamon, 1966).

9. Deschamps, G.A. "Part II - Geometrical representation of the polarization of a plane electromagnetic wave." Proc. IEEE, 39 (1951) 540-544.

10. Kennaugh, E.M. "Polarization properties of radar reflectors." Ohio State University Antenna Laboratory, Project Report 389-12 (AD2494) (RADC, AF28(099)-90, 1952).

11. Sinclair, G. "The transmission and reception of elliptically polarized waves." Proc. IEEE. 39 (1951) 535-540.

12. Copeland, J.R. "Radar target classification by polarization properties." Proc. IRE, 48 (1960) 1290-1296.

13. Huynen, R.J. Phenomenological Theory of Radar Targets (Drukkerij Bronder, 1970).

14. Kurokawa, K. "Power waves and the scattering matrix." IEEE Trans. Microwave Theory and Techniques, MTT - 13 (1965) 194-202.

15. Boerner, W.M., El-Arini, M.B., Chan, C.Y. and Mastoris, P.M. "Polarization dependence in electromagnetic inverse problems." IEEE Trans. Antennas and Propagation, AP-29 (1981) 262-270.

16. Jacobi, J.H. Larsen, L.E. and Hast, T.C. "Water immersed microwave antennas and their application to microwave interrogation of biological targets." IEEE Trans. MicrowaveTheory and Techniques, MTT-27 (1979) 70-78.

17. Ruck, G.T., Burrick, D.E., Stuart, W.D. and Kirchbaum, C.K. Radar Cross Section Handbook, Vols. I and II (Plenum, 1970).

18. Rao, S.P., Santosh, K. and Gregg, E.C. "Computer tomography with microwaves." Radiology, 135 (1980) 769-770.

19. Larsen, L.E. and Jacobi, J.H. "Microwave interrogation of dielectric targets. Part I: by scattering parameters." Medical Physics, 5 (1978) 500-508.

20. Larsen, L.E. and Jacobi, J.H. "Microwave scattering parameter imagery of isolated canine kidney." Medical Physics, 6 (1979) 394-403.

21. Larsen, L.E. and Jacobi, J.H. "The use of orthogonal polarization in microwave imagery of isolated canine kidney. " IEEE Trans. Nuclear Science, NS-27 (1980) 1184-1191.

22. Adam, S.F. Microave Theory and Applications (Prentice Hall, 1969).

23. Jacobi, J.H. and Larsen, L.E. "Microwave interrogation of dielectric targets. Part II: by microwave time delay spectroscopy." Medical Physics, 5 (1978) 509-513.

24. Jacobi, J.H. and Larsen, L.E. "Microwave time delay spectroscopic imagery of isolated canine kidney." Medical Physics 7 (1980) 1-7.

25. Bernstein, R. "Digital image processing of earth observation sensor data." IBM J. Res. and Develop., 20 (1976) 40-57.

26. Rifman, S.S. and McKinum, D.M. "Evaluation of digital correction techniques for ERTS images." TRW Corporation Final Report, TRW 20634-6003-TU-00 (NASA, GSFC,1974).

27. Simon, K.W. "Digital image reconstruction and resampling for geometric manipulation" Digital Image Processing fr Remote Sensing (R. Bernstein, Ed.) pp. 84-94 (IEEE Press, (1978).

28. Gonzales, R.C. and Wintz, P. Digital Image Processing (Addison-Wesley, 1977).

29. Brenner, B.M. and Rector, F.C., Jr. The Kidney. Vols. 1 and II (Saunders, 1976).

30. Pitts, R.F. Physiology of the Kidney and Body Fluids, 3rd Edition (Yearbook Medical Publishers, 1974).

31. DeWardener, H.E. " The Control of sodium excretion." Am. J. Physiol., 235 (1978) F163-F173.

32. Foti, S.J., Flam, R., Aubin, J., Larsen, L.E. and Jacobi, J.H. "Water immerged phased array system for biological target interrogation". Proc Conf Electromagnetic Dosimetric Imagery (Larsen, L.E. and Jacobi, JH. Eds.) (in press, 1981).

TIME-OF-FLIGHT METHOD FOR POSITRON TOMOGRAPHIC IMAGING AND
STATE-OF-THE-ART OF DETECTOR TECHNOLOGY FOR EMISSION TOMOGRAPHY

R. ALLEMAND[*], R. CAMPAGNOLO[*], P. GARDERET[*], R. GARIOD[*],

M. LAVAL[*], M. MOSZYNSKI[**], E. TOURNIER[*], J. VACHER[*].

[*] C.E.A. - C.E.N.G. - L.E.T.I.
[**] from the Institute of Nuclear Research, Swierk-Otwock, Poland

1. INTRODUCTION

Positron computed tomography (P.C.T) is a very promising tool
for research and clinical applications in nuclear medicine.
P.C.T. consists in yielding images representing the distribu-
tion of positron emitting radionuclides (^{11}C, ^{13}N, ^{15}O, ^{18}F...).
The selected labeled molecule is administered to the patient
and the P.C.T. allows to obtain its distribution in several
transverse tomographic sections as a function of time. Many
molecules have been labeled with these radionuclides to investigate very important physiological and biochemical processes.

2. POSITRON TOMOGRAPHIC IMAGING

Carbon, nitrogen and oxygen, three elements of living matter
present a major interest for metabolic processes. Their associated positron emitting radionuclide (^{11}C, ^{13}N, ^{15}O) have a
short half-life, respectively T 1/2 = 20 min, 10 min and 2 min ;
so, they must be prepared in the near vicinity of the site of
their use, which requires the availability of a cyclotron.
Furthermore, that imposes to label the wanted molecules in a
very short time and to manipulate large quantities of radioactivity. Concerning the positron imaging, it means that the instrument must exhibit a very high counting rate capability and
that all the desired sections have to be handled simultaneously
in order to minimize the dose of radiation to the patient.
The basic concept of positron imaging consists in detecting
the two 511 KeV annihilation photons emitted 180° apart with
two opposing banks of detectors. The reconstruction method is

similar to those used in transmission computerized tomography :
each event is back-projected on the whole size of the image.
Scintillation detectors are well adapted for that application :
they exhibit a good detection efficiency for the 511 KeV γ rays,
and a fast timing characteristic can be obtained in order to
reduce random coincidences.
Different types of geometrical configurations have been tested
with suitable motions to make the linear and angular sampling.
[1] [2] [3].
A polygonal array or a ring shape with adaquate linear and
angular motions are the most used. Multislices capabilities
are provided in the most recent systems.

3. TIME-OF-FLIGHT TECHNIQUE (T.O.F.)

Time-of-flight technique consists in directly determining the
localization of each event (fig 1). That method supposes that
a very fast time-coïncidence technique should be obtained : a
time interval of 1 n sec corresponds to a point source position
variation of 15 cm.
G.Brownell [4] and more recently W.Dunn [5] suggested to use
T.O.F. information for positron tomographic imaging. A time
fluctuation of 180 psec (FWHM) was obtained by W.Dunn with very
fast plastic scintillators and with an energy threshold adjusted
to 300 KeV, but such a system provided a much too low sensitivy
to be used in a clinical way. [5].

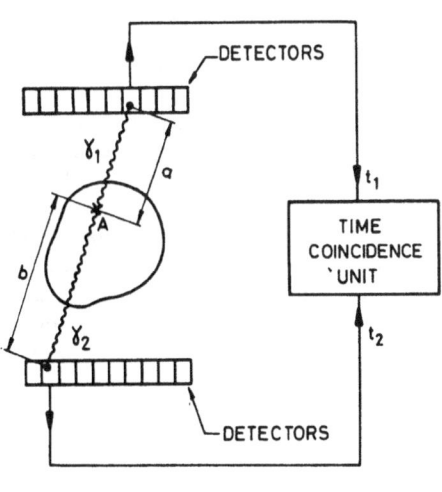

$$b-a = c \ (t_1 - t_2)$$

Fig. 1 : principle of the time-of-flight method

126

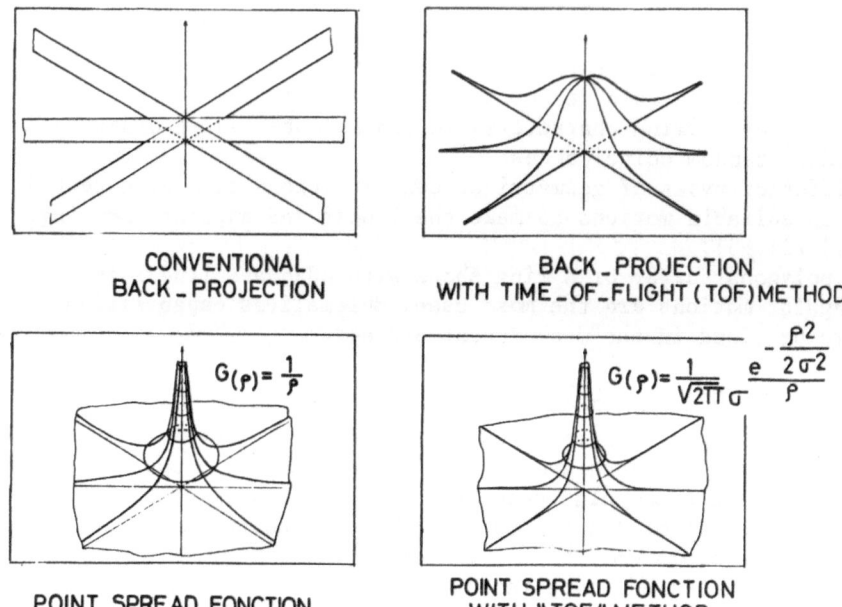

CONVENTIONAL
BACK _ PROJECTION

BACK _ PROJECTION
WITH TIME _ OF _ FLIGHT (TOF) METHOD

$$G(\rho) = \frac{1}{\rho}$$

$$G(\rho) = \frac{1}{\sqrt{2\pi}\ \sigma} \cdot \frac{e^{-\frac{\rho^2}{2\sigma^2}}}{\rho}$$

POINT SPREAD FONCTION

POINT SPREAD FONCTION
WITH "TOF" METHOD

Fig. 2 : basic difference between the conventional method and the
T.O.F. technique

4. PRINCIPLE OF THE PROPOSED METHOD

This method consists in combining the advantages of a fast and
efficient detection method providing the T.O.F. information
with those of the reconstruction method by backprojection [6][7]
In measuring the time distribution of the events with a far
greater accuracy than the transit time of a photon in the object,
a gaussian spatial distribution of each event can be determined.
The basic difference between the conventional method and the
proposed method is shown in fig 2. In the first case, the section of the point spread function is of the form $1/\rho$, where ρ
is the distance to the point source. In the second case, the
point spread function is a gaussian function whose section
$G(\rho)$ is given by :

$$G(\rho) = \frac{1}{\sqrt{2\pi}\sigma} \cdot \frac{e^{-\frac{\rho^2}{2\sigma^2}}}{\rho}$$

where : ρ is the distance to the point source
     σ is the standard deviation of the gaussian function.
Fig 2. shows the information is much more concentrated close to
the point source in the T.O.F. technique than in the conventional method because the information is back-projected on a
length only a fraction of the image size.

5. COMPARISON BETWEEN THE CONVENTIONAL METHOD AND T.O.F. TECHNIQUE

That comparison may be expressed by a sensitivity gain defined as the ratio of the number of counts needed to obtain the same signal to noise ratio with the two methods.

5.1. Theoretical estimation

That approach has been carried out in assuming that the T.O.F. measurement may be modelized as a linear filter with gaussian spread function (whose σ is the standard deviation). The comparison was made in estimating the signal to noise ratio in the central area of an uniform activity phantom ($\emptyset$ in diameter) as a function of σ. The different steps of the reconstruction method used for that evaluation are the following :

- the histogram of the T.O.F. data along each coïncidence path is back-projected after smoothing with a gaussian impulse response (whose σ is the standard deviation). Variance of noise can be then calculated.
- the back-projected image is obtained by the data accumulation from all the paths, and the associated variance of noise is deduced.
- the final image is obtained through a bi-dimensional filtering using a filter matched to the T.O.F. accuracy. In order to allow the noise comparison, the apodisation function has been adjusted to provide the same global spread spatial function as in conventional reconstruction.

The variance of noise is then calculated as a function of σ and for various object diameters. The results, expressed in terms of sensivity gain are plotted in fig. 3.

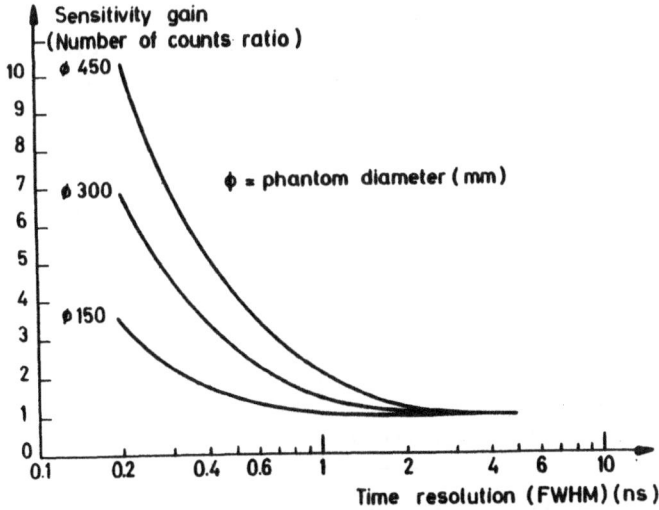

Fig. 3 : sensitivity gain as a function of the F.W.H.M. time resolution

As σ is increased, the variance approaches that obtained with conventional method. That approach assumes an infinite number of coïncidence events. It may not be optimal for medical positron imaging because the number of events is relatively poor, and then the statistical fluctuation in timing data become significant. A second approach, taking into account these statistical aspects, is investigated by another group [8].

5.2. Experimental approach

An experimental approach has been carried out with a cylindrical phantom moved in translation and in rotation between two opposite detectors. First results are promising but the advantages of the T.O.F. technique have not been yet quantified. In a first step, a qualitative comparison with the conventional method shows a statistical noise reduction and a better outlines perception of the spots for the T.O.F. technique. A quantitative comparison will be published shortly.

6. FAST COINCIDENCE TIMING DETECTION

Inorganic scintillator detectors are the most suitable ones for our purpose because they combine three major advantages = a high stopping power, a fast coïncidence timing, and a large scintillator volume availability.

Historically, activated sodium iodide NaI(Tl) and bismuth germanate (BGO) have been widely used for positron imaging but they are not convenient for T.O.F. because they exhibit too long a light decay time. More recently, our group suggested to use cesium-fluoride (CsF) [6] and this approach has been followed by other groups [8] [9].

6.1. Cesium-fluoride characteristics

Up to now, CsF appears to be the most suitable scintillator for our purpose because it combines a relatively high atomic number,

CHARACTERISTICS	NaI(Tl)	B.G.O.	CsF
Density (g/cm^3)	3.67	7.13	4.61
Atomic numbers	11,53	82,32,8	55,9
Linear attenuation coefficient at 511kev (cm^{-1})	0.34	0.92	0.44
Scintillation peak wavelength (nm)	413	480	390
Index of refraction at peak wavelength	1.85	2.15	1.48
Relative scintillation output	100	8	6
Scintillation decay time (nsec)	230	300	3

Table 1   Main physical properties of inorganic scintillators for positron imaging

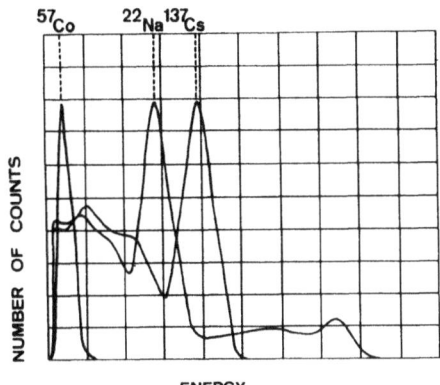

Fig. 4 : γ rays energy spectra from ^{137}Cs (660 KeV)
^{57}Co (122 KeV) and ^{22}Na (main peak at 511 KeV) with a
23 mm in diameter and 40 mm long CsF scintillator coupled to a XP 2020 fast photomultiplier.

a high density, and a sub-nanosecond coincidence resolving time
capability. Table 1 summarizes the main physical properties of
these three inorganic scintillators.

Fig. 4 shows the energy spectra of γ rays from ^{137}Cs (660 KeV),
^{57}Co (122 KeV) and ^{22}Na (photoelectric peak at 511 KeV) sources
with a 23 mm in diameter and 40 mm long CsF scintillator coupled
to a XP 2020 fast photomultiplier. The F.W.H.M. energy resolution
is better than 20 % at 511 KeV.

Fig. 5 shows the emission spectrum of a CsF scintillator measured
under X-ray irradiation by means of a monochromator and a XP 2020
Q photomultiplier (quartz window). A U.V. component at 335 nm has
been found, which seems to take a significant part in timing characteristics. That assessment is based on the fact that a better
timing was obtained with photomultipliers having a U.V. glass window. The contribution of the optical coupling with the photomultipliers has been pointed out in measuring the light yield of a CsF
sample with and without soft glass window. It was found that 12 %
more light are obtained with direct coupling. That difference is
explained by a better optical matching and by a U.V. photons absorption inside the window, but the quantitative contribution of
each effect has not been established yet.

Fig. 6 shows the time distribution of the light pulse shape of a
CsF scintillator (diameter 23 mm and 40 mm long) under γ ray irradiation. This study has been performed by means of the single
photon method [10] as show in fig. 7. The CsF crystal is irradiated by 511 KeV annihilation photons from 68 Ga source. The timing
reference detector is the XP 2020 photomultiplier coupled with a
fast plastic scintillator. The coincidence is made with a HR 400
microchannel plate photomultiplier which receives attenuated light
so that only single photons are detected. The light pulse shape
is obtained by measuring the time distribution of the detected
single photoelectrons. No low component has been found ; thus CsF
exhibits a very high counting rate capability and this property

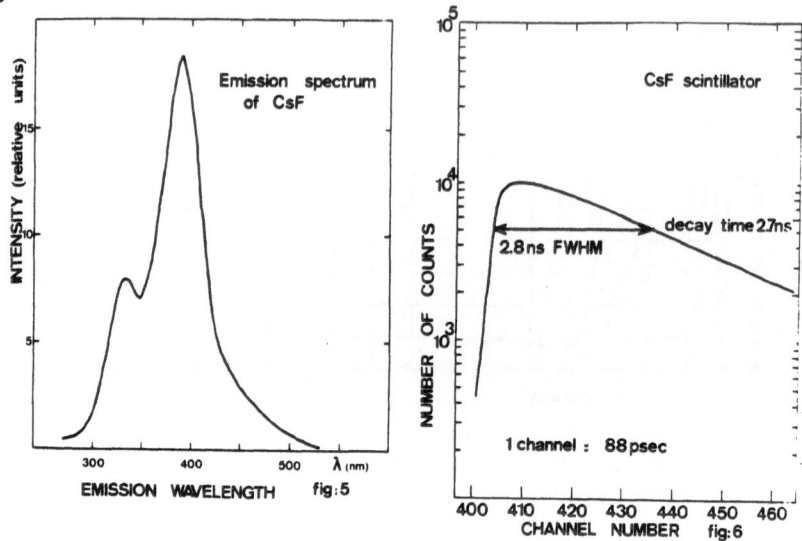

Fig. 5 : emission spectrum of CsF scintillator

Fig. 6 : time distribution of the light pulse shape of a 23 mm
in diameter and 40 mm long CsF scintillator under γ ray
excitation

has already been applied for positron imaging without using T.O.F.
information [1].

Table 2 gives the T.O.F. accuracy as a function of the crystal
lenght. It shows that the length is strongly linked to the timing
characteristic. As the coïncidence detection efficiency is also
dependant of the length, a figure of merit can be defined which is
the ratio of efficiency on T.O.F. A 40 mm long direct coupled
scintillator gas been chosen for our P.C.T. design, but this value
does not represent a sharp optimum.

Concerning the light yield, significant improvements have been
reached. In a previous paper [6], the relative scintillation output of the first samples* was measured to be 5 % of NaI(Tℓ)'s.
Now, 8 % is usually obtained with the new samples.

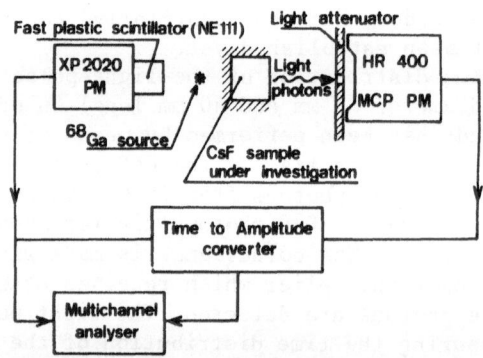

Fig. 7 : principle of the single photon method

*Manufactured by Harshaw Chemical Company and by L.E.T.I.

CRYSTAL LENGTH (cm)	TIME OF FLIGHT [*] (ps)	THEORETICAL COINCIDENCE DETECTION EFFICIENCY [**] (%)	FIGURE OF MERIT (EFFICIENCY/T.O.F.)
1.5	325		
3	375	53	0.14
4	435	69	0.16
4.4	470	74	0.16
5	520	79	0.15

[*] for a threshold at 140 Kev

[**] $\mu : 0.44$ cm^{-1}

Table 2 Detection figure of merit as a function of crystal length

Furthermore, the influence of the crystal coating on the timing characteristics has been established. A diffusing coating gives about 15 % more light than a reflecting one, but the light pulse rise time is almost 1.5 shorter for the reflecting one. As the time pick-off is based on the first photons emission, the final result is that a reflecting coating appears to be better than a diffusing one. In the same conditions, an improvement of 30 psec of the 470 psec FWHM time resolution has been obtained.

6.2. Photomultiplier
A very fast photomultiplier is needed in order to keep negligible the timing P.M. tube contribution. Fast commercially available P.M. tubes are two inches in diameter and the corresponding spatial resolution for a P.C.T. would be very poor. A one inch diameter P.M. tube seems to be a good trade-off for a whole body P.C.T. Time measurements were performed with 1"1/8 diameter P.M. type 1992[***] and R 1398[****]. The best results were obtained with this last one. It yields about 25 % more photoelectrons due to a better window transparence at the U.V. component (U.V. glass instead of soft glass for P.M. 1992)and a better collection of the most energetic photoelectrons [12]. As previously shown by M. MOSZYNSKI and B. BENGTSON [13] a better timing can be obtained in picking the last dynode signal. The main results are summarized in table 3 in which the figures represent mean values from tests with several samples.

6.3. Overall timing characteristics
A 40 mm long and 23 mm in diameter scintillator directly coupled to a P.M. 1398 has been chosen for our P.C.T. design. That represents a trade-off between a lot of parameters and particularly : the sensivity, the spatial resolution and the T.O.F. accuracy. The

[***]Manufactured by Radiotechnique Compelec
[****]Manufactured by Hamamatsu

132

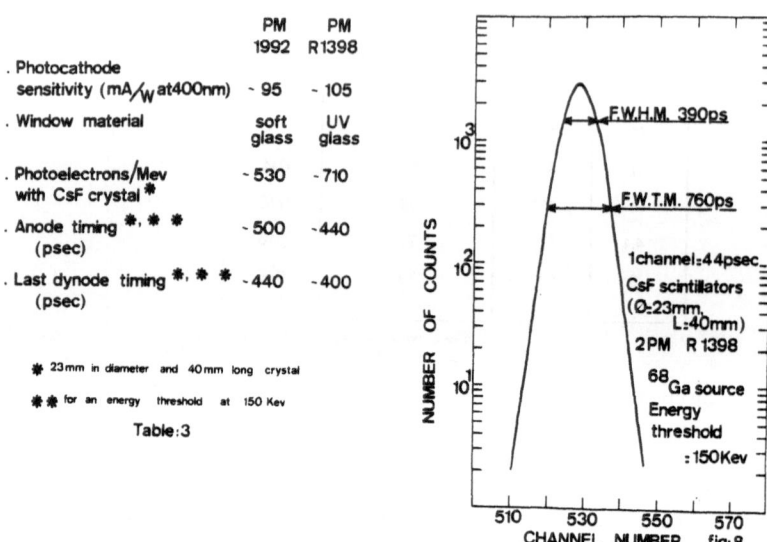

	PM 1992	PM R1398
. Photocathode sensitivity (mA/$_W$ at400nm)	~ 95	~ 105
. Window material	soft glass	UV glass
. Photoelectrons/Mev with CsF crystal *	~ 530	~ 710
. Anode timing *,** (psec)	~ 500	~440
. Last dynode timing *,** (psec)	~ 440	~ 400

* 23 mm in diameter and 40mm long crystal

** for an energy threshold at 150 Kev

Table : 3

F.W.H.M. 390ps

F.W.T.M. 760ps

1channel:44psec
CsF scintillators
(∅:23mm,
L:40mm)
2PM R 1398
68Ga source
Energy
threshold
:150Kev

NUMBER OF COUNTS

CHANNEL NUMBER   fig:8

Table 3   Comparison between photomultiplier tubes type 1992 and
R 1398

Fig. 8 : time spectrum of coïncidences of 511 KeV annihilation
photons measured with two CsF scintillators (23 mm in
diameter and 40 mm long) and two PM R 1398

energy threshold choice has also to be considered. All other parameters being unchanged, the timing is 400 psec with a threshold
at 150 KeV and 330 psec at 400 KeV, but the detection efficiency
of the photopeak fraction is only a half of that at 150 KeV, due
to the radiation scattering inside the detector itself. That leads
to choose a 140 KeV threshold, because a loss of a factor 4 in
coïncidence sensitivity would not be compensated by the T.O.F.
sensitivity gain. The fig. 8 shows the time spectrum of coïncidence of 511 KeV annihilation radiation measured with two CsF
scintillators (∅ 23 mm, L : 40 mm) and two P.M. R 1398, the timing signal being picked on the last dynode. A 390 psec FWHM time
resolution has been obtained with a single pair of detectors tu-
ned in a laboratory environment. It represents an optimal value,
but other tests have been carried out with several probes representing a bank of detectors and a 500 psec time resolution (FWHM)
seems to be a realistic figure for an operational machine.

7. SENSITIVITY COMPARISON WITH B.G.O. P.C.T.

The figure n° 3 shows a sensitivity gain of about 4 compared to
a CsF conventional P.C.T. for a 450 mm diameter object.
With the same scintillator size, a B.G.O. machine would give 20 %
more detection efficiency at the center which means an overall
sensitivity gain of 3.2 for the T.O.F. method.
It has to be noticed that this advantage of CsF would be lower
with smaller crystals due to the efficiency losses by packaging,

a higher fraction of γ ray scattering, and a poorer angular response. Neverless, this last parameter is not really a disadvantage because the measured activity distribution for an uniform phantom is several times higher on the edge than at the center ; thus the statistical accuracy is minimum at the center and the sensitivity comparison in this area is the moste significant one.

Conclusion

Positron imaging is essentially a method for studying dynamic phenomena and positron emitters are characterized by a short life which allows to inject a high activity. This means that a high counting-rate capability is a major feature of a P.C.T.; furthermore, a high resolving time permits the reduction of random coïncidence events which yield a low spatial frequency background, reducing the contrast of the image and introducting an error for quantitative measurements. For these points of view, CsF appears to be the most suitable scintillator.
Its fast light emission allows to reach a time-of-flight information which improves the signal to noise ratio of the image. That advantage is a function of the object size and the T.O.F. accuracy. Now, a 500 psec time resolution (FWHM) seems to be a realistic characteristic for an operational machine.
The comparison between the conventional method and the T.O.F. technique has been expressed in terms of sensitivity gain which is the ratio of the number of events needed to obtain the same signal to noise ratio. A sensitivity gain of 4 has been theoretically estimated with a 500 psec timing and for a 450 mm diameter phantom. This evaluation seems to be in a good ageement with the first experimental results. This work has to be considered only as a suitable way to make a quantitative comparison ; the image perception is complex and a more significant comparison has to be made with an operational T.O.F. machine.
It has to be noticed that the T.O.F. method advantage is closely linked to the object diameter. In the present state-of-the-art of detectors timing, it is obvious that the choice of the T.O.F. method is more justified for a whole-body P.C.T. than for a brain one, but further significant improvements in timing accuracy can be expected, giving then a wider field of applications. It has to be added that the future of this technique will be also dependant on the state-of-the-art in very high speed analog and digital data manipulative methods. As a first step, the importance of CsF is remaining for a P.C.T. design without the use of T.O.F. technique, the CsF high counting-rate capability being a major advantage for fast dynamic studies with short lived emitters.
A four rings T.O.F. whole body positron tomograph is under construction in LETI. It will be set up in the service hospitalier Frederic Joliot à ORSAY.

134

Acknowledgments

This paper summarizes the present status of a joint work of different LETI groups. The authors wish to thank C. JANIN and R. ODRU
for their extensive assistance and to point out the helpful contribution of M. MOSZYNSKI (from the Institute of Nuclear Research-
Swierk-Otwock-Poland and visitor in LETI) for his large experience
in fast timing techniques.

This work has been mainly supported by l'Institut de recherche
fondamentale (C.E.A.). The whole-body T.O.F. P.C.T. design has
been undertaken with the help of service hospitalier Frederic
Joliot à ORSAY (FRANCE) and all the LETI participants at this design wish to thank Dr. D. COMAR and F. SOUSSALINE for their very
helpful discussions and clinical informations.

Informal but efficient connections with M. TER-POGOSSIAN
(Washington University Medical School, St. Louis, MISSOURI) on
common interest technical problems merit to be noticed.

REFERENCES

[1] Ter Pogossian MM, Mullani NA, Hood JT, Higgins CS,
     Ficke DC = design considerations for a positron emission
     transverse tomograph (PETT V) for imaging of the brain.
     J. Comput. Assist. Tomogr. 2 : 539-544, 1978.

[2] Phelps ME, Hoffman EF, Sung-cheng Huang, Kuhl DE : design
     considerations in positron computed tomography.
     I.E.E.E. Trans. Nucl. Sci. N.S 26 n° 2 : 2746-2751, 1979.

[3] Budinger T.F. : instrumentation trends in nuclear medicine.
     Semin Nucl. Med 7 : 285-297, 1977.

[4] Brownell GL, Burnham CA, Wilensky S : New developments in
     positron scintigraphy and the application of cyclotron
     produced positron emitters. In Medical Radioisotope Scin-
     tigraphy. Vol. 1 . Proceedings of a symposium Salzburg,
     August 6-15, 1968 - Vienna, I.A.E.A, 1969, p466.

[5] Dunn WL : Time-of-flight localization of positron emitting
     isotopes. Thesis in Physics . Vanderbilt University,
     Nashville, TN, 1975.

[6] Allemand R, Gresset C, Vacher J. : Potential advantages
     of a Cesium fluoride scintillator for a time-of-flight
     positron camera.
     J. Nucl. Med. 21 (2) : 153, 155, 1980.

[7] Campagnolo R, Garderet P, Vacher J : Tomographie par emet-
     teurs positrons avec mesure de temps de vol. Colloque in-
     ternational sur le traitement du signal. Nice, Mai 1979.

[8] Ter Pogossian MM, Mullani NA, Ficke DC, Markham J,
     Snyder DL : Photon time-of-flight assisted positron emis-
     sion tomography.
     J. Comput. Assist. Tomogr. 5(2) : 227-239, 1981.

[9] Mullani NA, Ficke C, Ter Pogossian MM : Cesium fluoride :
     A new detector for positron emission tomography. I.E.E.E.
     Trans. Nucl. Sci NS 27 : 572-575, 1980.

[10] Moszynski M, Vacher J, Odru R.
     Nucl. instr. and meth. (to be published).

[11] Ter Pogossian MM : Private communication on CsF positron
     emission transverse tomograph (PETT VI).

[12] Moszynski M, Allemand R, Laval M, Odru R, Vacher J : Recent
     progress in fast timing with CsF scintillators in applica-
     tion to time-of-flight positron tomography. (Submitted to
     J. Nuel instr. and meth) May 1981.

[13] Bengtson B, Moszynski M. Nucl. instr. and meth. (to be
     published).

SCANNED PROJECTION RADIOGRAPHY

Walter L. Robb, Ph.D.
Vice President and General Manager
General Electric Company
Medical Systems Operations
Milwaukee, Wisconsin U.S.A.

William R. Brody, M.D., Ph.D.
Associate Professor of Radiology and
   Electrical Engineering
Director, Research Laboratories
Stanford University Medical Center
Palo Alto, California U.S.A.

The field of diagnostic radiology has incorporated many exciting new procedures and technical developments during its 85-year history since the discovery of the x-ray in 1895. But no period has been more fruitful, perhaps, than the last decade when developments have appeared at a remarkable pace. Through all these changes, however, the fundamental goals of diagnostic radiology have remained unaltered. Basically, these goals are:

o To develop increasingly less-invasive procedures;

o To obtain the maximum diagnostic information possible at a given dose, or the necessary information at the minimum dose;

o To increase the flexibility and convenience of various methods in obtaining diagnostic information;

o To accomplish these objectives in a cost-effective manner.

The imminent appearance of clinical digital radiography systems is fully compatible with these objectives. Rather than merely moving the field of diagnostic radiology in a radically new direction, the application of digital technology to radiography and fluoroscopy promises significant advances toward achieving the goals of radiology. The most appealing benefits of digital radiography are:

o Improved low contrast detectability;

o Capability for accurate and interactive processing of the detected information;

o Synchronization of diagnostic procedures;

o Flexible image display;

o Digital storage of raw data and images.

BACKGROUND

Digital radiography is a direct consequence of the needs of diagnostic radiology, combined with technological advances in digital electronics. As the technology of digital processors and memories have progressed and the cost of such devices declined, digital techniques have been introduced into various areas of medical imaging. Computers were first applied to nuclear medicine procedures about 15 years ago. However, the appearance of the computed tomography scanner in 1972, marked the popular acceptance of computers and digital techniques in medical imaging. The impact of the digital computed tomography image, as well as the results of some direct comparisons between prototype digital systems and conventional systems, all served to accelerate the interest in digital radiography.

Digital radiographic systems can be defined as those systems in which the detected x-ray information is converted into digital form and is available for processing prior to display. It is convenient to differentiate digital radiographic systems by the geometry of the x-ray beams variously employed, such as pencil beams, fan beams and area beams. However, it now appears that area beam and fan beam systems, due to the requirements for short scan times, excellent low contrast detectability and reasonable cost, are the two most promising geometries for practical clinical systems.

DIGITAL FLUOROGRAPHY

Area beam digital radiographic systems span a range of architectures, including the digitizing of the output of an image intensifier/TV chain; reading an exposed selenium plane with scanning electrometers and then digitizing the output; and even digitizing standard radiographs and processing the data. But the most common area beam devices are the so-called "digital fluorography" systems, also known as "digital fluoroscopy" systems. They essentially consist of an x-ray image intensifier, a high-quality television camera whose output is converted into a digital format, a digital processor and a display.

Digital fluorography is clearly a descendent of TV fluoroscopy and has even more directly evolved from efforts to obtain subtraction images from TV fluoroscopic systems. In the early 1970s, a group at the University of Wisconsin, led by Charles A. Mistretta, Ph.D., developed a system for K-edge subtraction fluoroscopy using analog methods. Subsequently, the availability of digital technology at reasonable cost led to the development of a digital system for both K-edge imaging and temporal subtraction. Independently, a research group at the University of Arizona developed a digital fluorographic system. Both these experimental systems generated substantial interest in digital fluorography technology.

One of the major advantages of digital fluorography is short data acquisition times. The entire projection image is acquired in just a few milliseconds, making it feasible to acquire a number of sequential images for temporal subtraction studies. Intrinsic system noise is primarily generated by the television camera. But since current camera designs are capable of achieving signal-to-noise ratios approaching one thousand to one, visualization for most clinical applications is primarily limited by quantum noise. In very low contrast studies with relatively high x-ray intensity at the detector, the additive intrinsic system noise will represent the performance limit.

Since the entire subject volume is irradiated simultaneously, digital fluorographic systems may suffer some image degradation from x-ray scatter. This problem can be minimized if thin anatomical portions are studied and/or if geometric magnification and scatter-reducing techniques (i.e. grids) are employed. Additional image degradation can occur from light scatter within the x-ray image intensifier called "veiling glare".

SCANNED PROJECTION RADIOGRAPHY

Fan beam digital radiography systems are referred to by the term "scanned projection radiography", or "SPR". Alternatively, they are sometimes called "line-scanned" systems. For purposes of this discussion, we will employ the former term to refer to digital radiography with a fan beam system.

Different detectors have been investigated for fan beam geometries, including xenon ionization chambers, scintillators with photomultiplier tubes or photodiodes, intensifying screens with photodiodes, and others. The most familiar scanned projection radiography devices are the localization systems employed on computed tomography scanners which use the CT detector and electronics to generate a "computed radiograph" of the anatomy. Such images are produced by mechanically translating the patient through a narrowly collimated x-ray fan beam, sequentially exposing a single line to form an image containing multiple lines of information. The tube and detector both remain stationary during acquisition of image data, while the patient is advanced through the x-ray beam. This imaging technique sharply contrasts to conventional radiographic imaging systems and digital fluorography systems which simultaneously acquire the entire projection image.

Crude SPR localization devices were originally developed both to aid the technologist in choosing the CT slices to be imaged and to aid the radiologist in retrospectively localizing a slice of interest and referencing it to other anatomical features. But it was immediately apparent that these digital radiographs might have diagnostic value. A comparison of the CT/T ScoutView system with a conventional film/screen system supports this contention. Using a special phantom containing four sets of pre-drilled holes of various diameters in each of four quadrants of varying radiographic contrast, it was determined that this early form of SPR had significantly better low contrast detectability (below 5% contrast) than standard radiography.

Consequently, General Electric developed a prototype scanned projection radiography system based upon the CT/T scanner. Called the RadView system, this unit went into operation in 1978, under a collaborative agreement with Stanford University Medical Center.

A significant feature of SPR is the substantial scatter rejection of this geometry. The collimated detector receives photons transmitted through the section being irradiated, thus effectively eliminating scattered radiation. Adjacent sections are not irradiated, and thus do not contribute to the scatter. The residual scatter in this configuration is negligible. Such an SPR system also facilitates the use of high quantum efficiency detectors which can be applied directly to data acquisition systems. Such detectors are relatively free of noise and make efficient use of the radiation dose. Another important feature is the "focal plane shutter" effect. This allows scans of dynamic structures to be taken in a few seconds and be virtually free of motion blurring. Since the scan lines are acquired sequentially, each portion of the image represents a different time interval. Therefore, as long as each line is acquired in a few milliseconds, the image will be free of motion blurring. The image will, however, have a subtle distortion which should not inhibit diagnosis. A horizontally moving vessel, for instance, will be reproduced slightly aslant, though it will be in good focus throughout its length.

SPR VS. DIGITAL FLUOROGRAPHY

Both scanned projection radiography and digital fluorography have relative advantages and disadvantages.

Area Beam Devices

Area beam devices are generally used in conjunction with a conventional image intensifier and, thus, have a potentially high compatibility with existing systems. When used for digital subtraction with larger-than-normal fluoroscopic exposures, such systems have high contrast sensitivity at potentially real time image rates. Such a system is ideally suited to temporal subtraction and, depending on the permissable degree of background scatter and veiling glare, may also be useful for energy subtraction techniques.

Fan Beam Devices

Fan beam devices offer several distinct advantages over area beam systems, though they are achieved at the expense of image repetition rate and x-ray tube heat loading. The low image repetition rate can also restrict applications of temporal subtraction and may preclude the use of SPR for some procedures. However, good scatter rejection, coupled with high intrinsic signal to noise ratios, allow the SPR device to achieve a particular image quality with less exposure than the area beam. Subtraction images are primarily x-ray quantum limited. Scatter rejection is especially important in energy subtraction. Generally, the different spectra have unequal scatter fields. With the fan beam geometry, the detected scatter fields are small, so their degrading effects on energy subtraction are minimized. In addition, since SPR has evolved directly from CT, there exists a very high potential for compatibility with advanced CT scanners or, in some cases, with existing CT localization systems.

SUBTRACTION TECHNIQUES

The main advantage of digital radiographic systems over conventional systems is that the digital system can provide improved low contrast detectability with increased dynamic range. Clinically, the goal is to be able to use this improved performance for intravenous arteriography, as well as analysis of soft tissue structures. In general, the low contrast structures of interest are surrounded by soft tissue, bone, or air-filled structures that are of little interest, but can mask the desired detail. Even though the detector may have sufficient low contrast sensitivity to provide information about the structure of interest in the images, the viewer often needs assistance to visually separate these signals from the background. In other words, the low contrast structures of interest must be made more conspicuous.

In CT, this is accomplished by the reconstruction process. Overlying and underlying structures are separated from those of interest when the cross-sectional image is produced. CT, thus, largely owes its excellent ability to visualize subtle structures to this "depth subtraction" capability. The function of the subtraction process in digital radiology is similar: to remove or suppress the potentially confusing effects of uninteresting overlying and underlying structures, thereby enhancing the detectability of the structures of interest.

Two types of subtraction -- temporal and energy -- are being investigated:

Temporal Subtraction

Temporal subtraction, also called "mask mode" subtraction, is a technique that can be employed to remove overlying and underlying structures when the object of interest is enhanced by an administered contrast agent. It is similar in concept to film subtraction, since images are acquired with and without contrast, and subtracted from each other.

Theoretically, temporal subtraction offers a very high signal-to-noise ratio for imaging iodinated contrast materials. The techniques for performing temporal subtraction are simple. However, limitations do exist, the principal one being its susceptibility to misregistration artifacts caused by patient motion between the time the pre-contrast image is acquired and when the contrast image is acquired. Temporal subtraction is also not suitable for contrast studies in which considerable time elapses between administration and contrast visualization; for example, the gallbladder. Misregistration can occur even when pre- and post-contrast images are separated by only several seconds. However, careful patient positioning, multiple subtraction pairs, and relative translation of images in a subtraction pair can help minimize such errors.

Temporal subtraction is further limited in that administered contrast material must be used and changes in contrast must occur rapidly.

Acquisition of multiple images helps assure that at least one image is taken at the peak of the contrast bolus, thereby producing the image with the maximum low contrast detectability.

Energy Subtraction

Energy subtraction is less susceptible to motion artifacts since this technique exploits the differences in attenuation properties between the contrast material and the surrounding soft tissue and bone. This graph shows the energy dependence of the mass attenuation coefficients of iodine and soft tissue.

In this example, images are made at energies E_1 and E_2 slightly below and above the K-edge -- the large discontinuity in the attenuation of iodine at 33 keV These images are then subtracted. Because the attenuation coefficient of soft tissue changes only slightly for the two energies, soft tissue shadows will be virtually can-

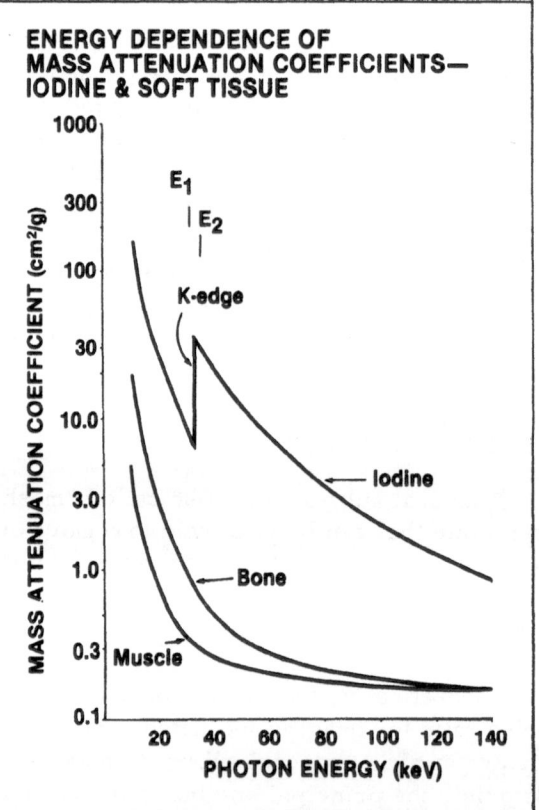

celled in the difference image. On the other hand, because the iodine attenuation coefficient undergoes a significant change, its image will be preserved. The relative ratio of contrast between the iodine and soft tissue is thereby increased.

Energy subtraction using two x-ray beams is termed "dual-energy" imaging. It need not be confined to energies just above and below the iodine K-edge. In fact, insufficient x-ray tube output at K-edge energies, for instance, and patient exposure considerations make the use of higher energies preferable in most circumstances. Methods using these high energies are called "non-K-edge" energy subtraction.

A characteristic of both K-edge and non-K-edge energy subtraction is that in addition to logarithmic processing, the subtraction must also be weighted. This means that prior to subtraction, the high energy image must be multiplied by a factor different from the factor applied to the low energy image. This is different from temporal subtraction in which the weights applied to the two presubtraction images are the same.

Energy subtraction employs the different relative attenuation characteristics of fat, soft tissue, bone and iodine, depending upon the energy of the incident x-ray beam. These differences arise because the two dominant processes which attenuate the x-ray beam -- photoelectric absorption and Compton scattering -- behave differently for low and high atomic number materials. For example, iodine attenuates x-rays predominately by photoelectric absorption throughout the entire diagnostic x-ray energy spectrum, while fat is predominately a Compton scatterer.

RadView uses a method to separate the photoelectric component of attenuation from that due to Compton scattering, making it possible to selectively identify or remove certain materials. Rather than express the attenuation of materials directly in terms of their photoelectric and Compton components, it is possible to represent the attenuation as a combination of plastic and aluminum components. From knowledge of the plastic and aluminum portions, it is always possible to recalculate the actual photoelectric and Compton weights. The attractiveness of this method is that plastic and aluminum are physical materials and can be readily used for calibration.

The imaging sequence in SPR is first to obtain the images from the low and high kVp beams, then combine them to generate the plastic and aluminum components of the object being imaged. Then, beam hardening corrections are made to improve image uniformity. Once the plas-

144

tic and aluminum components are determined, any material can be cancelled in the energy difference image, depending on the weights applied to the plastic and aluminum components.

The major technical requirements for an energy subtraction imaging system include several that are shared with digital fluorography systems, plus additional requirements unique to dual-energy systems. Common requirements are:

o Adequate intrinsic signal-to-noise ratio so that the image quality is primarily limited by the quantum statistics of the transmitted x-rays and not system limitations;

o The number of digital levels per pixel should be selected to not significantly degrade the intrinsic signal-to-noise ratio and dynamic range of the system;

o Subtraction should be performed on the logarithm of the measured intensity to prevent image contrast in an artery of constant diameter and contrast agent concentration from varying as a function of the amount of material overlying and underlying the artery;

o The system should be able to amplify the difference image to fill the dynamic range of the display and storage device;

o Image repetition rate should be suitable for the target organ of interest;

o The x-ray exposure time for each image should be short enough to prevent significant loss of spatial resolution due to physiological motion.

Additional requirements for dual-energy systems are:

o High and low energy x-ray beams should be generated with minimal spectral overlap.

o The system should provide a method to rapidly switch between the high and low energy x-ray beams to minimize spatial registration problems characteristic of temporal subtraction;

o An efficient means should be provided to reject
scattered radiation. This is more critical for
energy subtraction than for temporal subtraction, since the scattered radiation fields are
likely to be different for the high and low
energy beams;

o The quantum detection efficiency should be
comparable for the two energy beams.

SPR CLINICAL APPLICATIONS

Clinical applications of digital radiography fall into three distinct
areas, including intravascular contrast studies, non-vascular contrast
studies, and non-contrast studies. We will discuss each area as it
specifically relates to scanned projection radiography systems.

Intravenous arteriography is a particularly appealing application
for digital radiographic techniques since it holds the promise of providing low-risk arteriographic screening on an outpatient basis. Current research is concentrating on carotid and peripheral arteriography,
thoracic and abdominal aortography, pulmonary arteriography and
ventriculography. Future applications may encompass intracerebral
and coronary arteriography.

Energy-dependent subtraction methods are particularly attractive
for intravenous arteriography because of their ability to provide images
free from motion effects. With energy subtraction, only a single post-
contrast image is necessary since it contains both the low and high
energy components. Depending upon the method of implementation,
the low and high energy components of the image can be acquired
simultaneously, or in rapid succession, so that there will be no significant relative motion between the two components. In comparison,
the pre- and post-contrast images with temporal subtraction methods
must, by definition, be separated by the time interval necessary for
intravenously-injected contrast media to transit the region of interest,
usually some 5-10 seconds.

Using a prototype SPR system based upon a modified CT/T computed
tomography scanner, some 100 patients received intravenous arteriographic studies using either temporal subtraction, dual energy sub-

traction, or both. This system, called RadView, employs a fan-beam CT/T 8800 scanner in which the x-ray source and detectors remain stationary while the patient is mechanically translated through the gantry. For dual energy scanning, the x-ray source emits alternating pulses of low and high energy x-rays as the patient is advanced. Each pulse is 5.5 milliseconds in duration and alternates between 85 kVp and 135 kVp. Because the pulsing rate is fast compared to the velocity of patient translation (which varies from 20-50 mm per second), the dual energy images produced by this technique are perfectly registered and not subject to motion artifact. The low and high energy images are combined using a computer algorithm to cancel soft tissue or bone, selectively.

Patients selected to receive intravenous arteriography had all recently undergone catheter arteriography of the carotid artery or thoracic aorta. A #16 gauge intravenous cannula was inserted into the basilic or cephalic vein in the antecubital fossa. Radiographic contrast media in the form of Renografin-76 was injected using an automatic injector at a rate of 8-12 milliliters per second for a total volume of 0.67-1.0 milliliters per kilogram of body weight. One to three dual-energy images were obtained following contrast injection, resulting in a patient exposure of approximately 130 milliroentgens per image.

Intravenous arteriography using film subtraction techniques was used for many years until supplanted over the last two decades because of the superiority of images obtained with the more invasive catheter techniques. The resurgence of interest in intravenous arteriography can be credited to three developments:

     o Development of inexpensive digital electronic
       circuitry with the capability of storing multiple
       images and performing the subtraction process
       rapidly;

     o Improvements in electronic x-ray detectors
       having the accuracy and precision necessary
       for subtraction imaging;

     o Refinements in therapeutic vascular procedures
       which require detection of disease in the patient
       with minimal symptoms.

Disadvantages of performing intravenous arteriography with conventional film subtraction methods included the need to use large amounts of contrast, the cumbersome nature of the film subtraction process, and the inability to remove the artifacts generated by patient motion. As a result, this technique was rarely used in most centers, except for those patients in whom selective arterial catheterization was impossible or prohibitively hazardous.

Current applications of intravenous arteriography include screening for atherosclerotic disease in the extracranial carotid, iliac and femoral arteries; evaluation of the thoracic and abdominal aorta; pulmonary arteriography; and cardiac ventriculography. The use of this technique for detection of renal artery stenosis, visualization of arterial bypass grafts, and for detection of intracerebral aneurysms has recently been reported. Substantial improvements in the spatial resolution and subtraction methods are required, however, before intravenous arteriography can be routinely applied to study the coronary arteries and the intracerebral vessels.

Finally, it should be recognized that there is a tradeoff in image quality with intravenous arteriography compared to selective catheter arteriography. Superior images can be obtained with the latter if greater risk, discomfort and cost are acceptable. For outpatient studies, however, intravenous arteriography may provide diagnostic images at lower cost and lower risk to the patient. The development of balloon angioplasty procedures, and the increasing sophistication of vascular surgical procedures, have improved the results of treatment of various manifestations of arteriosclerotic disease. To detect these disease processes earlier, the need for less invasive diagnostic screening procedures has become apparent. Catheter procedures will continue to be necessary to provide high resolution images in patients with known disease where the therapeutic decision-making process requires this increased detail and warrants the small but finite risk associated with catheter angiographic procedures.

Contrast and non-contrast dual-energy studies have been variously used to image the chest, skeletal, kidney, liver, gallbladder, bowel and vascular systems. Protocols for more detailed evaluations of the diagnostic effectiveness of dual-energy radiography for different disease states are underway.

Dual-energy SPR images of the gallbladder, kidney and chest are very useful. For abdominal imaging, the use of selective soft tissue cancellation provides effective removal of bowel gas shadows. Visualization of the gallbladder, especially when obscured by bowel gas shadows, can be enhanced by soft tissue subtraction. This allows the gallbladder to be displayed at much higher contrast.

An intravenous pyelogram performed on a patient with lymphoma demonstrated the value of eliminating the confusing bowel gas shadows which obscure the contrast-filled kidneys and collecting systems with soft tissue subtraction. This particular patient had received water-soluble contrast in the GI tract for a prior CT scan. While this contrast was not particularly apparent on the unsubtracted image, the distal colon was well-demonstrated on the soft tissue cancelled image. The perirenal and other retroperitoneal fat planes were also enhanced by the subtraction process. This enhancement was achieved because of the difference in chemical composition between fat and lean body tissues.

In the chest, the use of dual-kVp imaging allows selective cancellations of either bone or soft tissue shadows. A chest radiograph of a patient with prostate carcinoma and known bony metastases showed some of the rib lesions, but obscured the diffuse involvement of the spine. The unsubtracted SPR image at 85 kVp showed similar features. However, a selective soft tissue subtraction image demonstrated the bony metastases clearly with rib and spine involvement. In addition, the bone-cancelled image highlighted the extra-osseous soft tissue shadows associated with some of the rib metastases.

The improved skeletal detail which results from soft tissue subtraction is also apparent to the knowledgeable observer.

Finally, application of soft tissue subtraction to determine calcification of pulmonary nodules was demonstrated. A large pulmonary nodule located adjacent to the left hemidiaphragm was seen with the SPR image. The presence of lesion calcification was suspected on plain film chest radiography, but could not be confirmed with an unsubtracted image, even when edge enhancement algorithms were applied. On the other hand, the soft tissue subtraction image unequivocally showed the crescentic calcification around the periphery of the nodule.

Dual-energy SPR provides selective cancellation or enhancement of materials of any specified average atomic number. While non-K-edge dual-energy techniques have been proposed before, attempts to produce subtraction images have been impaired for two reasons:

> o Other methods using film/screen systems for
> x-ray detection may have been limited by the
> non-linearities and limited dynamic range of
> film detectors, and by the energy-dependent
> scatter accepted by these area detectors;

    o The lack of rapid energy-switching x-ray
generators or alternate means of producing
Compton and photoelectric images makes the
subtraction method highly susceptible to motion artifacts when in-vivo subtraction studies
are performed.

With the rapid-switching generator used in the current study, the
low and high kVp images are in perfect spatial registration, so that
motion effects are minimized.

While any desired atomic number material may be cancelled by this
technique, the selective soft tissue subtraction and the bone subtraction
with the residual space occupied by the bone filled with an equivalent
thickness of soft tissue (which is called bone mimic tissue subtraction)
were most useful. Soft tissue subtraction images remove soft tissue
variations. In the chest and abdomen, for instance, this technique can
isolate the skeletal structures from confusing superimposed shadows
without the administration of contrast. Abdominal and retroperitoneal
fat planes, having a lower average atomic number than water, become
negative shadows on the tissue-cancelled image. The soft tissue subtraction also appears useful for the detection of calcification in soft
tissue lesions, such as pulmonary nodules.

With the administration of urographic or cholecystographic contrast
media, the soft tissue subtractions enhance kidney and gallbladder
images. The removal of confusing bowel gas shadows may alleviate
the need for conventional tomography, which is otherwise often required for satisfactory studies. In addition, the subtraction may be
useful in small and large bowel imaging, either with water-soluble
contrast media or with barium.

The bone subtraction, and especially the bone mimic tissue subtraction, were found most useful in the chest where the confusing rib
shadows are eliminated for unimpaired views of the pulmonary paren-
chyma. Because of the high incidence of unrecognized pulmonary
nodules lying under the ribs, it has been postulated that bone removal
will improve nodule detection. In addition, these studies show that
bone mimic tissue images enhance visualization of air-tissue interfaces, such as the mediastinal pleural reflections, the pleural surfaces,
the larynx, trachea and bronchi.

The use of tissue or bone subtraction with dual-energy techniques
leads to images in which lesion detection is limited by signal-to-noise
ratio and, hence, by dose. In the unsubtracted images, as with con-

ventional radiography, lesion detection is more often limited by interference from superimposed high contrast structures than by dose.
With subtraction, these interfering tissues can often be removed, allowing one to see low contrast lesions by increasing the contrast of the displayed image up to the limits imposed by the signal-to-noise ratio.

PENDING DEVELOPMENTS

Both SPR and digital fluorography show promise of becoming clinically
important tools. As current research progresses, areas for additional
research and development become apparent. To extend the performance
of scanned projection radiography, several system performance parameters are being addressed. Three specific performance factors --
spatial resolution, signal-to-noise ratio, and scan speed -- must be
enhanced if a truly valuable clinical system is to be developed:

Spatial Resolution

The spatial resolution of an SPR system in the lateral direction is
primarily determined by the detector cell spacing. In the longitudinal
direction, it is primarily determined by the width of the fan beam. The
most direct approach to improving lateral resolution is to make the cells
smaller and pack them closer together. There are three factors that
provide practical limits to this approach.

> o Individual detector output. As the cell size
> decreases, the magnitude of the current out-
> put also decreases. This places more stringent
> requirements on the electrical amplification cir-
> cuitry with respect to noise contribution. In
> the extreme case, the intrinsic system noise
> limits the performance of the system.
>
> o The plates separating the individual detector
> cells. As the active area of the cell decreases,
> the ratio of plate thickness to cell active area
> increases. Since x-ray photons that hit the
> plates are not converted to electrical output,
> the quantum detection efficiency of the detec-
> tor decreases in proportion.

o <u>Field of view</u>. As the cell spacing decreases, the field of view also decreases. If it is desired to maintain the same field of view, the number of channels must be increased. This can prohibitively affect the complexity and cost of an SPR system.

As the detector cell spacing is decreased, resolution is ultimately determined by the focal spot. Generally, cell spacing is not reduced sufficiently for this to be a consideration.

Longitudinal spatial resolution is determined by the width of the fan beam. By placing lead collimators at the output of the x-ray tube, the fan beam width can be reduced up to a certain point. Beyond that, there is a "pinhole camera" effect which causes the beam width to be determined solely by the size of the focal spot on the anode of the x-ray tube. Further improvements in longitudinal spatial resolution can only be achieved by reducing the focal spot size if a single-line detector is used. Smaller focal spots imply a reduced instantaneous power capability in the x-ray tube. As a result, beyond a certain point, there is a tradeoff between longitudinal spatial resolution and signal-to-noise ratio.

<u>Signal-to-Noise</u>

For the SPR configurations using CT-type detectors and electronics, the signal-to-noise ratio in an x-ray image is governed mainly by x-ray statistics. The signal-to-noise ratio can only be improved by an increase in the number of detected x-ray photons. There are two ways in which this signal-to-noise can be improved with no increase in scan times:

o An increase in the instantaneous tube output;

o and an improvement in the quantum detection efficiency of the detector.

The limit to increasing instantaneous tube output is the melting point of the target anode, and is determined by the focal spot size and other details of the tube design. Quantum detection efficiency of the detector can be increased somewhat by a design optimized for scanned projection radiography.

Scan Speed

It is desirable to complete a scan as quickly as possible in order to image the bolus of contrast media while it is still in the vessel of interest. The scan speed can be increased by increasing the relative speed between the patient and the pulsed fan beam. This has the effect, however, of degrading longitudinal spatial resolution as well as low contrast sensitivity. The effect can be alleviated to some extent by increasing the viewing rate. Collecting more views per unit of time places greater demands on the data acquisition system, however. The accuracy, linearity, gain and offset parameters of the data acquisition system are all adversely impacted.

SUMMARY

Increased information on a per dose basis is inherent in scanned projection radiography devices that incorporate low-noise CT detectors and data acquisition systems. Selective tissue and contrast cancellation using energy subtraction techniques has been demonstrated by SPR. As a result, energy subtraction methods appear to have a potential use in intravenous arteriography, as well as non-vascular and non-contrast applications.

The emergence of digital x-ray represents a new plateau in diagnostic imaging where the skills of the medical profession and the technical capabilities of industry can combine to move radiology closer to its goals.

Photoelectronic imaging and optical recording

G.J. Arink
Philips Medical Systems Division
Eindhoven, The Netherlands

Abstract

The management of diagnostic images and patient records
which at present is done by filing films and paper
documents is subject to improvement. Especially, with
the growing variety and intensity of use of digital
imaging modalities the need for communication of images
and for computer compatible mass storage has drastically
increased.
The traditional film files have associated with them
problems of slow access, loss of images, virtually no
possibility for interaction with the stored information,
large space requirements, and manual clerical work.
The images made by digital modalities are archived
by means of CRT hardcopy films and by recording the
digital image data on magnetic tape and diskettes.
This is done because the CRT camera cannot accurately
represent the large contrast resolution available in
the digital image data.
Moreover, the increasing number of digital imaging
modalities necessitates integration and fast access to
all the available diagnostic information of a patient
during examination planning and treatment, which cannot
be offered by existing filing systems.
Newly emerging optical disk systems more adequately
perform archival storage because they offer large capacity random access, and have only a fraction of the media
cost.
The digital optical recorder is a computer peripheral

154

which stores 1000 M bytes of user data on each side of
an optical disk with a diameter of 30 cm (12 inches).
The user data rate of recording is in the range of
0.25 to 1 M byte/second. The bit error rate is better
than 10^{-12}, and the archival life is longer than 10 years.
Taking into account the requirements of a 500 bed hospital
a ten year image file is stored on about 3000 optical
disks, occupying a small office room.
Realisation of a digital image management system requires
interfaces to the image generating systems and to diagnostic viewing consoles.
Inclusion of large area radiographs is done by a high
resolution film digitizer. Output of diagnostic images
is done mostly on high-resolution CRT displays.
Elective hardcopy film output is provided by a computer
compatible hardcopy unit.
These elements as well as the database architecture and
transmission network demand a detailed study of performance
requirements and system planning of the user interfaces.
The concepts and solutions developed in the Picasso
project (Picture Computation and Storage System) of the
Philips' Research Laboratories in Hamburg and in the
Megadoc project of the Philips' Research Laboratories in
Eindhoven demonstrate the feasibility of diagnostic image
management systems.

Introduction

The management of diagnostic images and patient records
receives renewed attention, especially, because the
digital modalities add new complications to the already
existing problems of film filing. Innovative solutions to
digital image management aim to satisfy new user needs,
e.g. integration of medical information, fast access,
improved radiological operations, and cost savings by
lower storage media cost, reduction of filing space and
reduced effort. A number of design studies and pilot projects carried out at several institutes aim at identification of adequate system concepts and development of the
technological basis for these solutions.
The subject will be introduced by a summary of the
existing problems with traditional filing systems,
extended through a discussion of the new requirements
imposed by digital modalities, and concluded with a
brief description of electronic systems which might help
to find a solution to some of the problems of diagnostic
image management in the future.

The existing image management situation

Storage, retrieval and communication of medical diagnostic
images are intertwined very closely with imaging and
viewing methods and procedures. In traditional X-ray
imaging continuous improvements of imaging equipment and
medical X-ray film have created a system which from the
standpoint of the user has many advantages including simplicity, ability to record a large amount of information,
ease of interrogation, good archival properties, and
relatively high insurance against loss of information
due to mishandling and artifacts.
However, the use of film has a number of disadvantages,
the most important of which are,e.g.,slow access to
films of old examinations, loss due to misfiling and
unrecorded loans, virtually no possibility to interact
with the recorded information, relatively large space
requirements for storage, considerable physical effort
for routine retrieval of master folders and increasing
cost and locked-up silver value of the films. These
aspects will be examined after a look at the basic reasons
for archiving.
There are three reasons for archiving medical images. First,
radiographs are considered an indispensible part of
legal record keeping requirements.
The length of the legal period is different in various
regions. The American College of Radiologists recommends
a period of 7 years and accepts a minimum of 5 years. In
some states the films of pediatric patients must be
kept untill the age of maturity. In Europe the archiving
period generally is 10 years. This is also the case in
Germany, but here the liability of radiologists extends
over a period of 30 years.
The second reason, of course is the need to have comparison
images available when the patient returns for a new
examination after a period of time and in the course
of a treatment.
Finally, nearly all diagnostic departments keep teaching
files with copies of selected radiographs and multiformat
camera films.
In 1977 Vosburgh reported a study based on a survey of
300 hospitals which showed that 95 % of the U.S. hospitals
routinely retrieve patients' old radiographs at the time
of a new radiographic examination.
The same study noted that almost all archiving solutions
were fully manual and reasonably uniform among hospitals
with 100 beds or more.
The general pattern of diagnostic film use is shown in
Figure 1.

After quality approval the films are read, in most cases via a prereading file, and the resulting findings are documented, The films are used in the report discussion and put on loan. Later they are collected and kept in an active file. When they have not been used during some years they are finally moved to a permanent file for the remainder of the legal period. The characteristics of daily file, active file and permanent file are summarized in Figure 2.

For subsequent examinations the patient's master folder containing the films is retrieved and made available for the new examinations or the pre-reading file.

The master folder with the new films added is usually colour-coded corresponding to the date of most recent use. If space requirements so dictate the master folders in the permanent file are moved off-premises. Whereas master folders in the active storage are routinely retrieved at each patient visit, retrievals from permanent storage are usually made on special request only.

The recall rate of images is highest during the first 3 to 6 months.

Typically about 60 percent of the images is retrieved at least once during this period. The recall rate drops markedly after the first year, and for films over three years old, it amounts to only 0.5 percent per year.

The traditional filing method described above has some problems associated with it which motivate a search for better solutions.

First, due to manual retrieval operations and sometimes remote storage locations the access to stored films is slow.

For cases with a more complex examination plan it may be difficult to have images of various types of examinations available for combined diagnosis within a reasonably short period.

Loss of images due to poor identification, misfiling and unrecorded loans is a much quoted problem (Darlak, 1982). The method of manual film filing, colour-coding and retrieval of masterfolders requires a considerable physical effort. Also, it has been reported (Vosburgh, 1977) that only a fraction of the master folders which are routinely retrieved contain films that are relevant for a new examination.

As an archiving medium film does not allow direct interaction with the recorded information. More diagnostic information is extracted if the radiographic image is manipulated or processed in order to compensate for the characteristics of the imaging system or to bring the image information into the range of optimum visualisation of the eye (Trussel, 1981).

FIGURE 1

RADIOGRAPHIC DATA FLOW

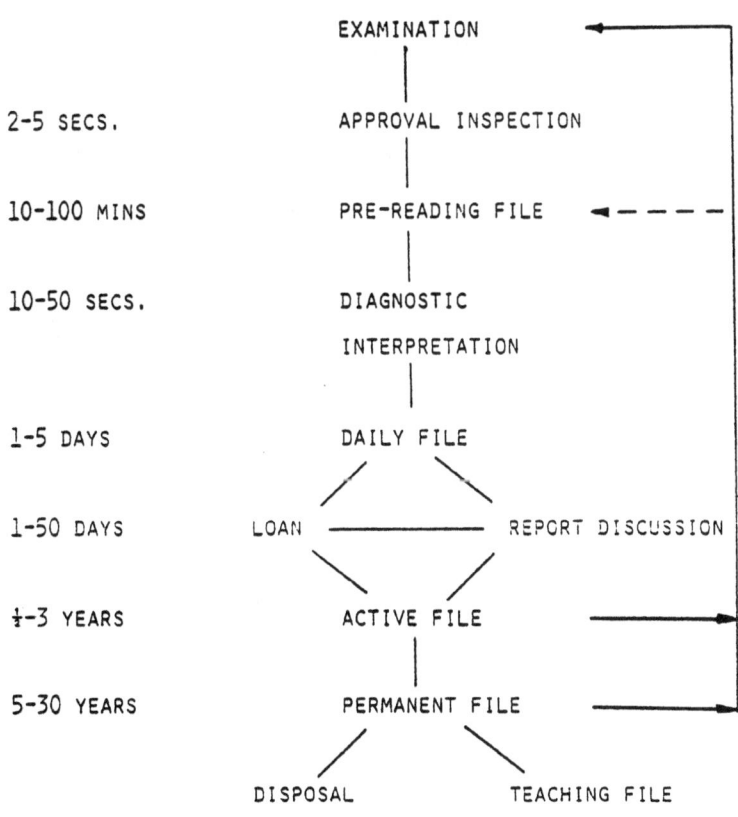

Figure 2

Characteristics of three types of film files

Type	Archival period	Access speed	Number of film folders	Frequency of access	Typical location
Actual (working file)	Some months	Seconds	Thousands	Many times per examination	Within X-ray department
Short-term (Active file)	Some years	Minutes	Some hundred thousand	Once per examination	Outside X-ray department
Long-term (Permanent file)	5 to 30 years	Hours	Hundreds of thousands	Only upon explicit request	Often outside hospital

Finally, the current film files have associated with them
large space requirements. The typical film production of
a 500 bed hospital with 50 000 patients per year requires
about 100 meters of shelf space per year. About one-third
of American hospitals are reported to have serious radiographic storage and retrieval problems, and a lack of
space is cited as the most prominent complaint (Vosburgh,
1977).
Frequently, extra space is already desired for expansion
of diagnostic services and placement of new equipment.

Archiving needs for new imaging devices

The new and emerging digital imaging modalities have
added an entirely new and different element to the in-
adequately solved problems of film-based departments, i.e.
the management of images generated in digital electronic
form.
In film-based practice the film was the final document on
which the diagnostician based his impression. Digital modalities do not directly produce diagnostic images but,
generate arrays of numbers, i.e. digital images, which must
be manipulated and processed prior to conversion into an
analog display image. Also, it is likely that the
diagnosis is not based on one but on several or possibly
many display images (Angus, 1981).
The final permanent document for virtually all digital
modalities has been hardcopy film generated from an
electronic display device.
Because the video signals from which these films are made
do not have the same contrast resolution as the digital
images only a part of the information is shown. It is
desirable to save the digital data as well; at least for
the period of most intensive use. For this purpose the
image data are recorded on magnetic tape or diskettes.
These media cause extra cost and effort if they are used
in traditional filing operations. Magnetic tape requires
periodic data maintenance operations and has the disadvantage of slow and sequential access.
Moreover, tape reels are incompatible with film storage
and retrieval practice.
Diskettes are used as a medium for image communication
and viewing on separate consoles. Mostly, they are re-
used after a period of time.
The majority of diagnosticians intuitively reject the
notion of destroying the digital images while maintaining
for the permanent file only photographic copies of

display images. Therefore,it seems inevitable that electronic generation of diagnostic images will make it necessary and probably possible to replace filing on film by electronic means. This will make the file of images more accessable and more suitable for combining and interfacing with an increasing number of imaging modalities.
The magnitude of this problem continues to grow.
Whereas in 1960 nearly all diagnostic imaging was done by medical X-ray film, the number of images made by digital modalities in 1982 is roughly equal to the number of X-ray films; Figure 3.
However, due to the moderate spatial resolution of digital images there still is a large difference in the required storage capacity in comparision with the digital representation of large area radiographs. Inclusion of radiographs in a digital image management system still poses the most stringent requirements on storage capacity and access speed.
An increase in the number of digital modalities in X-ray imaging could change this situation in the course of time. The availability of large area image intensifiers with high-resolution video systems and the research possibilities of imaging detector arrays will impact radiology and is expected to partly eliminate X-ray film (Capp, 1981). The use of digital storage formats in these imaging systems has associated with it additional advantages, e.g. transmission of images over large distances without adding noise, and processing to better visualize diagnostic information.

Analysis of system requirements

The amount of image data to be stored is tremendous, especially if large area exposures are to be incorporated. An estimate of the image production is derived from the number of examinations and films generated as a function of hospital size and per specialisation. As has been mentioned earlier the data volume presently produced by large area radiographs is the major factor and this will be considered in the subsequent discussion.
A typical 500 bed hospital performs about 6000 X-ray examinations annually. For different types of examinations the number of exposures and films as well as the size of films differs considerably (Figure 4).
However, a parameter which is remarkably constant over large geographical regions is the area of film consumed per examination which is between 0.25 and 0.4 m^2, in average 0.3m^2.

Figure 3

Archiving requirements of a moderately large hospital

	Image matrix	No. of M bits per image	No. of patients per day	No. of images per examination	No. of images per year	G bits per year
X-ray film (24X30 cm equiv.)	5 lp/mm resolution	56	250	4	250.000	14.000
C.T. images	512^2X16	4	40	16	160.000	640
Nuclear Medicine						
static	256^2X8	0.5	15	5	20.000	10
dynamic	128^2X8	0.125	15	16	60.000	7.5
Ultrasound						
B-scan	512^2X8	2	40	3	30.000	60
real-time	512^2X8	2	40	8	80.000	160

Figure 4

Number of X-ray exposures and films per type of examination

	PERCENTAGE OF EXAMI- NATIONS	AVG. NUMBER OF FILMS PER EXAMINATION	AVG. NUMBER OF EXPOSURES PER EXAMINATION	MAJOR FILM SIZES USED (CM)
SKELETON	48	2-3	2-3	18 x 24, 24 x 30
COLON	2	8	13	24 x 30
OTHER DIGESTIVE TRACT	12	4-5	10-11	24 x 30, 18 x 24
RESPIRATORY TRACT	28	1-2	1-2	35 x 35
URO-GENITAL	5	6	6	24 x 30, 30 x 40
OTHER E.G. NERVOUS SYSTEM, HEART AND VESSELS, MAMMOGRAPHY, TOMOGRAPHY.	5	8-10	8-10	35 x 35, 24 x 30, 30 x 40

The number of bits required to express the information
content of the X-ray film depends on the physical parameters of image formation, e.g., number of photons, detec-
tive quantum efficiency, energy distribution of the X-rays,
and Compton scattering in the subject. The spatial and
contrast resolution must be adequate to visualize all the
required contrast/detail of the anatomy and pathology.
For X-ray films all significant information is contained
in the range of spatial frequencies below 10 lp/mm
(Takaya and Pollack, 1978), and in most cases 5 lp/mm
is a reasonable upper limit considering the MTF of the
imaging system. Frequently, even a lower spatial resolution suffices to accurately depict the required anatomical
detail.
For radiographs of 24X30 cm (9X12 inches) this means that
7 Mbytes of data is generated, if each pixel is expressed
in 8 bits. At this level of resolution the average film
area per examination generates about 30 Mbytes of uncompressed image data.
For the digital imaging modalities the spatial resolution is more moderate, e.g. 512^2 or 1024^2, but the contrast
resolution is higher, i.e. 10 to 12 bits, and the number
of images per examination is relatively large, usually
about 15. This results in 45 to 180 Mbits per examination
or 5.6 to 22 Mbytes of uncompressed data when "bit
packing" is applied, e.g. putting two 12 bit words into
three bytes.
The storage capacity requirements of the diagnostic
imaging department of a moderately large hospital have
been estimated. These estimates indicate an annual storage
requirement of approximately 10^{13} bits. If the data must
be maintained for a period of 10 years, the storage
capacity increases to 10^{14} bits.
These tremendous quantities of data emphasize the need
for a detailed evaluation of the diagnostically required
spatial resolution and point out the need for data
compression techniques. Data compression for grey scale
images, a method for optimizing the coding of pixel values
to reduce the number of bits to be filed without losing
essential information, has been demonstrated to produce a
compression ratio up to about 8. Adaptive techniques
are able to give a compression ratio up to 25 (Wendler and
Meyer-Ebrecht, 1982).
It is thought that the data capacity can be reduced by a
factor ten through judicious selection of the image
sampling aperture and by application of data compression.
This gives a total data capacity of approximately 10^{13} bits
to be stored for the archival period.

Technology for digital image management

Until recently the only possibility for digital storage of
large amounts of data was provided by magnetic recording
media, e.g. magnetic disks and tape. The high cost of these
media as well as handling and maintenance, i.e. short
archival life, made them unattractive for mass storage of
medical image data.
New means of mass storage like the digital optical recorder
(DOR) for the first time offer the capability to start
realizing computer compatible long-term image archiving.
Digital image management is based on a system design for
acquisition of images, an image database, a transmission
network, and display viewing stations and hardcopy film
output devices. The essential elements of digital image
management are shown in Figure 5. The diagram also indicates
a possible interface with departmental and hospital information systems which contain patient data and related
medical records. All image sources must be considered in
the systems concept.
Naturally, digital imaging devices can be compatible with
digital mass storage. Also, video images can be digitized
and stored electronically.
The problem in all digital imaging devices is the high
bandwidth which is required for real-time acquisition
and direct viewing of the images just obtained. As in
present computed tomography and subtraction angiography
systems this capability is realized through the use
of solid state memories and magnetic disk systems on
which a number of images are stored. Buffering the image
production of examinations in foreground storage leaves
them available for rapid diagnostic viewing and reduces
the bandwidth for transmission to archival storage. This
can be used in combination with data compression coding to
lower the average data rate further and make a more economical use of the storage media.
X-ray film is included in a digital image management system
by scanning and conversion to a digital format.
This can be done immediately after film processing or
later at any convenient moment. The films can continue to
be used during the active file period, e.g. up to 3 or
6 months.
The recorded images are retrieved by querying the database and retrieving examination data, findings and the
desired image files. The retrieved images are viewed
on a display monitor or reproduced on hardcopy film.
The hardcopy film is viewed on a lightbox providing a
user interface which is compatible with existing viewing
practice.

165

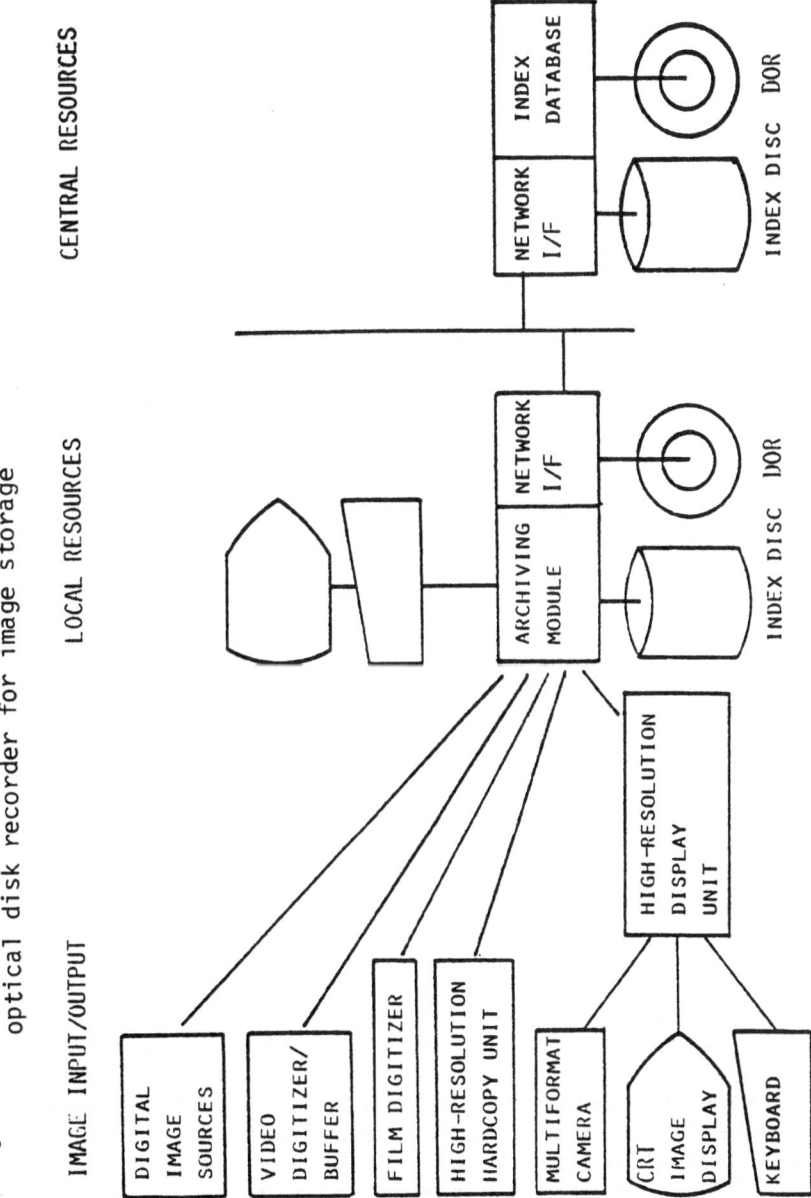

Figure 5 Essential elements of a digital image management system using the optical disk recorder for image storage

For image retrieval of digital modalities use is made of
the softcopy display and CRT camera functions which are
integrated in these imaging devices and in the diagnostic
viewing consoles available for these systems. Multi-
modality viewing of images stored in an integrated database
is one of the new capabilities offered by digital image
management.

The desired access time to the file will vary according
to the functional requirements. Retrieval of images from
the active file requires a response time of a few seconds.
For images of 30 to 50 Mbits this is a formidable requirement, which is lowered somewhat if the images are stored
and transmitted in a compressed format.

The technology for high-speed data transmission has been
realized in modern local area networks between distributed
computer systems. These are either baseband or broad-
band communication networks which make use of coaxial
cable or fiber optic links (Electronic Design, April 16,
1981). The problem here resides in the fetching of data
from the storage medium and in the terminal electronics
that connects to the network.

Retrieval from the permanent file may be allowed to take
a few minutes.

Therefore, it will probably be better to transfer each day
to a temporary file the image data of patients who are
scheduled for examination.

This file can also be used to store the day's production
of new images until diagnostic viewing and interpretation
has been completed. Afterwards, the patient files and
the new image information can be stored in the permanent
file.

Digital mass storage

The storage and retrieval function is advantageously
based on the digital optical recorder (DOR) which is
expected to become a widely used component in office
automation systems. There is a large market for archival
storage in commercial and banking transactions, legal
document processing, and image recording in industrial
and medical applications.

The DOR is excellently suited for random access storage and
retrieval of relatively large volumes of images, facsimile
documents and text pages.

One digital optical disk can store about 500.000 A-size
typed pages, roughly 25.000 high resolution facsimile

documents, 10.000 encoded CT images or 500 to 1000
digitized and encoded radiographs.
Some years ago, Philips announced the feasibility of
digital optical recording (Bulthuis, 1979).
At that time prototype optical recorders were used which
had a helium neon gas laser and an external optical modu-
lator.
A major breakthrough was reached with the introduction
of the solid state diode laser, which made the recorder
less complex and smaller in size. The diode laser
consists of a small AlGaAs chip mounted in a transistor
housing with an optical window. The device produces a
light output of 20 mW and higher. About 12 mW are used to
write data onto the DOR disk, and 8 mW are sufficient
to read data from the disk.
The DOR is designed to be compatible in data rate and
error protection with computer systems (Dinklo, 1980).
The DOR disk is a sandwich of two glass plates separated
by spacers which form an air space. The diameter of the
disk is 30 cm (12 inches). The inner side of both plates
is covered with a thin plastic coating in which a spiral
track is made by a premastering process. Deposited on
the coating is a tellurium layer with a thickness of
approximately 350 Angströms.
The pitch of the track is 1.5 microns and the total
number of revolutions of the track is about 36 000.
The pregrooved track already includes the headers of the
sectors into which the data are written.
The header consists of the track number, sector number,
and bit and word synchronisation codes.
The data are recorded along the track in a modulated
pattern of ones and zeroes which is formed by burning
holes with a diameter of about one micron in the tellurium
layer.
The principle of optical recording is shown in Figure 6.
The light emitted by the diode laser is collected by a
lens and deflected towards the disk by a polarizing beam
splitter. It passes a quarter lambda plate and is
focussed onto the disk by a servo-controlled objective
lens.
The light reflected by the disk falls through the quarter
lambda plate again and passes now the polarizing beam
splitter. A fraction of the light impinges on the photodiode which serves as the tracking detector for keeping the
lightbeam in the track. Another part of the light falls
on the second photodiode element and is used for focusing
the objective lens and for detection of the recorded data.
Immediately after recording the data are read by a second
laser system. The read data are compared to the write
data and if an error is found the data are written again

168

Figure 6

Principle of optical recording

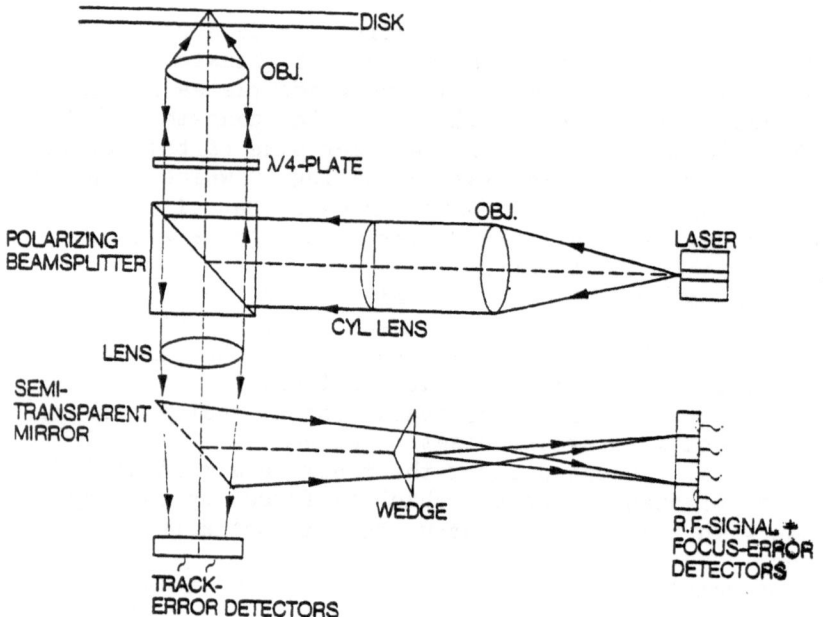

in the next sector. This is called "direct read after
write".
The capacity of the disk is 1000 Mbytes of user data per
disk side.
The user data rate of recording and reading is 2 Mbits per
second.
The average access time of a data sector is 150 milliseconds.
For application as a computer peripheral a bit error rate
of 10^{-12} is required. This has been demonstrated in
extensive test programs. The low bit error rate is obtained
by adding error detection and correction bits intermixed
with the data stream.
The optical disk is a write-once medium for data archiving.
By means of accelerated testing the archival life of
recorded disks is defined as longer than 10 years.
As a new technology the ultimate capacity of optical recording is not yet fully exploited in the initial product designs. In principle the data rate of writing and reading
can be about 10 Mbits/second. Even higher data rates
of 100 Mbits/second have been reported for experimental
designs (Nadan, 1982). However, standard computer systems
associated with the digital optical disk drive do not
support such a high rate.
Optical recording has an advantage compared to magnetic
recording because the intertrack distance is very small,
and the information density is much higher, i.e. by a
factor of 10 to 100. Therefore, optical disk storage can
be more economical than magnetic storage.

System structure and configuration

In the general structure of an image management system
two types of data can be distinguished,i.e. image data
including keys and directories recorded on DOR disk,
and index data consisting of patient and examination
data, reports, image descriptors, and location codes of
the images on DOR disk.
The data recorded in the index database is permanently on-
line whereas for image data only the DOR disks placed on
recorder drives are on-line and the remainder is either
located in a disk cabinet or in a jukebox cartridge box
which holds a moderate number of disks. The jukebox
mechanically retrieves DOR disks and positions them on
recorder or player drives.
The system structure for implementing the index and image

database functions can be either distributed or central.
In a distributed system the archiving nodes serve a
limited number of imaging devices all of which can access
the stored image data directly. This configuration is
better adapted to individual variations in workload,
compared to a central system. A central system would
have a considerable overhead for image data communication.
A distributed system configuration can show attractive
modularity characteristics both in functions and capacity.
Functional advantages are gained because special functions
can be dealt with by dedicated peripherals and processors.
Dedicated processors often have performance/price ratios
over those of general-purpose computers.
Concerning capacity advantages are obtained because
relatively small system additions can be realized to
match the system closely to the user requirements.
Extensions that are required at a later date can be made
without changing the basic architecture. In a new area
like image management this is an essential point.
The technology of a distributed image database system will
require in addition to the DOR a number of peripherals
and processing devices which perform rapidly and flexibly
the various processing tasks which occur in the system.
General purpose computers are flexible but far too slow.
Dedicated hardware development for each specific processing
task will provide speed but is impractical and uneconomic.
In the Picasso project (Picture Computation and Storage System) carried out by the Philips' Research Laboratories in
Hamburg a possible solution to the problem of system architecture and dedicated processors is investigated. The project
aims to bridge the gap between fast but specialized hardware and flexible but slow general-purpose computers.
The Picasso picture computer is thought of as an elemental
computer which handles a whole picture, e.g. 512^2 pixels,
just as a normal computer handles a single word. Consequently, its registers are of megabit size; Figure 7
(Wendler, 1982).
The equivalent of the arithmetic logic unit of the computer is a bank of processing elements which is specialized
for a distinct class of picture operations in order
to achieve maximum speed. Data transfers from registers
to processing elements are done word sequentially.
Hence, overall speed largely depends on the organization
of this data transfer. Here advantage is taken of the
regularity with which image matrices are processed.
Since a common feature of image operations is the
sequence of accesses to the register, each processing
element has its own address generator specialized to a
particular address sequence.

171

Figure 7   Architecture of the modular Picasso picture processor

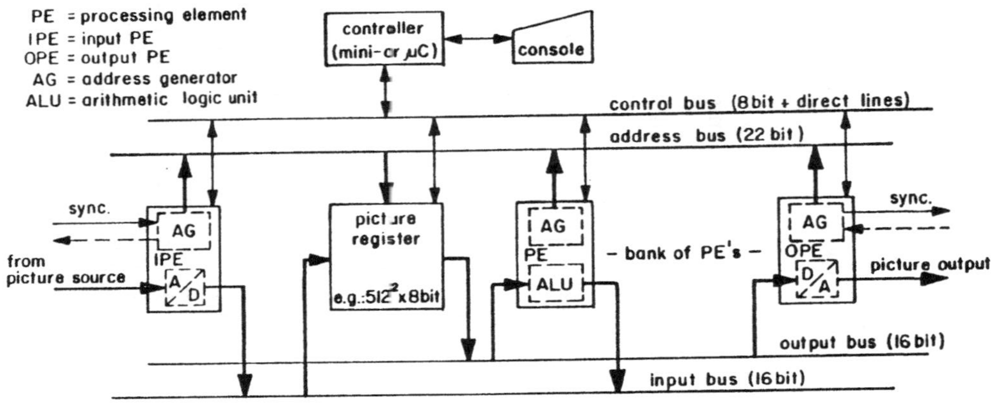

PE = processing element
IPE = input PE
OPE = output PE
AG = address generator
ALU = arithmetic logic unit

In a similar way input and output functions are designed to interface peripherals, backup memory devices and transmission channels. These specialized processing elements form the modules from which dedicated image input, output and archiving stations are assembled. These principles can be used in a design shown in Figure 8. Several diagnostic imaging systems are interfaced to a dedicated image base by means of a high-speed link for transmission of image data and commands. The data rate of transmission is kept within reasonable limits because the image input and output devices have their own data buffers. The buffer size may be sufficient to cover the first few days of on-line diagnostic use of the images.

The total system is formed by several image base stations and a patient database for alphanumeric data. The elements of this system can be distributed over a diagnostic imaging department including a file room and remote sub-units.

These and other concepts developed in the Picasso-project (Picture Computation and Storage System) of the Philips' Research Laboratories in Hamburg, and in the Megadoc project of the Philips' Research Laboratories in Geldrop (Eindhoven) demonstrate the feasibility of diagnostic image management systems (Meyer-Ebrecht, 1980; de Vos, 1981).

Concluding remarks

The digital optical recorder (DOR) offers a near-term solution for storage and retrieval of medical images. The application needs have to be carefully defined. For replacement of a film file (radiographs, spotfilm and multiformat films) the requirements can be calculated based on current filing operations. For real-time fluorographic imaging and new digital modalities the workload and communication pattern is more difficult to predict.

From the start of system design the economy of the solutions has to be taken as a goal. The DOR disk is expected to provide markedly lower archiving medium costs, compared to digital magnetic media. The system cost is not determined by the DOR but, depends mainly on the interfaces and peripheral devices for image input and output. Image processing is an integral part of nearly all system elements providing image data compression, data preprocessing and display processing. New photo-electronic and digital imaging devices will need a unified form for data formats, storage and retrieval interfaces, and image data communication.

Figure 8   Distributed digital image management system based on
a modular processor architecture

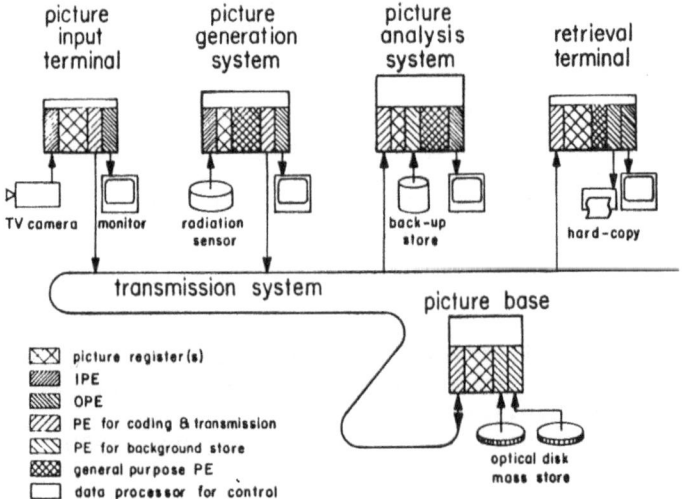

References

(1) William M. Angus, M.D. Ph. D
     Diagnostic image management today and the future
     In: Digital Subtraction Angiography: An Application
     of Computerized Fluoroscopy
     C.A. Mistretta a.o., Eds.
     Year Book Publ., Chicago, 1982

(2) K. Bulthuis, M.G. Carasso a.o.
     Ten billion bits on a disk
     IEEE Spectrum, August 1979; 26-33

(3) M.P. Capp
     Radiological imaging - 2000 A.D
     Radiology 138: 541-550, March 1981

(4) J.J. Darlak
     Nonfilm radiographic image transmission and storage
     with remote and random access
     Proc. PACS Conf., Jan. 18-21, 1982
     SPIE Vol. 318 part I, p. 186-192

(5) J.A. Dinklo
     Digital optical disk systems
     In: The computer in the Doctor's Office; O. Rienhoff
     and M.E. Abrams,Eds.
     North-Holland Publishing Company, 1980

(6) Local Networks
     Electronic Design, Vol 29, No. 8, April 16, 1981,
     p. 89-140

(7) D. Meyer-Ebrecht
     The management and processing of medical pictures:
     An architecture for systems and processing devices
     1980 IEEE Workshop on Picture Data Description and
     Management
     August 27-29, 1980 Asilomar Conference Grounds,
     Pacific Grove, California, USA

(8) J.S. Nadan
     Recent advances in digital optical recording
     Proc. PACS Conf., Jan. 18-21, 1982
     SPIE vol 318 part I, p. 32-35

(9) T. Takaya and V. Pollack
     Laser scanning system for the digital transmission
     of X-ray pictures over voice-grade telephone
     channels
     Medical and Biological Engineering and Computing,
     May 1978, Vol 16, p. 316-322

(10) H.J. Trussell
     Processing of X-ray images
     Proc. IEEE, Vol 69, No. 5, May 1981, p. 615-627

(11) J.A. de Vos
     MEGADOC - A document archiving system based on
     digital optical recording
     Symposium Outlook for Optical and Video Disk Systems
     and Applications
     The Institute for Graphic Communication
     July 27-29, 1980
     Carmel, California, USA

(12) K.G. Vosburgh
     Storage and retrieval of radiographic images
     Radiology, 123; 619-624, June 1977

(13) Th. Wendler a.o
     Modular multiprocessor picture computer architecture
     for distibuted picture information systems
     Proc. PACS Conf., Jan. 18-21, 1982
     SPIE Vol 318 part I, p. 125-132

(14) T. Wendler and D. Meyer-Ebrecht
     A proposal standard for variable format picture
     processing and codec approach to match diverse
     imaging devices
     In: Proc. Picture Archiving and Communication Systems,
     Jan. 18-21, 1982 SPIE Vol 318 part I, p. 298-305

COMPTON TOMOGRAPHIC IMAGING: DESIGN ASPECTS AND PERFORMANCE

RICCARDO GUZZARDI, MARGHERITA ZITO, MAURIZIO MEY

C.N.R. Institute of Clinical Physiology
Via Savi, 8   56100 PISA, ITALY

Introduction

Since 1959 (1) Lale proposed the use of scattered radiation in the examination of internal electron density of tissues, using high energy gamma rays.
The advantages of using the detection of photon scattering comes, mainly, for two reasons:
a) as shown in figure 1, the detected photons contain precise and direct positional information which is dependent, at a given irradiation geometry, on the scattering angle, and detector position;
b) the number of detected photons is linearly proportional to the electron density of the target. In fact, according to Battista (2), for a monoenergetic, non-polarized source, the fluence of photons singly scattered by an infinitesimal volume at B, and reaching the detector collimator, is given by:

$$dN = \Phi_0 f_1 f_2 \left[\int_{\alpha-\Delta\alpha}^{\alpha+\Delta\alpha} \frac{d\sigma}{d\Omega} (E_0,\alpha) \, d\Omega \right] \rho \, dS \, dz$$

with

$$f_1 = \text{EXP}\left[-\int_B^A \mu(E_0,z)\ dz\right]$$

and

$$f_2 = \frac{\displaystyle\int_{\alpha+\Delta\alpha}^{\alpha-\Delta\alpha} \frac{d\sigma}{d\Omega}(E_0,\alpha)\ \text{EXP}\left[-\int_l \mu(E_1,l)\ dl\right]d\Omega}{\displaystyle\int_{\alpha+\Delta\alpha}^{\alpha-\Delta\alpha} \frac{d\sigma}{d\Omega}(E_0,\alpha)\ d\Omega}$$

Φ_0 = photon fluence rate of the incident beam ($cm^2 s^{-1}$).
dS = infinitesimal cross-sectional area of the incident beam (cm^2).
Δz = infinitesimal thickness of the scattering volume (cm).
ρ = electron density at B (e cm^{-3}).
α = photon scatter angle (deg).
$d\sigma/d\Omega$ = klein-Nishina differential cross section for a non polarized incident beam.
l = scattered photons path length (cm).
f_1 = primary beam attenuation factor.
f_2 = scattered beam mean attenuation factor.

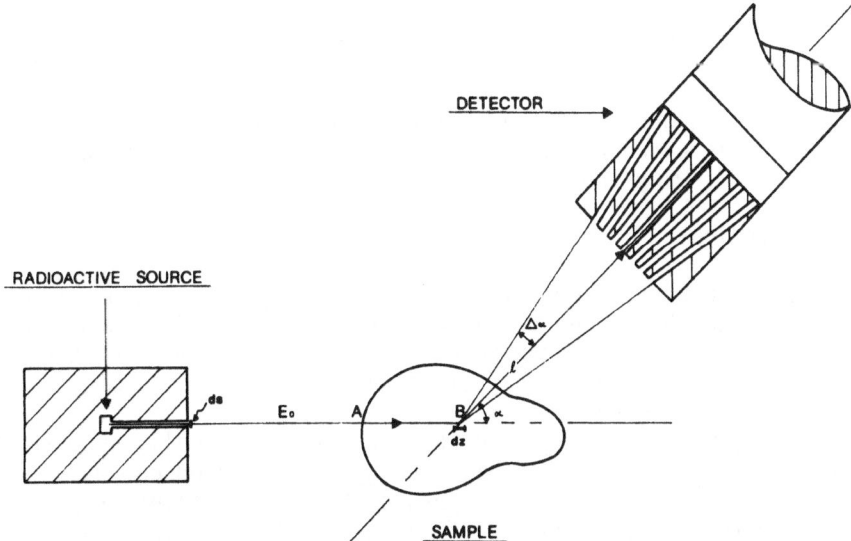

Fig. 1. Source and detector arrangement for Compton Scattering measurement (see text). A pencil beam coming from a collimated radioactive source irradiates a target along the line AB. The photons scattered at an angle α are detected using a collimator focusing in B.

Finally the total system single scatter fluence rate is given by:

$$N = \int_0^{\Delta S} \int_{\frac{1}{2}(-\Delta z)}^{\frac{1}{2}(\Delta z)} dN$$

For a constant incident fluence rate Φ_0 and in a fixed geometry (α, f_1, f_2 constant), N will be modulated only by the electron density at B. This is the basis for fixed point densitometry. This approach has been used by different authors to measure the density of an apriori selected internal volume of bone or lung, associating the scattering technique with transmission measurements (3,4,5): the transmission measurement is used for correcting the mentioned attenuation factors f_1 and f_2. In fact, a second detector is placed in line with the incident beam, to take the transmission, and a second source, emitting photons of energy equal to that of the previous scattered beam, is placed in line with the original detector.
The previously described approach permits the absolute measurement of the electronic density of the internal volume of interest, however, it does not permit precise location of the target volume within the body with respect to the different internal structures. The production of tomograms can be achieved with the scattering techniques; however, in this case, both f_1 and f_2 are no longer constant, and their point-by-point effect must be carefully considered. In general, the imaging methodologies can be classified in three main categories, as it will be described in the next section, following the design principle and the scanning mode.

Systems design.

Different approaches and different systems capable of generating density images have been developed and evaluated. Following the scanning approach, they can be classified in three main categories depending upon the number of simultaneous volume elements being scanned, figure 2.
a) Point-by-Point Imaging: In this approach originally proposed by Lale (1), a fine beam of high energy x-rays, produced by a 5.6 MeV linear accelerator, is passed through a patient; rays scattered from a small volume of tissues (2.5 cm thick) are accepted by a large focusing collimator, behind the patient, and reach a liquid scintillator tank. Images can be obtained by scanning; however, this approach did not find further application in this form by other investigators. Later, Clarke (6,7,8) proposed and built an apparatus to be used for clinical purposes. In this design the source was constituted by a well collimated

beam of Co-60 gamma rays (29.6 TBq = 800 Ci) and the detector consisted of a focusing collimator and large blocks of scintillating plastic coupled to photomultipliers accepting a mean scattering angle of 45°. Even in this design, images are generated through scanning by movement of the patient bed.
Compton backscatter also has been used for quantitative measurements of lung function in children (9): a source of Cs-137 irradiates the patient's chest with a narrow beam; the scattered radiation is observed during inspiration and expiration, at a medium angle of about 110° by means of a scintillator and a focusing collimator. This method was not originally developed for imaging purposes even if, in principle, it can be done.

b) Line-by-Line Imaging: This is a different imaging modality having, as fundamental requirement that of generating the spatial information, simultaneously along a selected transverse body line. This is the volume defined by the primary incident beam within the body. Originally, this approach was developed by Farmer (10). In this design the radiation beam was constituted by a pencil beam of Cs-137 (1.4 TBq = 40 Ci) and the scattered radiation was detected by a Germanium crystal coupled to a diverging fan collimator. In this way the angle-energy relationship of the detected scattered radiation permits the easy reconstruction of the density distribution of the irradiated volume. Furthermore, a set of parallel scans permits the reconstruction of the image of an entire coronal or transverse section.

COMPTON IMAGING

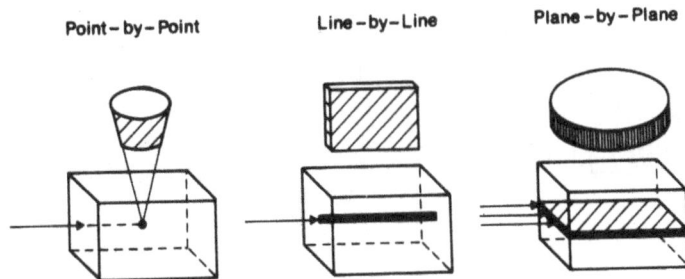

Fig. 2. Designs for Compton Imaging:
a) Point-by-Point requiring a 2-D scanning through mouvement of the target or of both source and detector;
b) Line-by-Line requiring only linear scanning;
c) Plane-by-Plane requiring only static measurements.

180

More recently, a system using a linear detector sensitive to the position, the CGR Scanicamera, has been developed by Moretti (11). The radiation source was, in this approach, a twin of collinear and collimated sealed point sources of Ir-192 (5.5 GBq each) irradiating in opposite directions but on the same line, the patient chest. Images were, even in this scan, obtained by linear scanning c) Plane-by-Plane Imaging: The main feature of this approach is that of the simultaneous production of the picture of the density distribution over a large area, for example, a brain or chest section. In this case, the scattered photons are detected by a large-field-of-view detector.

All different authors using this methodology have always used the most common and easily available detector, the gamma camera. They all use a geometry in which the irradiation plane defining the tomographic volume is always parallel to the detection plane. In fact, Mirrel (12) exploited a system mainly suited for brain tomography and consisting of a circular collimated source of 185 GBq of Tc-99m. The images are acquired using a gamma camera equipped with a low-energy parallel collimator. Multislice imaging was obtained by translation of the irradiation plane. The short half-life of the Tc-99m requires, of course, a frequent loading and high operational cost.

Later Okuyama (13) proposed a system for breast imaging using a gamma camera with a parallel hole or a pinhole collimator (to get image magnification). The radiation source was, in this approach, constituted by a fan beam of gamma rays generated by a collimated point source of about 3.7 GBq of Tc-99m or Cs-137. The choice of the radioisotope poses, however, severe limitations in the choice of the collimator, for the oblique forward high energy penetration.

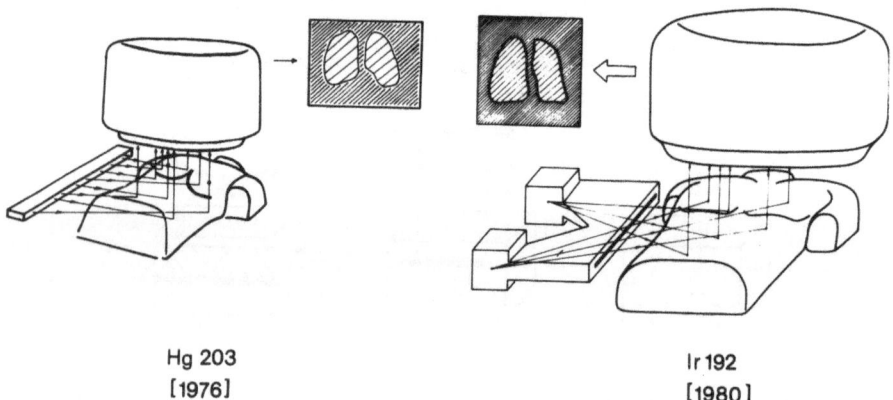

Hg 203
[1976]

Ir 192
[1980]

Fig. 3. Schematic design of 90° Compton Scattering Tomography (CST) of the lung using the gamma camera. The main difference between the two designs relies in the modality (source and geometry) used to generate the collimated radiation beam irradiating a selected chest section.

Finally, the authors of this work have designed and realized an imaging approach specifically suited for lung studies (14,15,16, 17).

Figure 3 schematizes the principle of the 90° Compton Tomography of the lung whose results and applicative possibilities will be described in detail in this work.

As shown in the scheme, the technique has proceeded since 1976 with some modification in the design of the irradiating system, both source and geometry, in order to increase scattering yields and simplicity of use. In both cases the image of the density distribution of the irradiated chest section is obtained through the detection, with the gamma camera equipped with a parallel hole collimator, of the radiation scattered at 90° by the selected chest section. This approach does not require computers except for quantitative data analysis or for correction of the attenuation of both primary and secondary beam. Table 1 shows the main design characteristics between the two mentioned approaches. Basically, the use of the Hg-203 source, in a linear distribution, offers the advantage of a completely monochromatic radiation while the Ir-192 one has that of increased scattering yield, longer half-life, safe loading. This for the use of sealed sources. The more complex energy spectrum of the Ir-192 with respect to the Hg-203 produces an increased detection of multiply scattered photons but, however, this is compensated by the possibility of simul-

DESIGN ASPECTS OF THE COMPTON SCATTERING IRRADIATOR

RADIONUCLIDE		^{203}Hg	^{192}Ir
ACTIVITY	(GBq)	55,5	2 x 74
HALF-LIFE	(DAYS)	47	74
INCIDENT ENERGY	(KeV)	279	296,308 317,468
SCATTERING PEAK	(KeV)	180	191;245
SOURCES DISTANCE	(CM)	80(LINEAR)	40(TWIN)
COLLIMATOR CHANNEL	(CM)	13	20
SLIT WIDTH	(MM)	3	3
PHOTON FLUENCE	(RELATIVE)	1	1,8

Table 1. Design specifications of the 90° CST for the chest considering both approaches of linear source (Hg-203) and twin point sources (Ir-192).

taneous generation of two images at different photon energies generated from the same section. This information can be used for correcting the attenuation of the secondary scattered beam. Figure 4 shows the picture of the TomoCompton, (manufactured by the C.G.R.) the mobile irradiating system for Compton Tomography of the chest. The mechanical design permits an accurate positioning of the radiation beam and its translation following the specific chest sections to be irradiated. Furthermore, the mobility of the irradiator permits it to be removed when the study is completed or to be used with other gamma cameras, particularly mobile. This last possibility is of great interest because it would permit to move the technique at the patient bed to be used, for example, for monitoring purposes in acute patients.

90° CST of the lung: performance.

In this section the physical performance of the system for lung tomography will be examined and evaluated in relation to their implications for clinical quantitative imaging:
a) density linearity and multiple scattering: in a previous paper (18), the performance of the Hg-203 system has been examined. Figure 5 shows the results using the Ir-192 system and plots the photon efficiency (cpm/cc/Ci) vs. the mass density of the target.

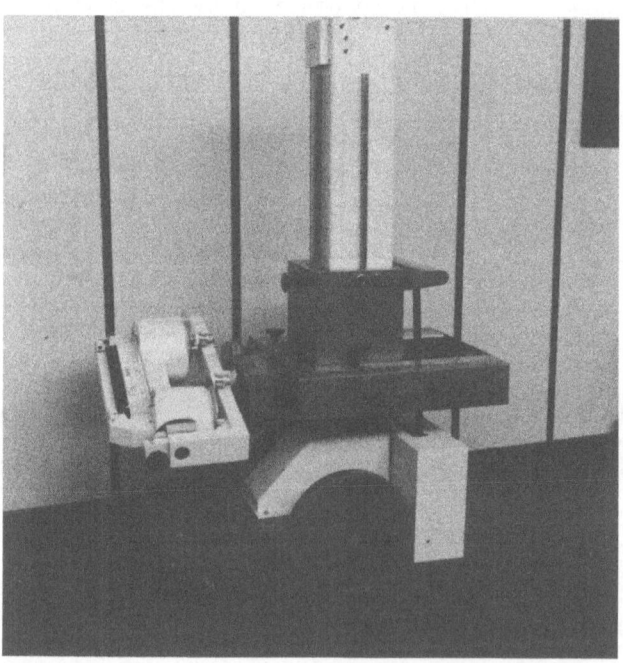

Fig. 4. Picture of the TomoCompton, the mobile irradiator containing the sources of Ir-192. The mechanical support permits a controlled and accurate positionning of the radiation beam.

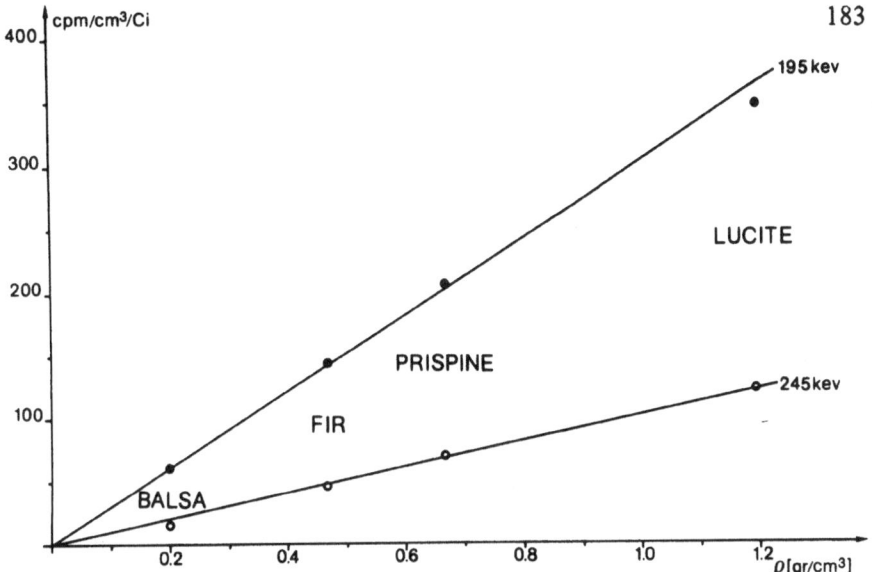

Fig. 5. Scattering yield and density linearity using targets mate
rials of increased density. The energy window on both 195 KeV and
245 KeV scattering peaks was 20%. The target was positionned at 1
cm distance from the High Resolution-Medium Energy collimator at
19 cm distance from the irradiating slit.

It is important to notice the good linear relationship of the
counts-density curves reflecting the pure Compton effect. These
measurements were obtained in air, i.e., in ideal conditions without diffusing medium surrounding the target itself. However, in
the real situation, of in vivo measurements, the scattering yield
value is affected by the problem of the additional noise, origin-
ating mainly by the detection of multiple scattering. This effect
comes mainly from the poor energy resolution of the NaI(Tl) detector (19). The amount of multiple scattering present in the
energy window used was evaluated through an experimental approach
similar to that suggested by Battista (2) and schematized in figure 6. The method consists of measuring the multiple scattering
contribution, evaluating, experimentally and with separate measurements, the scattering counts from an internal target. This
experiment gives the possibility to evaluate the amount of multiple scattering superimposed to the singly scatterd fluence. We
did the experiment using the balsa as target material, a 10% energy
window and the HR-ME collimator. The multiple scattering contribution was measured as 18%. This is a value which can be considered
as a reference within the lung, while as the density increases this
kind of noise increases and, for example, in the heart the multiple
scattering contamination will be much higher. Furthermore, this
influence depends on the chosen energy window: a 20% window gives
a 24% of noise; on the other side, the sensitivity gain will be
much higher than the noise (18).

184

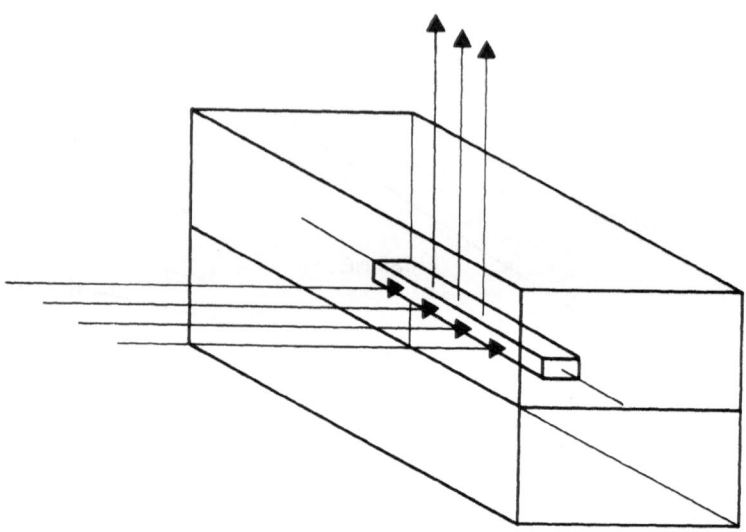

Fig. 6. Scheme for multiple scattering measurement: the 90° Compton scattering is detected from a target internal to a larger diffusing medium; comparison with the measurements of the same target in air (see text) permits to evaluate the multiple scattering contributions.

This effect is important in the quantitative evaluation of the absolute density of the chest. Various measures can be taken to correct for it using an additional energy window at lower energy (2) or an apriori evaluation based on the subtraction of a fixed percentage of the detected scattering, assuming the encountered structure and density.
b) Spatial Resolution: The spatial resolution (FWHM) of the system was evaluated using the previously mentioned collimator, figure 7. The slight discrepancy between the measured and the calculated values arises from the fact that the latter were evaluated considering only the intrinsic resolution of the gamma camera crystal at 191 KeV and the geometrical resolution of the detector collimator, without taking into account the effect of the penetration of the collimator septa at the detected energy, specially from the high energy peaks of the Ir-192. The collimator choice is of crucial importance in Compton imaging with external sources, particularly during in vivo measurements. In fact, as photons scatter at any angle, it is important that a given direction of scattering, falling in the detector field of view, the amount of lead, from the collimator septa, crossed by the scattered photons be sufficient to stop angles different than 90°.

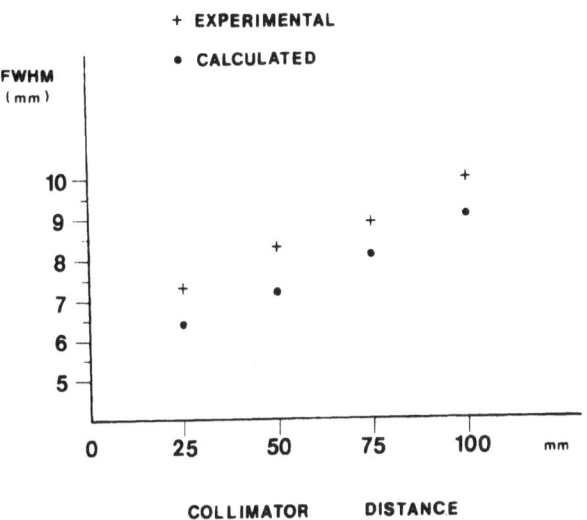

Fig. 7. FWHM (mm) in air and at different distances from the colli‑
mator.
High Resolution-Medium Energy (HR-ME) collimator characteristics:
2x2 mm² Hole size, 1 mm septal thickness,47 mm lenght.

In fact, even if energy windowing is used, penetration of forward
scattered photons results in a Compton noise superimposed to the
true signal. This disturbing effect has been observed with low
energy collimators. Once the previous requirement is satisfied
the parallel hole collimator can be optimized according to the re‑
quirements needed by the specific clinical or pathological situa‑
tion to be investigated, lung tumors or edema for example, balanc‑
ing the statistical noise σ, the spatial resolution R and the
density resolution D. These parameters can be related as follows:
$\sigma^2 \alpha \ R^{-2} D^{-1}$. A more detailed description of this problem was given
in a previous paper (18).
c) Tomographic Resolution: The tomographic performance of the
system was evaluated in several ways using both simple phantoms
to get quantitative results and realistic chest phantoms to assess
the in vivo performance. Figure 8 shows the picture of the Lucite
phantom used to quantify the possibility of detecting the size of
circular disks, 1 cm thick, at different distances from the colli‑
mator. In the experimental condition the phantom was positioned

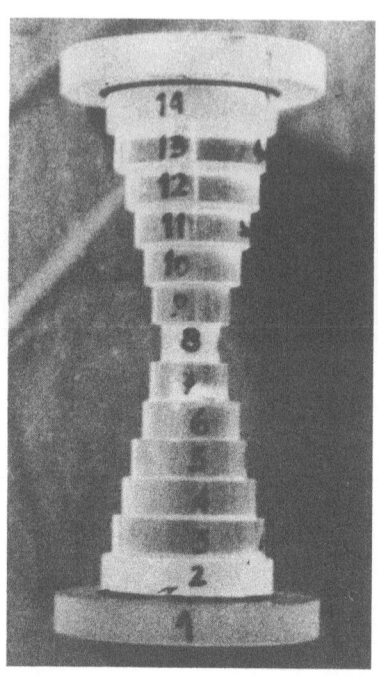

Fig. 8. Tomographic lucite disk
phantom 1 cm. thick each and of
different diameters.

on the collimator face with one of the largest size of the disk;
the different sections were irradiated by the incident beam at
different levels corresponding to the planes of the individual
disks. The results of the performed measurements are plotted in
figure 9 and compared to the actual values: the agreement was
really good and demonstrated the tomographic capability of the
method giving no geometrical distortion at the different levels,
except for the decreased accuracy moving far from the collimator
face and due to the deterioration in spatial resolution.
The possibility of detecting the various structures of the chest
was evaluated using a realistic chest phantom, the Humanoid, constituted by a bony thorax embedded in an opaque tissue equivalent
material. It incorporates dog lungs, fixed in the inflated state
and an anatomically realistic mediastinum. The component material
and the distribution of the different chest structures, including
large vessels, permits both to really evaluate image quality and
tomogrpahic performance in a standard format and an easier comparison with other methodologies. Figure 10 shows a standard x-ray
picture of the phantom, in the A-P projection, where the usual
chest structures are clearly visualized. This phantom, of course,
is not affected by respiratory motion, then the image quality is
better than during the in vivo measurements where the expected
blurring effect will be clearly manifest. Using that phantom and
the 90° CST, a set of frontal tomographic section has been obtained
as shown in figure 11. The images were corrected for the attenua-

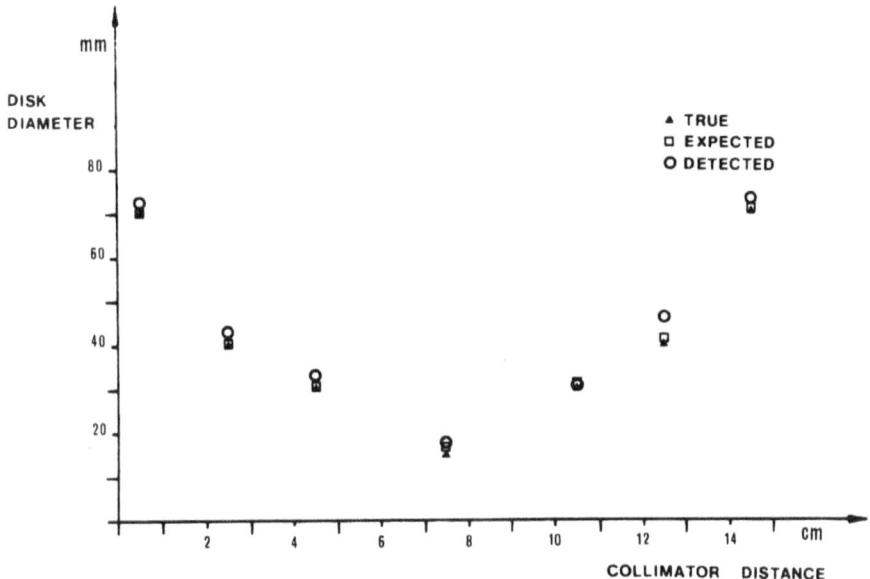

Fig. 9. Tomographic phantom results: the detected values (o) of the disk diameters at different tomographic levels of irradiation, are plotted, and compared with the true values (Δ), and the expected ones (□). These were calculated considering the geometrical va riation in resolution at different distances from the collimator face.

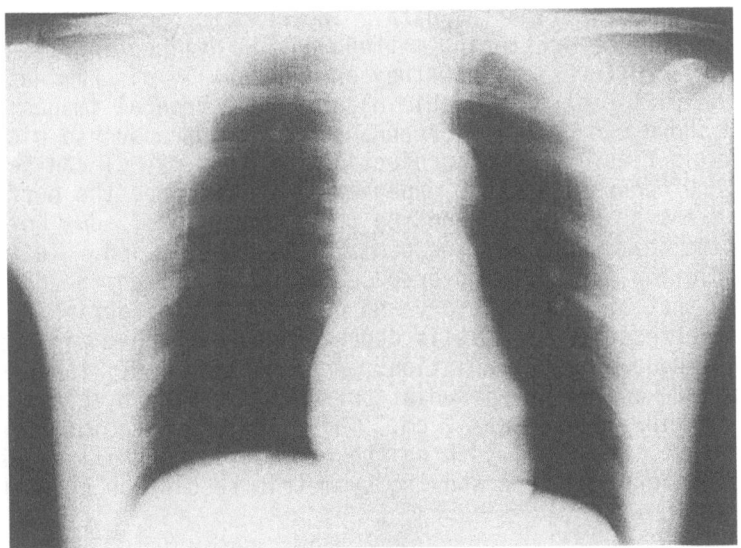

Fig. 10. A-P radiograph of the Humanoid chest phantom.

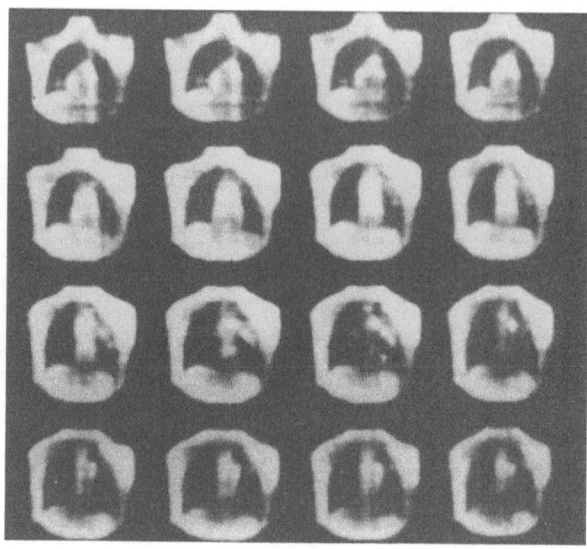

Fig. 11. Series of 16 frontal Compton Tomographic sections of the phantom in fig. 10 (left-right-top-bottom) showing the different chest structures. A tumor is visualized behind the heart in the first row of pictures.

tion of the primary incident beam using an algorithm which will be described in detail in a different paper. In practice the correction procedure acts completely automatic through the detection of the regions showing homogeneous density, and then the original image is corrected for an attenuation coefficient determined by a fitting of the experimental data. The results demonstrate the capability of the scattering methodology in delineating the different chest structures and how they are regionally discriminated along the different tomographic planes. The frontal images previously shown can be easily rearranged to get transverse pictures, as shown in figure 12, and projections as in x-ray CT can be obtained. Of course, in this experimental situation, the performance in the transverse plane cannot be the same as in CT, due both to the finite beam width and the gamma camera resolution. In fact, the resolution of the transverse section depends, on the horizontal axis, by that of the detector, and on the other direction by the slice thickness. This last is dependent on both beam width and spatial frequency of irradiation. In our experiment, the distance between each one of the irradiation planes (center-by-center) during the irradiation was 1 cm. This distance is comparable to what we have, as pixel width on the other axis, permitting us to get a transverse picture showing symmetric resolution on both directions.

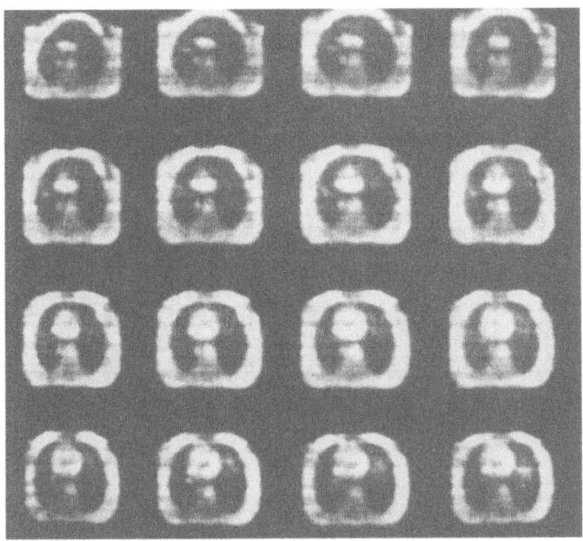

Fig. 12. Transverse pictures, after data rearrangement, of the fron
tal images shown in figure 11 starting from a superior chest section.

Discussion.

The technique of 90⁰ Compton Scattering Tomography for lung studies
described in the previous paragraphs represents a simple and inexpensive tool for the morphological and functional investigation of
the lung state and, particularly, of its density.
As shown in the section describing the system's performance, these
are mainly dominated by the detection apparatus, the gamma camera
and its collimation, particularly for sensitivity, spatial resolution and density resolution. Then, the great simplicity of the
method is balanced by the intrinsic performance on the detection
system. In principle, better and more effective designs could be
realized: use of two opposite and collinear radiation beams in
order to increase scattering yield for unit time and reduce the
attenuation effect; use of a solid state area detector to improve
the energy resolution, a key factor as far as multiple scattering
rejection is concerned; use of much more intense radiation sources
in order to significantly increase the scattering rate and strongly
reduce the acquisition time. This last possibility would require
heavier shielding of the irradiator for radioprotection problems.
It is interesting to observe that this technique, being used with
a widely available detector, i.e., the LFOV gamma camera, is easily
applicable and can be used as a complementary tool in nuclear medicine studies. In fact, where 2-D conventional lung emission
studies are performed, 90⁰ CST can be used without moving the
patient to delineate the lung volume; furthermore, an interesting
and also useful possibility of application, is that of Single
Photon Tomography using rotating gamma cameras, as shown in
figure 13.

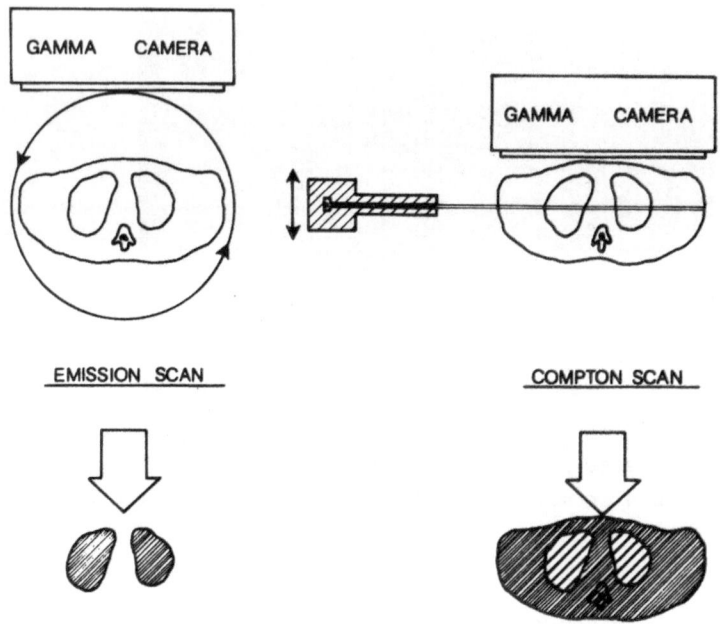

Fig. 13. Scheme for complementary use of both Single Photon Tomography with rotating gamma camera and Compton Tomography, as a tool for correcting the attenuation in the emission tomography of the chest.

One of the problems present in this technique is that of the attenuation correction when emission studies of the chest are performed. In fact, while attenuation correction is easily and effectively performed in the brain due to the relatively simple and uniform attentuation, the chest does not provide an acceptable solution due to the difficulty in getting the information on the distribution of the various attenuation coefficients. The lack of doing this, avoids the possibility to accurately quantitate the amount of labelled tracer distribution in the heart or in the lung. To this purpose, transmission methods have also been proposed (20,21) using point sources far from the crystal face or flood fields. It does seem, however, that the image quality and the accuracy in the determination of the attenuation coefficient will be superior with the scattering approach.
Other applications could be envisaged, as for example (22) 3-D morphological imaging of the chest in radiotherapy treatment planning to permit delineation of the exact location and size of the region to be irradiated.

However, the most important field of application of the described methodology, seems to be the diagnostic one. In fact, the unique possibility of moving the technique close to the patient bed to monitor and measure the evolution of the chest density, appears to be the most promising and important one, as in fact this information, presently, cannot be gathered using either x-ray CT or conventional radiological imaging.

References.
1) Lale P.G.: "The examination of internal tissues, using gamma ray scatter with a possible extension to megavoltage Radiography." Phys. Med. Biol., 4, (1959), 159-166.
2) Battista J.J., Santon L.W., Bronskill M.S.: "Compton Scatter imaging of transverse Sections: Correction for multiple scattering and attenuation." Phys. Med. Biol., 22, (1977), 229-244.
3) Garnett E.S., Kennett T.J., Kenyon D.B., Webber C.E.: "A photon scattering technique for the measurement of absolute bone density in man." Radiology, 106, (1973), 202-212.
4) Kennett T.J., Webber C.E.: "Bone density measurement by photon scattering II: inherent sources of errors." Phys. Med. Biol., 21, (1976), 770-778.
5) Kaufman L., Gamsu G., Swann S., Murphey L., Hiruska B., Palmer D.: "Measurement of absolute lung density by Compton Scattering densitometry." IEEE Trans. Nucl. Sci., MS-23, (1976), 599-605.

6) Clarke R.L., Van Dyk G.: "Compton scattered gamma rays in diagnostic radiography. In: Medical Radioisotope Scintigraphy." 1,
STI/PUB/193, (1959), 248-260.

7) Clarke R.L.: "A gamma ray scanner for diagnostic radiography."
Chalk River, Ontario, Canada A.E.C.L. 2270, (1965).

8) Clarke R.L., Milne E.N.C., Van Dyk G.: "The use of Compton scat
tered gamma rays for tomography." Invest. Radiol., 3, (1976), 225-
-235.

9) Reiss K.H., Schuster W.: "Quantitative measurements of lung
function in children by means of Compton Backscatter." Radiology,
102, (1972), 613-617.

10) Farmer F.T., Collins M.P.: "A new approach to the determination of anatomical cross sections of the body by Compton scattering of gamma rays." Phys. Med. Biol., 16, (1971), 577-586.

11) Moretti J.L., Mathieu E., Cavellier J.F., Roux G.: "90° Compton Scattering and its implementation by means of a bar detector
scintigraph." J. Nucl. Med. All. Sci., 24, (1980), 111-119.

12) Mirrel S.G., Anderson G.W., Blahd W.N.: "A tomographic brain
imaging system using Compton scattered gamma rays." In: IAEA Symposium on Medical Radionuclide Imaging, IAEA-SM-210/270, (1976),
255-262.

13) Okuyama S., Mishina H., Sera K., Matsuzawa T.: "Compton Soft-
tissue imaging and its capability expanded by direct magnification
and Shinozaky color TV system." Radiology, 131, (1979), 215-220.

14) Guzzardi R., Mey M., Pistolesi M., Solfanelli S., Giuntini C.:
"Tomography by 90° Compton Scattering." J. Nucl. Med. All. Sci.,
21, (1977), 72-77.

15) Pistolesi M., Guzzardi R., Mey M., Solfanelli S., Giuntini C.:
"Regional lung density imaging by 90° scattering of an external
gamma ray source." Proceed. 16th S. Diego Biom. Symp., J.I.Martin
ed., New York, Academic Press, (1972), 45-54.

16) Pistolesi M., Solfanelli S., Guzzardi R., Mey M., Giuntini C.:
"Pulmonary regional densitography by detection of the 90° scattered radiation from an external source of gamma rays." J. Nucl. Med.
27, (1977), 94-97.

17) Guzzardi R., Bottigli U., Mey M.,: "Sources for 90° Compton
Scattering Tomography of the lung." Nuklear Medizin, Suppl. 17,
(1980), 879-900.

18) Guzzardi R., Mey M.: "Further appraisal and improvements of 90°
Compton Scattering Tomography of the lung." Phys. Med. Biol., 26,
(1981), 155-161.

19) Guzzardi R., Mey M., Giuntini C.: "90° Compton Scattering To-

mography of the lung; detection characteristics and correction of the attenuation." J. Nucl. Med. All. Sci., 24,(1980), 163-169.

20) Budinger T.F., Gullberg G.T.: "Transverse section reconstruction of gamma-ray emitting radionuclide in parients. Reconstruction Tomography in diagnostic Radiology and Nuclear Medicine." (M. Ter Pogossian Ed. University Park Press, 1972).

21) Maeda H., Itoh H., Ishii Y., Mukai T., Todo G., Fujita T., Torizuka K.: "Determination of plural edge by gamma camera ray transmission Computed Tomography." J. Nucl. Med., 22, (1981), 815-817.

22) Battista J.J., Bronskill M. J.: "Compton scatter imaging of transverse sections: an overall appraisal and evaluation for radio therapy planning." Phys. Med. Biol., 26, (1981), 81-99.

Part III: *Clinical Imaging: Basic Principles of Acoustical NMR
and Transmission Tomographic Imaging*

ACOUSTICAL IMAGING: THEORY LIMITATIONS AND RELATIONSHIPS TO
OTHER IMAGING MODALITIES

P.N.T. Wells

Department of Medical Physics
Bristol General Hospital
Bristol BS1 6SY, United Kingdom

ABSTRACT.   The basic physics of ultrasound is reviewed. Ultrasonic diagnosis employs frequencies in the low megahertz range
which is generated and detected by piezoelectric transducers.
Pulse-echo information may be displayed as an A-scan, an M-mode
recording, as a two-dimensional B-scan (often obtained in real
time), or as a C-scan. The Doppler effect gives rise to audible
shift frequencies in ultrasound reflected from moving structures.
This can be used for flow studies and for imaging. Ultrasonic
methods, which are generally limited to the study of soft tissues,
provide information which may be complementary to that obtainable
with other diagnostic techniques; but they compete for financial
resources, and the technologies are continuously changing.

1 INTRODUCTION

Ultrasound is a form of energy which consists of mechanical
vibrations the frequencies of which are so high that they are
above the range of human hearing. The lower frequency limit of
the ultrasonic spectrum may generally be taken to be about 20 kHz.
Most biomedical applications of ultrasound employ frequencies in
the range 1-15 MHz. At these frequencies, the wavelength is in
the range 1.5-0.1 mm in·soft tissues, and narrow beams of ultrasound can be generated without excessive attenuation.
    This paper is intended to provide an overview of contemporary
ultrasonic, or "acoustical", imaging. The physical principles
are treated in more detail elsewhere (1), and references are
given only to newer or less well-known topics.

2 BASIC PHYSICS OF ULTRASOUND

Ultrasonic energy travels through a medium in the form of a wave.
Although a number of different wave modes are possible, almost all
biomedical applications involve the use of longitudinal waves.
The particles of which the medium is composed vibrate backwards
and forwards about their mean positions, so that energy is transferred through the medium in a direction parallel to that of the
oscillations of the particles. The particles themselves do not
move through the medium, but simply vibrate to and fro. Thus,
the energy is transferred in the form of a disturbance in the
equilibrium arrangement of the medium, without any bodily transfer
of matter.

The wavelength, λ, and the frequency, f, are related to the
propagation speed, c, according to the equation

$$c = f\lambda \qquad\qquad\qquad (1)$$

In most soft tissues, the speed is close to that in water (about
1 500 m s^{-1}); it is virtually independent of frequency (2). This
speed results in a wavelength of, for example, 1 mm at a frequency
of 1.5 MHz. The speed in gas and gas-containing structures is
lower (typically 300-600 m s^{-1}), and that in bone is higher
(2 500-4 000 m s^{-1}).

In any imaging system, the wavelength of the radiation used
to form the image is one of the factors which determines the
resolution. In typical ultrasonic imaging studies, it is
desirable to resolve structures of a few millimetres in size.
This determines that the minimum ultrasonic frequency needs to be
around 3 MHz, corresponding to a wavelength of 0.5 mm. The
maximum frequency is limited by the attenuation of ultrasound,
which increases with frequency, being about 1 dB cm^{-1} MHz^{-1} in
soft tissues. The attenuation in gas and bone is much greater
than that in soft tissues.

When a wave meets the boundary between two media at normal
incidence, it is propagated without deviation into the second
medium. At oblique incidence, the wave is deviated by refraction
unless the speeds in the two media are equal. The relationship
is

$$(\sin \theta_i)/(\sin \theta_t) = c_1/c_2 \qquad\qquad\qquad (2)$$

where θ_i and θ_t are the angles of incidence and transmission, and
c_1 and c_2 are the speeds in the two media. Note that refraction
can generally be ignored in soft tissues, in which the speeds are
nearly equal.

In any given medium, the ratio of the instantaneous values
of particle pressure and velocity is constant. This constant
value is called the "characteristic impedance", Z, of the medium,

and it is equal to the product of the corresponding density and speed; thus

$$Z = \rho c \qquad (3)$$

If the characteristic impedances of the media on each side of the boundary are equal, the wave travels across the boundary unaffected by the change in the supporting medium. If the characteristic impedances are unequal, however, the incident energy is shared between the waves reflected and transmitted at the boundary. At normal incidence, the fraction, R, of the incident energy which is reflected is given by the equation

$$R = \left[(Z_2 - Z_1)/(Z_2 + Z_1) \right]^2 \qquad (4)$$

Thus there may be small reflexions at boundaries between soft tissues, which have similar speeds and densities. There are large reflexions, however, at the boundaries between soft tissue and gas (which has a low characteristic impedance) and between soft tissue and bone (which has a high impedance).

In general, medical ultrasonic imaging is restricted to studies of soft tissues. It is unsuitable for investigating gas-containing structures and bone, because of large differences in speed (causing refraction and making it difficult to measure distance, large differences in characteristic impedance (causing large reflexions), and high attenuation.

The somewhat idealised situation in which an ultrasonic wave is reflected by an extensive flat surface is called "specular reflexion". For example, the smooth surface of a normal heart valve leaflet may be considered to approach a specular reflector; although the surface is curved, the radius of curvature is quite large in relation to the wavelength.

It is important to realise that the results of calculations of refraction and reflexion conditions at a plane boundary may not apply to a similar characteristic impedance discontinuity at a rough interface or small obstacle. The specular component of reflexion is replaced, by an amount that depends on the geometric characteristics of the discontinuity, by components of scattered energy. This effect becomes important when the dimensions of the discontinuity are in the order of the wavelength or less. If the scattering dimensions are of wavelength order, however, the situation is much more complicated, and the intensity of the wave scattered in any particular direction depends on the orientation and shape of the obstacle. This is the situation at many of the boundaries in biological tissues, and the scattering problem is not amenable to theoretical solution for two reasons: the geometry is not well defined, and the ultrasonic characteristics of the tissue components are not accurately known.

The frequencies of the reflected and incident waves are equal if the reflecting boundary is stationary. Movement of the reflector towards the source, however, results in a spatial compression of the wavelength of the reflected wave, and vice versa. The phenomenon is called the "Doppler effect".

At normal incidence, if f is the frequency of the incident wave, and v is the velocity of the reflecting boundary towards the source, the Doppler shift, f_D, in the reflected frequency which occurs in the reflected wave ($f_D = f' - f$, where f' is the received frequency) is given by

$$f_D = 2\ vf/c \tag{5}$$

provided that v << c, as is generally the case in diagnostic applications. In these applications, it often happens that the direction of the motion of the reflecting boundary is at an angle, γ, with the incident wave, although the incident and reflected wave are effectively coincident. This is commonly the situation in the transcutaneous measurement of blood flow velocity in peripheral vessels. Then

$$f_D = 2\ v\ (\cos \gamma)\ f/c \tag{6}$$

so that it is necessary to know γ in order to calculate v.

3   GENERATION AND DETECTION OF ULTRASONIC WAVES

At megahertz frequencies such as are employed in diagnostic applications, ultrasound is both generated and detected by the piezoelectric effect.

Although there are many natural crystals which are piezoelectric (the best-known is quartz), the most commonly used transducer material is the synthetic ceramic lead zirconate titanate. This material is polarised during manufacture to make it strongly piezoelectric.

Disc transducers are commonly used in diagnostic applications. In the steady state, if I_0 is the intensity at the surface of the transducer, and I_z is the intensity at a distance z from the transducer along the central axis, then

$$I_z/I_0 = \sin^2\{(\pi/\lambda)[(a^2 + z^2)^{\frac{1}{2}} - z]\} \tag{7}$$

where a is the radius of the disc. Moving along the central axis towards the disc, the intensity increases until a maximum is reached at a distance z'_{max} from the disc, given by

$$z'_{max} = a^2/\lambda \tag{8}$$

provided that $a^2 >> \lambda^2$. The position of this maximum may be considered to separate the ultrasound into near and far fields. The beam in the near field is roughly cylindrical, although it

may be focused either by a lens, by using a curving transducer, or
by an array. Deep in the far field, the directivity function is
given by

$$D_s = \frac{2 J_1 \ (ka \ sin \ \theta)}{ka \ sin \ \theta} \qquad (9)$$

where θ is the angle relating D_s to the central axis of the beam,
and J_1 is the first order Bessel function. Thus the main lobe of
the beam diverges at angle $\pm$ θ about the central axis, given by

$$\theta = sin^{-1} \ (0.61 \ \lambda/a) \qquad (10)$$

If the transducer produces (or responds to) a transient
ultrasonic disturbance, the ultrasonic field is modified because,
at any particular point in the field, the contributions from the
different elementary parts of the source surface may not be equal.
As a result, the sharply defined inhomogeneities of the steady
state become increasingly smeared and homogeneous as the pulse
length is reduced.
     The construction of an ultrasonic transducer designed for
pulse-echo operation is shown in Figure 1.

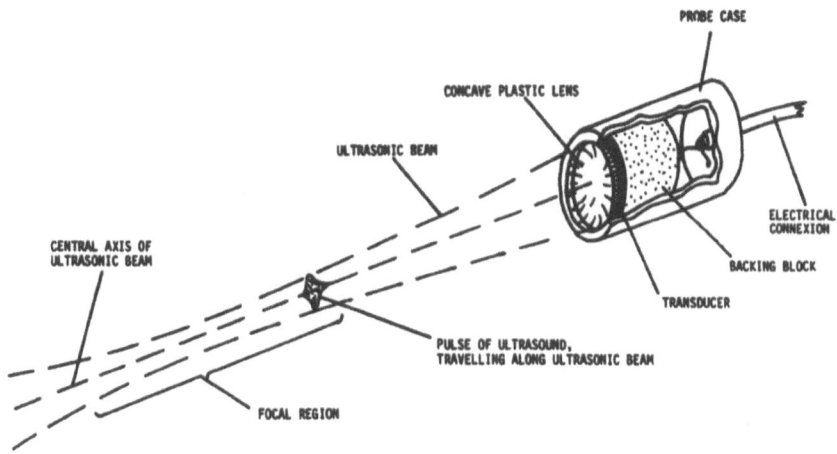

Fig. 1. Construction of a typical transducer for pulse-echo
operations, showing beam and pulse shapes.

4   PULSE-ECHO DIAGNOSTIC METHODS

An ultrasonic pulse is reflected when it strikes the boundary
between two media of differing characteristic impedances, and the

time delay that occurs between the transmission of the pulse and
the reception of its echo depends on the propagation speed and the
path length. It is generally assumed that, in soft tissues, there
is a constant relationship between time and distance; ultrasound
travels 10 mm in about 6.7 μs.

Pulse-echo ultrasonic instruments range in complexity from
the simple distance-measuring A-scope, through the time-position
recording system and the static two-dimensional B-scope to real-
time systems gathering data from two-dimensional planes within
three-dimensional volumes.

4.1   The A-Scope

The basic elements of the simplest type of pulse-echo system for
medical diagnosis, called the "A-scope", are illustrated in Figure
2. The rate generator simultaneously triggers the transmitter, the

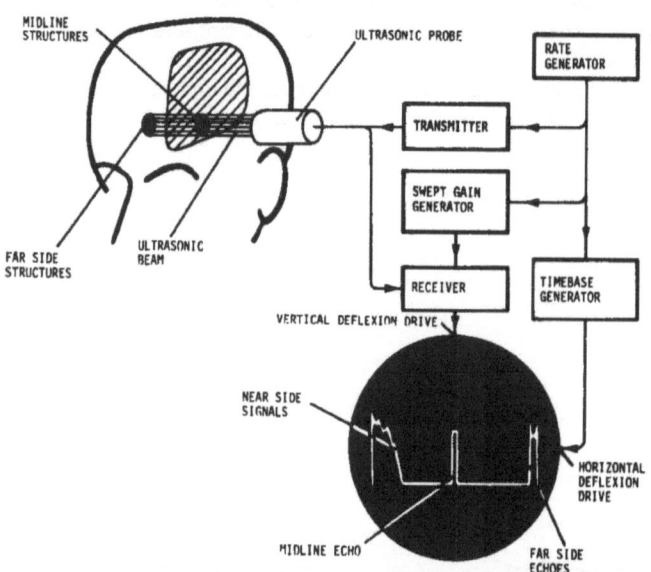

Fig. 2. Basic elements of the A-scope, shown here
being used for brain midline localisation.

swept gain generator (which increases the gain of the receiver
with time, to compensate for the increasing attenuation of echoes
from deeper structures), and the timebase generator. Vertical
deflexions of the horizontal timebase occur at positions corresponding to echo-producing targets along the ultrasonic beam
within the patient. Rapid repetition of the process (typically
1 000 times per second) results in a flicker-free display.

4.2 Time-Position (M-Mode) Recording

The information obtained with a pulse-echo system is a combination
of range and amplitude data which can simply be presented as an
A-scan (section 4.1). The same information, however, may alternatively be displayed on a brightness-modulated timebase, in such
a way that the brightness increases with echo amplitude; this type
of display is called a B-scan.

A time-position recording of structure position along the
ultrasonic beam may be generated from a B-scan as shown in Figure
3. The recording is composed of many separate B-scan lines lying
side-by-side. Conventionally, increasing distance into the
patient is represented by more downward deflexion on the recording,
and earlier time, horizontally towards the right. The time

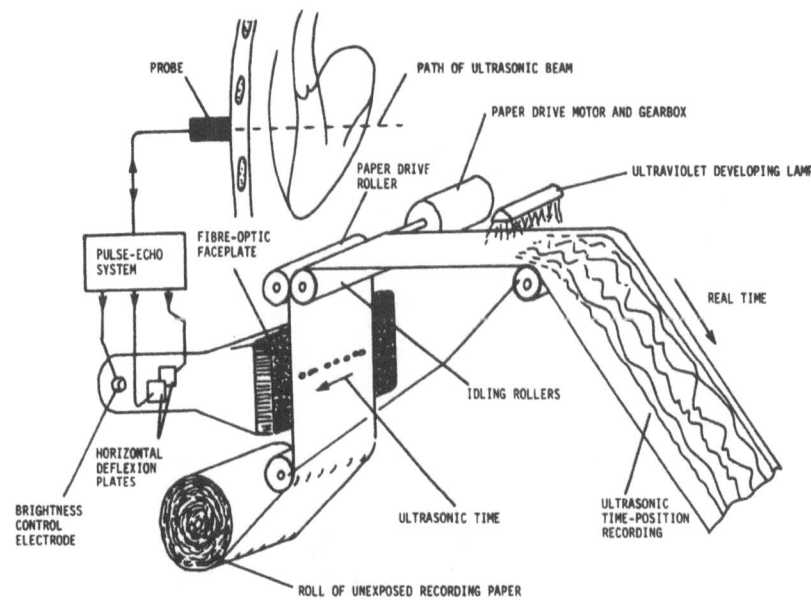

Fig. 3. Time-position recording system using a continuous strip
of photographic paper sensitive to ultraviolet light, shown here
being used for mitral valve motion study.

required to form a single B-scan line depends on the depth of
penetration; for example, a time of 133 µs corresponds to a depth
of 100 mm. Structures within the body do not move significant
distances during so short a time, so that (provided that the
pulse repetition rate is fast enough) the movements of structures
such as heart valves may be studied.

4.3   Two-Dimensional B-Scanning

The production of an image of a cross-section through soft tissue
structures of the body may be accomplished by relating the
positions of registrations on the display to the positions of the
corresponding echo-producing structures within a defined two-
dimensional plane in the patient.

The first type of two-dimensional scanner, and one which is
still in common use, is the so-called "static" B-scan instrument.
Figure 4 is a block diagram showing a typical arrangement. The

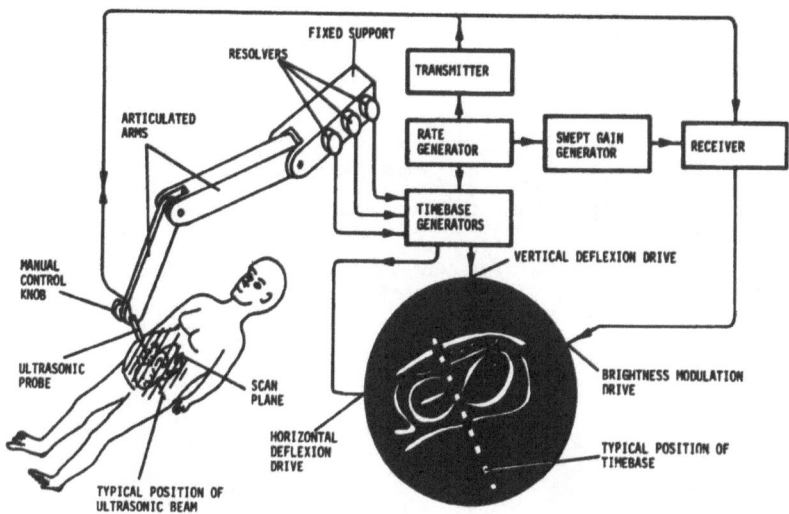

Fig. 4.   Basic elements of static two-dimensional B-scope, shown
here being used for an obstetric study.

horizontal (x) and vertical (y) deflexion circuits are driven by
separate ultrasonic timebases, simultaneously triggered by the
rate generator. The x and y coordinates of the start of the
timebases which form the images are controlled by the resolvers
in the scanner, and these resolvers also control the direction of
the resultant timebase across the display. Thus the output from
the receiver, arranged to brightness-modulate the display,
produces registrations on the resultant timebase in positions
corresponding to the echo-producing targets in the patient. A
two-dimensional image is built up by moving the probe so that the
part of the anatomical cross-section which it is desired to
visualise is scanned by a sufficient number of discrete ultrasonic
lines. The image is stored on a scan converter, which has two
distinct functions: it acts as an image memory, and it converts
from the ultrasonic scan format to a TV-raster format to allow
the image to be viewed on a suitable cathode-ray tube monitor.

Although analogue scan converters have the advantage of high
resolution and dynamic range, they are prone to drift; nowadays,
digital scan converters (typically 512 x 512 pixels with 5 bit
words) are almost always used. Moreover, digital scan converters
allow line-by-line refreshment of the image during continuous or
intermittent scanning movements (3).

Static scanners have extensive clinical applications,
particularly in abdominal investigations. It is often useful,
however, to have a real-time imaging capability, in which the
image frame rates are fast enough to allow movement to be followed.
Ultimately the frame rate is limited by the speed of ultrasound.
If, for example, a penetration of 150 mm is required, the time
which elapses between the transmission of the ultrasonic pulse and
reception of the echo from the maximum range is equal to 200 µs
(taking the speed to be 1 500 m s^{-1}). The corresponding maximum
pulse repetition rate is 5 000 s^{-1}. Thus the maximum image line
rate is 5 000 s^{-1}, equal to the product of the number of lines
per frame and the number of frames per second. Thus, at 40 frames
s^{-1}, there could be 125 lines per frame, and so on.

Some of the many methods of rapid scanning to produce real-
time images are illustrated in Figure 5.

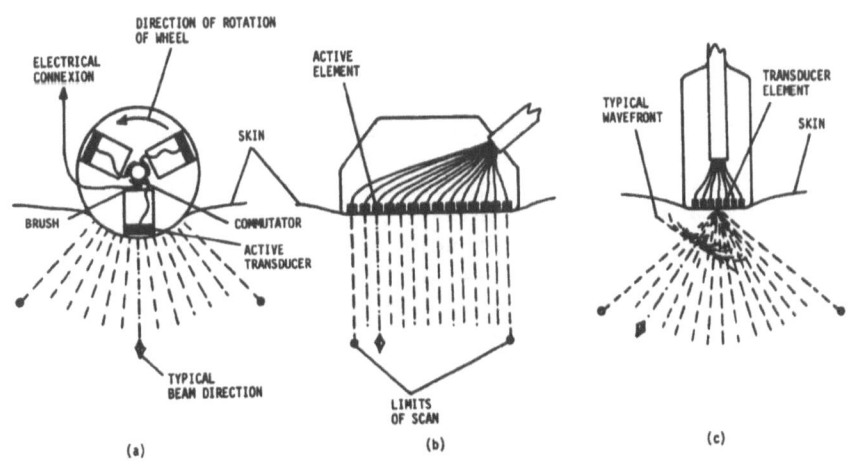

Fig. 5. Methods of real-time scanning.

In the arrangement shown in Figure 5a, a conventional single-
element transducer, or group of single-element transducers, is
mechanically driven to form images in real time but otherwise
similar to those made by conventional "static" two-dimensional
scanners. Figures 5b and 5c show two arrangements - an
electronically addressed linear array and an electronically
steered array - which produce real-time scans with static

transducers.

The principles of the electronically addressed linear array type of real-time scanner are illustrated in Figure 6.

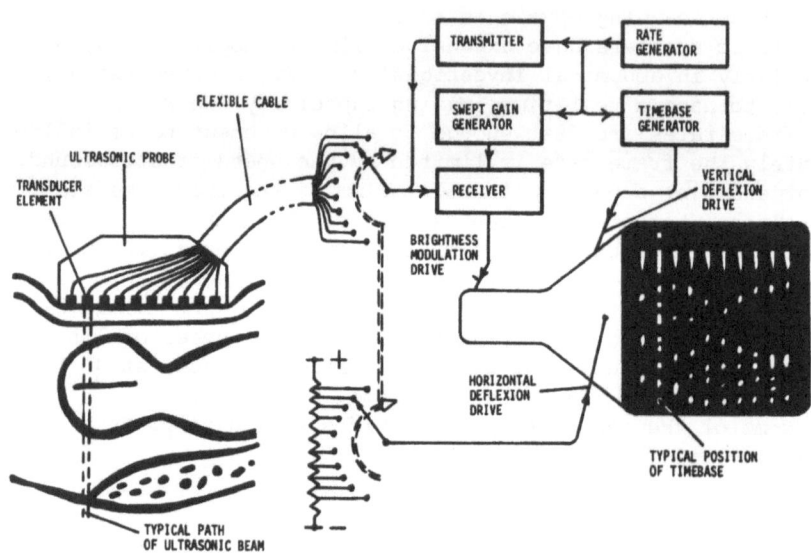

Fig. 6. Basic elements of electronically addressed linear array real-time scanner.

In this diagram, the probe contains 10 separate transducer elements (in a practical system, the number is usually between 20 and 128). The rate generator, typically operating at a prf of 2 000 s^{-1}, triggers the transmitter. In this simple example, the transmitter pulse is applied, through a sequencing switch, to one of the transducer elements. (Again, in a practical system, this sequencing switch, and the second switch operating synchronously with it, is usually electronic and not mechanical.) Simultaneously, the rate generator triggers the time-base generator connected to the vertical deflexion plates of the cathode ray tube display. Echoes returning from within the patient are detected by the transducer element which emitted the original pulse, fed through the sequencing switch, and amplified (under swept gain control, triggered by the clock), to brightness-modulate the display. Each element is rapidly addressed in sequence, and a two-dimensional image is built up by the second sequencing switch applying appropriate horizontal deflexion voltages to the display.

In the earliest linear array systems, the transducer elements were addressed one at a time. In this situation, a compromise is necessary. On the one hand, it is desirable to have a large number of lines in the image, and this requires a large number of transducers. On the other hand, it is desirable to have good resolution, which depends on having a non-divergent (or even focused) beam of ultrasound. Unfortunately, the beam divergence in the far field increases as the transducer is made more narrow. The difficulty can be circumvented by having an array of many narrow transducers (so that the objective of high line density can be achieved) operated in groups to ensure an adequate aperture (so that the resolution is acceptable). A common arrangement is to have 64 elements operated in groups of 4, stepped one element between lines, thus giving 61 lines of ultrasonic information.

The second type of electronically-controlled real-time scanner makes use of the beam steering capability of an array. Consider the array, consisting of four long narrow elements, illustrated in Figure 7. The introduction of appropriate time

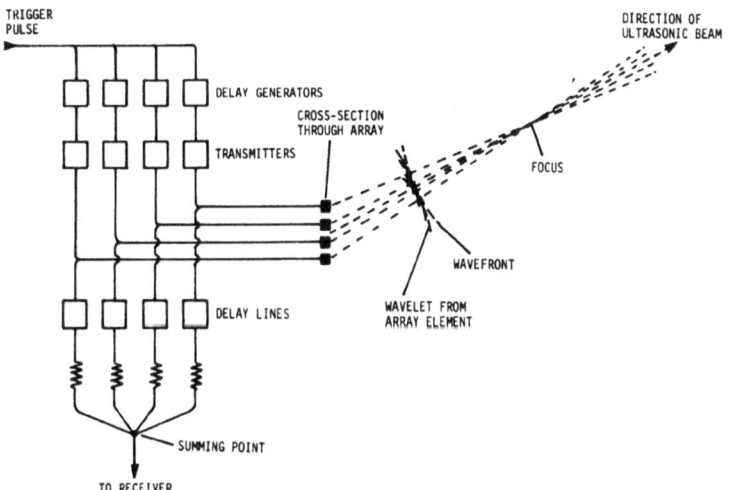

Fig. 7. Principles of electronic beam steering. The transmitting and receiving delay times of each array element are equal, and the time grading across the array determines the direction of the ultrasonic beam.

delays in the signal paths allows the beam to be directed through any desired angle (within certain limitations), and also to be focused. Moreover, on reception the position of the focus may be swept continuously to coincide with instantaneous range of the target; this technique is also valuable with linear array scanners. Typically, electronically steered arrays have around 20 elements, and the external dimensions of the probe are similar to those of a conventional single-element transducer probe.

4.4   C-Scanning

The C-scan is a two-dimensional display of a plane normal to the

direction of the ultrasound within the patient. It can be
generated by scanning the transducer in a regular pattern (usually
through a water bath) over the surface of the patient. At each
position of the transducer, the echo signal detected from an
electronically gated region at constant depth is arranged to
brightness modulate the display. The scanning speed is
necessarily slow, because only one pixel is obtained with each
transmitted pulse. The value of the method is that it can make
it easier to interpret anatomical relationships in certain
situations.

4.5   Resolution in Pulse-Echo Systems

Within the limitations imposed by noise and by the maximum per-
missible transmitted power, the maximum useful dynamic range of
the echoes received in conventional medical diagnostic pulse-echo
systems is about 100 dB. This dynamic range is shared between the
variations in echo amplitude at particular ranges, and the
attenuation of echoes which increases with distance. In practice,
at any particular range, an echo amplitude variation of about 30
dB is the maximum which may usefully be employed, since the
azimuthal resolution is unlikely to be acceptable with a larger
dynamic range. Therefore, around 70 dB is available to provide
swept gain compensation for attenuation. An attenuation of 1 dB
cm^{-1} MHz^{-1} corresponds to 0.15 dB per wavelength, or to 0.3 dB per
wavelength of penetration (taking account of the go-and-return
path). With 70 dB of swept gain, a penetration of 200 wavelengths
is a reasonable compromise.

The resolution cell is the volume of material within which
the interaction providing the data takes place. The length of the
resolution cell depends on the duration of the ultrasonic pulse,
and is typically equal to two wavelengths. Its width is about
five times its length, although the two may be roughly equal where
the beam is focused from a typical aperture.

4.6   Speckle

Modern ultrasonic scanners have gray scale displays which produce
images with a range of tonal values. The strongest echoes correspond to specular reflexions from major boundaries. Lower level
echoes originate from small scatterers within "homogeneous"
tissue, and several of these scatterers may lie within the
resolution cell. The echo amplitude from such an ensemble depends
on the spatial relationships of the scatterers, and so it also
depends on the direction of the ultrasonic beam (4). This
phenomenon is analogous to laser speckle, and arises because of the
coherent nature of the imaging process.

4.7   Multiple Reflexion Artifacts

A serious limitation of the pulse-echo method is due to the
multiple reflexions, or reverberations, that the ultrasonic pulse
may suffer during its propagation. For example, in Figure 2
echoes returning to the probe from within the patient are themselves partially re-reflected at the probe surface, and these
pulses themselves act as if they were transmitter pulses, relatively small in amplitude and appropriately delayed in time.
Echoes of these small pulses produce registrations, if they are
large enough to be detected, at positions corresponding to twice
the distances at which the true echoes are registered. These
"multiple reflexion" artifacts may often be quite easily recognised
because of their regular spacings. Those due to gas and bone are
generally inconveniently large, and they are a fundamental
limitation of ultrasonic diagnosis.

5   DOPPLER DIAGNOSTIC METHODS

Ultrasonic Doppler methods are nowadays both widely used and of
established value in the study of moving structures in clinical
diagnosis (5). The Doppler shift in frequency of an ultrasonic
beam reflected from a moving structure (or ensemble of scatterers)
is used to provide information about the velocity of the structure
(or ensemble), either for interpretation by ear, or for analysis
by instrument. This convenient situation arises because it happens
(see Equations 5 and 6) that targets within the body, which move
at velocities of up to about 200 mm s^{-1}, give rise to Doppler
shift frequencies in the audible range when irradiated with low-
megahertz frequency ultrasound.

The choice of the ultrasonic frequency depends on the clinical
application. A compromise is necessary between the penetration,
the variation of Doppler shift frequency for a given variation in
target velocity, the sensitivity to small reflectors, and the size
and shape of the ultrasonic field. In obstetrics and cardiology,
the optimal frequency is generally 2-3 MHz, but in blood flow
studies, it may be as high as 10 MHz.

The same restrictions and limitations (such as the necessity
to maintain good ultrasonic coupling, and the inability to
operate successfully through gas) which apply to ultrasonic pulse-
echo methods, also apply to ultrasonic Doppler methods.

5.1   Continuous Wave Doppler Systems

The block diagram of a continuous wave Doppler system is shown in
Figure 8. The transmitter operates continuously, providing an
output of constant amplitude and frequency. The ultrasonic probe
contains separate transmitting and receiving transducers. (These
are generally necessary because it is important to minimise the

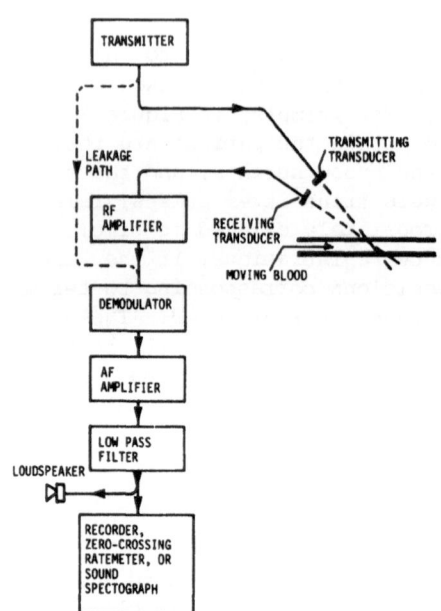

Fig. 8. Basic elements of
continuous wave Doppler
system, shown here being used
to study blood flow.

direct transfer of energy from the transmitter to the radio
frequency amplifier, in order to avoid overloading the receiver.)
The output from the rf amplifier consists of a mixture of signals,
some of frequency equal to that of the transmitter (these are due
to reflexions from stationary structures in the ultrasonic field,
and electrical leakage), and some of frequencies shifted by the
Doppler effect. These signals are mixed in the demodulator, the
output from which contains the difference frequencies between the
transmitted ultrasonic wave and the Doppler shifted received waves.
The output from the demodulator is filtered to allow these
difference frequencies to pass, whilst unwanted (higher) frequencies are stopped. The difference frequencies, which in general
fall in the audible range, are amplified, and either an operator
listens to them, or they are analysed electronically. In clinical
applications, the Doppler shifted signals do not consist of a
single frequency, but they extend over a frequency spectrum (since
the beam simultaneously interrogates structures moving at different
velocities). For this reason, measurements of Doppler shift
signals made by ratemeters, such as the zero-crossing frequency
meter, need to be interpreted with caution. In most investigations
with Doppler techniques, it is generally very much safer to subject the Doppler signals to frequency spectrum analysis; this may
be done by on-line or off-line instruments.

5.2   Pulsed Doppler Systems

A block diagram of a typical pulsed Doppler system is shown in
Figure 9. The pulse repetition rate is controlled by the clock,
which triggers the monostable to open the gate to allow the

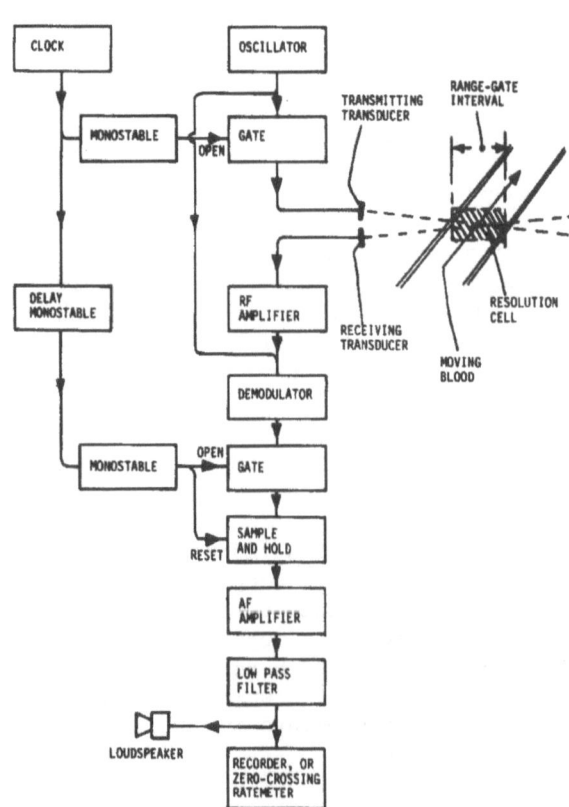

Fig. 9. Basic
elements of pulsed
Doppler system.

transmitting transducer to be excited for a period corresponding
to the width of the target volume which it is desired to study.
Echoes returning from within the patient are amplified, and mixed
in the demodulator with the signal from the oscillator (equal in
frequency to that which was transmitted). The delay monostable
triggers the monostable controlling the receiver gate, so that
the gate opens to allow a voltage, which is in effect a sample
corresponding to the Doppler shift due to motion in the target
volume, to be stored in the sample-and-hold circuit. The sample-
and-hold is reset immediately prior to being updated by a new
sample resulting from the following ultrasonic pulse. The output
from the sample-and-hold is thus a rectangular wave with a long
"mark" and a short "space", the envelope of which is an audible
signal representing the Doppler shifted information from the
target volume. The upper frequency limit (which is related to the

maximum value of target vector velocity which can be measured)
which can be detected without ambiguity depends upon the sampling
rate. The maximum sampling rate is limited by the ultrasonic
transit time to and from the target of interest, and by the
reverberation decay time. It is well known in information theory
that if a signal waveform has frequencies in its spectrum extending from zero to an upper frequency f_{max}, it is possible to convey
all the information in the signal provided that the sampling
frequency is at least 2 f_{max}. This sets an upper limit to the
maximum unambiguously measurable velocity vector at any given
penetration for a given ultrasonic frequency.

5.3   Directionally Sensitive Doppler Systems

Simple Doppler systems merely measure the magnitude of the
frequency difference between the transmitted and received ultrasonic signals, and not the sign of the difference. This sign
carries the information about the direction of the movement of the
target, either towards or away from the probe. This directional
information is vital in some diagnostic situations.

   If the signal always consists, at any instant in time, of
movement (or flow) in only one direction, a detector capable of
switching a logic circuit to indicate whether the movement is in
the forward or reverse direction would be satisfactory. (This is
the method employed in many commercially-manufactured systems.)
Almost invariably, however, in practice the Doppler signal consists, at least for some of the time in each periodic cycle, of
simultaneous signals from targets moving in opposite directions.
Logic circuits are then inappropriate, and there is really no
substitute for the sound spectrograph as a display device. Other
directionally-sensitive detection arrangements include single
sideband and superheterodyne techniques.

5.4   Two-Dimensional Doppler Imaging

In many clinical situations, adequate diagnostic information can
be obtained with a hand-held Doppler probe. It is necessary,
however, for the investigator to know the anatomy of the structure
being studied in order to interpret the results.

   In studies of the vascular system it is often useful to have
a two-dimensional map showing the position of blood vessels. The
ultrasonic Doppler shifted signals from flowing blood are sufficiently characteristic to allow their presence to be identified
by logic circuitry. This capability is exploited in the two-
dimensional scanner shown in Figure 10. The probe is mounted on a
two-dimensional coordinate-measuring scanner, the resolvers of
which provide data enabling computation of the x and y voltages
that control the deflexion circuits of a direct-view electronic
storage tube. The probe is arranged so that the ultrasonic beam
is at least slightly inclined to the direction of flow in the

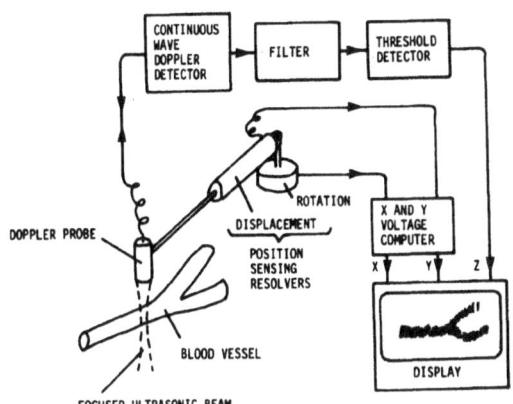

Fig. 10. Basic elements
of continuous wave two-
dimensional Doppler
imaging system.

vessels to be visualised. When the beam passes through moving
blood the Doppler detector generates an output which is filtered
(to remove artifacts due to low velocity movements such as those
of the probe over the skin) and, provided that the output exceeds
a preset threshold level, it switches on the electron beam of the
display. A two-dimensional map showing those regions in which
flow has been detected is constructed on the display by scanning
the probe over the area of skin overlying the vessel. Since
arteries and veins often lie close together, a directionally-
sensitive circuit is arranged to inhibit the display when flow is
detected in the opposite direction to that in the vessel under
study.

A two-dimensional scan of a blood vessel made with a continu-
ous-wave Doppler instrument is essentially a plan view, representing the projection of the blood vessel onto the skin surface along
the line-of-sight of the ultrasonic beam. The same type of image
can be obtained with a pulsed Doppler scanner range-gated to a
constant depth (or even to a variable depth, under the control of
the operator) within the blood vessel. Because the pulsed-Doppler
scanner is capable of measuring range (as well as velocity), and
thus of displaying the depth of detected flow, cross-sectional
and longitudinal images of the blood vessel lumen can also be
produced. Typically a pulsed Doppler scanner has 32 serial gates,
each representing flow in a 1 mm increment along the ultrasonic
beam, and the system operates at 5 MHz and is directionally-
sensitive. Furthermore, in appropriate anatomical situations, it
is possible to determine the orientation, lumen cross-sectional
area, and flow velocity profile, by means of pulsed-Doppler scanning, and thus to estimate blood flow volume.

5.5   Resolution in Doppler Systems

The lateral resolution of a Doppler system at any particular distance from the transducer depends on the effective width of the ultrasonic beam. This in turn depends on the beam profile, and the signal processing arrangements including the detector threshold level.

The range resolution of a continuous wave Doppler is, in effect, such that any detectable target gives a signal; the penetration is limited by attenuation. Pulsed Doppler systems have range resolution determined by the effective length of the ultrasonic pulse, and in principle the situation resembles that in a conventional pulse-echo system.

6   COMBINED PULSE-ECHO IMAGING AND DOPPLER MEASUREMENT

The combination of pulse-echo two-dimensional imaging of blood vessels (or of structures suspected of being blood vessels, or of the heart) with pulsed Doppler measurement of blood velocity in defined volume elements in the image is becoming established as a powerful technique. It may be expected to be further refined.

7   RELATIONSHIP OF ULTRASOUND TO OTHER IMAGING MODALITIES

Diagnostic imaging techniques should not be considered in isolation, since they each can contribute different clinical information. Traditional radiographic imaging is still used with photographic film for the bulk of investigations, although other detection methods, such as xeroradiography, are possible. Digital radiography will become important, especially in intravenous arteriography. Computed tomography is well-established for head investigations, but its role in body scanning remains to be defined. Radionuclide imaging demonstrates physiological function, and gamma cameras are widely used in abdominal and dynamic cardiac studies. Emission computed tomography leads to easy differentiation of anatomical structures, and the clinical potential of the use of short-lived cyclotron-produced radioisotopes is attractive although expensive. Ultrasonic imaging of soft-tissue structures is vital in obstetrics and in cardiology, and very important in abdominal and small-parts studies. Real-time scanning is both economical and informative. Doppler scanning of blood vessels promises to be a valuable method. Thermographic imaging, in which surface temperature is mapped, has a limited role. Nuclear magnetic resonance imaging of proton distributions and relaxation times is potentially important because it may give tissue characterisation, there is no scan plane restriction, and it seems to be safe.

The relationships of ultrasound to the other main contemporary imaging modalities are set out in Table 1. It is important to remember two key points. Firstly, ultrasound competes with the other techniques for the financial resources which make its

Imaging method	Hazard	Property imaged	Clinical specialities in which applicable
Ultrasound	Probably none	Density, elasticity, movement and flow	Obstetrics, cardiology, internal medicine, and all others excluding gas and bone
Radiography	+ to ++	X-ray attenuation	All but obstetrics
Computed tomography	++	X-ray attenuation	Neurology, all others excluding obstetrics
Radioisotopes	+ to ++	Physiological function	Neurology, internal medicine, cardiology, endocrinology and all others
Thermography	o	Surface temperature	Burns, vascular disease, surface tumours
Microwave imaging	Probably none	Dielectric properties	Not yet established
NMR imaging	Probably none	Proton and other nuclide properties	Potentially all

Table 1. Comparison of features of imaging modalities.

provision possible, and it is clinical relevance which should decide between the success or failure of any particular investigation. Secondly, rapid progress is being made in the development of every existing technology, and new ones are beginning to emerge, so the situation will certainly not remain static.

REFERENCES

1. Wells, P.N.T. *Biomedical Ultrasonics* (London: Academic Press, 1977).
2. Wells, P.N.T. "Absorption and dispersion of ultrasound in biological tissue." *Ultrasound in Medicine and Biology* 1 (1975) 369-376.
3. Robinson, D.E. and Knight, P.C. "Computer reconstruction techniques in compound scan pulse-echo imaging." *Ultrasonic Imaging* 3 (1981) 217-234.
4. Wells, P.N.T. and Halliwell, M. "Speckle in ultrasonic imaging." *Ultrasonics* 5 (1981) 225-229.
5. Wells, P.N.T. "Ultrasonic Doppler equipment." In: *Medical Physics of CT and Ultrasound*, ed. Fullerton, G.D. and Zagzebski, J.A. (New York: American Institute of Physics, 1980, 343-366).

214

NUCLEAR MAGNETIC RESONANCE (NMR) IMAGING: AN OVERVIEW

A. Everette James, Jr. 1)

Department of Medical Imaging & Radiological Sciences
Vanderbilt University School of Medicine
Nashville, Tennessee

The first nuclear magnetic resonance (NMR) experiments were performed about thirty-five years ago (1-3). NMR subsequently became a significant method for chemical analysis. The use of NMR for imaging purposes, however, was not realized until the first NMR zeugmatograms were produced by Lauterbur in 1972 (4). In past months, resolution on NMR studies has improved to the point that the images have sufficient anatomical information to rival those that are achieved by x-ray computed tomography (5-8). It has become apparent that NMR imaging can be utilized in clinical practice because of recent improvements in data acquisition time and spatial resolution (5,8).

Additionally, those signals utilized to produce NMR images also contain unique tissue contrast information reflecting chemical and structural composition. NMR may represent a diagnostic technique of greater potential than the new imaging developments in digital radiography, pulsed Doppler real-time ultrasound, positron emission tomography (PET), or computed x-ray tomography (CT). A schematic diagram for a total-body NMR imaging system is shown in Figure 1.

---

1. Additional authors are listed following the Acknowledgments of this chapter.

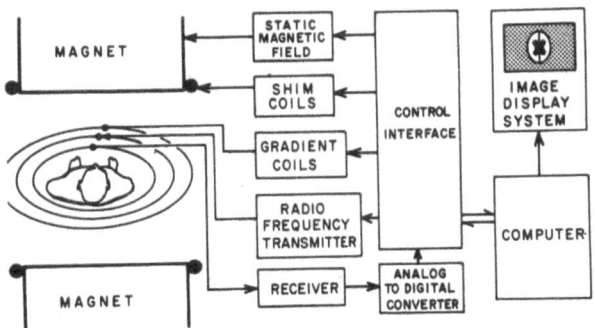

Figure 1. Schematic of an NMR image system. The aperture between the large resistive magnets is sufficient to accommodate the human torso. The gradient, RF and receiver coils are seen transversely. An image display system (IDS) is shown with a projected "brain scan" to illustrate the dual function of the imaging device.

THE NMR TECHNIQUE

Certain properties of atoms should be reviewed to place present developments in the technique in perspective. Nuclei of atoms with odd mass numbers have a spin which produces an associated magnetic field or moment. These nuclei essentially behave like tiny magnets. If placed in a static magnetic field, these nuclei will experience a force (torque) and will tend to align their axes in the direction of the field. This effect is similar to several tiny magnets that are placed in the field of a larger magnet. Some of these nuclei line up parallel to the magnetic field since it is the orientation of lowest inherent energy. Other nuclei will be aligned in an antiparallel direction corresponding to an excited state. The nuclei also exhibit a characteristic moment resembling that of a spinning top as it rotates in the gravitational field of the earth. This rotational movement is termed "precession" (Figure 2).

The frequency at which the spinning nuclei rotate about their axis is called the Larmor frequency, ω_0. The Larmor frequency is specifically determined by the magnetic field strength (B_0) and a constant, the gyromagnetic ratio (γ). The gyromagnetic ratio is a constant that is characteristic for each nuclear species. This relationship is expressed mathematically as:

$$\omega_0 = \gamma B_0. \tag{1}$$

The important point of this relationship is that the frequency is directly proportional to the magnetic field strength.

216

In NMR analysis, the nuclei to be studied are irradiated (energized) with an electromagnetic (radiofrequency) pulse of the same frequency as the Larmor frequency. Provided the RF is at exactly the same frequency as the characteristic precession frequency for the nuclei, energy absorption or resonance can occur. An observable RF signal will be produced when the excited nucleus returns to the ground state in a process called relaxation. The description of this process as <u>nuclear magnetic resonance</u> is derived by the process of matching the radiofrequency and the Larmor frequency.

When the RF pulse is at the Larmor frequency, the nuclei to be studied will absorb the interrogating energy. These nuclei will then change in their position relative to the applied magnetic field. The position alteration is directly related to the pulse duration. Following the interrogating (RF) pulse, these nuclei will possess surplus energy. Once the RF pulse has ceased, the nuclei will radiate to their surroundings this acquired energy as they assume their natural energy level and position. A complex signal is emitted which will die away at a characteristic rate. The nuclei thus "relax" to their original alignment in the magnetic field and, in the process, re-emit at the resonant frequency. The choice of exciting pulse duration and spacing are important to the imaging process.

Relaxation times are parameters that characterize the ability of nuclei to transfer their acquired energy to their immediate

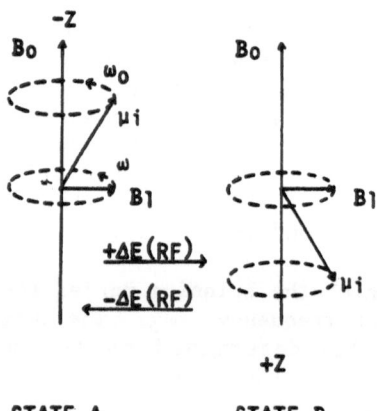

STATE A   STATE B

Figure 2. Precession of a magnetic moment, μ, and an angular velocity, ω, about a static magnetic field, B, in the Z direction is depicted. STATE A depicts the low energy state in which μ is oriented parallel to B_o. STATE B is the high energy state oriented opposed to B_o. The RF field (B_1) is applied at 90° with respect to B_o.

environment. The NMR signal diminishes exponentially with a characteristic decay (Free Induction Decay, FID). The re-emitted energy provides a signal that can be subsequently detected by receiver coils, measured, and subjected to analysis. The length of time required for relaxation is related to the nuclei of interest and their coupling to the general nuclear environment. The greater facility to pass energy to neighboring nuclei or their environment, the more rapidly those irradiated nuclei can return to their original state (relax).

The release of energy by an excited nucleus is called relaxation. Nuclei may relax by two processes. If this energy is transmitted into the environment, then the relaxation mechanism is called longitudinal or spin-lattice relaxation. Energy may also be exchanged by an excited nucleus transferring its energy to another nucleus in the ground state by a process called transverse or spin-spin relaxation. These relaxation mechanisms are expressed by their respective time constants: the longitudinal or spin-lattice relaxation time, T_1 and the transverse or spin-spin relaxation time, T_2.

T_1 represents the time required for the nuclei interrogated by the RF pulse to reach thermal equilibrium with the bulk material (the general nuclear environment). It may be detected by changing the direction of the net magnetic moment $180°$ (π RF pulse) and waiting a sufficient time interval (τ) (Figure 3A). The transverse relaxation time is a parameter used to characterize the effects of similar nuclei on those that produce the FID signal which is measured after RF interrogation. T_2 is related to the time required to dephase individual nuclear precessions and is manifested by linewidth broadening. The measurement of T_2 is illustrated in Figure 3B.

Another important parameter is the nuclear density (ρ) which is a major determinant in which nuclei can be used to produce an image. The nuclear density represents the relative number or, possibly more important, the concentration of nuclear spins. If a nucleus is not sufficiently abundant, it cannot be imaged because of insufficient signal strength.

One should regard nuclear density, T_1 and T_2 as parameters that characterize the nuclei to be analyzed and the environment in which these nuclei exist. The NMR signal, depending upon the pulsing and detection sequence, may provide information about nuclear density, T_1 and T_2 measurements or ratios and combinations of these parameters. A characteristic feature of NMR is that the information provided by the study can be controlled from the selection of the NMR experimental design. Although this is a virtue of great potential, it does make NMR a rather complex method of inquiry.

218

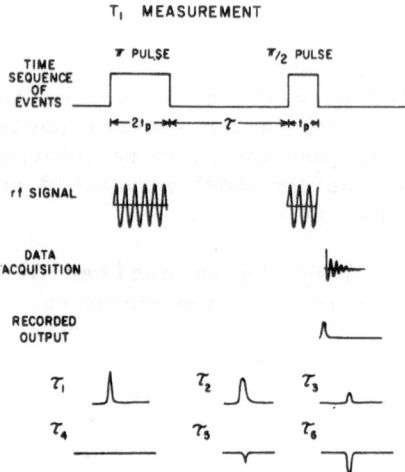

Figure 3A. A schematic description of a technique for measuring T_1. A trace of the RF signal is compared with the data as acquired.

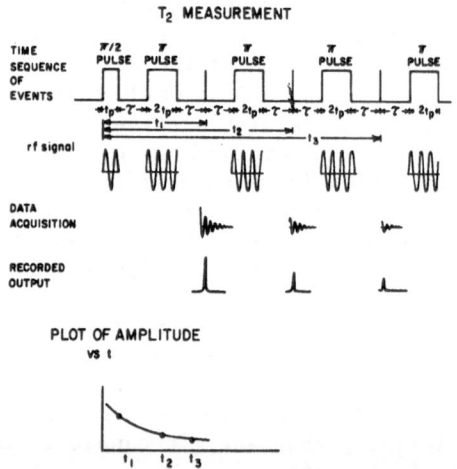

Figure 3B. A schematic description of a technique for measuring T_2. An amplitude plot demonstrates the relation to time.

In the classic chemical NMR experiment there is no spatial information because of the circumstance that all areas of the sample are subjected to the same magnetic field and have the same resonant frequency. Spatial information has been achieved with NMR imaging techniques by a number of different mechanisms and approaches, each with certain virtues and limitations (5,9-13).

NMR IMAGING

The engineering of NMR devices suitable to create images of the distribution of certain nuclei (mainly protons) in the human body has presented a rather formidable challenge. Acquiring accurate information in the spatial domain may be achieved by a number of techniques. The most common technique has been the employment of a field gradient. This means that there will be a change in the magnetic field strength as one proceeds in a certain direction. If a field gradient is applied to a static magnetic field so that there is a linear increase or decrease of the field that is spatially dependent, the nuclei located at different areas in the field will experience slightly weaker or stronger fields than similar nuclei located elsewhere and will thus resonate at a slightly different frequency. When the RF pulse is swept through the area to be imaged, the energy absorbed and signal emitted will be related in a known fashion to the imposed field gradient. Nuclei in a weaker area will absorb and re-emit the RF energy at a lower frequency than the emissions from nuclei in the area of the stronger field gradient. In this manner, information is obtained regarding the position of the signal from these frequency differences. Therefore, spatial determinations can be made. Because determination of spatial definition results from the coupling of radiofrequency radiation and magnetic fields, the technique has been described as "zeugmatography," translating from Greek and following the concept of "joining together to form a picture" (12).

Gradients can be applied at fixed angles with the static field (B_o) or may be fixed at an optimum orientation with the static field and another gradient swept electronically through the area to be imaged. This flexibility and potential for rapid data acquisition should prove significant in clinical application. These devices should have little mechanical constraint in their use.

Using these techniques, it then becomes possible to produce an image of either the distribution of relaxation times (T_1, T_2) or the nuclear density or some combination of these parameters. The linear magnetic field gradients combine vectorally; thus, any desired gradient may be created by adjusting the electrical current in the individual coils (gradient coils) that encircle the object to be studied. With this arrangement, linear gradients can be established in the desired (x,y or z) directions to determine the imaging plane without mechanical motion of the apparatus or patient. The multi-planar imaging capability of NMR is of great clinical significance. In fact, the ability to view an area from a number of different orientations may result in anatomical detail from the composite NMR images that contains greater useful information than x-ray computed tomography.

For water and simple fluids, T_1 and T_2 are approximately 5 seconds and are considered to be equal. For soft tissues and solids, T_2 is appreciably shorter than T_1; a difference in relaxation times that can be advantageously used in NMR imaging of biological tissues. The relaxation time differences will allow creation of an image with different appearance of the various tissue composition and structures of the human body, much as x-ray attenuation is employed to reflect density differences in computed tomography. One should recall, however, that attenuation of radiation is a property that reflects little of the body composition and that in NMR the signals reflect atomic and chemical information at the cellular level. Thus, NMR images potentially represent a much more fundamental and important expression of health and disease than a property such as energy attenuation.

The nucleus most commonly studied in nuclear magnetic resonance imaging is hydrogen (^{1}H, the proton), as we have noted. Progress is being made in the use of surface coils for sensitive signal detection of other nuclei. It is doubtful, however, that images generated from the NMR signals of nuclei other than ^{1}H will be utilized clinically in the near future. However, other nuclei have a much lower signal and/or have a lower biological abundance than ^{1}H, making imaging with these nuclei extremely difficult.

The use of field gradients and the technique of reconstruction from projections is the most commonly employed method for NMR imaging and has been used by many laboratories following the initial activity in this area in the mid 1970's (4). The signal is first obtained by the field gradient method and a frequency analysis is performed using the Fourier transform which will then provide the necessary spatial information. In this manner, a profile is generated which represents a projection in a single dimension of the proton distribution in the tissue to be analyzed. If the magnetic field gradient is then rotated through a series of angles and at each location a projection is obtained, then by using filtered back projection one can reconstruct an image of the object. The images created in this fashion will reflect the intensity distribution of the proton NMR signal in the specific location. Thus, the static field spatial dependence, as a result of the application of gradients, will allow the measurements to be be used to create images of proton distribution and relaxation times. Whether the images are of T_1, T_2 or a combination of parameters is at the election of the individuals performing the NMR experiment.

The NMR imaging technique of reconstruction by filtered back projections has been utilized by the majority of groups in the field (12,14,15). A number of scanning modes besides projection reconstruction, however, are possible with NMR. One technique confines the effective NMR response to a single point which can be moved through the magnetic field or the patient can be moved through the point (11,16). This sensitive point technique can be extended to include an entire line of points which can be scanned simultaneously. Several methods have extended this technique to collect data points within an entire plane without the use of projection reconstruction.

Images of single slices can be stacked to build a complete three-dimensional array similar to methods currently used in CT. With NMR, however, the complete three-dimensional array can be scanned simultaneously. This technique represents the most efficient use of the NMR signal and allows the extraction of multiple imaging planes from the data without repeating the scan.

As noted, the unique feature of NMR imaging when compared with conventional radiographic techniques is that experimental design can significantly change the character of the data acquired. The choices of the experiment related to measuring T_1, T_2, and proton density will also change the appearance of the images. Although this complexity may prove to be a constraint in user understanding, it provides an opportunity to acquire image contrast in a totally unique manner.

Certain physical limitations associated with the characteristics of the magnet employed, RF coil configuration, and patient gantry design will determine what type of information can be derived from the NMR experiments. The image contrast depends upon the NMR parameters chosen for the image. In proton imaging, image contrast will clearly delineate gray and white matter which is not differentiated nearly so well on CT or radionuclide brain scans (Figure 4). The apparent differences in gray and white matter appearance are thought to be due to the water and lipid content of the various components of the neurophil. Tomographic proton images may also be generated in multiple orthographic or oblique angles (Figure 5).

Selection of the magnet to be used for the static field is an important consideration in the design of an NMR imaging device. Iron-core magnets, in general, do not have the necessary pole gap to accommodate the human torso. The weight of such a magnet will also produce certain problems in room construction and location in the health care facility. Air-core and superconducting magnets can be made with a sufficient aperture for patient use, but considerations of expense and requirements of field uniformity may dictate the choice of instrumentation. Without excessive shimming

222

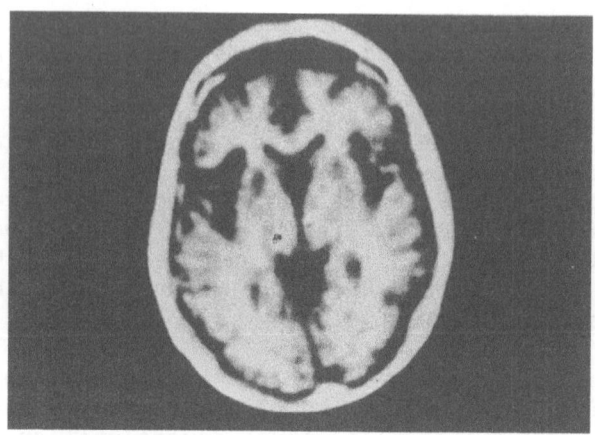

Figure 4. **Transverse NMR brain scan. Note** gray and white matter contrast and anatomical differentiation. (Courtesy of John Gore, Medical Physics Department, Hammersmith Hospital, London, England.) This image was recorded in the first quarter of 1981 and begins to approach the anatomical depiction of those achieved by CT. The soft tissue contrast is believed to be a result of differences in water and lipid content in various constituents of the neurophil.

procedures, a practical field uniformity with variance of approximately 1 part in 10^4 can be achieved with air-core magnets. Field non-uniformity, however, can be partially compensated by using a steep field gradient. The effect of field non-uniformity can also be diminished by employing a high RF power for the interrogating pulse. These high RF power requirements are somewhat difficult to achieve but may be necessary to provide the spatial information needed in clinical use.

Usually, the air-core NMR units that have been used in the initial clinical trials have a modified Helmholtz configuration. The magnet consists of two large central coils with two coils of smaller diameter outside of the larger ones, connected in series. This instrument design results in an open form of construction without the presence of iron. Thus, the apparatus is lighter in weight due to the absence of the iron but is not as efficient in magnetic field generation. This requires greater radiofrequency input to produce the magnetic field. The larger space between the central coils has several advantages. Of fundamental importance is accommodation of the human body as well as space for the subsidiary gradient systems and the RF coil. With the air-core systems, iron objects nearby can degrade magnetic field homogeneity. This circumstance may require construction of some type of shield. These air-core magnets have a low initial cost in comparison with the superconducting magnets. Operating costs,

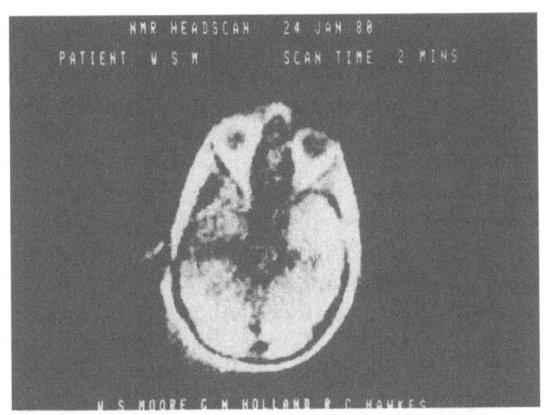

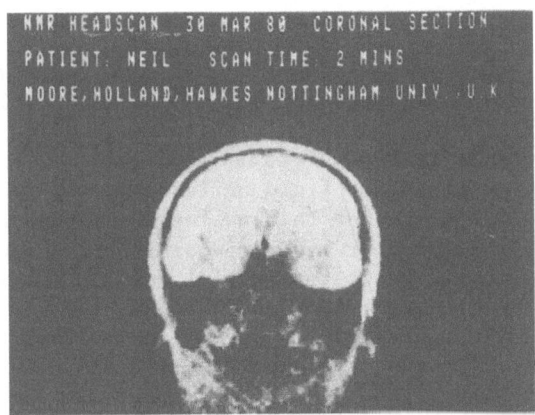

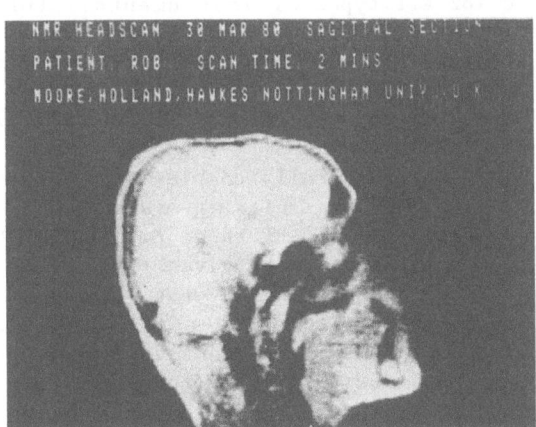

Figure 5. Tomographic NMR images. (A) Transverse view, (B) Coronal view, (C) Sagittal view. (Courtesy of G. Neil Holland, Department of Physics, University of Nottingham, Nottingham, England.) The ability to select and change imaging planes electronically without patient or instrument movement is a significant feature for clinical practice.

however, may be considerable with air-core magnets because of the much greater demand for electrical power and the use of large volumes of water for magnet cooling.

Superconducting magnets offer the advantage of improved magnetic field homogeneity and inherent stability. These magnets are able to provide fields with a uniformity of 1 part in 10^6 when fully shimmed. Superconducting magnets require some type of cooling (usually liquid helium) with attendant requirements for housing and room construction. The cost of a superconducting magnet, at present, is several hundred thousand dollars. Again, operational costs may provide some savings to offset the large initial investment when compared with other types of magnets.

There is no present agreement as to which magnet configuration will eventually become the most clinically appropriate design. This decision will depend greatly upon the method chosen for image generation, information anticipated from the study, and the patient population in a particular hospital. Most investigators agree that field uniformity is, in general, a desirable feature; but whether this uniformity should be 1 part in 10^4 or some lesser or greater level of tolerance remains to be determined. The requirements for spatial resolution shown to be necessary during clinical trials will be a very important determinant of instrument requirements. The aperture between the magnets and RF coils should be approximately 40 cm or larger to accommodate the human torso. The requirement for aperture size does not mean that there exists magnetic field uniformity over the entire 40 cm disc for all types of instruments. For example, a technique that samples at a designated point will require uniformity and stability in the location that is being sampled. Speed of data acquisition must be accommodated within the constraints of physiological motion and patient acceptance.

The human body is structurally complex and inhomogeneous. It behaves as a complex conducting mass in response to electromagnetic radiation in the RF range employed in NMR imaging (17-19). The effect of tissue depth gives rise to the phenomenon of attenuation of the interrogating RF wave. The signals returned to the receiver coils experience phase shift of the RF field as they pass through body tissues; analogous in some respects to the phenomenon of "beam hardening" in x-ray computed tomography. The RF interrogating pulse in an NMR experiment has certain strength requirements if one wishes to achieve appropriate penetration into tissue at depth. Preliminary calculations and clinical experience suggest that the RF pulse should be kept below approximately 20 MHz for NMR intracerebral studies and approximately 10 MHz for abdominal imaging. These estimated guidelines are preliminary and clinical use may obligate the imaging specialists to other limits of frequencies. Obviously, this is an area where additional data will be of great significance. We would believe that activity in this area will increase markedly in the next several years.

Medical trials will be necessary to document which particular NMR experiments record those parameters (ρ, T_1, T_2), ratios, or combinations that provide meaningful data in pathophysiological rather than anatomical terms. Certain investigations have demonstrated that specific parameter NMR images will provide a particular type of tissue discrimination. This can be observed in certain NMR images, especially those intracranial studies which demonstrate excellent gray and white matter differentiation. One would anticipate that this ability would be very important in examining the tissues of various "solid" organs, such as the liver and pancreas. To express the tissue discrimination in clinically meaningful terms regarding health and disease states, however, awaits correlation with known medical abnormalities. NMR signals from fluids, soft tissue, and fat are stronger than those from bone. The signals from human muscle and tendons have been shown to be of intermediate strength. Since achieving a "tissue signature" from transmission or reflected ultrasound waves and x-ray computed tomographic numbers have been only partially successful, this form of tissue characterization by NMR has profound clinical implications. Bone and air pose little difficulty for NMR imaging as opposed to ultrasound. The most peripheral signal in NMR images will be from the skin. Familiarity with the normal response will require the same type of orientation and learning process as was experienced with x-ray computed tomography in the early to mid 1970's. We would anticipate that these images will be compared with plain and contrast conventional radiographic studies, nuclear medicine radionuclide images, x-ray computed tomographic images and those acquired by ultrasound.

The anatomical resolution achieved by NMR images is dependent upon a multitude of factors. As an example, if the T_2 value is long, then the field gradient should be large enough to insure that in the static field (B_0), the difference between data points will exceed the intrinsic resonance width. In liquids, T_2 is sufficiently long but NMR imaging of soft tissues poses more rigid requirements in creating spatial data. The resolution of discrete points of an NMR image is related to the matrix size of the picture elements. The pixel size will determine the limit of resolution. Voluntary patient movement, physiological motion, as well as physical parameters such as non-linearity of field gradient, phase errors, and non-uniformity of either the RF pulse or B_0 magnetic field will tend to degrade resolution in NMR images. Methods to overcome or compensate for these constraints are varied. The ability to create images conveniently in many different planes without either patient or mechanical movement of the instrument offers a significant advantage for NMR imaging.

The information provided by NMR experiments is fundamentally different from attenuation of x-ray energy as in computed tomography, radiopharmaceutical localization as in positron emission, reflection of high frequency sound waves and conventional nuclear medicine studies. The fact that the NMR signal may represent a composite of nuclear density, the effect of like nuclei upon those being specifically studied (T_2) and the influence of the general nuclear environment (T_1) should be emphasized and appreciated. The complexity of NMR investigation requires understanding by the user and investigator of the methods employed to generate the image. This will be especially important initially when the clinical efficacy of this method is being established.

Traditionally, states of health and disease have been regarded in patho-anatomical terms. Classic studies in pathology, histology, and anatomy have provided guidelines to determine abnormal and normal states of body tissues. Analysis using NMR techniques will allow investigation of normal and abnormal in chemical/physiological terms. The concept that chemical and physiological alterations precede changes in histology or anatomy makes NMR potentially a sensitive diagnostic method to detect disease in very early stages.

The relaxation times of malignant tissues generally differ significantly from those parameters in normal human tissues of the same histologic type (16,20,21). Results to date have generally indicated that malignant tissues tend to have longer relaxation times than normal tissue. Hopefully, NMR images will utilize the variation in T_1 to produce images of high contrast between normal and malignant tissue.

Analysis of disease states by correlating the pathophysiology with the metabolic status as an expression of chemical alteration is a major area where NMR imaging offers promise. These considerations are particularly important for conditions involving compromised blood flow, diminished oxygenation, and alterations in water content of tissues. NMR imaging may be improved by increasing the concentration of other paramagnetic atoms and not just protons. This would be the equivalent of "contrast" injection. NMR studies using ^{31}P determinations may allow specific evaluation of the location and extent of muscle injury and even document the time course of metabolic impairment. This type of inquiry offers a unique method to assess directly and noninvasively the basic metabolic functions at the site of organ or structure injury (22). NMR may afford a method of diagnostic analysis to determine the efficacy of therapy or to document the presence of irreversible tissue damage.

Blood flow has been imaged and measured by several groups using NMR techniques (23). Comparing this information with analysis of metabolic function in the framework of an anatomical image offers a myriad of possibilities for diagnostic inquiry in the future.

NMR instrumentation offers certain advantages over conventional imaging modalities. Several of these advantages include: multi-planar imaging capability, no ionizing radiation, no moving parts, flow measurement, greater soft tissue contrast, and potentially greater pathophysiologic significance. Positron emission tomography (PET) systems will require the proximity of a cyclotron. Therefore, PET is expensive and more complex to perform clinically. The ability to study multiple planes in x-ray computed tomography (CT) requires either reconstruction and integration of multiple planes or a combination of instrument and patient reorientation. CT also involves the use of moving parts which lead to a greater chance of mechanical failure and increased maintenance expense.

Data acquisition time, at present, poses somewhat of a problem with NMR imaging. At present, the standard computed tomographic images (under 5 seconds) are acquired in a more timely fashion than NMR images (2-3 minutes). These accommodations will necessarily be translated into realistic compromises and efficacy judgements in the initial clinical trials. Because the contrast information is so unique and the facility to acquire data in several orientations, these resolution and time constraints may not be as significant in clinical practice. Resource commitments and distribution guidelines for NMR devices will probably follow the x-ray computed tomography prototype.

NMR will undoubtedly be compared with other modalities in medical imaging and comparisons and correlations will be the subject of intense future investigation. To consider NMR as merely an anatomical imaging technique represents failure to appreciate the true potential of this methodology. The value of this type of chemical analysis will provide fundamental measurements of disease processes at the cellular level. The challenge will be for the users to maximize these advantages, i.e., superb anatomical detail and biochemical characterization, which are not present together in other types of investigative techniques (24,25).

ACKNOWLEDGMENTS

Drs. William Moore and Robert Hawkes at the University of Nottingham provided many of the insights in this communication, as did the participants of the Vanderbilt University Symposium on NMR

Imaging (1980) (24,25). The encouragement of Dean John Chapman and Vice President Roscoe Robinson to continue work in the field of NMR has been of supportive significance. The support of the Vanderbilt Center for Medical Imaging Research (CMIR) was quite helpful. We wish to dedicate this effort to the late M. D. Ingram, the Executive Director of CMIR.

AUTHORS (continued from title page)

Ronald R. Price
Robert Stewart
C. Leon Partain

Department of Medical Imaging and Radiological Sciences
Vanderbilt University School of Medicine
Nashville, Tennessee

Stephen Harms

Department of Radiology
State University of New York, Stoneybrook
        and
University of Arkansas, Little Rock

with the assistance of:

John Gore

Department of Medical Physics
Royal Postgraduate Medical School
Hammersmith Hospital, London, England

G. Neil Holland

Department of Physics
University of Nottingham
Nottingham, England

F. David Rollo
James A. Patton
Jon J. Erickson

Department of Medical Imaging and Radiological Sciences
Vanderbilt University School of Medicine
Nashville, Tennessee

REFERENCES

1. Bloch, F. Physics Review 70 (1946) 460.
2. Bloch, F. Physics Review 70 (1946) 474.
3. Purcell, E.M., Torres, H.C. and R.V. Pound. Physics Review 69 (1946).
4. Lauterbur, P.C. "Image formation by induced local interactions: Examples of employing nuclear magnetic resonance." Nature 242 (1973) 190-191.
5. Moore, W.S. and G.N. Holland. "The NMR CAT scanner – a new look at the brain." Journal of Computer Assisted Tomography 4 (1980) 1-7.
6. Holland, G.N., Hawkes, R.C. and W.S. Moore. "Nuclear magnetic resonance tomography of the brain: Coronal and sagittal sections." Journal of Computer Assisted Tomography 4 (1980) 429-433.
7. Mallard, J., Hutchison, J.M.S., Edelstein, W., Ling, R. and M. Foster. "Imaging by nuclear magnetic resonance and its bio-medical implications." Journal of Biomedical Engineering 1 (1979) 153-160.
8. Hawkes, R.C., Holland, G.N., Moore, W.S. and B.S. Worthington. "Nuclear magnetic resonance tomography of the brain: A preliminary clinical assessment with demonstration of pathology." Journal of Computer Assisted Tomography 4 (1980) 577-586.
9. Crooks, L.E., Grover, T.P., Kaufman, L., et al. "Tomographic imaging with nuclear magnetic resonance." Investigative Radiology 13 (1978) 63.
10. Mansfield,P. and A.A. Maudsley. "Medical imaging by NMR." British Journal of Radiology 50 (1977) 188-194.
11. Damadian, R. "Field-focussing nuclear magnetic resonance (FONAR) and the formation of chemical scans in man." Philosophical Transactions of the Royal Society London (1980).
12. Lauterbur, P.C. and C.M. Lai. "Zeugmatography reconstruction from projections." IEEE Transactions on Nuclear Science 27 (1980) 1227-1231.
13. Hinshaw, W.S., Andrew, E.R., Bottomley, P.A., et al. "Display of cross-sectional anatomy by nuclear magnetic resonance imaging." British Journal of Radiology 51 (1978) 273-280.
14. Shepp, L.A. "Computerized tomography and nuclear magnetic resonance." Journal of Computer Assisted Tomography 4 (1980) 94-107.
15. Brooks, R.A. and G. DiChiro. "Theory of image reconstruction in computed tomography." Radiology 117 (1975) 561-572.
16. Damadian, R. "Tumor detection by nuclear magnetic resonance." Science 171 (1971) 1151-1153.
17. Barnothy, M.F., ed. Biological Effects of Magnetic Fields, vol. 2 (New York: Plenum Press, 1969).

230

18. Budinger, T.F. "Thresholds for physiological effects due to RF and magnetic fields used in NMR imaging." IEEE Transactions on Nuclear Science 26 (1979) 2821-2825.

19. National Radiological Protection Board. "Exposure to nuclear magnetic resonance clinical imaging." (1980) (available from The Secretary, NRPB, Harwell, Oxon. OX11 ORQ, United Kingdom).

20. Hollis, D.P., Economon, J.S., Parks, J.C., et al. "Nuclear magnetic resonance studies of several experimental and human malignant tumors." Cancer Research 33 (1973) 2156-2160.

21. Mansfield, P., Morris, P.G. and R. Ordidge. "Carcinoma of the breast imaged by nuclear magnetic resonance (NMR)." British Journal of Radiology 52 (1979) 242-243.

22. Hollis, D.P., Nunnally, R.L., Taylor, G.J., et al. "Phosphorus nuclear magnetic resonance studies of heart physiology." Journal of Magnetic Resonance 29 (1978) 319-330.

23. Singer, J.R. "Blood flow measurements by NMR of the intact body." IEEE Transactions on Nuclear Science 27 (1980) 1245-1249.

24. Partain, C.L, Price, R.R., Rollo, F.D. and A.E. James, Jr. Nuclear Magnetic Resonance (NMR) Imaging (Philadelphia: W.B. Saunders, Co., in press).

25. James, A.E., Jr. and C.L. Partain, eds. "Proceedings: Vanderbilt University NMR Imaging Symposium, Oct. 1980." Journal of Computer Assisted Tomography 5 (1980) 285-305.

COMPUTERIZED TRANSMISSION TOMOGRAPHY:
CT AND DIGITAL VOLUME SCANNING

B. Pullan

University of Manchester
Department of Medical Biophysics

INTRODUCTION

The formation of radiographic images results from the interaction of X-ray beams with the tissue of a patient. The image which results is a representation of the distribution of interaction within the body. The degree of interaction can be determined by measuring and recording either the number of photons which are transmitted through a body or alternatively the distribution of scattered photons (1). In this paper only those methods which rely on transmission measurements will be considered. It will be shown that all high efficiency methods produce data with a very wide dynamic range which is difficult to transmit into the eye and brain of an observer. Computer tomography represents one solution to the problem and can be regarded as a method for compressing the dynamic range of relevant data. Other solutions are probably possible and the construction of versatile high efficiency X-ray systems which give most of the advantages of current C.T. systems should be possible. The basic arguments which lead to this conclusion will now be developed.

THE BASIC RADIOGRAPHIC PROCESS

X-ray sources with sufficient output for practical diagnostic radiology produce a broad spread of X-ray energies. If in the range of energies E to E + dE there are $N_o(E)dE$ photons in a beam entering an object as shown in Figure 1, the number of photons of energy E which will emerge unscattered will be

232

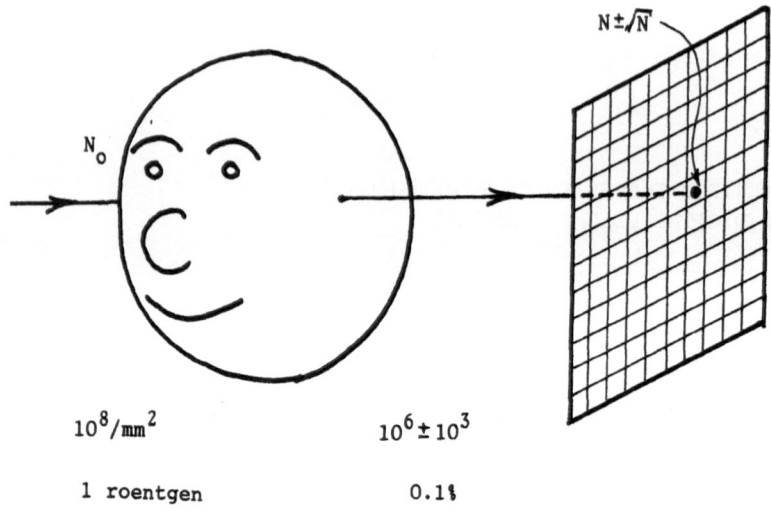

$10^8/\text{mm}^2$ $10^6 \pm 10^3$

1 roentgen   0.1%

Figure 1. An elemental beam traversing a head showing that the uncertainty in the numbers of photons transmitted is 0.1% for 1 roentogen exposure.

$$N(E) = N_O(E)e^{-\sigma(E)x} \tag{1}$$

Where x gm/cm^2 is the thickness traversed by the photons and $\sigma(E)$ is the mass attenuation coefficient at the energy E.

The total number of photons to emerge will be

$$N = \int_0^{Emax} N(E)\,dE \tag{2}$$

$$N = \int_0^{Emax} N_O(E)e^{-\sigma(E)x}\,dE$$

On the assumption that there is an effective energy $\bar{E}$ for the photons

$$N = N_O e^{-\sigma x} \tag{3}$$

Where N_o is the total number of photons entering the object, N is the total number to emerge unscattered and σ is the mass attenuation coefficient at the effective energy $\bar{E}$. The distribution of N for a particular set of beams which pass through an object from the source is recorded either directly as a radiograph on film or measured and stored for subsequent processing or display as a computed tomogram or digital radiograph. In all cases the process limiting the extent to which fine detail or small contrasts in tissue density can be visualised are basically the same.

The radiation exposure to the object at a particular X-ray energy is proportional to the number of incident photons per unit area. The ability to detect small changes in emergent photon flux, and therefore tissue composition and density, is limited by statistical fluctuations.

The variance in N can be shown to be

$$Var\ (N) = N(1 - N/N_o) \tag{4}$$

In the case where $N/N_o \ll 1$, Var (N)=N and the standard deviation of N is $\sqrt{N}$.

It is instructive to look at the relative size of these fluctuations in a radiographic system when the exposure to an object about 20 gm/cm^2 thick is one roentgen. Figure 1 shows a small elemental beam of radiation traversing a patient's head and being detected either by one element in an array of detectors or a small area of a film or film screen combination. If it is assumed that the detector element measures 1mm x 1mm and that the X-ray focus to patient distance is large, then at 1 roentgen exposure and at an effective energy of 60 Kev of the order of 10^8 photons will be incident upon each 1mm x 1mm element of the patient. Of these approximately 10^6 will emerge unscattered. The fluctuation or standard deviation will be $\sqrt{10^6}$ or 10^3. The relative uncertainty is therefore only 1 in 10^3 for an exposure of 1 roentgen, consequently changes in X-ray flux of the order of 0.1% should be detectable at 1 roentgen exposure.

This implies that at acceptable doses the dynamic range of the information carried in the radiation emerging from a patient is very wide and presents a significant display problem. This is illustrated in Figure 2 where the flux recorded in one line of elements is plotted. To make optimal use of the recorded information the contrast range has to be expanded so that the eye can just discern statistically seperable levels. With a good display

234

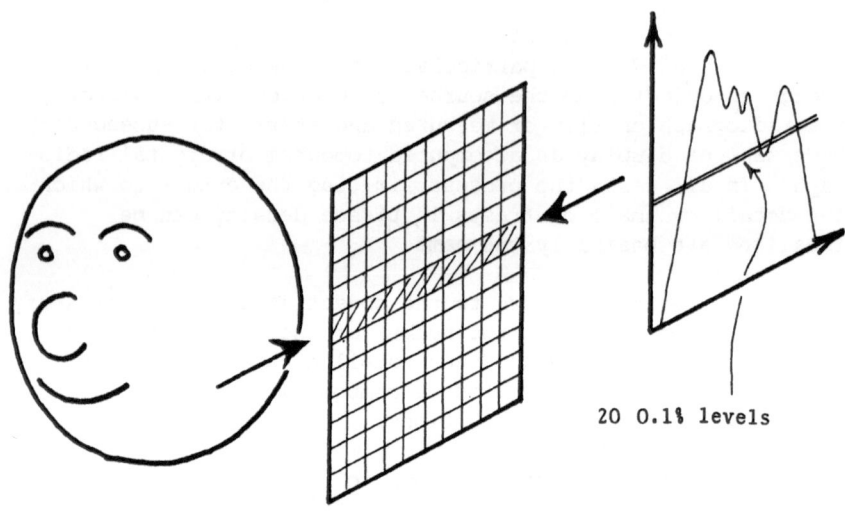

20 0.1% levels

Figure 2.   Only a small part of the dynamic range of
            radiographic data can be displayed directly.

the eye can just about discern 20 levels of illumination so that
as illustrated in Figure 2, only a very small part of the dynamic
range of the available data can be transmitted to the brain of the
observer. In any practical radiographic system which is to be
capable of the density resolution possible at 1 roentgen
exposure some means of dynamic range compression is required to
allow visual interpretation of the data recorded by the detectors.

DYNAMIC RANGE COMPRESSION

Introduction

     Computed tomography can be thought of as one means of
achieving the dynamic range compression required. The method
of computed tomography makes a series of measurements of X-ray
transmission through a slice of tissue as shown in Figure 3.
From these measurements the distribution of X-ray attenuation in
the cross section is calculated and displayed (2), (3). This is
equivalent to a plane radiograph of a slice of uniform thickness
taken from the patient as shown in Figure 4. Because the brain
is relatively uniform in attenuation the contrast of the display
can be increased so that changes of the order of 1 part in 1000
can be visualised whilst keeping the whole brain within the 20
display levels which the eye can perceive. The bone of the skull

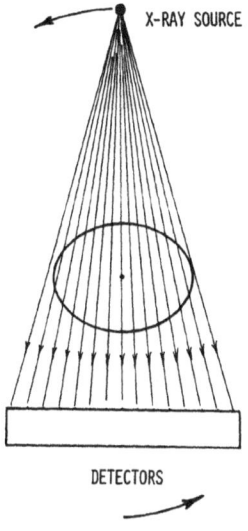

Figure 3.   The basic arrangement of one type of CT scanner
showing the method of making a large number of
transmission measurements through a slice of tissue.

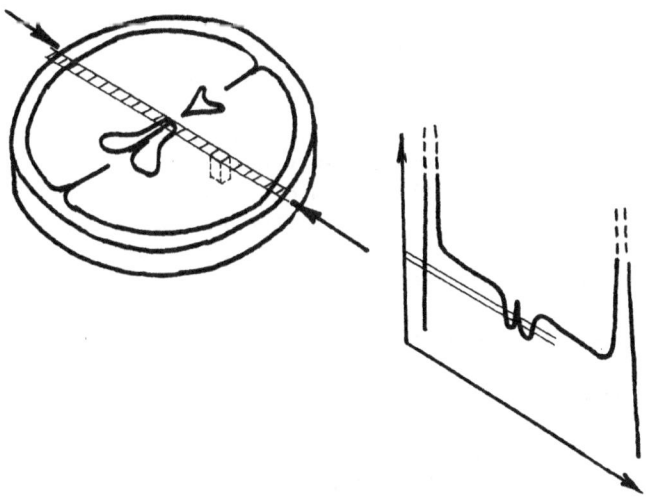

Figure 4.   The dynamic range of data in regions of interest is
compressed by using C.T. to synthesise a radiograph
of a slice of uniform thickness.

is of course well outside this range but because it is placed
around the edge of the brain it does not affect the visualisation
of small changes in the brain.

As well as being a means of contracting the dynamic range
of data the production of a picture of a slice has the further
advantage that, in the case of complicated objects, overlying
structures which would normally confuse the observer are removed.
For simple objects such as the brain the reduction of the dynamic
range of relevant data is however an important reason for the
success of computed tomography.

There are a number of alternative approaches to the problem
of dynamic range compression. The first of them is illustrated
in Figure 5 which shows one line of data from a radiograph where
the range of data is compressed by only displaying edges. The
resulting image or radiograph would look like a xerogram but if the
edge extraction is done by image processing in a computer there
is much more control over the edge detection and enhancement process
and in addition the original image is still available for subsequent
processing. Little work has been done on this approach but it is
worthy of further investigation where relevant information lies
in edges or sharp features.

An alternative approach is illustrated in Figure 6 where a
change has been made which results in small but meaningful
differences between two radiographs taken under different conditions.
Subtraction of the two radiographs leads to data with a low dynamic
range which can easily be displayed and perceived by the eye and
brain. Two procedures have been proposed by which meaningful
changes can be brought about. (4), (5), (6). Macovski (4) has
proposed a method in which X-ray energy changes produce the necessary differences either with or without the use of contrast media.
Ovitt, Capp et al (5) and also Kruger, Mistretta et al (6) have
demonstrated subtraction of radiographs taken before and after
intraverous contrast infusions.

In the limiting case in which all the photons which emerge
from the patient are recorded and no significant noise is added
by the recording system the above methods are capable of a high
sensitivity to contrast media. It will be shown later that 1mm
diameter vessels should theoretically be visualisable by a high
efficiency recording and subtraction method with a contrast
concentration of only 2 mg/ml at an exposure of 1 roentgen.
Animal experiments show that concentrations of upto 20 mg/ml can
be achieved by intravenous rather than intra-arterial injectons

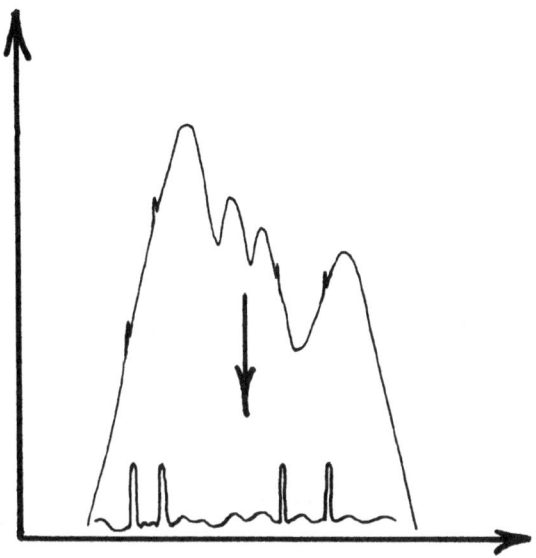

Figure 5. Dynamic range contraction by edge enhancement.

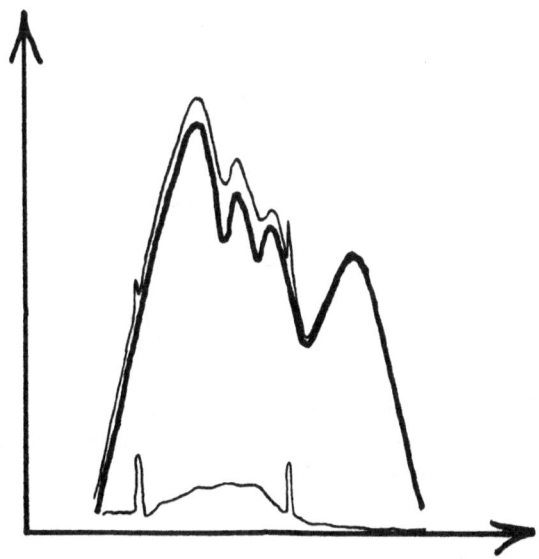

Figure 6. Dynamic range contraction by subtraction.

Dynamic Range Contraction by Subtraction

Consider two beams of radiation of energy E and geometric cross section a x a as shown in Figure 7. One beam traverses tissue of thickness x gm/cm^2 and mass attenuation coefficient $\sigma(E)$. The other beam traverses a similar piece of tissue but containing an additional thickness x_a gm/cm^2 of a material of mass attenuation coefficient $\sigma_a(E)$. This additional thickness being contrast medium in a blood vessel or organ.

If N_o photons enter the tissue the number of photons N_1 emerging unscattered from tissue alone is

$$N_1 = N_o e^{-\sigma(E)x} \tag{5}$$

If an equal number of photons enters the tissue to which contrast medium has been added, the number of photons emerging unscattered is

$$N_2 = N_o e^{-\sigma(E)x} e^{-\sigma_a(E)x_a} \tag{6}$$

The probability of detecting a difference in the number of emergent photons in the above two cases and thus visualising the difference as a vessel or region of relatively high contrast concentration is related to the difference between N_1 and N_2 divided by the uncertainty in this difference, the signal to noise ratio S/N. This can be defined as follows

$$S/N = \frac{N_1 - N_2}{\sqrt{N_1 + N_2}}$$

Substituting for N_1 and N_2 from (5) and (6) and assuming that $x_a \sigma_a \ll 1$

$$S/N = \sqrt{\frac{N_o e^{-\sigma(E)x}}{2}} \, (\sigma_a(E)x_a) \tag{7}$$

In practice it is desirable to collect radiographic data under conditions such that the maximum signal to noise ratio is obtained with the minimum radiation exposure.

The exposure $R = \dfrac{N_o}{a^2 K(E)}$ $\qquad\qquad$ (8)

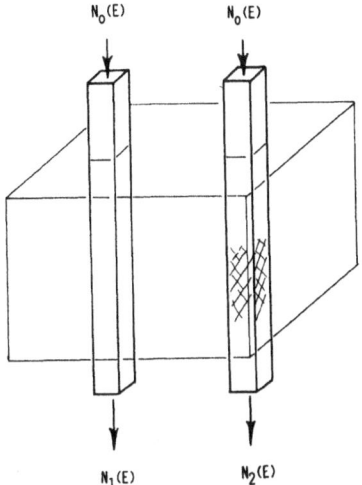

Figure 7. Volume of tissue traversed by two beams, one through
tissue alone and the other through a region containing
added contrast medium.

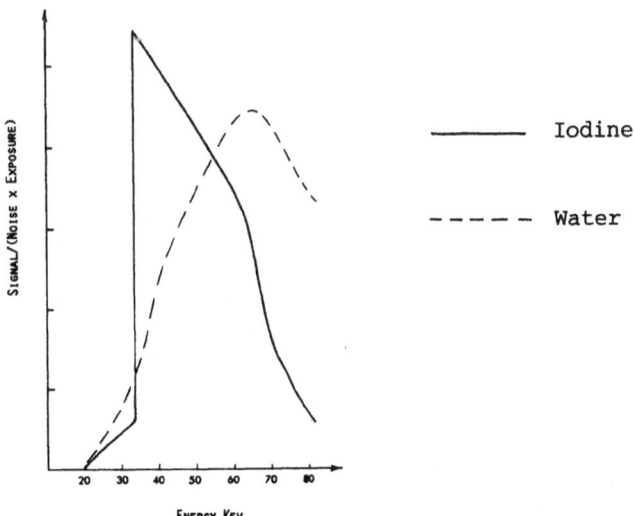

Figure 8. Variation of signal to noise ratio per roentgen exposure
with X-ray energy.

Table 1

Energy Kev	A(E) Iodine 1 mg/cm^2	Water 50 mg/cm^2	B(E)	(S/N)/R Iodine	Water
30	8.98 x 10^{-3}	16.0 x 10^{-3}	5.12	0.046	0.08
40	23.5 x 10^{-3}	11.5 x 10^{-3}	21.2	0.50	0.24
50	12.7 x 10^{-3}	10.5 x 10^{-3}	33.5	0.43	0.35
60	7.70 x 10^{-3}	9.5 x 10^{-3}	45.6	0.35	0.43
80	3.49 x 10^{-3}	9.0 x 10^{-3}	47.1	0.16	0.42
100	1.91 x 10^{-3}	8.5 x 10^{-3}	40.7	0.05	0.35

where K(E) is the number of photons per roentgen.

The signal to noise ratio per unit exposure can be calculated
from (7) and (8) and is

$$(S/N)/R = \left[\sigma_a(E) x_a \right]\left[K(E) \sqrt{e^{-\sigma(E)x}} \right] a^2 / \sqrt{2N_o} \qquad (9)$$

$$= A(E) B(E) \quad a^2 / \sqrt{2N_o} \qquad (10)$$

where A(E) and B(E) are the first and second bracketed terms in
equation (9). Values of A(E), B(E) and (S/N)/R are given in
Table 1 and are plotted in Figure 8 for the addition of 1 mg/cm^2
of iodine and also 50 mg/cm^2 of water. The thickness of the object
being radiographed is assumed to be 20 gm/cm^2. From Figure 8 it is
clear that there is an optimal energy at which to detect and
visualise changes. This is between 60 and 70 Kev when detecting
soft tissue changes and about 35 Kev when detecting the presence
of contrast media. It is of interest to note that computed
tomographic scanners tend to employ beams with an effective energy
between 60 and 70 Kev and are designed primarily to visualise soft
tissue changes. Clearly if a CT scanner is to be used for the
detection or visualisation of iodine containing contrast media
it should be operated with an effective beam energy of approximately 35 Kev for maximum dose efficiency.

The above data can be used to determine the concentration
of contrast medium which could just be visualised in a vessel
of a given size. Assuming that the added iodine is contained in

a vessel of internal diameter 1mm it is easy to show, using equation (9), that the concentration required to give a signal to noise ratio of 5 is of the order of 2 mg/ml when the effective beam energy is 40 Kev and the exposure is assumed to be 1 roentgen. As already pointed out this is a contrast level which can easily be achieved in arteries by intravenous infusion.

The calculations thus far have discounted the effects of scattered radiation and in effect made the assumption that the detectors are well collimated and do not respond to scatter. The effect of this scatter even, if detected, need not be severe and it can be shown as follows that scatter only makes a small difference to the signal to noise ratio.

Assume that each detector receives N_s scattered photons. The signal to noise ratio is consequently degraded to become

$$(S/N)_s = \frac{N_1 - N_2}{\sqrt{N_1 + N_2 + 2N_s}} \tag{11}$$

for $N_1 \approx N_2$, ie. small changes

$$(S/N)_s = \frac{N_1 - N_2}{\sqrt{2\sqrt{N_1} + N_s}} \tag{12}$$

Substituting N_1 and N_2 from equations (5) and (6) and assuming that $\sigma_a(E)x_a \ll 1$

$$(S/N)_s \approx (S/N)\left[\frac{1}{\sqrt{1 + N_s/N_1}}\right] \tag{13}$$

In many radiographic situations $N_s \approx N_1$ and consequently

$$(S/N)_s \approx (S/N)/\sqrt{2}$$

The scatter thus degrades the signal to noise ratio but only as a slowly varying function of the ratio of scattered to primary photons.

An alternative to subtracting radiographs taken before and after contrast infusion is to take both radiographs with the contrast present but at two different energies.

Consider again the two beams of radiation as shown in Figure (7). One beam traverses tissue alone and the other beam traverses an equal amount of tissue but with added contrast medium. The number of photons to emerge through tissue alone is $N_1(E)$.

where
$$N_1(E) = N_o e^{-\sigma(E)x} \qquad (14)$$

The number of photons to emerge through the region with added contrast medium is $N_2(E)$.

where
$$N_2(E) = N_o e^{-\sigma(E)x} e^{-\sigma_a(E)x_a} \qquad (15)$$

$$= N_1 e^{-\sigma_a(E)x_a} \qquad (16)$$

Assuming now that two radiographs are taken at energies E_1 and E_2 such that $N_1(E_1) = N_1(E_2)$ i.e, the soft tissue components of the image disappear when the two radiographs are subtracted. The signal to noise ratio for the detection of the contrast medium is now

$$S/N = \frac{N_2(E_2) - N_2(E_1)}{\sqrt{N_2(E_2) + N_2(E_1)}} \qquad (17)$$

Substituting for $N_2(E_1)$ and $N_2(E_2)$ from (14) and (16) and making the assumptions that $N_1(E_2) = N_1(E_1)$ and $\sigma_a(E)x_a \ll 1$

$$S/N \approx x_a \sigma_a(E_1) \sqrt{\frac{N_o e^{-\sigma(E_1)x}}{2}} \left[1 - \frac{\sigma_a(E_2)}{\sigma_a(E_1)} \right] \qquad (18)$$

This expression can be compared with (7) where the signal to noise ratio for subtraction with no energy change was derived for radiographs taken with and without contrast. Thus without energy change.

$$S/N \approx x_a \sigma_a(E_1) \sqrt{\dfrac{N_o e^{-\sigma(E_1)x'}}{2}} \tag{19}$$

For maximum sensitivity to iodine E_1 should be about 35 Kev and E_2 should be high enough for the photo-electric effect in iodine to be small. A suitable value for E_2 would be 60 Kev. For these two energies.

$$\frac{\sigma_a(E_2)}{\sigma_a(E_1)} = \frac{\sigma_a(60 \text{ Kev})}{\sigma_a(35 \text{ Kev})} \approx 0.1 \tag{20}$$

and $\qquad 1 - \dfrac{\sigma_a(E_2)}{\sigma_a(E_1)} \approx 0.9 \tag{21}$

The signal to noise ratio for energy subtraction would therefore be slightly lower than for a pre and post contrast subtraction. The overall dose efficiency of the energy subtraction method is however higher because of the increased penetration of the higher energy radiation and the larger number of photons required to produce a particular radiation dose.

This can be demonstrated as follows:

The exposure $\qquad R = \dfrac{N_o}{a^2 K(E)} \qquad$ for each radiograph $\tag{22}$

The total exposure from the two radiographs taken at different energies is

$$R_t = \frac{N_o(E_1)}{a^2 K(E_1)} + \frac{N_o(E_2)}{a^2 K(E_2)} \tag{23}$$

as $N_1(E_1)$ is assumed to equal $N_1(E_2)$

$$N_o(E_1)e^{-\sigma(E_1)x} = N_o(E_2)e^{-\sigma(E_1)x}$$

$$R_t = \frac{N_o(E_1)}{a^2}\left[\frac{1}{K(E_1)} + \frac{e^{-\left[\sigma(E_1)x - \sigma(E_2)x\right]}}{K(E_2)}\right] \tag{24}$$

In the case of pre and post contrast subtraction the total exposure

$$R_s = \frac{N_o(E)}{a^2}\left[\frac{2}{K(E_1)}\right] \tag{25}$$

As the signal to noise ratio is approximately the same for both methods under the assumptions which are made, the exposure ratio (r) for the same signal to noise ratio is given by

$$r = \left[\frac{1}{K(E_1)} + \frac{1}{K(E_2)}\left[\frac{e^{-\sigma(E_1)x}}{e^{-\sigma(E_2)x}}\right]\right]\frac{K(E_1)}{2} \tag{26}$$

Assuming the following values

$$K(E_1) = K(33Kev) = 150 \times 10^8$$

$$K(E_2) = K(60Kev) = 304 \times 10^8$$

$$\sigma(E_1) = \sigma(33Kev) = 0.32 \text{ cm}^2/\text{gm}$$

$$\sigma(E_2) = \sigma(60Kev) = 0.20 \text{ cm}^2/\text{gm}$$

$$x = 20 \text{ gm/cm}^2$$

The value of r is 0.5

Thus for the same signal to noise ratio the energy subtraction method is approximately twice as dose efficient as the pre and post contrast subtraction method.

GENERAL CONSIDERATION REGARDING SUITABLE EQUIPMENT

In the previous section an attempt has been made to demonstrate the idea that at acceptable radiation doses the dynamic range of radiographic data is very wide and that compression of this dynamic range is necessary for effective visualisation of normal structures and changes caused by disease processes. It was also suggested that computed tomography represents one of a set of possible range compression methods and that the same fundamental physical limits apply in the case of all methods. Some of these limits have already been explored in previous sections. Other limitations occur when equipment is considered to implement the various methods and these will now be considered.

Volume Scanning

For optimum imaging of iodine containing contrast media effective X-ray energies of approximately 35 Kev and 60 Kev are required for subtraction methods and 60 or 70 Kev for soft tissue imaging by non subtraction methods such as direct computed tomography or edge enhancement. At these energies the maximum sustained exposure that can be achieved at the surface of a patient using current X-ray tubes is of the order of 2 roentgens per second for focus to object distances of about one metre. The exposure required for vessel visualisation using contrast agents is of the order of 1 roentgen and at this exposure soft tissue changes of the order of 0.1% are detectable. After intravenous administration a bolus of contrast passes in a few tens of seconds and remains roughly constant in concentration for a few seconds. Even when bolus injections of contrast are not being used exposure times should be kept to a few seconds so that no significant movement occurs due to breathing or peristalsis. To visualise the heart, exposures as short as 0.1 sec are required.

It is clear therefore that for a practical radiographic system capable of gathering all the information available at a particular radiation dose, this dose has to be delivered to every image element in the required exposure time and the emergent photons from each element must be detected with as near to 100% efficiency as possible and no noise, additional to the fundamentally limiting statistical noise in the detected number of photons, should be added by the detecting system.

Figure (9) shows three possible radiographic schemes for making a series of X-ray transmission measurements through a volume of tissue. In 9 (a) a single beam and detector scan over the image area. If it is assumed that an exposure of 1 roentgen is to be achieved at every point then it would take 45,000 seconds to gather all the data in a 300 x 300 image matrix. The time taken to acquire data is significantly reduced by the scheme shown in 9 (b). In this case a linear array of detectors is scanned down the patient and the total data acquisition time is now reduced to 160 seconds. This would still be too long for a subtraction method using contrast agents or for direct visualisation of edges or soft tissue changes because of organ motion. Figure 9 (c) shows a more acceptable system in which an array of 300 x 300 detectors allows a data acquisition time of only 0.5 seconds.

The scheme shown in figure 9 (b) is used to obtain the transmission measurements required for a single C.T. slice and for scout view or scannergram images. A specially built scanning detector array has been built as Rad View by the General Electric Corporation (7) and is intended as a stand alone radiographic system without a computed tomographic facility. In this device an energy subtraction scheme is implemented for the visualisation of contrast agents. The device is however limited by the sustained output that can be achieved by X-ray tubes and the consequent long scan times for high sensitivity.

The arguments presented earlier indicate that any really practical system which is capable of producing a two dimensional projection of a volume of tissue should employ a two dimensional detector system which has close to 100% efficiency upto an effective energy of the order of 60 or 70 Kev.

The spatial resolution to be achievable in such a system should be of the order of 2 line pairs per millimetre or better to compete with conventional film screen combinations. Significantly greater resolutions could not in any case be used effectively for the visualisation of soft tissue changes of the order 0.1% or small blood vessels using intravenous contrast at acceptable radiation doses. Higher resolutions would of course be justified if large contrasts were being visualised as between soft tissue and bone.

A generally useful radiographic system would appear
possible if a two dimensional detector array could be produced
with a high efficiency for detecting radiation upto 60 or 70 Kev
effective energy and having a spatial resolution of the order of
2 line pairs per millimetre.

A number of attempts have been made to realise such a
detector system using X-ray image intensifiers coupled to low
noise television cameras. (3). (4). Whilst image intensifiers
have a relatively high quantum efficiency at energies appropriate
for pre and post contrast subtraction methods, they are not very
efficient at the higher energies. In addition even the best
current TV camera tubes are too noisy to be used directly and
have to be coupled through analogue to digital converters into
storage devices which sum a number of images so improving the
signal to noise ratio of the composite image so produced. This
technique has been used by the above workers (3), (4).

The rapid developments in charge coupled array devices could
provide the required low noise television camera. The very wide
dynamic range and low noise of these devices (8) allowing direct
integration of the light from an image intensifier (9).
Research is going on in many centres to produce efficient two-
dimensional detector systems and it is possible there will be a
choice of suitable detector systems in the near future.

To allow the data manipulation required for the various
dynamic range contraction stratagems it will be necessary to
digitise the outputs from detector arrays for storage and
subsequent processing in computers. A significant limitation on
the usefulness of digital data from arrays of detectors is the
current cost and bulk of suitable storage. Recent developments
in the home or domestic video market provide a solution to this
problem. Video discs with a projected storage capacity of
2×10^{10} binary bits, sufficient to store about 100, 14" x 17"
chest radiograph with no loss of information, are likely to be
available in the near future at a cost of a few tens of dollars
per disc. Writers for such discs are already available and this
new technology provides a real solution to the problem. Indeed
the availability of such a large storage capacity at such a low
cost will have a profound effect on the future development of
radiology.

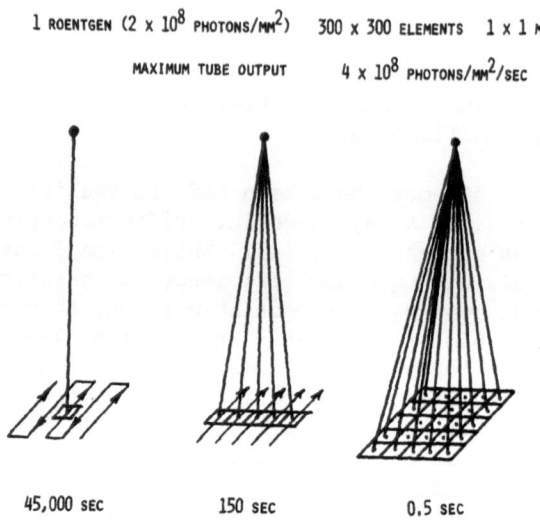

1 ROENTGEN (2×10^8 PHOTONS/MM^2)   300 x 300 ELEMENTS   1 x 1 MM^2

MAXIMUM TUBE OUTPUT 4×10^8 PHOTONS/MM^2/SEC

45,000 SEC   150 SEC   0.5 SEC

Figure 9.   Three methods of gathering transmission data for
volume scanning.

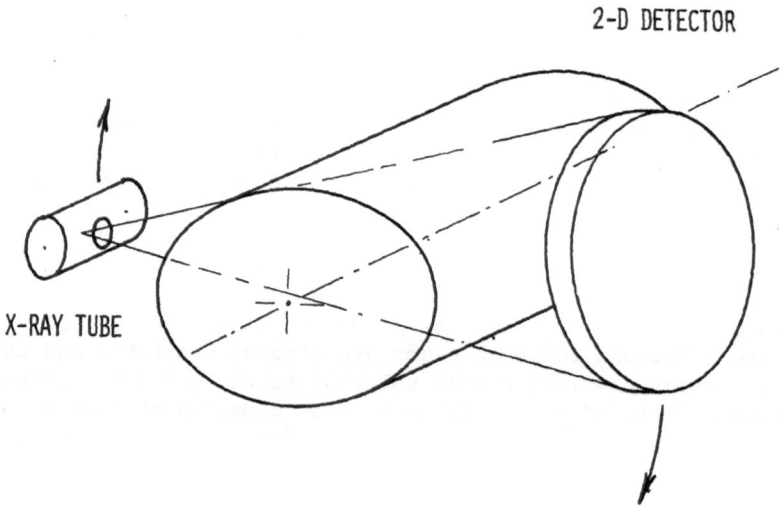

2-D DETECTOR

X-RAY TUBE

Figure 10.   A generally applicable radiographic apparatus
employing an X-ray tube and two dimensional detector
the positions and movements of which can be controlled
in a flexible manner.

Tomography

The principles of computed tomography have been extensively
reviewed in published works of widely varying complexity (10),
(11), (12) and it is purposeless to reproduce this material in
this paper. As already stated in an earlier section, tomography
has two beneficial effects. The first is in synthesising a
radiograph of a uniformly thick slice in which there can be a
high sensitivity to tissue change whilst all relevant data
is contained within a limited dynamic range. The second is in
removing overlying structures which in the case of complicated
objects, would cause confusion. Both these effects are beneficial
when displaying radiographic data and any generally applicable
volume scanning system should allow the tomographic principle to
be used. It is therefore of interest to examine the conditions
under which a general volume scanning apparatus with tomographic
facilities could be implemented.

The essential feature of a system would be a two dimensional
detector of high quantum efficiency and a limiting resolution of
the order of 2 line pairs per millimetre. This would allow low
dose imaging in high contrast situations such as chest and in
addition the visualisation of low contrasts by edge enhancement,
subtraction or tomography at higher doses. Such a system would be
capable of covering a significant fraction of the work load of a
radiology department, even without the tomographic facility.
A simple tomographic facility could be provided by implementing
the digital equivalent of conventional tomography. This would
comprise a simple back projection to the plane which contained
the axis of rotation of the tomographic system and would be
equivalent to the smearing which takes place for out of plane
detail in conventional tomography. Such a system would however
be highly dose inefficient. With a two dimensional detector, the
output of which can be digitised and stored for each position of
the tube and detector, it is possible to do far better than the
simple smearing of conventional tomography.

The system illustrated in Figure (10) would provide a series
of two dimensional projections of the object being radiographed.
Projections could be taken over a narrow range of angles in a simple
system or for a full rotation at the expense of greater complexity.
Tomographic cross sections can be computed using conventional
algorithms (13) for only a narrow range of projection angles.
Figure 11 shows a reconstruction using an EMI 5005 scanner. The
reconstruction is of an EMI test phantom lying within the machine
aperture but with its axis pointing vertically upward as shown
in Figure (12a). Projection values have been taken over a range
of $\pm 20^\circ$ and reconstructed using the EMI 5005 standard algorithms
but with all projection values outside the range $\pm 20^\circ$ set to the

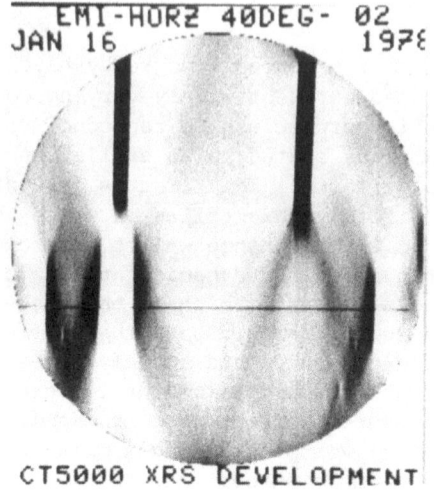

Figure 11.   Reconstruction of a phantom from projections
gathered over 40°. The phantom is cylindrical and
its axis lies vertically within the computed slice.

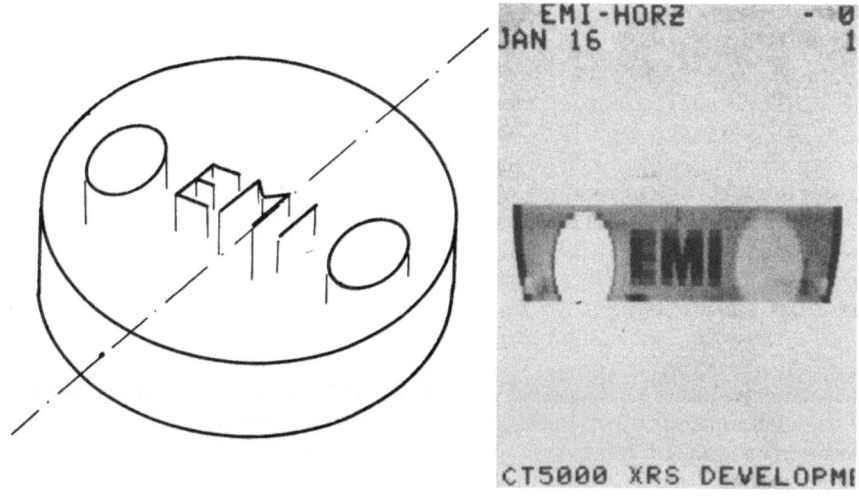

Figure 12.   (a)   Phantom position for the scan shown in Figure 11
(b)   A slice perpendicular to the axis of the phantom
assembled from a set of contiguous slice as shown
in Figure 11.

water calibration phantom readings. As expected the resolution in the vertical direction is poor and that in the horizontal direction good. This implies that a horizontal slice with good resolution in both directions could be synthesised from a series of narrow contiguous slices. Figure (12b) shows such a slice. There are probably better algorithms for narrow angle reconstruction than the one used (14) but this simple example serves to demonstrate the idea that the data gathering geometry of a tomographic scanner can be flexible.

A scanner employing a two dimensional detector and gathering data from only a narrow range of angles, whilst more versatile, is however likely to be less accurate in providing measures of the distribution of attenuation than conventional C.T. systems. It could however be argued that accurate absolute attenuation values provided by conventional C.T. scanners have not been of great value in clinical practice. In practice only relative values or differences between one region and another appear to be used for diagnostic purposes and consequently there would not be a significant penalty in clinical practice. Rather a significant gain would result through the availability of a general radiographic tool of much greater versatility than that provided by the rather limited and expensive current generation of C.T. scanners. If accuracy can be discarded a number of constraints on machine design are relaxed and simple algorithms which give adequate picture quality but poor accuracy become useable, so lowering demands on data handling and computing systems.

CONCLUSIONS

The availability of high quantum efficiency two dimensional detector systems should lead to a new generation of radiographic tools capable of gathering data at, or near to, the theoretical minimum dose. For high contrast objects this will lead to radiology at significantly lower doses than those currently experienced using conventional film screen combinations. For lower contrasts, detectable at higher doses, a number of processing and display methods can be implemented. Examples which have been considered are edge enhancement, pre and post contrast subtraction, energy subtraction and computed tomography.

Suitable detectors are being developed and image intensifiers combined with low noise television cameras are showing some considerable promise for this application. Computer technology is already adequate for the data handling and processing task. Recent development in memory technology in the form of the digital video discs promise a solution to the problem of the very large amount of data which has to be stored.

Given all these developments it appears reasonable to
assume that it will be possible for a versatile radiographic
system, with a tomographic as well as plane radiographic facility
to be available in the not too distant future. Such a device
would almost certainly surplant C.T. scanners in their present form.

REFERENCES

1. Battista J.J. and Bronskill. "Compton-scatter Tissue
Densitometry:Calculation of Single and Multiple Scatter Photon
Fluences." Phys. Med. Biol. 23 (1978) 1-23.
2. Hounsfield G.N. "Computerised transverse axial scanning
(tomography). Part 1. Description of system." Br.J.Radiol. 46
(1972) 1016-1022.
3. Newton T.H. and D.G.Potts. "Radiology of the skull and
brain:Technical aspects of computed tomography." Mosby (1981).
4. Macovski, A. "Iodine imaging using spectral analysis",
in Noninvasive Cardiovascular Measurements (eds. H.A.Miller,
E.V. Schmidt and D.C.Harrison), Society of Photo-Optical
Instrumental Engineers, Bellingham, Washington. (1978) 67-75.
5. Ovitt, T.W., Capp, M.P., Fisher, H.D., Frost, M.M.,Lebel,
J.L., Nudelman, S., and Roehrig, H. "The development of a
digital video subtraction system for intravenous angiography", in
Noninvasive Cardiovascular Measurements (ed. H.A. Miller,
E.V. Schmidt and D.C. Harrison), Society of Photo-Optical
Instrumentation Engineers, Bellingham, Washington. (1978) 61-65.
6. Kruger, R.A., Mistretta, C.A., Houk, T.L., Reiderer, S.J.,
Shaw, C.G., Goodsitt, M.M., Crummy, A.B., Zweibel, W., Lancaster,
J.C., Rowe, G.G., and Flemming, D. "Computerized fluoroscopy
in real time for noninvasive visualisation of the cardiovascular
system," Radiology, 130, (1979) 49-57.
7. Brody, W.R. Sommer F.G. et al, "Dual-Kvp radiography."
Proceedings of S.P.I.E. Vol 273. (1981) 239-243.
8. Tompsett, M.F. "Video-signal generation," in Electronic
Imaging (ed. T.P. McLean and P. Schagen), Academic Press London,
(1979) 55-101.
9. Walker, G.A.H. Buchholz V. et al. "Applications astronomiqu
des recepteurs d'images a response lineare". (ed. Duchesne and
Lelieure, Obs de Paris-Meudon) (1976) 24
10. Brooks R.A. Di Chiro G."Principles of computer assisted
tomography (CAT) in radiographic and radioisotope imaging." Phys.
Med. Biol. 21, (1976) 689.
11. Pullan B.R. "Basic principles of computed tomography:
Theory." Proceedings of Enrico Fermi summer school on Medical Physic
Verrena (1979).

12. Macovski A. Herman G.T. "Principles of reconstruction algorithms." Radiology of the skull and brain. Technical aspects of computed tomography, ed. Newton T.H. and Potts D.G. (The C.V. Mosby Company) (1981).

13. Dovas T. Dept. Medical Biophysics, University of Manchester. Personal Communication.

14. Myers M.J. "Computer processing in longditudinal isotope tomography." Information processing in scintigraphy ed. A. Todd-Pokropek (1975) 343-352.

SOME IMAGING CHARACTERISTICS OF THE DYNAMIC SPATIAL RECONSTRUCTOR
X-RAY SCANNER SYSTEM

T. Behrenbeck, L. J. Sinak, R. A. Robb, J. H. Kinsey,
and E. L. Ritman

Department of Physiology and Biophysics, Mayo Clinic,
Rochester, Minnesota 55905

INTRODUCTION

In late 1979, the Dynamic Spatial Reconstructor (DSR), a
multiple x-ray source, stop action, volume scanning imaging device
was installed (1,2). At present, the operational characteristics
and biomedical utility of the Dynamic Spatial Reconstructor (DSR)
are being evaluated. This research project involves scanning
experimental animals and carefully selected patients with cardiovascular and pulmonary pathology. The DSR scanner utilizes a computerized transaxial tomography principle to generate images of
transverse slices of the body. As illustrated in Figure 1, 14
x-ray tubes and 14 television cameras (of the 28 for which it is
designed) are attached to the scanner. The x-ray tubes are
arranged 12º apart along a semicircular array with television
cameras positioned opposite each x-ray source. As each x-ray tube
is pulsed for 350 microseconds, a 30 cm x 30 cm image is generated
on a fluorescent screen. The corresponding television camera is
gated on for 762 microseconds and the fluoroscopic image is
recorded on the image isocon target for subsequent readout and
recording on video disc. The patient or animal scanned is positioned inside the machine at the center of rotation as indicated
in the schematic in Figure 1. The data flow of the system is
illustrated in the schematic flow diagram in Figure 2. The 14
television images of the fluoroscopic images, generated by the 14
x-ray pulses over an 11 millisecond period, are recorded in multi-
plexed form on seven video disc channels at a repetition rate of
60 scans/second. Each of the upto 120 horizontal scan lines of
each of the 14 video fields can now be used to reconstruct the
image of a corresponding cross section. The video signal is

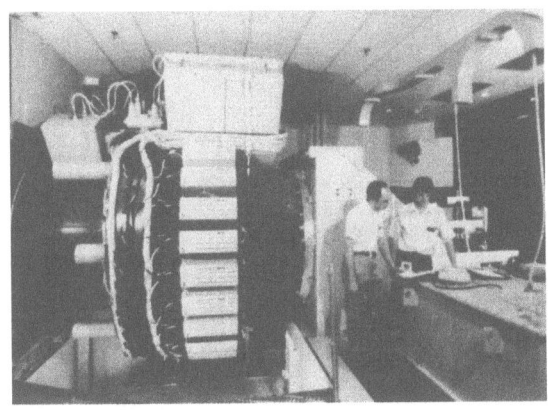

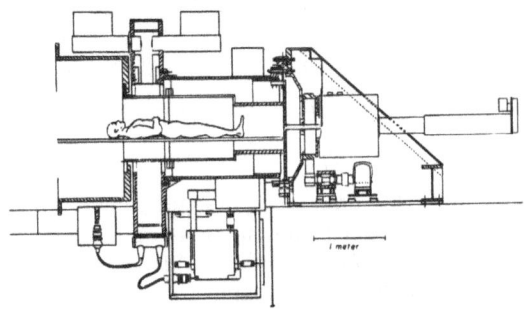

06/81/ELR

Figure 1. <u>Upper panel</u>: Dynamic Spatial Reconstructor scanner
assembly. The entire structure to the left of the men is cantilevered from the triangular base. Multiple image isocon t.v.
cameras and corresponding x-ray sources are arranged along a vertical plane. Rotation of the cantilevered section increases the
number of angles of view per scan in proportion to the programmed
duration of the scan. <u>Lower panel</u>: Midline longitudinal section
of the scanner shows relationship of human subject lying on table
and the surrounding gantry.

digitized with a real-time analog-to-digital converter and the
x-ray intensity data normalized for the non-uniform distribution
of the overall detection system. A "stack" of 120 cross section
images is generated (see Figure 3) for each 1/60 second of the
duration of a scanning sequence (upto 20 seconds).

An Alderson Rando phantom was used to evaluate the x-ray
exposure (3). At 100 KeV peak potential and 1000 mA for each
x-ray pulse (21 mAs), the radiation entrance dose for a 14 x-ray
tube system was 905 mR/second in the thoracic region of interest.
The thyroid region was exposed to somewhat less than 300 mR/
second, the eye 7 mR/second, and the gonads to somewhat less than

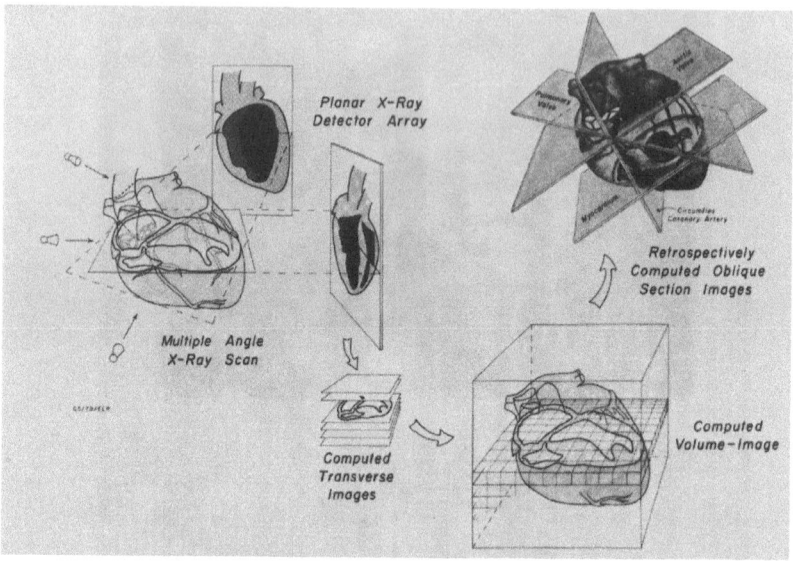

Figure 2. Schematic flow chart of the sequence of procedures performed by the Dynamic Spatial Reconstructor system for generation
of volume images which can be viewed following mathematical sectioning in arbitrary orientations and locations. X-ray images of
the chest and its anatomic contents (e.g., heart) are recorded
from many angles of view around the patient or experimental animal.
This information is used to generate the data ("stack" of images
of parallel transverse sections) required for a volume image using
a reconstruction algorithm. Synthesis from up to 240 parallel,
1 mm thick, cross sections of the chest and its contents results
in three-dimensional array of little cubic picture elements
(voxels) each with a grey scale value. The final panel illustrates the need for sectioning this volume image in arbitrary
orientations and locations. Parallel contiguous sections would be
required for measurement of regional myocardial wall thickness:
An oblique section would be required for measurement of pulmonary
valve area, many multi-oriented adjacent (and often intersecting)
contiguous sections may be required for visualization of coronary
artery cross sections along the length of tortuous multi-oriented
major branches of the coronary arterial tree. (Reproduced with
permission from Ritman et al., The Physiologist 22(6):39-43
(December) 1979).

1 mR/second. Consequently for a 4-5 second scan encompassing
several heart cycles which are required to evaluate ventricular
function during the passage of contrast agent through the myocardium and through the lung, total exposure in an adult of up to
5 R might be required.

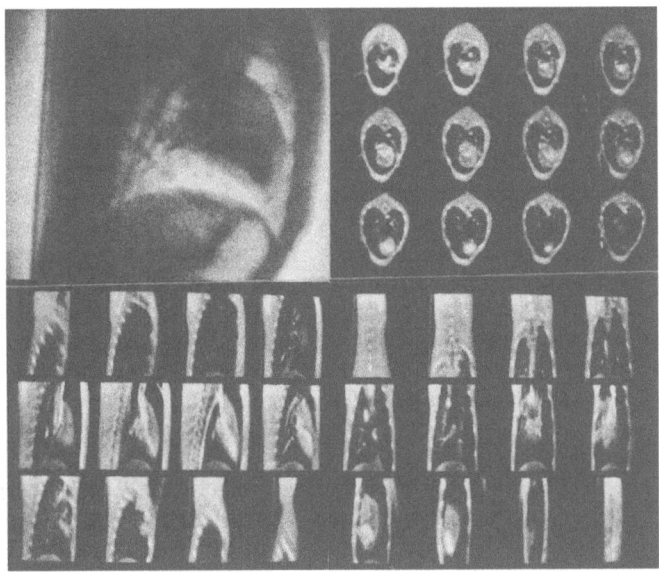

Figure 3. Upper left panel represents a single video profile of
a scan of a canine thorax from just one imaging system on the DSR.
Radiopaque contrast material (1 ml/kg body weight) was injected
into the inferior vena cava of the anesthetized dog several seconds
prior to commencing the scan so as to delineate the heart's left
ventricle. From the multiple cameras surrounding the animal it
was possible to reconstruct approximately 120 transverse sections,
12 of which are shown in the upper right panel. The sections are
arranged in descending order from the top left to the lower right
of this panel. Roentgen contrast agent in the blood of the left
ventricular chamber and various major blood vessels show as bright
areas in the section images. These imaged transverse sections were
mathematically re-sliced to produce images of sagittal and coronal
sections, illustrated in the lower two panels. (Reproduced with
permission from R. A. Robb, "High-Speed Three-Dimensional Computed
Tomography and Multi-Dimensional Display of the Heart, Lungs, and
Circulation. Medical Physics of CT and Ultrasound: Tissue Imaging
and Characterization. Medical Physics Monograph No. 6, AAPM,
pp 656-702, 1980).

     The philosphophy behind the design of the DSR has four major
aspects. First, a volume has to be scanned rather than a slice
in order to permit measurement of, for instance, muscle mass, chamber volumes and lung volumes. These values can only be obtained
from multiple cross sections through the region of interest.
Secondly, a volume has to be scanned because an accurate and meaningful (in a pathophysiological sense) measurement can often only

258

be obtained from an image of an oblique section through the body.
Such an oblique section, with the correct orientation (e.g., normal
to the vessel lumen) and location (e.g., through a valve orifice)
in the organ or structure of interest, can be computed with certainty only from a volume image. Thirdly, the volume has to be
imaged within a sufficiently brief period of time such that the
motion of the object of interest is less than about one resolution
element. The DSR is designed to have maximal spatial resolution
of approximately 1 mm in the heart. Fourthly, the images have to
be generated at sufficient repetition rate for a sufficient period
of time so that time varying motion can be quantitated. One cardiac cycle requires approximately 20 points for analysis (4) and
an indicator dilution curve, which might occur over several cardiac cycles, needs approximately 10 points per second for adequate
resolution.

These capabilities are illustrated in the following figures.
Figure 4 illustrates that the entire myocardium can be displayed
and measured with some accuracy as to its three-dimensional shape:

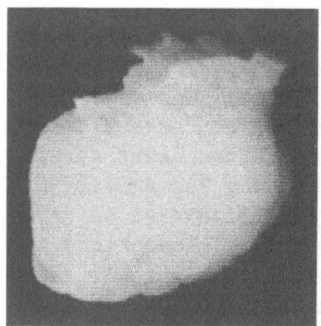 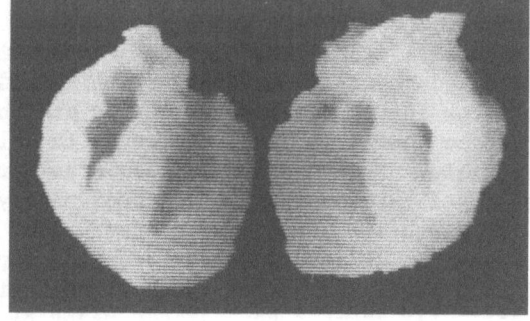

09/80/RAR

Figure 4. Computer-generated three-dimensional shaded surface
displays of isolated human heart determined from 50 reconstructed
cross sections of the heart obtained by the DSR. Epicardial and
endocardial boundaries in each cross section are automatically
recognized and synthesized into 3-D surfaces which are illustrated
by a simulated light source at eye of observer. Left panel shows
lateral-oblique view of heart. Ascending aorta can be seen at top
right. Right panel shows anterior-oblique view of heart after it
is mathematically opened into halves to permit viewing of internal
structures. Left ventricular chamber is larger of two chambers.
Both the right and left atria can be seen, as well as openings to
the superior vena cava, pulmonary artery, and aorta. (Reproduced
with permission from R. A. Robb, "X-Ray Computed Tomography: An
Engineering Synthesis of Multi-Scientific Principles", CRC Press
(In Press)).

total myocardial mass, regional myocardial mass, and wall thickness. A dynamic sequence of such data provides estimates of regional wall dynamics and volume dynamics of the heart. In the case where a two-dimensional or one-dimensional measurement is required, this can be obtained from a section image (5). The right upper panel of Figure 2 illustrates a number of instances in the heart where such oblique images might be required for such measurements. This need for randomly oriented oblique images requires that the spatial resolution of the three-dimensional or volume image be essentially the same in the axial and transverse directions.

In addition to dimension measurements, motion provides important indices of cardiac and pulmonary function. As illustrated in Figure 5, regional wall dynamics can be evaluated with this scanner. Regional wall dynamics has been demonstrated to be a good index of regional myocardial function (6). The magnitude

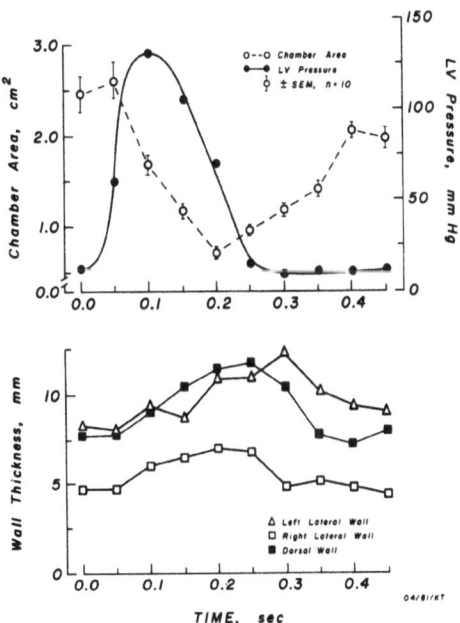

Figure 5. Data from a single transverse cross section of a dog's left ventricle imaged with the DSR. Each data point was measured from one transaxial image. These images were generated from 112 views, 1 mm thick and repeated 16 per second throughout one cardiac cycle. The dog was anesthetized with morphine and pentobarbital. Spontaneous heart rate was 120 beats/minute. Roentgen contrast agent, 1 ml/kg, was injected into the inferior vena cava. The scan was performed during the levo phase of this angiogram.

260

of the rate of myocardial wall thickening during the systolic phase decreases directly with impairment of myocardial perfusion. Finally, the passage of contrast agent along a blood vessel can be used to construct indicator dilution curves as illustrated in Figure 6. The contrast agent generated dilution curve can be used to compute flow by the Stewart-Hamilton principle. The passage of dye along a straight or an unbranched section of vessel can also be used to derive blood flow from the mean transit time of the bolus of contrast medium along a vessel. In principle, the extensive application of indicator dilution techniques in projection images (7) can be directly applied to the DSR generated CT images with the added advantage that superposition is not an obstacle.

Objective Evaluation of DSR Imaging Characteristics

The DSR is made up of independent components such as x-ray tubes, television cameras, electronic amplifiers, etc., all of which can be independently controlled and have their unique effects on image characteristics. Not surprisingly, therefore, there is variation of DSR image characteristics from scan to scan due to the independent setting of each component. Variability of

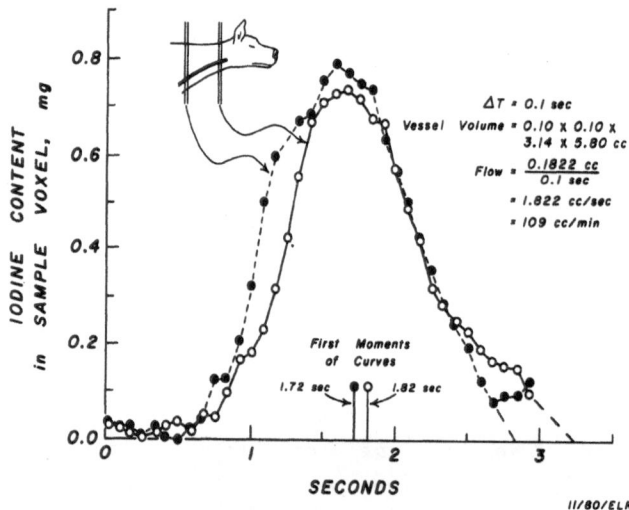

Figure 6. Neck of an anesthetized 22 kg dog was scanned during passage of 2 ml bolus of roentgen contrast medium. An electromagnetic flow meter at the distal end of the carotid artery provided independent estimate of carotid blood flow. Two dilution curves obtained by sampling the transaxial image brightness over the carotid artery region were used to compute blood flow by the Stewart-Hamilton and transit time methods. Independently estimated flow was 120 ml/min. These data were obtained at 100 KV, 10 mAs, and 0.083 second scan repetition intervals.

image quality during one scan of several seconds is minimal. The noise of the cross section images behaves in a stochastic manner as is suggested in Figure 7. One might conclude from these data that the noise of the images generated by the DSR would be minimized by adding up the signals generated by a number of adjacent video scan lines, that is, increasing imaged slice thickness. This, however, accentuates the problem of partial volume effects. The partial volume effect impairs accuracy due to blurring of edges at the expense of reduced noise.

As a consequence, it is important to first compute oblique sections from the stack of thin transaxial sections, followed by summing the thin oblique sections to enhance signal-to-noise to the extent that the partial volume effect will allow. As illustrated in Figure 8, if this sequence of analysis is followed, the imaged slices through a phantom held in an axial direction is quite comparable. For this phantom, the limiting high contrast spatial resolution is approximately 1.5 mm. Images such as these were used to compute a modulation transfer function (MTF) for the DSR, as illustrated in Figure 9. A limiting high contrast resolution of 1 mm is indicated under the conditions of the scan. The air to plexiglass roentgen density difference can be achieved <u>in vivo</u> if the iodine in blood concentration exceeds 30 mg iodine/ml.

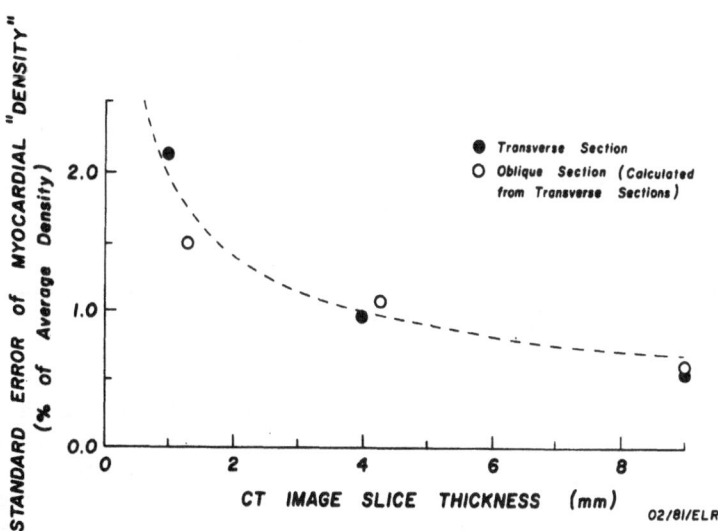

Figure 7. Variability of estimated myocardial roentgen opacity was evaluated in a 15 kg dog. Slice thickness of imaged transverse (and retrospectively computed oblique) section was increased as indicated along abscissa. Sampled area of 0.25 cm² contained 100 pixels. The dashed line is analytically computed square root function of slice thickness.

262

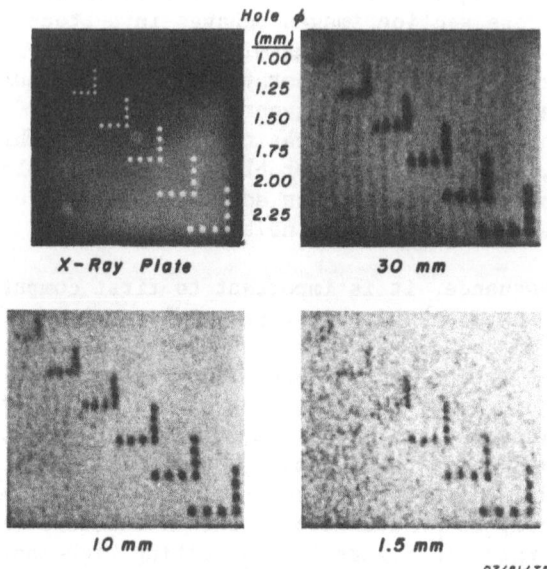

Hole φ
(mm)
1.00
1.25
1.50
1.75
2.00
2.25

X-Ray Plate   30 mm

10 mm   1.5 mm

07/81/TB

Figure 8. Plexiglass cube with air-filled holes was scanned with its plane to be imaged oriented in a transaxial, oblique, and axial direction. This figure shows an image computed from the multi-slice data obtained with the cube held in the axial direction. After retrospective computation of images of thin slices in the axial plane, images of adjacent axial planes were added to provide improved signal-to-noise. The scan was performed at 100 KV, 6 mAs, 120 angles of view around 180°. The reconstructed images are displayed with pixel size of 0.8 mm.

Such concentrations are readily achieved by bolus injections of contrast agent into vessels upstream to the anatomic site of interest.

To illustrate the conflict between increasing slice thickness on reducing noise and increasing the partial volume effect, the accuracy of estimates of coronary artery stenosis length and severity were examined. The dilemma is illustrated schematically in Figure 10. The study consisted of suturing contrast filled tygon tubing, with artificially created "stenoses", to the epicardium of a dog (8). An x-ray picture of these pseudo-coronary arteries is shown in Figure 11. This resolution problem is compounded by small size of coronary arteries. The limiting spatial resolution of the DSR cross section images is somewhat poorer than 1 mm and yet we are to evaluate some stenoses that are as small as 1.5 mm long and 0.6 mm in cross-sectional diameter. However,

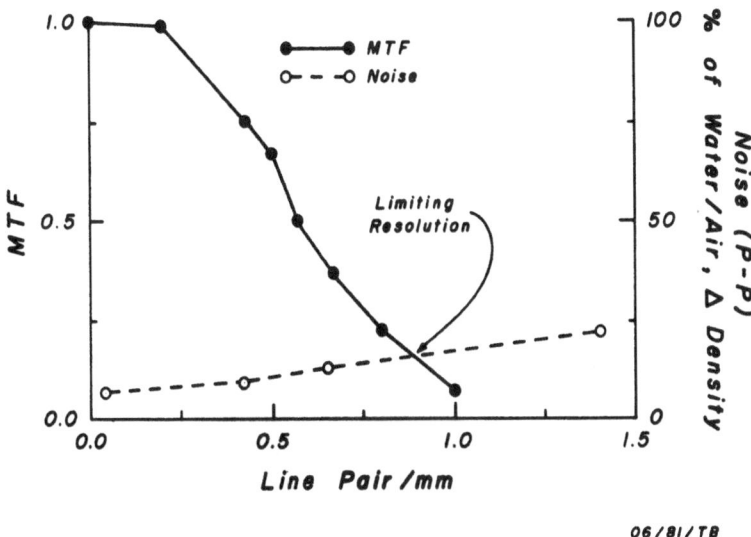

06/81/TB

Figure 9. Spatial resolution of high contrast phantom (see Figure 8) which was scanned with image plane in transaxial plane of DSR. Peak to peak noise was measured and sampling pixel size determined by the line pair resolution.

the total brightness in the blurred region of the lumen tends to remain linearly related to the cross-sectional area provided the concentration of contrast agent in the vessel lumen remains constant. This brightness x area product is measured and depicted in a manner illustrated in the schematic of Figure 12. The role of the number of slices and thickness of the slice in evaluating the stenotic region is illustrated in Figure 13. These data indicate that increased thickness of the slice impairs our ability to measure the severity of a stenosis. Increased concentration of contrast agent provides a more accurate index of stenosis severity as illustrated in Figure 14. These same data can also be used to estimate stenosis length as illustrated in Figure 15.

The partial volume effect rapidly becomes severe as the slice thickness approaches the size of the structure. This partial volume effect has to be weighed against the increased signal-to-noise that results from increased image slice thickness. Figure 16 illustrates that the sum of these opposing factors results in a minimum, that is, a point at which maximum accuracy is obtained due to minimized noise in the presence of tolerable partial volume effects. The conditions of this minimum must depend on the structure of interest as well as the scanning conditions and the amount of contrast agent present.

264

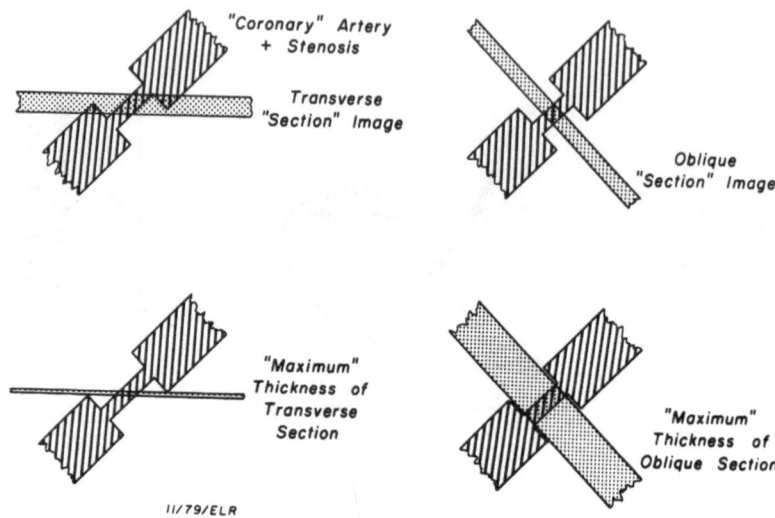

Figure 10. Schematic representation of the interrelationship between imaged slice thickness and orientation of imaged slice to a coronary artery stenosis. This schematic illustrates the capability of the DSR. Transaxial images must be thin (and contiguous) so as to permit computation of appropriately oriented and positioned thin oblique section. Images of these oblique sections can be summed to provide maximum signal-to-noise. The number of oblique images summed depends on blurring effect due to partial volume effect.

CONCLUSION

The DSR is a high temporal resolution system with the ability to provide randomly oriented oblique sections with minimal deterioration of spatial resolution. Optimal spatial and density resolution of the images of the oblique sections can be achieved by appropriate retrospective selection of slice thickness and positioning of the oblique slices relative to the anatomic structure or lesion of interest.

ACKNOWLEDGEMENTS

The authors express their thanks to Messrs. D. I. Erdman, C. R. Hansen, R. W. Roessler, and M. H. Rhyner for their work on the scanner, Messrs. D. P. Hanson and L. T. Thorson and Ms. S. K. Zahn for the programming and data processing, and Ms. M. C. Fynbo and Ms. J. A. Lauer for the preparation of this manuscript and illustrations.

This work was supported in part by research grants HL-04664 and RR-00007 from the National Institutes of Health, Bethesda, Maryland.

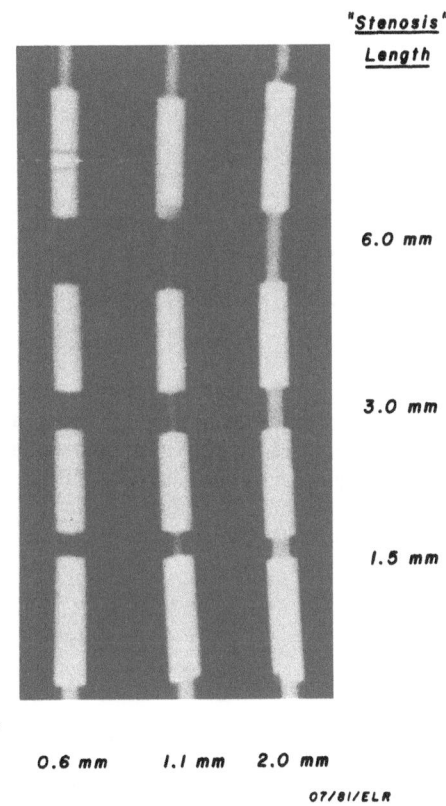

Figure 11. Roentgenogram of plastic tubing (3.2 mm diameter) filled with contrast medium. These tubes were sutured to epicardium of dog which was then scanned.

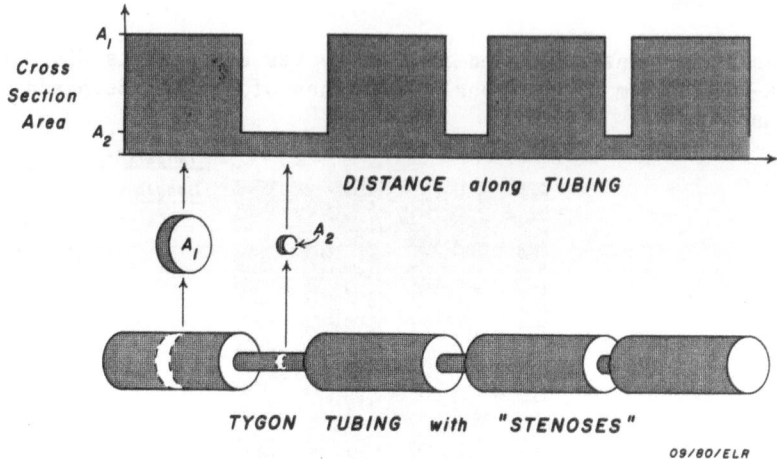

Figure 12. Schematic representation of computation of "brightness x area product" index from transaxial images of tubing sutured to epicardium (see Figure 11). This index is used to estimate change in vessel lumen cross-sectional area. This index requires that concentration of roentgen contrast agent is constant over extent of stenosis being evaluated.

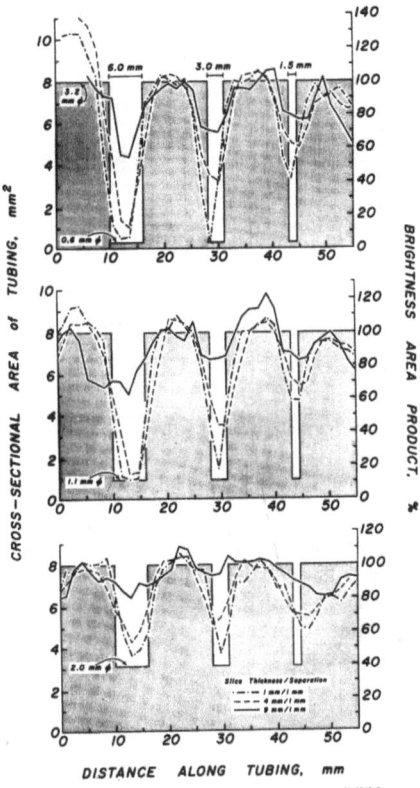

DISTANCE ALONG TUBING, mm

Figure 13. Role of image slice thickness in accuracy of estimated fractional "stenosis" in tygon tubing sutured to dog's epicardium. These data were generated with 310 mg iodine/ml in the lumen. Increase of slice thickness greater than 4 mm results in marked underestimate of stenosis greater than 3 mm in length. Even the 1 mm thick slice resulted in gross underestimate of stenosis when length of stenosis was less than 3 mm.

268

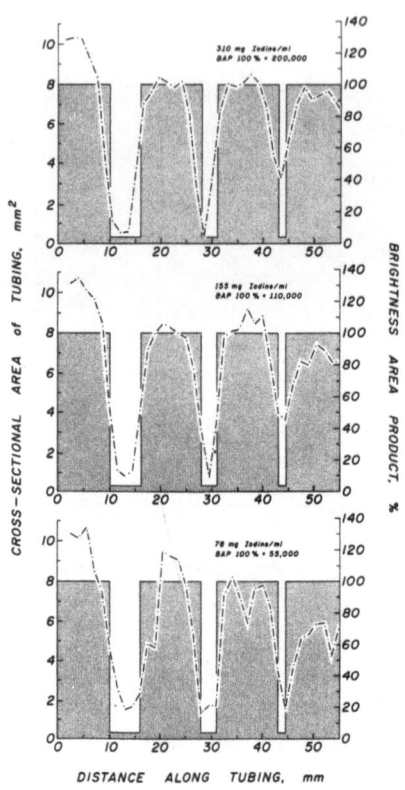

Figure 14. Similar data as in Figure 13. In this case, imaged
slice thickness is maintained at 1 mm and role of decreasing concentration of roentgen contrast agent is evaluated in one of the
tygon tubes. The main effect of decreasing concentration is the
loss of signal-to-noise in the brightness x area product. However,
even at 25% of maximum concentration, the 1.5 mm long stenosis was
detected – a concentration that would be readily achieved in the
coronary arteries following intra-aortic injection of contrast
agent.

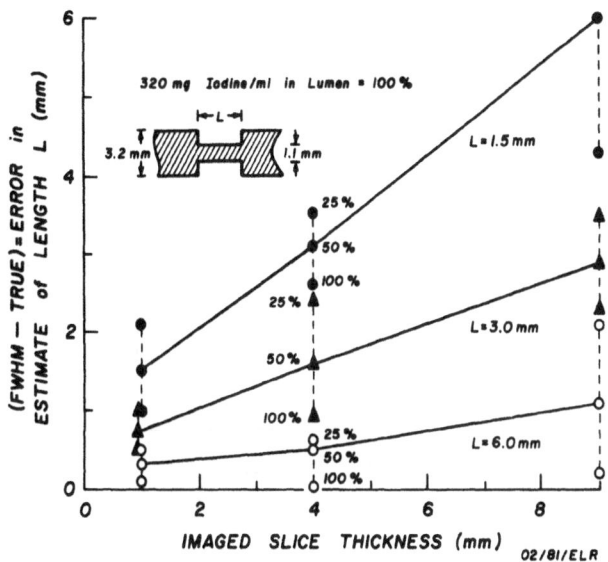

Figure 15. Accuracy of estimated length of stenosis (88% narrow-ing of 3.2 mm diameter lumen) as indicated by error of estimate decreases with imaged slice thickness. Slice separation remains 1 mm, i.e., for slices thicker than 1 mm there is overlap of slices. In all instances, the higher the concentration of roentgen contrast agent, the greater the accuracy.

270

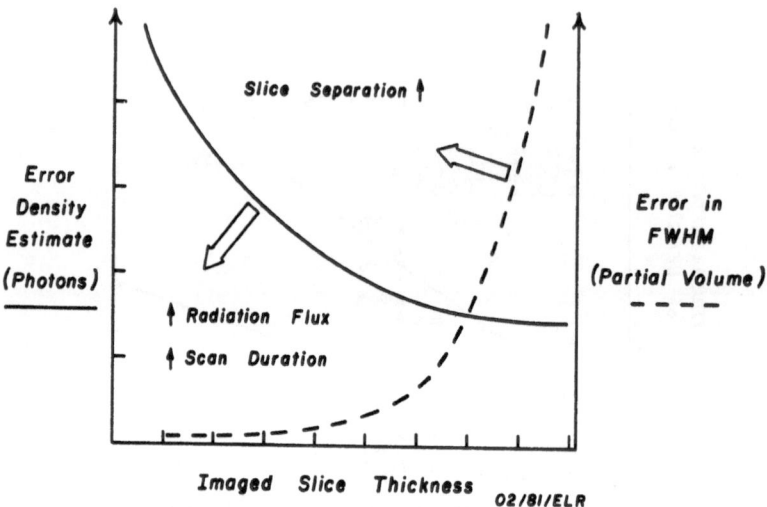

Figure 16. Synopsis of data presented in Figures 7 and 15. The
solid line indicates decrease in noise as slice thickness is
increased. Conversely, error in measurement due to partial volume
effect increases with slice thickness (dashed line). For a given
anatomic feature, the optimum tradeoff between these effects
depends largely on the dimensions and shape of the feature. Consequently, the capability for retrospective adjustment of imaged
slice location and thickness is highly desirable. The DSR image
data format provides this flexibility.

REFERENCES

1. Ritman, E. L., R. A. Robb, S. A. Johnson, P. A. Chevalier, B. K. Gilbert, J. F. Greenleaf, R. E. Sturm, and E. H. Wood. "Quantitative imaging of the structure and function of the heart, lungs, and circulation." Mayo Clinic Proceedings 53 (1978) 3-11.

2. Ritman, E. L., J. H. Kinsey, R. A. Robb, L. D. Harris, and B. K. Gilbert. "Physics and technical considerations in the design of the DSR: A high temporal resolution volume scanner." American Journal of Roentgenology 134 (1980) 369-374.

3. Kinsey, J. H. and A. L. Orvis. "High repetition rate volumetric x-ray CT scanning." IEEE Transactions on Nuclear Science NS-28(22) (1981) 1732-1735.

4. Bove, A. A., M. C. Ziskin, E. Freeman, J. L. Gimenez, and P. R. Lynch. "Selection of optimum cineradiographic frame rate: Relation to accuracy of cardiac measurements." Investigative Radiology 5 (1970) 329-335.

5. Harris, L. D., R. A. Robb, T. S. Yuen, and E. L. Ritman. "The display and visualization of 3-D reconstructed anatomic morphology: Experience with the thorax, heart, and coronary vasculature of dogs." Journal of Computer Assisted Tomography 3(4) (1979) 439-446.

6. Dumesnil, J. G., E. L. Ritman, R. L. Frye, G. T. Gau, B. D. Rutherford, and G. D. Davis. "Quantitative determination of regional left ventricular wall dynamics by roentgen videometry." Circulation 50 (1974) 700-708.

7. Heintzen, P. H. and J. H. Bürsch. Roentgen-Video-Techniques for Dynamic Studies of Structure and Function of the Heart and Circulation, 2nd International Workshop Conference (Georg Thieme Publishers, Stuttgart, 1976).

8. Scanlan, J. G., D. E. Gustafson, P. A. Chevalier, R. A. Robb, and E. L. Ritman. "Evaluation of ischemic heart disease with a prototype volume imaging computed tomographic (CT) scanner: Preliminary experiments." The American Journal of Cardiology 46 (1980) 1263-1268.

Part IV: Clinical Imaging: Basic Principles of Emission Tomography & Radiopharmaceutical Chemistry

POSITRON EMISSION TOMOGRAPHY (PET)

Michel M. Ter-Pogossian, Ph.D.

The Edward Mallinckrodt Institute of Radiology,
Washington University School of Medicine,
St. Louis, Missouri

Among emerging medical diagnostic imaging modalities,
positron emission tomography, often abbreviated to its acronym
"PET", belongs in the category of nuclear medicine. Indeed, the
image forming variable in PET is the distribution in the structure under study of a radionuclide administered systemically in
the form of a selected radiopharmaceutical prior to the imaging
procedure. Yet a number of specific features endow PET with a
distinct identity within the broader category of nuclear
medicine imaging.

The premise which provides the foundation of PET is that
any physiological activity results from and/or is accompanied by
biochemical changes in the organ from which the physiological
activity stems, and changes in physiological activity and
pathology are reflected by or stem from regional biochemical
changes which diverge from the norm. The objective of PET is to
study normal and abnormal organ physiology by detecting in these
organs, in vivo, regionally, and noninvasively biochemical
changes which are either known or suspected to be of importance
to the functional integrity of the organ studied. This general
goal falls within a broad definition of nuclear medicine imaging
and the distinctive features of PET in achieving this goal
consists of two components: 1. the limitation of the PET
imaging to radionuclides decaying by the emission to positrons;
and 2. their imaging by means of a computed tomographic
reconstruction process practically identical to that used in
conventional transmission computed tomography.

The reliance of PET upon the imaging of radionuclides
decaying by the emission of positrons stems from the

serendipitous combination of two highly propitious properties shared by certain radionuclides. 1. A small number of radionuclides possess chemical properties which render them particularly useful in the study of physiological processes. The most important of these radionuclides (sometimes referred to as "physiological" radionuclides) are carbon-11, nitrogen-13, oxygen-15, and fluorine-18. The potential usefulness of carbon-11, nitrogen-13, and oxygen-15 as radioactive indicators for physiological processes is probably obvious. Indeed, all organic material contains carbon, many metabolic processes essential to life are aerobic and therefore require oxygen, and a substantial percentage of human organs rely on nitrogen in their structure. Fluorine, chemically, is of much lesser importance in metabolic processes, but the chemical nature of that atom is particularly propitious for the labeling of metabolic analogs, the use of which has been well demonstrated to be convenient in the study of some metabolic pathways. 2. Carbon-11, nitrogen-13, oxygen-15 and fluorine-18 all decay through the emission of positrons.

Positrons which are positively charged electrons emitted by a limited number of radionuclides in their decay process, are a manifestation of antimatter and they have a fleeting existence in our universe. After a positron is emitted by a radionuclide it loses its kinetic energy in a manner similar to that of an electron in a series of excitations and ionizations and, usually after losing most of its kinetic energy, it interacts with a negatively charged electron. This interaction consists in the annihilation of the masses of the two particles and the energy thus made available appears in the form of two electromagnetic photons, the annihilation radiation, which are emitted nearly at 180° one from the other in nearly opposite directions. Each annihilation photon carries an energy of approximately 511 keV. After the administration of a positron-emitting radionuclide to a subject for imaging purposes, the positrons emitted by this radionuclide undergo annihilation within a couple of millimeters of their site of emission (this distance varies with the energy of the positrons emitted), and the annihilation photons escaping the subject under study can be detected externally, usually by means of scintillation detectors in a manner similar to that of conventional gamma rays.

The property which renders positron-emitting radionuclides useful for their medical imaging is the fact that the annihilation radiation consists of two photons emitted simultaneously and traveling nearly in opposite directions. This radiation can be effectively detected by a system of two radiation detectors connected to an electronic coincidence circuit in such a fashion that the system records an event only if both detectors are triggered simultaneously, presumably by the two annihilation photons resulting from the same annihilation event. Thus, the above system, when triggered, localizes the site of the annihilation event to a straight line joining the two detectors. This coincidence detecting of the annihilation radiation provides a method of "electronic" collimation which is more efficient and precise than the absorption collimation used in conventional nuclear medicine. Under the circumstances, the imaging of the distribution of positron-emitting radionuclides in vivo through the coincidence detection of the annihilation radiation yields potentially images of a higher quality than can be obtained by conventional nuclear medicine methods, such as, in the imaging of the distribution of technetium-99m. Thus, the two foundations of PET are contributed by 1. the favorable chemical properties of a handful of radionuclides which happen to decay by the emission of positrons; and 2. by the particularly favorable physical properties exhibited by positron-emitting radionuclides for their imaging through the detection of the annihilation radiation.

In PET, the approach utilized in providing images of positron-emitting radionuclides consists in detecting the annihilation radiation escaping from a transverse plane of the subject to be imaged and reconstructing from these measurements of a transverse tomographic image. This purpose is achieved by determining the distribution of the annihilation radiation at a number of angles around the object to be imaged with the proper resolution to permit the reconstruction of the image with the desired resolution by a reconstruction process identical to that used in CT. In most modern PET devices these measurements are carried out by means of an array of scintillation detectors placed around the object to be imaged which are often animated with proper motions to achieve the needed angular and linear sampling frequencies. After data acquisition the image is reconstructed from measurement profiles thus obtained through the application of a computer applied algorithm which consists essentially in a filtered back-projection technique identical to that used in CT.

State of the art PET devices provide images with a spatial resolution of a few millimeters, a contrast resolution of a few percent in a period of time of less than a minute. Some fundamental physical limitations contributed by the range of the positrons after their emission by the radionuclides and by the divergence of the emission of the annihilation photons from colinearlity establish a physical limitation to the resolution that can be achieved by this modality to a couple of millimeters. However, other physical and biological factors in practical PET examinations, particularly limitations imposed by the signal to noise ratio achievable with tolerable doses of radiation, have resulted in the inability to reach the maximum resolution. Efforts are presently being invested throughout the world to improve the quality of PET images by optimizing the design of imaging devices. Systems with smaller scintillation crystals are being developed to achieve a higher spatial resolution. Improvements in signal-to-noise ratio are sought either by multiplying the number of detectors accepting radiation from the same volume of tissue with the purpose of capturing a larger fraction of the annihilation photons or by utilizing photon time-of-flight information. In the latter approach, the time difference between the arrivals of the two photons at the two detectors operated in coincidence is measured and this information is utilized in positioning the annihilation event between the two detectors. Several time-of-flight systems are presently under construction and at least two of such devices will, in all probability, be in operation within the next few months.

Perhaps the main difficulty in the broad application of PET is contributed by the short half-lives (C-11, 20 min; N-13, 10 min; O-15, 2 min; F-18, 110 min) of the "physiological" radio-nuclides. With the exception of fluorine-18 the other "physio-logical" radionuclides must for all practical purposes, be generated either within the center where they are to be used, or in its immediate vicinity. At this time, the most practical method for preparing these radionuclides is by means of a cyclotron. The specifications of such an accelerator for the generation of the "physiological" radionuclides include the ability of accelerating protons to an energy of about 16 MeV and deuterons to 8 MeV, although less powerful and more powerful machines are used for that purpose. Such a cyclotron, which typically weighs approximately 20 tons requires several feet of concrete (or other material) shielding and its installation in a medical center requires a substantial financial and spatial investment.

A second hurdle contributed by the fleeting lives of the "physiological" radionuclides is their incorporation into useful radiopharmaceuticals. Indeed, in many instances the labeling of a desirable radiopharmaceutical might include several time consuming steps, the length of which is sometimes highly incom-patible with the rapid decay of the labels to be used. It is interesting to note that in the earlier days of PET this hurdle was regarded as a major impediment to the utilization of C-11, N-13, and O-15. In the past few year, however, a number of imagnitive chemists have either applied or developed rapid synthetic techniques specifically for PET utilization and now the number of either useful or potentially useful radiopharma-ceuticals labeled with the physiological radionuclides is sufficient for a large number of physiological studies and the number of useful radiopharmaceuticals labeled with short-lived positron-emitting radionuclides is steadily increasing.

So far, the applications of PET have been most numerous in the study of the brain and to the lesser extent of the heart, although other larger organs, such as the lungs, liver, pancreas, and kidneys, have also been studied by this methodology. PET has already permitted the precise assessment of some important physiological parameters which are either difficult or impossible to evaluate by other methods. Among such measurements are the regional determination of cerebral blood flow, oxygen, glucose and amino acid metabolism, and blood volume, myocardial metabolism and assessment of the extent of myocardial ischemic disease. A particularly promising application of PET is in the in vivo and noninvasive assessment of biochemical changes occurring in the brain concomittant to mental disease. In oncology, PET permits the assessment of a large number of factors potentially useful in the assessment of therapy such as blood flow, blood volume, and metabolic integrity of the tumor as well as tumor bearing tissues. Another area of application of PET is in the study of the distribution of certain drugs (particularly neuroactive drugs) and in the assessment of their effect on cerebral metabolism.

PET unfortunately is a complex and expensive modality. Not only does it require the availability of a cyclotron with ancillary equipment for the rapid labeling of radiopharmaceuticals and one or more PET devices for imaging them but also the effective utilization of this modality can be carried out only with the availability of a large and capable team including physicists, mathematicians, chemists, and physiologists and physicians. In spite of these demanding requirements, there are now approximately 45 centers in the world where the PET methodology has either been already implemented or which are committed to its implementation. It is probably safe to state that within the next few years PET will be a widely used modality in the assessment of disease and in clinical diagnostic applications.

CURRENT STATUS AND LIMITATIONS OF SINGLE PHOTON EMISSION IMAGING

T. F. Budinger

Donner Laboratory and Department of Electrical
Engineering and Computer Sciences, University of
California, Berkeley.

INTRODUCTION

Single photon tomography dates from the early 1960's when
the first transverse section tomographs were presented by Kuhl
and Edwards (1) using a rectilinear scanner and simple back-
projection methods. With the availability of computer systems
and the impetus of computer assisted tomography using transmitted X-rays, nuclear medicine instruments were modified and a
number of mathematical approaches to tomographic reconstruction
were developed in the early 1970's (2-8). Major activities of
the past few years have been in three distinct approaches to
instrumentation and methodology:

1. The use of specialized tomographic devices which give
single transverse sections with potentially good resolution or
multiple noncontiguous sections (9-22);

2. The use of single or dual gamma cameras for acquisition
of multiangular data (23-31);

3. The use of limited angular range devices involving
special collimators for commercial gamma cameras, e.g., time
coded aperture methods (32); multiple pinhole apertures (33-35);
Fresnel aperture (36,37); and the rotating quadrant slant hole
collimator (38).

The first two approaches involve the gamma camera or banks
of detectors surrounding the subject to collect a complete
angular range of data. The third approach involves the collection of data over a limited angular range and falls in the

category of longitudinal tomography such as is performed by the
Anger Tomoscanner (PHO CON, Searle Radiographics). Reconstructed sections from data collected over a limited angular range
(Fig. 1) have distortions and artifacts which are object-
dependent (39). Theoretical analyses and experimental data
(39-43) show that artifacts are produced by activity outside a
particular longitudinal plane being reconstructed and that the
techniques lack intraplane quantitative capability. In
addition, the spatial resolution is not uniform. These problems
of limited angle tomography occur with positron coincidence
detection schemes as well (44). For these reasons, there is
currently only moderate interest in coded aperture tomography.
The focus of this paper is on transverse axial tomography
wherein the angular sampling takes place around 360°. The
devices capable of acquiring these data are shown in Fig. 2.
The 36-camera device of Fig. 2f has not been developed.

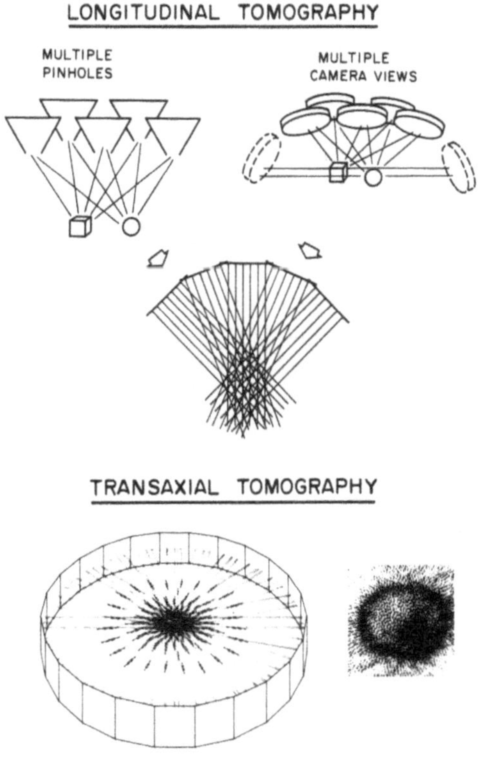

LONGITUDINAL TOMOGRAPHY

MULTIPLE
PINHOLES

MULTIPLE
CAMERA VIEWS

TRANSAXIAL TOMOGRAPHY

Fig. 1. The limited angular sampling from coded apertures leads
to non-uniform sampling and anisotropy in the point spread
function which is spatially variant. Complete angular sampling
around 360° is required to avoid these problems.

EMISSION (SINGLE PHOTON) TOMOGRAPHY

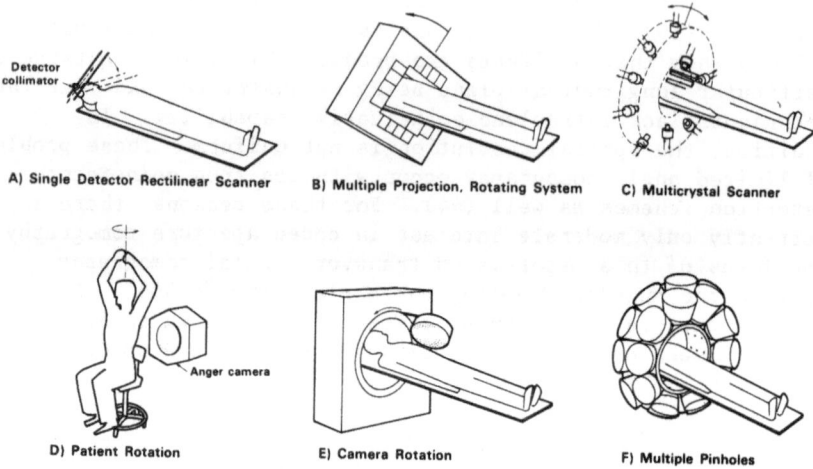

A) Single Detector Rectilinear Scanner   B) Multiple Projection, Rotating System   C) Multicrystal Scanner

D) Patient Rotation   E) Camera Rotation   F) Multiple Pinholes

Fig. 2. Instrument concepts used in single photon tomography.

Seven topics of single photon tomography technology are discussed below along with some comparisons to positron tomography. These are:

1. Reconstruction strategies
2. Attenuation compensation
3. Uniformity of spatial resolution
4. Scatter correction
5. Sensitivity
6. Dynamic emission tomography
7. Clinical applications.

SINGLE PHOTON TRANSAXIAL RECONSTRUCTION

Reconstruction Strategies

In emission tomography, we seek the position and strength of radionuclide distribution, and the mathematical algorithm must include some method to account for the attenuation between the unknown sources and the detectors. This task is far more difficult than that of x-ray tomography wherein the source position and strength are known at all times and only the attenuation coefficients need to be determined. The reconstruction algorithms are similar to those for X-ray CT with the exception of the incorporation of the attenuation compensation methods (2,45-47). At many centers, attenuation problems are ignored and the convolution method is used with results which, though not quantitative, are acceptable if the activity distribution is concentrated in the central portion of the subject. The usual strategy for gamma camera techniques is to organize the data into a series of slice projections, each corresponding to a section of 10 to 20 mm thickness. Each section is computed separately. Before reconstruction, compensation for field uniformity must be made (48,49), then one of several methods for attenutation compensation is employed.

Attenuation Compensation

The importance of methods used in compensating for attenuation is illustrated in Fig. 3. Projections from 3 bands of activity were used to reconstruct that activity with and without compensation for attenuation. The measured concentration at the center is 5 times lower than the true concentration for radionuclides with an attenuation coefficient of 0.15 cm^{-1} in a 20-cm diameter phantom.

Under conditions of constant attenuation coefficient distribution such as found in brain imaging, efficient methods have been developed (45,47). However, for situations of variable attenuation the only method which gives accurate results

DISTORTION OF EMISSION CT SECTIONS OF VARIABLE
SOURCE CONCENTRATIONS (20 cm disc of constant μ=0.15 cm^{-1})

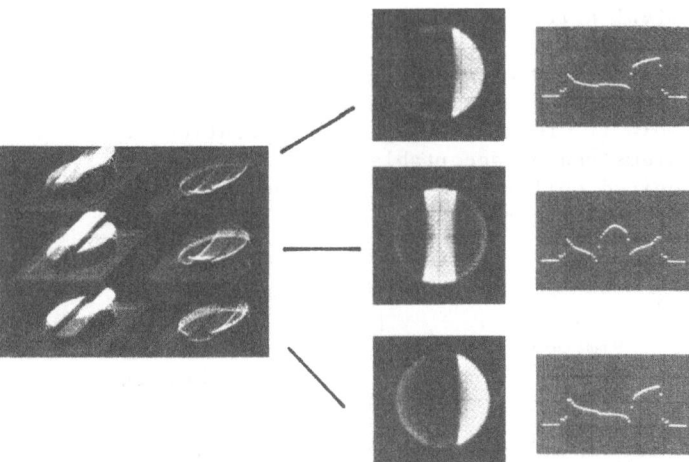

Fig. 3. Attenuation of the photons from sources in the subject cause major distortions in the reconstruction if conventional x-ray CT algorithms alone are used. If activity is concentrated mainly in the center of the attenuating medium, the artifacts do not seem to be important, but this is misleading. The measured concentration at the center of a 20-cm diameter disc will be in error by a factor of 5.

282

is the weighted least squares technique (2,46). Implementation
of this technique is practical but requires extensive digital
computation. The major difficulty is the need to acquire transmission data used to derive the attenuation coefficients before
proceeding to the emission reconstruction problem. The methods
for determining the attenuation coefficient distribution include
acquisition of transmission data or estimation of the
distribution using the emission data.

Methods for correcting for this attenuation error are easily
implemented in positron tomography because only the line
integrals of the attenuation coefficients are needed.

Spatial Resolution and Uniformity of Spatial Resolution

Because the region of object space which the collimator
"sees" varies with distance from a collimator, the point spread
function or resolution varies with distance as shown in Fig. 4.
Methods to compensate for this variation in the point spread
function include modification of the data by performing the
geometric mean of opposing projections (50) and a computational
approach which includes the point spread function in the reconstruction algorithm (51) which has not been satisfactorily
implemented because of the statistical limitations of the
available data in practical applications. Focusing collimator
systems can overcome this problem to some extent but not
entirely (16,48). Positron tomography has this problem to only
a small extent relative to the single photon systems.

The spatial resolution for single photon devices can be
11 mm FWHM with good sensitivity if special systems are used as
show in Table 1. Though the spatial resolution of the gamma
camera systems can be acceptable, the loss of sensitivity due
to the required collimation has resulted in commercial systems
with greater than 20 mm FWHM resolution.

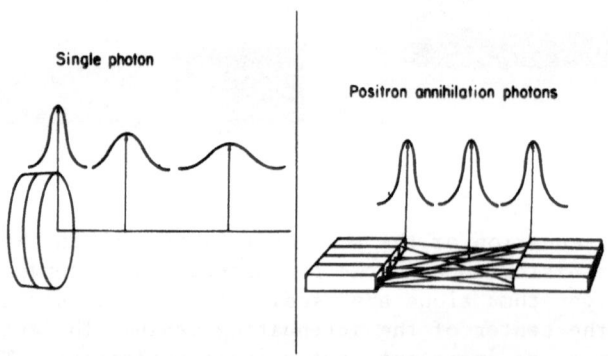

Fig. 4. Uniformity of resolution is generally poor with single
photon tomographic systems unless special collimation is used.

Table 1

Device	Sensitivity per plane (cts sec^{-1} μCi^{-1}cc^{-1})	Resolution	
		Transverse (mm)	Axial (mm)
Positron Tomographs (BGO)	50,000-75,000	7.5-9	15
Mark IV (9)	15,400	17	17
Harvard Scanning Multi-detector Brain System (16)	14,000	10	13
Harvard Scanning Multi-detector Body System (17)	4,600	26	33
Tomomatic-64 (20)	17,000	17	23
Headtome (22)	21,000	10	20
200-element HP Germanium System (24)	2,400[a]	20	20
Anger camera	~600	11	<11

[a] Estimated from 12,600 cps/μCi/cc in 1,640 cm^3 phantom.

Increased sensitivity is attained at the cost of resolution. The major impact of poor resolution is a loss of ability to quantitate the actual concentration in regions less than two times the dimension of the resolution in the reconstructed image as demonstrated in Figs. 5 and 6. A system with the resolution of 20 mm FWHM has only limited ability to give data representative of the true concentration.

Scatter

The contribution of scattered photons to the collected data in single photon tomography as well as in positron tomography can amount to as much as 30 percent of the total collected events. This means that a true void in a phantom or subject will have an observed activity of about 30 percent that of the activity in contiguous regions of the object. This problem has until recently been ignored, probably because the problems of uniform sensitivity in data collection and attenuation compensation were considered more important. Because this problem can

284

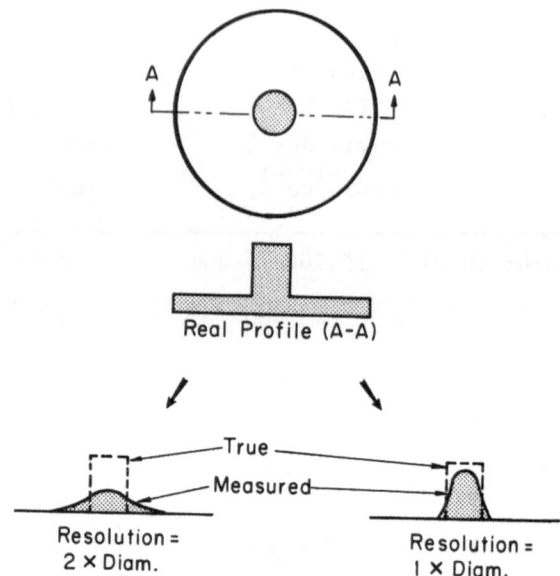

Fig. 5. System resolution defined as the full width at half maximum will not capture the true concentration of an object with similar or smaller dimensions.

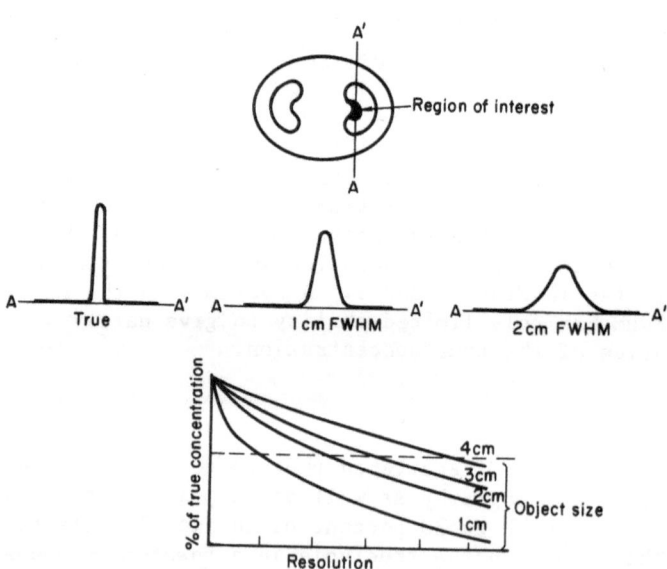

Fig. 6. Loss in quantitative recovery due to spreading out of activity from poor resolution systems.

lead to serious quantitative errors, the single photon
tomography procedure should include a scatter correction method.
The simplest method is to assume that the contribution from
scatter is constant or uniform across the image. If an estimate
of the scatter is made from phantom studies, then the reconstructed image can be corrected by subtracting the background.
Another method of recalculating the concentration ratios of
object to background assumes a constant scatter fraction (49).
These simple methods are not applicable generally because
Compton scattering depends on the shape of the scattering
material (the distribution of attenuation coefficients) and on
the distribution of the radionuclide. In addition, the scatter
contribution is very much dependent on the collimator and the
energy window. Some object dependent methods proposed for
scatter correction in positron tomography are also applicable
to single photon tomography (52). For example, using a phantom
with a large void it is possible to estimate what linear filter
and threshold will give the scatter contribution, then using
these parameters estimate the scatter image using the reconstructed image and the appropriate filter derived in the photon
study. An estimate of the true data is the difference between
the reconstructed image and the scatter image.

Sensitivity and Statistics

The major limitation of single photon tomography is the poor
statistics available for acceptable doses to the patient. The
problem lies in the need to collimate the photons to a small
region of a detector which results in a decrease of the solid
angle in proportion to the improvement (decrease) in resolution.
The decrease in solid angle means a decrease in statistics.
This channeling is not a problem for positron tomography because
electronic collimation is used. Even in positron tomography,
there is a need for more data because in both forms of emission
tomography there are about 1000 times fewer events collected
than in X-ray CT wherein 10^9 events are needed to calculate a
statistically reliable image. In emission tomography about
10^6 events per image are required for most studies of the
thorax and abdomen; however, this requires 26 minutes or more
for the rotating camera methods (26,53) and less time for the
single section systems, especially designed for tomography
(9,16,17).

An important aspect of the statistics problem is the fact
that the propagation of errors associated with the calculations
for correction of attenuation effects presents additional
statistical requirements. The usual method used for the
evaluation of RMS uncertainty in an image is to calculate
$1/\sqrt{N}$ where N is the number of events per pixel. For 1.2
million events, the result is five percent for 3000 resolution
elements (Fig. 7). Due, however, to the reconstruction, the
actual root-mean-squared (RMS) uncertainty is 44 percent. To

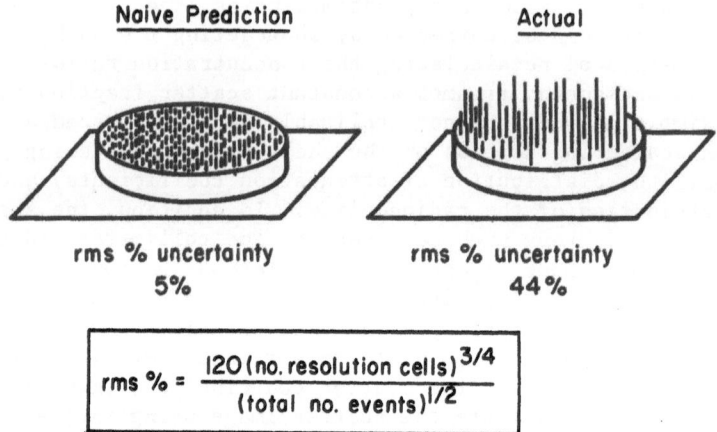

Total events − 1,200,000
Total resolution elements − 3000
400 events/element

Naive Prediction   Actual

rms % uncertainty   rms % uncertainty
5%   44%

$$\text{rms \%} = \frac{120\,(\text{no. resolution cells})^{3/4}}{(\text{total no. events})^{1/2}}$$

Fig. 7. Propagation of errors in reconstruction tomography leads to a decrease in quantitative certainty over that expected from Poisson statistics.

get better than 44 percent, one must have fewer resolution elements or more than a million events. This is the fundamental problem in the development of emission tomography.

Sensitivity involves the amount of detector material one can put around the patient and the efficiency of the detector material. The Union Carbide Cleon device (now called the Harvard Scanning Multidetector System) is an attempt to get more crystal material around the patient. Detectors are moved in and out and back and forth (Fig. 1c). The sensitivities of these systems are very good compared with that of a single gamma camera (Table 1). These devices produce images with artifacts primarily because the data set does not contain sufficient angular sampling and a form of aliasing occurs in the reconstruction. The present resolution for the head system is 11 mm and that for body machine is about 2.4 cm.

The statistical considerations of Fig. 7 are not entirely relevant to the actual imaging situations wherein there is a concentration of radionuclide in one portion of the transverse section rather than a more-or-less continuous distribution throughout the section. In practice the source distribution is localized to about 20 percent of the resolution elements, thus the effective number of resolution elements in a 3000 pixel image will lead to an RMS uncertainty of about 20 percent. This problem is dealt with analytically by considering the number of

resolution elements in a transverse section as the number of
elements in which the radionuclide is concentrated plus a
reduced number of background elements. The reduction factor is
based on the contrast. The basic equation for a uniform disc
distribution is (50):

$$\text{rms } \% = \frac{120 \, (n_t)^{3/4}}{(N_t)^{1/2}}$$

where n_t is the number of resolution cells and N_t is the
total number of detected events. The number of resolution cells
n_t is modifed by the expression for the effective number of
resolution cells:

$$n_t = M_t + \frac{M_b}{C}$$

where M_t is the number of cells in the target, M_b is the number in

the background, and C is the contrast. Thus, the operational equation

for a distribution with a uniform background and one target

concentration is:

$$\text{rms } \% = \frac{120 \left(M_t + \frac{M_b}{C} \right)^{3/4}}{(N_t)^{1/2}}$$

The importance of this modification can be appreciated by the
example of Fig. 8 wherein a comparison is made between heart
imaging with Tl-201 and heart blood pool imaging with Tc-99m
labeled red cells. A similar comparison using a Tc-99m radiopharmaceutical which concentrates in the myocardium (54) can
also be made. The gain in statistical uncertainty is due to
both the concentration of radionuclide in a few resolution cells
and the increase in amount of activity which can be injected,
if Tc-99m or I-123 are used instead of Tl-201. Measurements
made of the relative myocardial perfusion have shown good
sensitivity for detection of regions of low perfusion; however,
the resolution is only 20 mm FWHM, or greater. Thus, the true
quantitative ability will be poor (Figs. 5 and 6) until a system
with better resolution is used for the thorax of humans. New
heart seeking agents using Tc-99m will allow single photon

288

MYOCARDIUM   BLOOD POOL

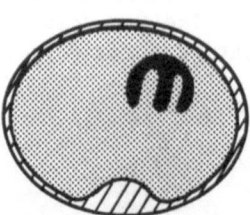 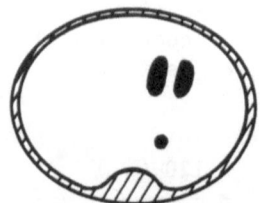

	(2 mCi Tl-201)	(20 mCi ^{99m}Tc-rbc)
Activity in section	15 µCi	250 µCi
Resolution cells	20 mm	20 mm
Effective number of resolution cells	1540	120
$(M_t + \frac{Mb}{c})$		

$$\text{RATIO*:} \quad \frac{\text{Myocardium rms uncertainty}}{\text{Blood pool rms uncertainty}} = \frac{(1540)^{3/4}}{(120)} \cdot \frac{(15)^{-1/2}}{(250)} = 28$$

Fig. 8. Comparison of the available statistics and difference in the effective number of resolution errors for two different single photon tomographic procedures.

tomography of the heart to become a practical procedure from a statistical standpoint, but variable attenuation compensation methods and systems with resolutions better than that presently available commercially are needed.

The arguments presented above regarding the importance of the effective number of resolution elements are in favor of imaging the heart but against imaging the distribution of radionuclides in the lungs as the lungs occupy most of the resolution elements. Thus, the effective number of elements is close to the actual number.

A single photon system having four detector banks arranged around the head (Fig. 9) has a sensitivity which is not very much less than that of a positron system for a resolution in the range of 20 mm FWHM (39). For a resolution of 10 mm full width half max or better the positron tomography sensitivity advantage is a factor of 10 or more than that of the single photon tomography (Table 1).

A single photon system for imaging the thorax or body has a very low sensitivity primarily because the sensitivity is inversely proportional to the radius squared for a single photon system. Here positron tomographic systems have a great

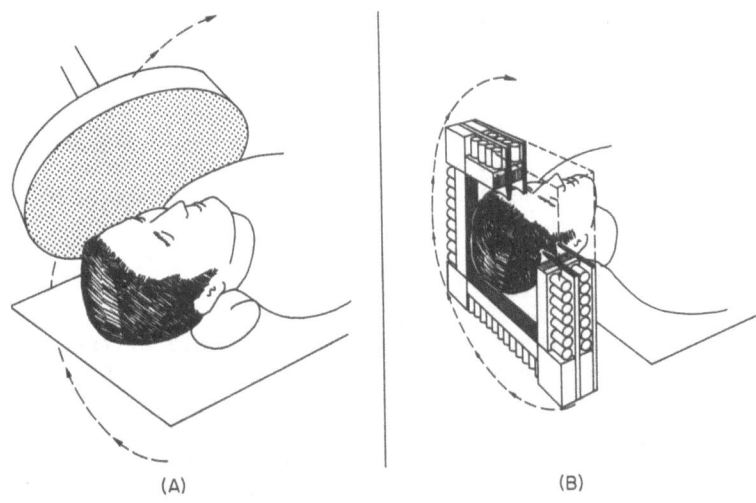

(A)   (B)

Fig. 9. A properly designed single photon tomographic instrument for the head can be 20 times more sensitive than a single gamma camera.

advantage because their sensitivity decreases only in proportion to the inverse in radius (39). Single photon tomography perspectives should not be based on statistical results from dog studies. The differences in the attenuation of data and this solid angle factor from a dog study to a human study are very great. From (50) we calculate that the available photons for a human abdomen study are one-half those from an animal study. The solid angle loss is a factor of 6 or greater depending on the size of the patient port. If the radionuclide is distributed in man's organs as it is in the dog, an additional loss factor must be taken into account because of the difference in organ size. Thus, we can expect an overall reduction in the statistics per slice to be a factor of 12 for a human body study compared to a dog study.

Specially designed single section machines do not give multiple continuous layers because shielding is used between layers to limit scatter and allow for better sensitivity in the collimator design. The high sensitivity of a single section, single photon device such as the Harvard multicrystal scanning device is not easily extended to a multisection instrument. An advantage of single photon tomographic systems employing gamma camera concepts is that multiple continuous sections can be obtained; however, this comes at the loss of sensitivity.

Whereas it is possible to obtain single photon tomographs using commercially available Anger cameras, specially designed devices will give a sensitivity improvement of a factor of 2-10 depending on the in plane resolution and slice thickness. Innovative collimator designs include the use of diverging collimators to improve sensitivity with the gamma camera (55,56). The design of Fig. 2f involves 36 gamma cameras and is highly impractical; however, some new device which incorporates modern digital gamma cameras or multicrystal arrays surrounding the patient is needed if practical whole body single photon tomography is to be performed.

Dynamic Emission Tomography

Dyanmic ECT refers to use of a time sequence of transverse sections from which uptake and washout kinetics can be deduced. The two major limitations to the application of dynamic computed tomography are the low statistics obtained and the necessity for rapid angular sampling. If motion of the detector assembly over about 45° is required, then imaging periods of about 10 sec are probably reasonable, and uptake kinetics might not be practical for single photon tomography. Washout kinetics, however, such as clearance from brain, heart, and kidney, can be obtained using single photon devices with which one can collect more than 100,000 events in 1 min or less. A single photon system with four banks of detectors arranged as shown in Fig. 9 has been developed recently. This system has the requisite resolution and can perform dynamic washout studies after inhalation of Xe-133 or Xe-127 (20,21). The Kuhl Mark IV scanner has high sensitivity as well (9). The Harvard Scanning multidetector system has adequate sensitivity, but must be modified to acquire more angles as has recently been shown (67).

Clinical Applications

Applications of single photon tomography for clinical studies preceded x-ray CT (9) and the first demonstration of quantitative physiological studies with single photon tomography was made in 1975 (57). At present the main interest in brain imaging is focused on the use of two approaches to measurement of brain blood flow. One approach involves rapidly sampling the change in activity using xenon-133 (20,21) and hopefully in the future xenon-127 where the dose advantage is a factor of 6. The second approach came as the result of the development of amines which(58-60)accumulate in the brain. The static measurement of the relative accumulation of the iodo-amphetamine compounds can be used to infer local cerebral metabolism (10,13; see also T. Hill et al. in this Symposium). The possibility for revival in brain imaging using emission tomography appears to be great because the new compounds concentrate in the brain in proportion to flow and can be imaged over short periods of time (5 minutes) with a resolution of 11 mm to 12 mm full width half max with appropriate instrumentation. Reviews of the promise of single photon tomography of the brain are found in Refs. 61-64.

Heart imaging over the past five years has been disappoint-
ing because the resolution of the commercial gamma camera
devices and the statistics available from the radiopharmaceuticals have not been adequate. With the advent of new compounds
which concentrate in the heart (54) there is renewed interest
in single photon tomography of the heart. Yet, a machine
designed specifically to do single photon tomography of the
heart is not yet commercially available.

Examination of liver and kidneys with single photon
tomography has been shown to be more specific and sensitive in
the detection of lesions than conventional projection imaging
(53). However, here, as in other parts of the body, the data
acquisition time is in the range of 30 minutes for available
devices because of the need for adequate statistics to implement
a reconstruction with distributed sources.

SUMMARY AND FUTURE PROSPECTS

1. Single photon tomography of the brain has an important
future, particularly through the advent of new radiopharmaceuticals (58-60) which appear to follow brain flow and can give
tranverse section images with scan periods of approximately 5
minutes (10-13).

2. The use of radiopharmaceuticals labeled with Tc-99m or
I-123 allows the injection of 10-20 millicuries which is 10-20
times more than the usual thallium-201 dose. This advantage
plus the statistical advantage which occurs when most of the
activity in a section is located in relatively few resolution
elements, makes single photon tomography of the thorax feasible
but improvement in instrumentation is needed. The resolution
will unlikely be better than 15 mm FWHM for studies of less than
30 minutes in body imaging.

3. Longitudinal tomography or tomography with coded
apertures involves limited angular sampling and gives artifacts
which are dependent on the orientation of the imaging system
relative to the geometry of the object being imaged. These
systems are not considered satisfactory alternatives to full
angular viewing around 360 degrees.

4. Methods for attenuation correction for constant
attenuation such as found in the head are available and
effective in reducing the single photon tomograph data to a
quantitative description. For variable attenuation the only
method available is that involving the incorporation of weighting factors in an iterative least squares approach which will
become practical with the advent of expanded computing
capabilities in small machines available to nuclear medicine
departments.

5. Data correction procedures need to be applied to compensate for

a) Non-uniformity of detector response
b) Attenuation
c) Variation in the point spread function
d) Scatter.

6. The greatest need is to develop a tomographic instrument which will meet the resolution and sensitivity requirements of the clinical situation. Though careful analyses are available (39,49,64,65) adequate instruments for head and body single photon tomography are not yet available.

ACKNOWLEDGMENTS

This work was supported by the U.S. Department of Energy and the National Institute of Heart, Lung and Blood under Grant P01 HL25840.

REFERENCES

1. Kuhl, D. E. and Edwards, R. Q. "Image separation radio-isotope scanning." Radiology, 80 (1963), 653-662.

2. Budinger, T. F. and Gullberg, G. T. "Three dimensional reconstruction in nuclear medicine by iterative least squares and Fourier transform techniques." IEEE Trans. Nucl. Sci., NS-21 (1974), 2.

3. Oppenheim, B. E. "More accurate algorithms for iterative three-dimension reconstruction." IEEE Trans. Nucl. Sci. NS-21 (1974), 72.

4. Todd-Pokropek A. E. "The formation and display of section scans." In: Proceedings of Symposium of American Congress of Radiology, 1971. Amsterdam, Excerpta Medica (1972), 545.

5. Bowley, A. R., Taylor, C. G., Causer, D. A., Barber, D. C., Kever, W. I., Undrill, P. E., Corfield, J. R., Mallard, J. R. "A radioisotope scanner for rectilinear, arc, trasnsverse section and longitudinal section scanner." (ASS--The Aberdeen Section Scanner). Br. J. Radiol. 46 (1973), 262-271.

6. Myers, M. J., Keyes, W. I., Mallard, J. R. "An analysis of tomographic scanning systems." In: Medical Radioisotope Scintigraphy, Vol. 1, Vienna, IAEA, SM-164/48 (1972) 331-345.

7. Tanaka, E., Shimizu, T., Iinuma, T. A. et al. "Digital simulation of section image reconstruction." Natl. Inst. Radiol. Sci. (Japan), Report NIRS-12 (1973) 3-4.

8. Keyes, J. W., Simmon, W. "Computer techniques for spatial (three dimensional) imaging." In: Sharing Computer Programs and Technology in Nuclear Medicine, (eds., Clark F. H., Maskewitz, B. F., Gurney, J. Oak Ridge, Tenn.), USAEC Report CONF-730627 (1973), 190-201.

9. Kuhl, D. E., Edwards, R. Q., Ricci, A. R., Yacob, R. J., Mich, T. J., Alavi, A. "The Mark IV system for radionuclide computed tomography of the brain." Radiology 121 (1976), 405-413.

10. Kuhl, D. E., Barrio, J. R., Huang, S. C., Selin, C., Ackermann, R. F., Lear, J. L., Wu, J. L., Lin, T. H., and Phelps, M. E. "Quantifying local cerebral blood flow by n-isopropyl-p-^{123}I-iodoamphetamine (IMP) tomography." J. Nucl. Med. 23 (1982), 250.

11. Stoddart, H. F., Stoddart, H. A. "A new development in single gamma transaxial tomography Union Carbide focused collimator scanner." IEEE Trans. Nucl. Sci. NS-27 (1979), 2710-2712.

12. Hill, T. C., Costello, P., Gramm, H. F., Lovett, R., McNeil, B. J., Treves, S. "Early clinical experience with a radionuclide emission computed tomographic brain imaging system. Radiology 128 (1978), 803-806.

13. Hill, T. C., Holman, B. L., Lovett, R., O'Leary, D. H., Front, D., Magistretti, P., Zimmerman, R. E., Moore, S. C., Clouse, M. E., Wu, J. J., Lin, J. H., and Baldwin, R. M. "Initial experience with SPECT (Single Photon Computerized Tomography) of the brain using n-isopropyl I-123-p-iodo-amphetamine." J. Nucl. Med. 23 (1982), 243-249.

14. Jarritt, P. H., Ell, P. J., Myers, M. J., Brown, N.J.G., and Deacon, J. M. "A new transverse-section brain imager for single-gamma emitters." J. Nucl. Med. 20 (1979), 319-327.

15. Holman, B. L., Hill, T. C., Wynne, J., Lovett, R. D., Zimmerman, R. E., and Smith, E. M. "Single-photon transaxial emission computed tomography of the heart in normal subjects and in patients with infarction." J. Nucl. Med., Vol. 20 (1979), 736-740.

16. Zimmerman, R. E., Kirsch, C. M., Lovett, R. D. et al. "Single photon emission computed tomography with short focal length detectors. In Single Photon Emission Computed Tomography and Other Selected Topics. Sorenson, J. A., Ed. New York, Society of Nuclear Medicine, (1980), 147-157.

294

17. Kirsch, C. M., Moore, S. C., Zimmerman, R. E. English, R. J., and Holman, B. L. "Characteristics of a scanning, multidetector, single photon ECT body imager." J. Nucl. Med. 22 (1981), 726-731.

18. Treves, S., Hill, T. C., Van Praagh, R. et al. "Computed tomography of the heart using thallium-201 in children." Radiology 133 (1979), 707-710.

19. Loken, M. K., Frick, M., COok, A. et al. "Evaluation of a single photon emission tomographic system. In: Emission Computed Tomography: The Single Photon Approach. (Ed., A Paras, E. Eikman), HHS Publication No. FDA 81-8177, Bur. Rad. Health, (1981), 252-267.

20. Bonte, F. J., Stokely, E. M. Single-photon tomographic study of regional cerebral blood flow in stroke. J. Nucl. Med. 22: 1049-1053, 1981.

21. Lassen, N. A., Henriksen, L., Paulson, O. Regional cerebral blood flow in stroke by 133-Xenon inhalation and emission tomography. Stroke 12: (1981), 284-288.

22. Kanno, I., Uemura, K., Miura, S. et al. HEADTOME: A hybrid emission tomograph for single photon and positron emission imaging of the brain. J. Comput. Assist. Tomogr. 5: (1981), 216-226.

23. Budinger, T. F., Cahoon, J. L., Derenzo, S. E., Gullberg, G. T., Moyer, B. R., and Yano, Y. "Three dimensional imaging of the myocardium with radionuclides. Radiology, 125 (1977), 433.

24. Keyes, J. W., Orlandea, N., Heetderks, W. J., Leonard, P. F., and Rogers, W. L. "The humongotron--A scintillation camera transaxial tomograph." J. Nucl. Med. 18 (1977), 381.

25. Jaszczak, R. J., Murphy, P. H., Huard, D., and Burdine, J. A. "Radionuclide emission computed tomography of the head with ^{99m}Tc and a scintillation camera." J. Nucl. Med., 18 (1977), 373.

26. Burdine, J. A., Murphy, P. H., and DePuey, E. G. "Radionuclide computed tomography of the body using routine radiopharmaceuticals. II. Clinical applications." J. Nucl. Med. 20 (1979), 209.

27. Keyes, J. W., Jr., Leonard, P. F., Brody, S. L. et al. "Myocardial infarct quantification in the dog by single photon emission computed tomography." Circulation 58 (1978), 227-232.

28. Keyes, J. W., Jr., Brady, T. J., Leonard, P. F., et al. "Calculation of viable and infarcted myocardial mass from thallium-201 tomograms." N. Nucl. Med. 22 (1981), 339-343.

29. Carril, I. M., MacDonald, A. F., Dendy, P. P. et al. Granial Scintigraphy: value of adding emission computed tomographic sections to conventional pertechnetate images (512 cases)." J. Nucl. Med. 20 (1979), 1117-1123.

30. Soussaline, F., Todd-Pokropek, A.E., Plummer, D., Comar, D., Loch, C., Houle, S., and Kellershohn, C. "The physical performances of a single slice positron tomographic system and preliminary results in a clinical environment." Eur. J. of Nucl. Med. 4 (1979), 237-249.

31. Ell, P. J., Jarritt, P. H., Cullum. "Detection of single photons with multidetector devices and a rotating gamma camera." In: Receptor-Binding Radiotracers, Vol. II. (ed. by W. C. Eckelman, CRC Press, 1982).

32. Koral, K. F., Rogers, W. L. and Knoll, G. F. "Digital tomographic imaging with a time-modulated pseudorandom coded aperture and an Anger camera." J. Nucl. Med. 16 (1975), 402-414.

33. LeFree, M. T., Vogel, R. A., Kirch, D. L. and Steele, P. P. "Seven-pinhole tomography - A technical description." J. Nucl. Med. 22 (1981), 48.

34. Vogel, R. A., Kirch, D. L., LeFree, M. T., and Steele, P. P. "A new method of multiplanar emission tomography using a seven pinhole collimator and an Anger scintillation camera." J. Nucl. Med. 19 (1979), 648.

35. Mathieu, L., and Budinger, T. F. "Pinhole digital tomography." Proceedings of the First World Congress of Nuclear Medicine, (1974), 1264-1266.

36. MacDonald, B., Chang, L.-T., Perez-Mendez, V. et al. "Gamma-ray imaging using a Fresnel zone-plate aperture multiwire proportional chamber, and computer reconstruction." IEEE Trans. Nucl. Sci. NS-21 (1974), 678-684.

37. Budinger, T. F. and MacDonald, B. "Reconstruction of the Fresnel-coded gamma camera images by digital computer." J. Nucl. Med. 6 (1975), 309-313.

38. Chang, W., Lin, S. L., and Henkin, R. E. "A rotatable quadrant slant hole collimator for tomography (QSH): a stationary scintillation camera based SPECT system." In: Single Photon Emission Computed Tomography and Other

Selected Computer Topics, (ed., J. A. Sorenson, 1980),
Society of Nuclear Medicine, New York 1980, 81.

39. Budinger, T. F.   "Physical attributes of single-photon
    tomography."   J. Nucl. Med. 22 (1980), 579.

40. Williams, D. L., Ritchie, J. L., Harp, G. D., Caldwell, J.
    H., and Hamilton, G. W.   "In vivo simulation of thallium-
    201 myocardial scintigraphy by seven-pinhole emission
    tomography."   J. Nucl. Med. 21 (1980), 821.

41. Rizi, H. R., Kline, R. C., Thrall, J. H., Besozzi, M. C.,
    Keyes, J. W., Jr., Rogers, W. L., Clare, J., and Pitt, B.
    "Thallium-201 myocardial scintigraphy: A critical
    comparison of seven-pinhole tomography and conventional
    planar imaging."   J. Nucl. Med. 22 (1981), 493-499.

42. Stokely, E. M., Tipton, D. M., Buja, L. M., Lewis, S. E.,
    DeVous, M. D., Sr., Bonte, F. J., Parkey, R. W. and
    Willerson, J. T.   "Quantitation of experimental canine
    infarct size using multipinhole single-photon tomography."
    J. NUcl. Med. 22 (1981), 55.

43. Tamaki, N., Mukal, T., Ishil, Y., Yonekura, Y., Kambera,
    H., Kawal, C. and Torizuka, K.   "Clinical evaluation of
    thallium-201 myocardial tomography using a rotating gamma
    camera: Comparison with seven pinhole tomography."   J.
    Nucl. Med. (1981).

44. Townsend, D., Peney, C., Jeavons, A.   "Objective
    reconstruction from focused positron tomograms."   Phys.
    Med. Biol. 23 (1978), 235-244.

45. Chang, L. T.   "A method for attenuation correction in
    radionuclide computed tomography."   IEEE Trans. Nucl. Sci.
    NS-25 (1978), 638-643.

46. Budinger, T. F., Gullberg, G. T., Huesman, R. H.   "Emission
    computed tomography. In: Topics in Applied Physics, Vol.
    32: Image Reconstruction from Projections; Implementation
    and Applications, (ed., Herman, G. T., Berlin, Springer-
    Verlag, 1979, 147-246).

47. Gullberg, G. T. and Budinger, T. F.   "The use of filtering
    methods to compensate for constant attenuation in single
    photon emission computed tomography."   IEEE Trans. Biomed.
    Eng. 2 (1981), 142-157.

48. Jaszczak, R. J., Chang, L. T., Stein, N. A., Moore, F. E.
    "Whole-body single-photon emission computed tomography
    using dual, large-field-of-view scintillation cameras."
    Phys. Med. Biol. 24 (1979), 1123-1143.

49. Jaszczak, R. J., Coleman, R. E., Whitehead, F. R. "Physical factors affecting quantitative measurements using camera-based single photon emission computed tomography (SPECT)." IEEE Trans. Nucl. Sci. NS-28 (1981), 69-80.

50. Budinger, T. F., Derenzo, S. E., Gullberg, G. T., Greenberg, W. L., and Huesman, R. H. "Emission computed assisted tomography with single-photon and positron annihilation photon emitters." J. Comput. Assist. Tomog 1 (1977), 131-145.

51. Ansari, A., Wee, W. G. Reconstruction from projections in the presence of distortion. In: Proceedings of the 1977 IEEE Conference on Decision and Control, Vol. 1, New Orleans, IEEE 77CH1269-OCS (1977), 361-366.

52. Derenzo, S. E., Budinger, T. F., Huesman, R. H., Cahoon, J. L., and Vuletich, T. "Imaging properties of a positron tomograph with 280 BGO crystals." IEEE Trans. Nucl. Sci. NS-28 (1981), 81-89.

53. Jaszczak, R. J., Coleman, R. E., Lim, C. B., Whitehead, F. R. "Lesion detection with single photon emission computed tomography (SPECT) and conventiunal imaging. J. Nucl. Med., 1982, in press.

54. Deutsch, E., Bushong, W., Glavan, K. A., Elder, R. C., Sodd, V. J., Scholz, K. L., Fortman, D. L., Lukes, S. J. "Heart imaging with cathionic complexes of technetium." Science (1981), 85-86.

55. Jaszczak, R. J., Chang, L-T., Murphy, P. H. "Single photon emission computed tomography using multi-slice fan beam collimators." IEEE Trans. Nucl. Sci. NS-26 (1979), 610-618.

56. Lim, C. B., Chang, L. T., Jaszczak, R. J. "Performance analysis of three camera configurations for single photon emission computed tomography." IEEE Trans Nucl. Sci. NS-27 (1980), 559-568.

57. Kuhl, D. E., Reivich, M., Alavi, A., Nyary, I., and Staum, M. M. "Local Cerebral Blood Volume Determined by Three-Dimensional Reconstruction of Radionuclide Scan Data." Circulation Research, 36 (1975), 610.

58. Sargent, T. S., Budinger, T. F., Braun, G., Shulgin, A. T., Braun, U. "An iodinated catecholamine congener for brain imaging and metabolic studies." J. Nucl. Med. 19 (1978), 71-76.

59. Kung, H. F., Blau, M. "Regional intracellular pH shift; a proposed new mechanism for radiopharmaceutical uptake in brain and other tissues." J. Nucl. Med. 21 (1980), 147-152.

60. Winchell, H. S., Horst, W. D., Braun, L., Oldendorf, W. H., Hattner, R., Parker, H. "N-Isopropyl-[^{123}I] p - Iodoamphetamine: single-pass uptake and washout; binding to brain synaptosomes; and localization in dog and monkey brain." J. Nucl. Med. 21 (1980), 947-952.

61. Hill, T. C., Lovett, R. D., and McNeil, B. J. "Observations on the clinical value of emission tomography." J. Nucl. Med., 21 (1980), 613-616.

62. Cowan, R. J., Watson, N. E. "Special characteristics and potential of single photon emission computed tomography in the brain." Semin. Nucl. Med. X (1980), 335-344.

63. Oldendorf, W. H. "Nuclear medicine in clinical neurology: an update." Ann. Neurol. 10 (1981), 207-213.

64. Budinger, T. F. "Revival of Clinical Nuclear Medicine Brain Imaing." J. of Nucl. Med. 22 (1981) 1094-1097.

65. Flower, M. A., Rowe, R. W., Webb, S., and Keyes, W. I. "A comparison of three systems for performing single-photon emission tomography." Phys. Med. Biol. 26 (1981), 671-691.

66. Rusinek, H., Reich, T., Youdin, M. "An ultrapure germanium detector array for quantitating three-dimensional distribution of a radionuclide: a study of phantoms." J. Nucl. Med 21, (1980), 777-782.

67. Moore, S. C., Parker, J. A., Zimmerman, R. E., Budinger, T. F., and Holman, B. L. "The effect of angular sampling on image quality of the Harvard multi-detector ECT brain scanner." Third World Congress of Nuclear Medicine, Paris (1982).

BIOCHEMICAL CONSIDERATIONS IN THE DESIGN
OF RADIOPHARMACEUTICALS

David R. Elmaleh, E. Livni and S. Levy

Massachusetts General Hospital, Boston, MA 02114

The goal of radiopharmaceutical chemistry is to design and
develop radiotracers targeted to an organ or function whose
activity kinetics in tissue can be detected externally by a gamma
or a positron device. Three years ago, Eckelman and Reba (1)
divided radiopharmaceuticals into the general categories of
specific and non-specific agents. The specific radiopharmaceuticals are the tracers that follow a biochemical pathway or are
involved in a particular interaction, for example metabolic
substrates, drugs or analogs, and antibodies. Non-specific
radiopharmaceuticals include radiolabeled liposomes, cells,
microspheres, perfusion agents, inert gases, ethers, alcohols or
thallium-201. The design and development of both types of
radiopharmaceuticals are important. In the case of myocardial
imaging agents, a perfusion agent that will enable differentiation of various stages of ischemia and infarction is as essential
as a specific tracer that will reflect metabolism since both
perfusion and metabolic functions change with injury.

This paper will focus on trends in the design of specific
agents. The greatest advantage of a specific metabolic substrate
is its biochemical rationale, whereas for the non-specific radiopharmaceuticals the rationale is more general in its nature
(charge, lipophilicity, size, etc.). The best radionuclides for
the development of specific tracers are the positron emitting
nuclides: carbon-11, nitrogen-13, oxygen-15 and fluorine-18.
Three of these nuclides are the building blocks of organic
molecules and as such they can be introduced into a metabolite
or organic molecule skeleton without altering its chemical
structure so that metabolic or biochemical pathways can be

followed. Fluorine-18 can be exchanged for a hydrogen atom in a molecule, and in many instances this does not significantly change the behavior of the organic or metabolic radiotracer. Other radionuclides such as iodine-123 or bromine-75 may also play an important role in labeling analogs for use in nuclear medicine.

The factors affecting the selection and design of radio-pharmaceuticals are: (a) the nature of the information required, such as static images for localization, data on transport, metabolism, or receptor binding sites and their properties, animal biodistribution studies or human clinical studies. (b) the chemical basis or biochemical rationale for the development of the radiopharmaceuticals. (c) the availability of a radio-nuclide with specific physical properties and of the chemical route for preparation of the radiolabeled agent.

Several recent reviews deal with the production of the positron radionuclides and their incorporation into biologically active molecules (2-9). We will discuss briefly some of the general aspects associated with labeling procedures.

GENERAL CONSIDERATIONS IN THE DESIGN OF RADIOPHARMACEUTICALS

Strategy of labeling with short-lived radionuclides

The short half-life of the positron emitting carbon-11, nitrogen-13, oxygen-15 and fluorine-18 radionuclides imposes some constraints on labeling strategies. It is essential to introduce the radionuclide in the latest possible stage of the synthesis. The stable precursors can be prepared and stored. Most of the reactions for labeling must be completed in less than three half-lives of the radionuclide from the end of bombardment (3). A mixture of labeled and unlabeled products are obtained and fast methods of separation, such as gas chromatography for gases or volatile compounds and liquid chromatography for others, should be adopted. The best approach for separation depends on the chemical characteristics of the preparation and should be simple in nature, e.g., solution separations of non-polar from polar compounds. If any final liquid chromatography purification is required, the preferred eluent should be water or an isotonic non-toxic buffer so that for in vivo studies the compounds can be administered in approximately isotonic solution.

Stereochemical effects

In many instances the biologic activity is related to the stereochemistry of the substrate molecules which may exist in two or more isomeric forms, geometrical or optical isomers. For example, the L-amino acids are the active forms, whereas the

D-forms are non-active or toxic; ortho- meta- and para- isomers of fluorophenyl-L-alanine (as analogs of L-phenylalanine) have different biological activity (10). When a single stereo-isomer of a labeled compound is required, a synthetic sequence with 100% stereospecificity should be adopted if possible, e.g., enzymatic syntheses with $^{13}NH_3$ were developed for several amino acids. Alternatively, an epimeric or racemic mixture may be generated and a procedure of resolution applied to the following step, e.g., the synthesis of some ^{18}F amino acids (10).

Specific activity

The specific activity is an important consideration for all radiopharmaceuticals produced. Fowler and Wolf (11) have commented on the confusion in the reporting of specific activity and have suggested the following nomenclature in order to eliminate misunderstanding: CF, carrier-free; NCA, no-carrier-added; and CA, carrier added. A high specific activity is essential in some central nervous system research. When receptor site mapping and quantitation are investigated, activities should be in the mCi/pmol range, since with specific activities in the mCi/mg range saturation problems may be encountered. Metabolic analogs, especially those containing ^{18}F are usually toxic due to their inhibition of the biochemical pathway, and a carrier-free or no-carrier-added high specific activity preparation should be considered. Methods of preparation that do not introduce stable fluorine into the reaction should be used when possible.

Table 1 lists the calculated specific activities for some radionuclides. It is clear that those with the more attractive properties are carbon-11, nitrogen-13, fluorine-18, iodine-123 and bromine-75.

Advantages and disadvantages of substrates and their analogs

When an analog is used as a metabolic substrate, the following must be considered in the interpretation of the data: (a) There are differences in the transport properties of the analog compared with the metabolite. (b) The enzyme affinities of the analog in different species may vary more than those of the natural substrate. (c) The correction for differences between metabolites and analogs may be more difficult when the organ of interest is in a diseased state. (d) The analog may have a toxic effect if it is an enzyme inhibitor or alters the metabolic pathway. (e) The radiation dosimetry may have a significant impact on the study designed.

Table 1

Physical Properties and Calculated Maximal
Specific Activities of Some Isotopes

ISOTOPE	HALF-LIFE	γ-ENERGIES KeV	CALCULATED MAX. SPECIFIC ACTIVITY Ci/mmole
Carbon-11	20 min	511	9,340,000
Fluorine-18	110 min	511	1,700,000
Bromine-75	95.5 min	511 286	1,955,400
Bromine-76	16.1 h	511 559 < OTHERS	193,300
Bromine-77	57 h	239 520	54,000
Bromine-82	35.5 h	554 619 < OTHERS	88,000
Iodine-123	13.3 h	159	234,000
Iodine-125	59.7 d	35	2,200
Iodine-131	8.1 d	364	16,000
Selenium-75	120 d	136 265 280	1,000

The use of a metabolite also presents certain problems in studying metabolism or drug pharmacokinetics, since the metabolite enters a chemical pathway which may lead to the degradation of the molecule and the elimination of its radioactivity, and the introduction and incorporation of the activity into other molecules. This necessitates alteration in the model of tracer kinetics to reflect washout and changes of activities in tissue, recirculation in plasma and reextraction as other metabolites. Some of these problems can be corrected when fast and meaningful sampling is possible. However it is not clear whether the transport properties and enzyme kinetics of the metabolite itself are altered in diseased states.

USE OF SPECIFIC RADIOPHARMACEUTICALS

This section is a brief summary of some recent radiotracers designed on the basis of their biochemical rationale.

Metabolites

Many known metabolites and their analogs have been used for the measurement of oxygen utilization, protein synthesis and metabolism, glucose metabolism in the brain, and glucose and fatty acid metabolism in the myocardium.

Oxygen-15 has been administered by the equilibrium inhalation method (12) to measure oxygen utilization in the brain. Ackerman et al.(13,15) have quantitated and correlated cerebral blood flow and oxygen metabolism in acute and chronic stroke and stroke prone patients. They suggest that measurements of oxygen metabolism and blood flow actually will enable the discrimination of viable from non-viable tissue and the staging of the severity of a stroke lesion for therapeutic purposes. Indications are that blood flow alone is not clinically so important as oxygen metabolism ($CMRO_2$) or oxygen metabolism in relation to cerebral blood flow. Baron et al. (16) have demonstrated a depression of blood flow and metabolism in the cerebral hemisphere contralateral to a cortical ischemic infarction. Frackowiak et al. (17) and Lenzi et al. (18) have found that when $CMRO_2$ falls below 1.2cc per 100 gram per minute, the clinical outcome is poor. Also, they have shown in their data a mismatch of cerebral blood flow and oxygen utilization in regions of cerebral neoplasm.

Amino acids

Two recent reviews deal with the introduction of N-13, C-11 and F-18 into amino acids by an enzymatic or chemical procedure (10,19). Labeled amino acids are important tracers for determining the metabolic pathways of specific amino acids in tissues or organs. In general, amino acids follow many common pathways; however, some are true indicators of protein synthesis. Methionine is an excellent donor of a methyl group for protein synthesis. This concept was utilized by Bustany et al. (20) in preliminary studies defining protein sythesis in the brain of baboons and patients with dementia.

The pancreas is an active site for the utilization of amino acids and the production of proteins. Many investigators have developed labeled amino acids as possible agents for pancreatic imaging (10,19). The use of ^{75}Se-selenomethionine has remained the only radiopharmaceutical that is routinely used in the clinic, despite its long biological and physical half-life. Carbon-11 labeled valine, tryptophan and methionine (21-24) have been employed in conjunction with the positron emission technique (PET) and have proved to be better agents for the study of this organ.

Studies of the heart using nitrogen-13 labeled amino acids has been reviewed recently by Gelbard et al. (19). Nitrogen-13-glutamate showed remarkable myocardial uptake in baboons and humans. This agent was also utilized in diagnostic studies of cell sarcoma in man and for following responses to chemotherapy (25-27). Henze et al. (28) are investigating a group of amino acids that are metabolized primarily in skeletal and myocardial muscle. Further, the rate of oxidation of branched-chain amino acid in the heart has been shown to increase in the presence of fatty acids. It may be possible to study this phenomenon in vivo using C-11 or F-18 labeled analogs of leucine or isoleucine.

The external monitoring of brain function with PET technique and positron radiotracers has permitted a preliminary description of cerebral amino acid metabolism and changes in neuronal structure associated with brain amino acid disorders. Comar et al. (29,30) evaluated C-11-methionine in phenylketonuric children and studied the effect of high levels of phenylalanine in the blood on the brain uptake of C-11-methionine in these patients.

Garnett et al. (31) employed 5-fluorine-18-3-4-dihydroxy-phenylalanine (F-18-DOPA) as a dopamine precursor in monkeys and described a three compartment model to quantitate the fractional rate of formation of dopamine in the brain. Other groups utilized C-11-D,L-DOPA for the detection of areas enriched with dopadecarboxylase (32).

Dihydroxyphenylalanine is also known to be a substrate in the biosynthetic conversion of L-tyrosine to melanin (33). On the basis of this observation F-18 or C-11 labeled DOPA was suggested as a probe for the detection of melanoma deposits (34, 35). Tyrosine a less proximate precursor for melanin biosynthesis had been proposed earlier (35). However, its selective incorporation into melanoma cells was far less than that of DOPA (36).

"Artificial" amino acid or non-metabolized amino acids have been suggested for studies of transport and for the detection of malignant neoplasm. Carbon-11-aminocyclobutane (ACBC) and amino -cyclopentane (ACPC) carboxylic acids (37,38) have been used as chemotherapeutic agents. They were labeled and used in imaging studies of neoplastic tissue. Carbon-11 alpha-aminoisobutyric acid was also suggested for transport and cancer studies (39).

Sugars

Glucose, the main energy substrate for the brain, was labeled with C-14 and C-11 and used with C-14 for measuring glucose metabolism in rat brain (40). Carbon-11-glucose was proposed as a label for the in vivo measurement of glucose metabolism (41,42). However, because of its rapid metabolism and the translocation of activity from the tissue, fast measurements are required to perform such studies. The generation of cameras that will enable such data collection are available (see Section by Ter-Pogossian).

A second technique (first proposed by Sokoloff and Reivich (43)) utilizing an analog of glucose enabled the in vivo measurement of glucose metabolism. 2-Deoxy-D-glucose (2DG) differs from glucose only by the lack of an hydroxyl group on the second carbon of glucose. This small change in the molecular structure causes substantial alteration in its behavior. Glucose is metabolized very quickly to CO_2 and H_2O, whereas 2-deoxy-D-glucose is phosphorylated in the first steps to 2-DG-6-phosphate, which intermediate is recognized by the enzyme system, and not further metabolized. Using C-14 and F-18-2DG and recently ^{11}C-2-DG (45) its fixation in brain tissue has been shown to reflect glucose metabolism (44-46). This concept was modified by Phelps et al. (47) to adjust for the egress of activity caused by the relatively slow dephosphorylation process. 2-Fluoro-deoxyglucose was used in patients with seizure disorders (48,49) in schizophrenics (50), in patients with Huntington's disease (51) and in stimulation studies (52-55). Glucose metabolism as measured in these studies and expressed in mg/100g tissue/min seems altered significantly from the normal.

In many instances there are different analogs which could be used in radiopharmaceutical design. For example for the glucose metabolic studies there are many possible deoxyglucose analogs that could be labeled on the 6-carbon of the glucose molecule. However, most of them were eliminated because of inappropriate chemical or biochemical properties (56,57), and only 2-DG, 3-DG and their fluoro analogs were proposed as possible agents (56). The final decision can be made only by in vivo determination of their behavior. Elmaleh et al. (57,58) performed comparative studies of these analogs and showed the advantages of 2-FDG over 3-FDG as a marker of glucose.

Fatty acids

Fatty acids (FA), the main source of energy for the heart muscle, have been labeled with ^{11}C and used as "physiological" substrates (59,60). Studies have also been performed with many radiohalogenated analogs (61-63) and analogs containing other radioactive heteroatoms (64). The washout activity from the myocardium is fast due to beta-oxidation of the ^{11}C-"physiological" substrates. In addition the radiohalogenated FAs suffer from enzymatic dehalogenation.

However, recently Livni and Elmaleh (65) have suggested a new approach for studying fatty acid metabolism in the heart, employing an analog that will be partially metabolized but trapped in the myocardial tissue in a predictable step, similar to 2-DG and 2-FDG. A review of fatty acid metabolism suggests a possible metabolic inhibition in the β-oxidation process. The step producing the corresponding β-ketoacylSCoA derivative could be inhibited chemically by introducing a methyl group on the β -carbon. According to their preliminary reported studies, the activity extracted by the heart is retained for a period longer than one hour.

Drugs

A wide spectrum of therapeutic drugs could be listed under this group. For convenience of discussion we will divide the drugs into two subgroups: drugs designed on the basis of the receptor ligand interaction, and all other drugs.

Receptor binding agents. The interaction of receptor and ligand is one of the most exciting areas of investigation (1). The determination of receptor populations utilizing labeled ligands is becoming a major focus of many groups.

In vivo studies of the dopaminergic or opiate receptors using labeled dopamine precursors or high affinity ligands to these receptors have been initiated. Morphine, heroin (66) and etorphine have been labeled with C-11 (67). Haloperidol labeled with F-18 and spiroperidol labeled with C-11 and F-18 have

been reported recently and some evaluation of their in vivo behavior commenced (68-70). The use of the [77]Br-analog of spiroperidol was reported by Friedman et al (71).

Successful preliminary in vivo study of the benzodiazepine
receptors was reported using ^{11}C-flunitrazepam (72) in the baboon
brain and of the muscarinic receptors with the ^{11}C-muscarinic
antagonist methiodide quinuclidinyl benzylate in the myocardium
(73).

Katzenellenbogen et al. (74) proposed the estrogen receptor
ligand interaction as the basis for radiopharmaceuticals for the
detection of estrogen responsive breast tumors (74). These
investigators described a method for predicting the selectivity
of many designed radiolabeled estrogens and analogs based on in
vitro affinity and lipophilicity studies of the drugs.

Eckelman and Reba used in vitro assays and a biomolecular
model for calculating target to blood ratio for many designed β-
adrenergic or muscarinic cholinergic blocking agents for myocardial radiotracers (75).

Studies involving neurotransmitters were discussed earlier
under amino acids.

Scheme 1 underlines the complex pattern of receptor-ligand
interactions. These pilot studies are just a beginning attempt
to delineate the processes involved.

The most useful radionuclides for labeling ligands are
carbon-11, nitrogen-18, fluorine-18, iodine-123 and bromine-75
because of the high specific activities that can be achieved with
them (see Table 1). The in vivo stability of the radiohalogenated
ligand must be demonstrated in each case.

Scheme 1

Possible Mode of Ligand Distribution

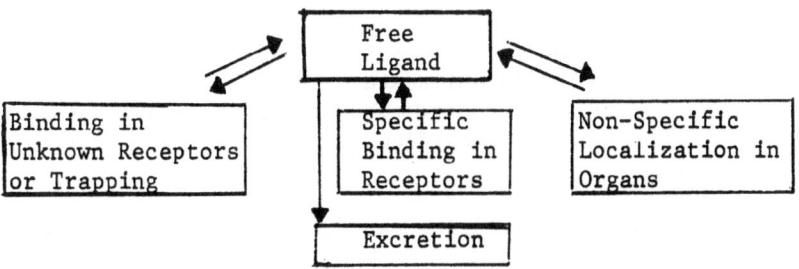

Other general factors affecting ligand distribution.

1. Specific Activity   2. Radionuclide Decay
3. Isomerism   4. Agonist Antagonist
                                         Effect

Other drugs. In this section we include drugs that have rationales other than receptor ligand interactions for their development.

In the amino acid section we have already mentioned C-11-alpha-aminoisobutyric acid, ACBC and ACPC. The latter chemotherapeutic agents labeled with C-11 exhibited good properties as tumor scanning agents (37-39).

Recently, Kung and Blau (76) described some agents dependent on regional intracellular pH shifts for uptake in the brain and other tissues. The selenium-75 labeled di- β-(morphoholinoethyl)-selenide (MOSE) and di- β-(piperidinoethyl)-selenide (PIPSE) have shown pronounced brain uptake in rats suggesting their use as cerebral perfusion agents.

The concept of enzyme inhibitors could be used in the design of drugs. Methyltrexate is a cancer chemotherapeutic agent and is also a dehydrofolate reductase inhibitor; 5-fluorouracil is also used in cancer chemotherapy and is a thymidylate synthetase inhibitor (77).

In addition to the use of labeled melanin precursors, there have been other approaches to the design of drugs that will bind melanin. A radioiodine labeled quinoline derivative (78,79) labeled chlorpromazine (80) have been tested. The rationale is the affinity of these compounds for melanin in vitro and in vivo. Chlorpromazine, for example, is an electron donor while melanin is thought to serve as an electron trap.

Recent developments in the design of adrenal medullary imaging agents has focused on radioiodinated analogs of the anti-hypertensive guanethidine. This drug is a neuron blocking agent. It is able to deplete peripheral tissues of their catecholamine stores by direct action on the adrenergic nerves (81). Wieland and Beierwaltes reported the development and the use of its radioiodinated analogs the iodo-aralkylguanidines. Meta-iodo-benzylguanidine could clearly delineate monkey adrenal medulla and human adrenal medullary tumors. This agent is also in preliminary trials for imaging myocardium, endocrine glands, spleen and lung (82-84).

N-isopropyl-p-iodoamphetamine was designed as a blood flow

indexing agent (85,86). This agent was used by Kuhl et al. (87) and Hill et al. (see other section in this book), in studies involving single photon tomography.

Antigen antibody reaction

The labeling of antibodies with radioiodine was suggested many years ago (88). However, this technique did not yield remarkable results because of the multiple binding of the antibodies to many antigens. With the development of the monoclonal antibody which has great specificity and can be readily available, this diagnostic approach may become a fruitful one.

The labeling of purified antibodies can be achieved in two ways: (a) by radioiodination of antibodies as reported in the case of antimyocin antibody (89,90). These labeled proteins will always be subject to in vivo deiodination and must be individually evaluated. (b) by the use of bifunctional chelating agents. This approach enables an amide bond of the antibody to the chelating agent and in addition to a radiotracer such as indium, gallium and possibly Tc-99m. The chelation of the specific protein fragments does not cause a major change in the protein molecule activity. The bifunctional chelating method was reported first by Sundberg with a diazonium salt (91). Later Krejcarek et al. used a mixed carboxycarbonic anhydride of DTPA (92). This approach was reviewed recently by Goodwin et al. (93) for the labeling of other molecules. Protein coupled by this method requires exhaustive purification by dialysis for several days to remove the free DTPA produced by hydrolysis (94).

Eckelman utilized a cyclic anhydride for the labeling of some amino compounds (95). This concept was adopted by Hnatowich et al. (96) for protein labeling. Due to its simplicity compared to all of the previous approaches and the stability of the cyclic anhydride this method has a high potential for success as the basis for labeling human serum albumin, antibodies, and some drugs. This approach is also under investigation at the MGH in collaboration with Harvard Medical School for tumor and myocardial imaging.

In summary, the increased availability of many radionuclides, together with new improved instrumentation for gamma and positron detection, have brought about the development of rapid labeling techniques for new types of radiopharmaceuticals which can yield functional as well as anatomical information. Because of the potential of this relatively new direction radiopharmaceutical development should be encouraged, and some effort should be made to draw the biochemist and the physiologist into collaboration in order to produce well designed radiopharmaceuticals based on biochemical pathways.

REFERENCES

1.   Eckelman, W.C. and R.C. Reba. "The classification of radiotracers." J. Nucl. Med. 19 (1978) 1179-1181.

2.   Wolf, A.P. and C.S. Redvanly. "Carbon-11 and radio-pharmaceuticals." Int. J. Appl. Radiat. Isotopes 28 (1977) 29-48.

3.   Wolf, A.P., D.R. Christman, J.S. Fowler and R.M. Lambrecht. "Synthesis of radiopharmaceuticals and labelled compounds using short-lived isotopes." In Radiopharmaceuticals and Labeled Compounds, vol. I (Vienna: IAEA, 345-379, 1973).

4.   Welch, M.J., J.O. Eichling, M.G. Straatmann, M.E. Raichle and H.M. Ter-Pogossian. "New short-lived radiopharmaceuticals for CNS studies." In H.J. DeBlanc, Jr. and J.A. Sorensen, eds., Noninvasive Brain Imaging: Computed Tomography and Radionuclides (New York: Society of Nuclear Medicine, 1975).

5.   Welch, M.J. and S.J. Wagner. "Preparation of positron-emitting radiopharmaceuticals." In J.H. Lawrence and T.F. Budinger, eds., Recent Advances in Nuclear Medicine, vol. 5 (New York: Grune and Stratton, 1978).

6.   Robinson, G.D., Jr. "Prospect for ^{18}F radiopharmaceuticals." In G. Subramanian, B.A. Rhodes, J.F. Cooper, V.J. Sodd, eds., Radiopharmaceuticals (New York: Society of Nuclear Medicine, 1975).

7.   Palmer, A.J., J.C. Clark and R.W. Goulding. "The preparation of F-18 labelled radiopharmaceuticals." Int. J. Appl. Radiat. Isotopes 28 (1977) 53-65.

8.   Straatmann, M.G. "A look at ^{13}N and ^{15}O in radiopharmaceuticals Int. J. Appl. Radiat. Isotopes 28 (1977) 13-20.

9.   Wolf, A.P. and J.S. Fowler. "Organic Radiopharmaceuticals: Recent Advances." In Radiopharmaceuticals II: Proceedings 2nd International Symposium on Radiopharmaceuticals, March 19-22, 1979.

10.   Elmaleh, D.R., M. Zalutsky, D. Comar, M.M. Goodman and G.L. Brownell, "C-11 and F-18 amino acids." In R.P. Spencer, ed., Radiopharmaceuticals, Structure Activity Relationships (New York: Grune and Stratton, 1981).

11.   Fowler, S.J. "Organic Radiopharmaceuticals Recent Advances." In Advances in Emission Tomography, ICG Conference, October 24-26, 1979.

12.   Subramaniam, R., N.M. Alpert, B. Hoop, Jr., G.L. Brownell and J.M. Taveras. "A model for regional cerebral oxygen distribution during continuous inhalation of $^{15}O_2$, $C^{15}O$ and $C^{15}O_2$." J. Nucl. Med. 19 (1978) 48-53.

13.   Ackerman, R.H., J.A. Correia, N.M. Alpert, J.C. Baron, A. Gouliamos, J.C. Grotta, G.L. Brownell and J.M. Taveras. "Positron imaging in ischemic stroke disease using compounds labeled with oxygen-15. Initial results of clinicophysiologic correlations." Arch. Neurol. 38 (1981) 537-543.

14. Ackerman, R.H., N.M. Alpert, J.A. Correia. "Importance of monitoring metabolic function in assessing the severity of a stroke insult (CBF: an Epiphenomenom?)." Cereb. Blood Flow Metab. 1, suppl. 1 (1981) 502.

15. Ackerman, R.H., S.M. Davis, J.A. Correia. "Positron imaging of CBF and metabolism in patients with cerebral neoplasma." J. Cereb. Blood Flow Metab. 1, suppl. 1 (1981) 575.

16. Baron, J.C., M.G. Bousser, D. Comar. "Crosses cerebellar diachisis: A remote functional depression secondary to supratentorial infarction of man." J. Cereb. Blood Flow Metab. 1, suppl. 1 (1981) 500.

17. Frackowiak, R.S.J., C. Pozzilli, N.J. Legg. "A prospective study of regional cerebral blood flow and oxygen utilization in dementia using positron tomography and oxygen-15." J. Cereb. Blood Flow Metab. 1, suppl. 1 (1981) 453.

18. Lenzi, G.L., R.S.J. Frackowiak and T. Jones. "Regional cerebral blood flow (CBF), oxygen utilization ($CMRO_2$), and oxygen extraction ratio (OER) in acute hemispheric stroke. J. Cereb. Blood Flow Metab. 1, suppl. 1 (1981) 504.

19. Gelbard, A.S. "[13]N-labeled Amino Acids," in R.P. Spencer, ed., Radiopharmaceuticals, Structure Activity Relationships (New York: Grune and Stratton, 1981).

20. Bustany, P., T. Sargent, J.M. Sandubray, J.F. Henry and D. Comar. "Regional human brain uptake and protein incorporation of ^{11}C-L-methionine studies in vivo with PET." J. Cereb. Blood Flow Metab. 1, suppl. 1 (1981) I-9, S-17.

21. Washburn, L.C., B. Wieland, T.T. Sun, R.L. Hayes and T.A. Butler, "[1-^{11}C]DL-Valine, a potential pancreas-imaging agent." J. Nucl. Med. 19 (1978) 77-83.

22. Washburn, L.C., T.T. Sun, B.L. Byrd, R.L. Hayes and T.A. Butler. "D,L-(carboxyl-^{11}C)tryptophan, a potential agent for pancreatic imaging: Production and preclinical investigations. J. Nucl. Med. 20 (1979) 857-864.

23. Syrota, A., D. Comar, M. Cerf, D. Plummer, M. Maziere and C. Kellershohn. "[^{11}C]methionine pancreatic scanning with positron emission computed tomography." J. Nucl. Med. 20, (1979) 778-781.

24. Kirchner, P.T., J. Ryan, M. Zalutsky and P.V. Harper. "Positron emission tomography for the evaluation of pancreatic disease." Semin. Nucl. Med. 10, (1980) 374-391.

25. McDonald, J.M., A.S. Gelbard, L.P. Clarke, T.R. Christie and J.S. Laughlin. "Imaging of tumors involving bone with ^{13}N-glutamic acid." Radiology 120 (1976) 623-626.

26. Gelbard, A.S., R.S. Benua, J.S. Laughlin, G. Rosen, R.E. Reiman and J.H. McDonald. "Quantitative scanning of osteogenic sarcoma with nitrogen-13-labeled L-glutamate." J. Nucl. Med. 20, (1979) 782-784.

27. Rosen, G., A.S. Gelbard, R.S. Benua, J.S. Laughlin, R.E. Reiman and J.H. McDpnald. "^{13}N-glutamate scanning to detect the early response of primary bone tumors to chemotherapy." Proc. Am. Assoc. Cancer Res. 20 (1979) 189.

28. Henze, E., J. Egbert, J. Barrio, F. Baumgartner, M. Phelps, D. Kuhl, H. Schelbert. "Myocardial energy metabolism evaluated by single pass uptake and positron emission computed tomography of N-13 and C-11 labeled amino acids." J. Nucl. Med. 22 (1981) p. 10.

29. Comar, D., - Cyclotron progress report. Service Hospitalier Frederíc Joliet Department de Biologie, 1978.

30. Soussaline, F., A.E. Todd-Pokropek, D. Plummer, D. Comar, C. Loch, S. Houle and C. Kellershohn. "The physical performances of a single slice positron tomographic system and preliminary results in a clinical environment." Eur. J. Nucl. Med. 4 (1979) 237-249.

31. Garnett, E.S., G. Firnau, C. Nahmias. "Blood brain barrier transport and cerebral utilization of dopa in living monkeys." Am. J. Physiol. (1980) R318-R327.

32. Korf, J., S. Reiffers, H.D. Beerling-Van Der Molen, J.P.W.F. Lakke, A.M.J. Paans, W. Vaalburg and M.G. Woldring. "Rapid decarboxylation of carbon-11 labeled DL-DOPA in the brain: A potential approach for external detection of nervous structures." Brain Res. 145 (1978) 59-67.

33. Fitzpatrick, T.B. "Mammalian melanin biosynthesis." Transactions St. John's Hospital Dermatol. Soc. 51 (1965) 1-26.

34. Van Langevelde, A., H.D. Beerling-Van Der Molen, J.G. Journee-de Korver, A.M.J. Paans and W. Vaalburg. "C-11 labeled melanin precursors as radiopharmaceuticals for the detection of eye melanoma." J. Nucl. Med. 22 (1981).

35. Meier, D.A., W.H. Beierwaltes and R.E. Counsell. "Radio-activity from labeled precursors of melanin in mice and hamsters with melanoma." Cancer Res. 27 (1967) 1354-1359.

36. Wick, M.M. and E. Frei III. "Selective incorporation of L-3,4-dihydroxyphenylanine by S-91 Cloudman melanoma in vitro." Cancer Res. 37 (1977) 2123-2125.

37. Hubner, K.F., G.A. Andrews, L. Washburn, B.W. Wieland, W.D. Gibbs, R.L. Hayes. T.A. Butler and J.D. Winebrenner. "Tumor location with 1-aminocyclopentane (^{11}C) carboxylic acid: Preliminary clinical trials with single-photon detection. J. Nucl. Med. 18 (1977) 1215-1221.

38. Washburn, L.C., T.T. Sun, B.L. Byrd, R.L. Hayes and T.A. Butler. "1-aminocyclobutane[^{11}C] carboxylic acid, A potential tumor-seeking agent. J. Nucl. Med. (1979) 1055-1061.

39. Schmall, B. and R.E. Bigler, "Radiolabeled Drugs: Use of positron-emitting radionuclides." In R.P. Spencer, ed., Radiopharmaceuticals, Structure Activity Relationships (New York: Grune and Stratton, 1981).

40. Hawkins, R.A., A.L. Miller, J.E. Cremer and R.L. Veech. "Measurement of the rate of glucose utilization by rat brain in vivo." J. Neurochem. 23 (1974) 917-923.

41. Raichle, M.E., K.B. Larson, M.E. Phelps, R.L. Grubb, Jr., M.J. Welch and M.M. Ter-Pogossian. "In vivo measurement of brain glucose transport and metabolism employing glucose-[11]C." Am. J. Physiol. 228 (1975) 1936-1948.

42. Raichle, M.E., M. Welch, R.L. Grubb, Jr., C.S. Higgins, M.M. Ter-Pogossian and K.B. Larson. "Measurement of regional substrate utilization rates by emission tomography." Science 199 (1978) 986-987.

43. Sokoloff, L., M. Reivich, C. Kennedy, M.H. DesRosiers, C.S. Patlak, K.D. Pettigrew, O. Sakurada and M. Shinohara. "The (^{14}C) deoxyglucose method for the measurement of local cerebral glucose utilization: theory, procedure and normal values in the conscious and anesthetized albino rat." J. Neurochem. 28 (1977) 897-916.

44. Gallagher, B.M., J.S. Fowler, N.I. Gutterson, R.R. MacGregor, C.N. Wan and A.P. Wolf. "Metabolic trapping as a principle of radiopharmaceutical design: Some factors responsible for the distribution of [^{18}F]2-deoxy-2-fluoro-D-glucose." J. Nucl. Med. 19 (1978) 1154-1161.

45. Fowler, J., A.P. Wolf, D.R. Christman. Private communication.

46. Kassis, A.I., S.J. Adelstein, J.S. Fowler and A.P. Wolf. "Uptake and radiotoxicity of F-18-2-fluoro-2-deoxyglucose in mammalian cells." J. Nucl. Med. 22 (1981) p. 45.

47. Phelps, M.E., S.C. Huang, E.J. Hoffman, C. Selin, L. Sokoloff and D.E. Kuhl. "Tomographic measurement of local cerebral glucose metabolic rate in humans with (F-18)2-fluoro-2-deoxy-D-glucose: Validation of method." Ann. Neurol. 6 (1979) 371-388.

48. Kuhl, D.E., M.E. Phelps, A.P. Kowell, E.S. Metter, C. Selin and J. Winter. "Effects of stroke on local cerebral metabolism and perfusion: Mapping by emission computed tomography of [18]FDG and [13]NH$_3$." Ann. Neurol. 8 (1980) 47-60.

49. Kuhl, D.E., J. Engel, Jr., M.E. Phelps and C. Selin. "Epileptic patterns of local cerebral metabolism and perfusion in humans determined by emission computed tomography of [18]FDG and [13]NH$_3$." Ann. Neurol. 8 (1981) 455.

50. Widen, L., M. Bergstron and G. Blomquist. "Glucose metabolism in patients with schizophrenia: Emission computed tomography measurements with 11-C-glucose." J. Cereb. Blood Flow Metab. 1, suppl. 1 (1981) 455.

51. Kuhl, D., M. Phelps, C. Markham. "Local cerebral glucose metabolism in Huntington's disease determined by emission computed tomography of ^{18}F-fluorodeoxyglucose." J Cereb Blood Flow Metab. 1, suppl. 1 (1981) 459.

314

52. Greenberg, J.H., M. Reivich, A. Alavi, P. Hand,
A. Rosenquist, W. Rintelmann, A. Stein, R. Tusa, R. Dann,
D. Christman, J. Fowler, B. MacGregor, A. Wolf. "Metabolic
mapping of functional activity in human subjects with the [18F]-
fluoro-deoxyglucose technique." Science 212 (1981) 503-516.

53. Mazziotta, J.A., M.E. Phelps, J. Miller and D.E. Kuhl.
"Tomographic mapping of human cerebral metabolism: Normal
unstimulated state." Neurology 31 (1981) 503-516.

54. Phelps, M.E., J.C. Mazziotta, D.E. Kuhl, M. Nuwer,
J. Packwood, J. Metter and J. Engel, Jr. "Tomographic mapping of
human cerebral metabolism: Visual stimulation and deprivation."
Neurology 31 (1981) 517-529.

55. Phelps, M.E., J.C. Mazziotta, J. Engel, Jr. "Metabolic
response of the brain to visual and auditory stimulation and
deprivation." J. Cereb. Blood Flow Metab. 1, suppl. 1 (1981)
467.

56. Tewson, T.J., M.J. Welch, M.E. Raichle. "[18F]-labeled
3-deoxy-3-fluoro-D-glucose: Synthesis and preliminary biodistribution data." J. Nucl. Med. 19 (1978) 1339-1345.

57. Goodman, M.M., D.R. Elmaleh, K.J. Kearfott, R.H.
Ackerman, B. Hoop, Jr., G.L. Brownell, N.M. Alpert and W.H.
Strauss. "F-18 labeled 3-deoxy-3-fluoro-D-glucose for the study
of regional metabolism in brain and heart." J. Nucl. Med. 22
(1981) 138-144.

58. Elmaleh, D.R., K.J. Kearfott, M.M. Goodman. "A comparison of 18F-sugar analogs." In V. Nanto and E.M. Soulinna,
eds., Animals in Medical Application of Cyclotrons, vol I1
(Turku Yliopisto, 1981).

59. Goldstein, R.A., M.S. Klein, H.J. Welch and B.E. Sobel.
"External assessment of myocardial metabolism with 11C-palmitate
in vivo." J. Nucl. Med. 21 (1980) 342-348.

60. Ter-Pogossian, M.M., M.S. Klein, J. Markham. "Regional
assessment of myocardial metabolic integrity in vivo by PET with
11C-palmitate." Circulation 61 (1980).

61. Feinendegen, L.E., K. Vyskak, C.H.R. Freundlieb, A.
Hock, H.J. Machulla, G. Kloster and G. Stocklin. "Noninvasive
analysis of metabolic reactions in body tissues, the case of
myocardial fatty acids." Eur. J. Nucl. Med. 6 (1981) 191-200.

62. Van der Wall, E.E., W. den Hollander, G.A.K. Heidendal,
G. Westera, P.A. Majid and J.P. Roos. "Dynamic myocardial
scintigraphy with 123-I-labeled free fatty acids in patients
with myocardial infarction. Eur. J. Nucl. Med. 6 (1981) 383-
389.

63. Otto, C.A., L.E. Brown, D.M. Wieland and W.H. Beierwaltes. "Radioiodinated fatty acids for myocardial imaging:
Effects of chain length." J. Nucl. Med. 22 (1981) 613-618.

64. Knapp, F.F., Jr. "Selenium and tellurium as Carbon
Substituents." In R.P. Spencer, eds., Radiopharmaceuticals,
Structure Activity Relationships (New York: Grune and Stratton,
1981).

65. Livni, E., D.R. Elmaleh, S. Levy, et al: "[1-C-11]-β-methylheptadecanoic acid: A new approach for assessing myocardial metabolism with positron tomography technique. J. Nucl. Med. in press.

66. Kloster, G., E. Roder, H.J. Machulla. "Synthesis, chromatography and tissue distribution of methyl-^{11}C-morphine and methyl-^{11}C-heroin." J. Labelled Comp. Radiopharm. 16 (1979) 441-448.

67. Maziere, M., G. Berger. J.M. Godot, C. Prenant and D. Comar. "Etorphine [11]C- : A new tool for "in vivo" study of brain opiates receptors." J. Labelled Comp. Radiopharm. 18 (1981) 291-295.

68. Tewson, T.J., M.E. Raichle and M.J. Welch. "Preliminary studies with [^{18}F]-haloperidol: A radioligand for in vivo studies of the dopamine receptors. Brain Res. 192 (1980) 291-295.

69. Maeda, M., T.J. Tewson and M.J. Welch. "Synthesis of high specific activity ^{18}F-spiroperidol for dopamine receptor studies. J. Labelled Comp. and Radiopharm. 18 (1981) 102-103.

70. Arnett, C.D., A.M. Findley, A.P. Wolf, J.S. Fowler and R.R. MacGregor. "Specific receptor labeling in vivo with C-11 spiroperidol." J. Nucl. Med. 22 (1981) p.13.

71. Friedman, A.M., C.C. Huang, H. Kulmala, R. Dinerstein, R. SO, M. Simonovic and N.Y. Mettzer. "([77]Br- -bromo-spiro-peridol as a dopamine receptor marker." J. Labelled Comp. and Radiopharm. 18 (1981) 104.

72. Menini, Ch., G. Arfel and R. Naquet. "Visualization of ^{11}C-flunitrazepam displacement in the brain of the live baboon." Nature (Lond), 280 (1979) 329-331.

73. Maziere, M., C. Cepeda, G. Berger, J.M. Godot, B. Guibert, J. Sastre, M. Crouzel, R. Naquet and D. Comar. "11-C-Muscarinic antagonist (MQNB) visualizes heart "In Vivo" by positron emission tomography. J. Nucl. Med. 22 (1981) p. 77.

74. Katzenellenbogen, J.A., K.E. Carlson, D.F. Heiman and J.E. Hoyd. "Receptor binding as a basis for radiopharmaceutical design." in R.P. Spencer, ed., Radiopharmaceuticals, Structure Activity Relationships, (New York: Grune and Stratton, 1981).

75. Eckelman, W.C., R.C. Reba, R.E. Gibson, W.J. Rzeszotarsei, F. Vieras, J.K. Mazaitis, B. Francis. "Receptor-binding radiotracers: A class of potential radiopharmaceuticals." J. Nucl. Med. 20 (1979) 350-357.

76. Kung, H., M. Blau. "Regional intracellular pH shift: A proposed new mechanism for radiopharmaceutical uptake in brain and other tissues." J. Nucl. Med. 21 (1980) 147-153.

77. Young, D. and W. Wolf. "QLAR of 5-Fluorouracil," in R.P. Spencer, ed., Radiopharmaceuticals, Structure Activity Relationships (New York: Grune and Stratton, 1981).

78. Packer, S., C. Redvanly, R.M. Lambrecht, A.P. Wolf and H.L. Atrins. "Quinoline analog labeled with iodine-123 in melanoma detection. Arch. Opthalmol. 93, (1975) 504-508.

316

79. Bockslaff, H., E. Jahns and H. Hundenshagen - "Keonena Szintigraphie mit einm doppellochinterakularet tumoren." Radioabe. Isot. Klinik. Forgch 13 (1978) 341-349.

80. Packer, S., R.G. Fairchild, P.K. Watts, D. Greenberg and S.J. Hannon. "Melanin binding radiopharmaceuticals." In R.P. Spencer, ed., Radiopharmaceuticals, Structure Activity Relationships (New York: Grune and Stratton, 1981).

81. Weiland, D.M. and W.H. Beierwaltes: A structure-distribution relationship study of adrenomedullary radio-pharmaceuticals in R.P. Spencer, eds., Radiopharmaceuticals, Structure Activity Relationships (New York: Grune and Stratton, 1981).

82. Gross, M., M. Frager, T. Volk, R. Kline, J. Sisson, D. Swanson, D. Wieland, N. Thompson, M. Tokes and W. Beierwaltes. "Localization of pheochromocytomas with I-131-M-iodobenzyl-guanidine (I-131-MIBG)." J. Nucl. Med. 22 (1981) p.5.

83. Wieland, D.M., L.E. Brown, D.D. Marsh, T.J. Mangner and W.H. Beierwaltes. "The mechanism of m-IBG localization: Drug intervention studies." J. Nucl. Med. 22 (1981) p. 20.

84. Wieland, D.M., L.E. Brown, W.L. Rogers, K.C. Worthing-ton, I-L. Wu, N.H. Clinthorne, C.A. Otto, D.P. Swanson and W.H. Beierwaltes. "Myocardial imaging with a radioiodinated norepinephrine storage analog." J. Nucl. Med. 22 (1981) 22-31.

85. Winchell, H.S., R.M. Baldwin and T.H. Lin - "Develop-ment of I-123-labeled amines for brain studies: Localization of I-123 iodophenylalkyl amines in rat brain. J. Nucl. Med. 21 (1980) 940.

86. Winchell, H.S., W.D. Horst, L. Braun, W.H. Oldendorf, R. Hattner and H. Parker. "N-isopropyl-[123I]-p-iodoamphetamine: single pass brain uptake and washout, binding to brain synapto-somes, and localization in dog and monkey brain. J. Nucl. Med. 21 (1980) 947-952.

87. Kuhl, D.E., J.L. Wu, T.H. Lin, C. Selin and M. Phelps. "Mapping local cerebral blood flow by means of emission computed tomography of N-isopropyl-ρ-(123I)-iodoamphetamine (IMP). J. Nucl. Med. 22 (1981) p. 16.

88. Pressman, D. and G. Keighley. "The zone of activity in antibodies as determined by the use of radioactive tracers: The zone of activity of nephritoxic antikidney serum." J. Immunol. (1948) 59. 141-146.

89. Khaw, B.A., G.A. Beller, E. Haber and T.W. Smith. "Localization of cardiac myosin specific antibody in myocardial infarction." J. Clin. Invest. 58 (1976) 439-446.

90. Beller, G.A., B.A. Khaw, E. Haber and T.W. Smith. "Localization of radiolabeled cardiac myosin-specific antibody in myocardial infarcts. Comparison with technetium-open stannous pyrophosphate." Circulation 55 (1977) 74-78.

91. Sundberg, M.W., C.F. Meares, D.A. Goodwin and C.I. Diamanti. "Selective binding of metal ions to macromolecules using bifunctional analogs of EDTA." J. Med. Chem. <u>17</u> (1974) 1304-1307.

92. Krejcarek, G.E. and K.L. Tucker. "Covalent attachment of chelating groups to macromolecules." Biochem. Biophys. Res. Comm. <u>77</u> (1977) 581-585.

93. Goodwin, D.A. and C.F. Meares. "Bifunctional chelates for radiopharmaceutical labeling." in R.P. Spencer, ed., in Radiopharmaceuticals, Structure Activity Relationships. (New York: Grune and Stratton, 1981).

94. Wagner, S.J. and M.J. Welch. "Gallium-68 labeling of albumen and albumen microspheres." J. Nucl. Med. <u>20</u> (1979) 428-433.

95. Eckelman, W.C., S.M. Karesh and R.C. Reba. "New compounds: Fatty acid and long chain hydrocarbon derivatives containing a strong chelating agent." J. Pharm. Sci. <u>64</u> (1975) 704.706.

96. Hnatowich, D.J., L. Warren. Private communication.

Part V: Image Processing & Autoradiography

IMAGE PROCESSING AND DISPLAY

A. Todd-Pokropek

Dept. of Medical Physics
University College London
Gower St., London WC1 UK

1. INTRODUCTION

The aim of this paper is to present a brief review of image processing, as employed in the field of medical imaging, and to include a discussion of the problems of display including that of 3-dimensional objects. The improvements in technology that have occured in the areas of CT, ultrasound (US) and single photon and positron emission CT, (SPECT and PECT), have resulted in a considerable expansion of the number and complexity of medical images, and the advent of other imaging procedures (NMR, digital radiology etc) is likely to further this trend. While medical images used to be exclusively two dimensional, the appearance of 3-D data has now become common, although the third dimension can be in space, or time, or even some other derived parameter (such as tissue character).
This paper will try to overview the subject in the following order:

1) Classical image processing (restoration)
2) Non-linear image processing
3) Quantitation of medical images
4) Creation of functional or parametric (derived) images
5) 2-D display
6) 3-D display

However, the overlap between these various topics is considerable, and rigid distinctions will not be enforced. Image processing in nuclear medicine will be the source of many examples but where possible the use of such techniques in the other areas of medical imaging (notably CT and US) will be indicated. The references given in the text are by no means complete and the interested reader is recommended [1] for further information on tomography, [2] on image processing in nuclear medicine, and [3] on image processing in general.

2. IMAGE PROCESSING FOR RESTORATION

In the initial period of growth of image processing techniques in medical imaging (and in particular, in nuclear medicine), there was considerable interest in various image restoration operations, that is, methods to unblur the blur introduced by the imaging system (e.g. [4,5].

Following the approach given by Andrews and Hunt [6], together with some ideas from Pratt [3], a general algebraic solution is presented, together with some specific implementations. The non-mathematical reader is recommended to skip to the summary at the end of this section.

Let $f(x,y)$ be the object that is being imaged, and $g(x,y)$ be the image that is obtained, then if $h(x,y)$ is the 'transfer function' of the imaging system, we may write:

$$g(i,j) = \sum_{k=0}^{N-1} \sum_{l=0}^{N-1} f(k,l).h(i-k,j-l) + n(i,j)$$

where $n(x,y)$ is an additive noise term. Note that, while noise is not in general additive, it may be 'whitened' by using the Anscome transform [7].
Let the convolution operator $\circledcirc$ be defined as:

$$f(x,y) \circledcirc h(x,y) = \int\int_{-\infty}^{\infty} f(x',y') . h(x-x',y-y') \, dx' \, dy'$$

If the Fourier transform is represented by $F\{\}$ such that $F\{g(x,y)\}$ is equal to $G(u,v)$ the Fourier transform of $g(x,y)$ then in the absence of noise:

$$g(x,y) = f(x,y) \circledcirc h(x,y)$$

and therefore:

$$G(x,y) = F(u,v) . H(u,v)$$

or:

$$f(x,y) = F^{-1}\{ G(u,v) / H(u,v) \}$$

where $F^{-1}\{\ \}$ indicates the inverse Fourier transform. This is the classical form for expressing deconvolution. However, the use of matrix notation is more supple and leads to a general solution which includes (albeit additive) noise.

Let f,g and n be expressed as column vectors of the form:

$$\tilde{g} = [\ g(0,0)\ g(1,0)\ \ldots\ g(N-1,0)\ g(1,0)\ g(1,1)$$
$$\ldots\ g(N-1,N-1)\ ]$$

and H is a matrix of size N^2 x N^2 composed of N^2 submatrices of form:

$$H = \begin{bmatrix} [H_0] & [H_{N-1}] & \ldots & [H_1] \\ [H_1] & [H_0] & \ldots & [H_2] \\ \ldots\ldots\ldots\ldots\ldots\ldots \\ [H_{N-1}] & [H_{N-2}] & \ldots & [H_0] \end{bmatrix} \text{ and } [H_j] = \begin{bmatrix} h(j,0) & h(j,N-1) & .. & h(j,1) \\ h(j,1) & h(j,0) & .. & h(j,2) \\ \ldots\ldots\ldots\ldots\ldots\ldots \\ h(j,N-1) & h(j,N-2) & .. & h(j,0) \end{bmatrix}$$

Then:

$$\tilde{g} = H \cdot \tilde{f} + \tilde{n}$$

where H is block Toeplitz and block circulant. Then a solution for finding an estimate $\hat{f}$ of the object distribution exists, using Lagrangian methods, being:

$$\hat{f} = (\ H^{*'}\ H + \gamma\ Q'\ Q\ )^{-1}\ H^{*'}\ g$$

where Q is a linear operator on f minimising $/Qf/^2$ such that $/g - H\ f/^2 = /n/^2$, and γ is equal to $1/\lambda$, and related to usual Lagrangian multipliers. The symbols * and ' represent the complex conjugate and transpose respectively.

There are a number of special cases of this solution:
Let Q be the identity matrix I, then:

$$\hat{f} = (\ H^{*'}\ H + \gamma\ I\ )^{-1}\ H^{*'}\ g$$

Let γ be equal to zero then, from the property that circulant matrices can be diagonalised by a Fourier transform, this corresponds to the (trivial) solution $F(u,v) = G(u,v)\ /\ H(u,v)$ given above.

Let Q be a finite difference operator, having a Fourier transform $P(u,v)$. In this case, the corresponding Fourier solution is:

$$\hat{F}(u,v) \ = \ \frac{G(u,v) \ . \ H^*(u,v)}{/H(u,v)/^2 \ + \ \gamma \ /P(u,v)/^2}$$

An example of this solution is that used by Boardman [8], with Q as a Laplacian operator, although in fact any order operator may be chosen.

Another alternative solution (or should it be called implementation) is where Q is given by:

$$Q \ = \ r_n^{1/2} \ / \ r_f^{1/2}$$

where r_f and r_n are the covariance matrices of f (the signal) and n (the noise) respectively. Let R_x be the power (Wiener) spectrum of x, then if γ is set equal to unity, a traditional Wiener filter is obtained such that:

$$\hat{F}(u,v) = \frac{H^*(u,v) \ . \ G(u,v)}{/H(u,v)/^2 \ + \ R_n(u,v)/R_f(u,v)}$$

As Andrews and Hunt [6] have stated: "the use of the Wiener filter to give 'optimal' restoration is part of the 'folklore' of image processing...". It may be 'optimal' in a least squares sense over a large series of images, but there is no guarantee that it is optimal for a specific image, or, even more so, for a region within an image.
However, consider the following operation:

$$\hat{f} \ = \ (\text{inverse filter})^k \ . \ (\text{parametric Wiener filter})^{1-k} \ . \ g$$

Thus:

$$\hat{f} \ = \ [\ (H^{*'}H)^{-1} \ H^{*'} \ ]^k \ . [(H^{*'}H + \gamma \ r_f^{-1}r_n)^{-1}H^{*'}]^{1-k} . g$$

Or:

$$\hat{F}(u,v) = \{\frac{H^*(u,v)}{/H(u,v)/^2}\}^k \ \{\frac{H^*(u,v)}{/H(u,v)/^2 + \gamma R_n(u,v)/R_f(u.v)}\}^{1-k} \ . G(u,v)$$

Take one particular solution, when k=1/2. This gives so-called homomorphic filtering, which is in fact the geometric mean of the inverse and Wiener filters such that:

$$\hat{F}(u,v) \ = \ \frac{G(u,v)}{(\ /H(u,v)/^2 + R_n(u,v)/R_f(u,v) \ )^{1/2}}$$

In summary, most of (classical) conventional image processing as it has been applied to medical images can be contained in the framework given above. For more specific details see [6]. What does this mean in terms of the value of image processing of medical images? Some, but not all, of the techniques described above have been applied to various types of images, with what must be called limited success. There have been a few evaluations using simulated and phantom data (e.g. [9,10]) and a few clinical trials (for example [11]). However, most publications have presented results in hearsay terms, showing a few 'striking' examples. With the improvement in imaging technology, interest in 'image processing' as such seems to have declined. But, in fact, as imaging procedures have become increasingly digital, or digitized, such techniques have merely become commonplace, and form essential parts of more complex procedures. For example, all CT reconstructions, in the form of filtered backprojections, require suitable filters or windows to be defined, and the framework given above may be used. All 'functional image' techniques require some image processing to obtain acceptable signal to noise ratios. Linear image processing of medical images can now be considered as a basic tool. In addition, up to now, limitations in computer power have resulted in the use of computationally cheap approximations to the image processing operations desired, on small matrices and with poor displays. The increasing availability of array processors (and good displays) could change this dramatically.

3. NON-LINEAR RESOLUTION RECOVERY

There have been many attempts to extend the theory given above by inclusion of some non-linear constraint, of which the most obvious is that of positivity, which also turns out to be rather powerful. Most images to be manipulated are by definition (only) positive. A suitable form of such a constraint is given in the expression:

$$g(x,y) = f(x,y)^2 \otimes h(x,y)$$

where a solution for $f(x,y)$ is required which by definition must be positive. Biraud (e.g. [12]) and others [13] have found suitable algorithms. Unfortunately, a closed form solution does not exist. Alternatively, a solution for $\log(f(x,y))$ may be sought which gives rise to various 'maximum entropy' formulations. Such a positivity constraint has been used in tomographic reconstruction [14]. Another simple implementation of the positivity constraint in CT is a modification of ART (Algebraic Reconstrution Technique), where the image being reconstructed is compared to the data observed, and an error term generated. When this error correction is not added to the pixels of the image being reconstructed (Additive ART) but is multiplicative, this ensures that pixel values will always remain positive.

There have also been a number of heuristic techniques, for example based on the use of Bayes Law [15]. This states that:

$$P[A/B] = \frac{P[B/A] \cdot P[A]}{\sum_C P[B/C] \cdot P[C]}$$

where P[A/B] is the conditional probability of A given that B has occured, and P[A] is simply the probability of A. Following Ortendahl et al [15], suppose that $f(i,j)$ is the i,j th value of the object (real) distribution, and $g(i,j)$ is the i,j th value of the observed image distribution then using Bayes Law:

$$P[g(i,j)/f(k,l)] = \frac{P[g(k,l)/f(i,j)] \cdot P[f(i,j)]}{\sum_m \sum_n P[g(k,l)/f(m,n)] \cdot P(f(m,n))}$$

Thus, expression the above in terms of a nuclear medicine image, $P[f(i,j)]$ is the a priori probability of an event at i,j and is equal to $f(i,j)/N$ where N is the total no. of events (photons) detected. Similarly, $P[f(i,j)/g(k,l)]$ is the probability of an event at i,j given that an event was observed at k,l. $P[g(i,j)/f(k,l)]$ is fairly obviously the system transfer function $h(i,j;k,l)$ or, if stationary, $h(k-i,l-j)$. But since:

$$f(i,j) = \sum_k \sum_l P[f(i,j)/g(k,l)] \cdot g(k,l)$$

Then if f^n is the nth iteration in the following equation:

$$f^n(i,j) = \sum_k \sum_l \frac{h(k-i,l-j) \cdot g(k,l)}{\sum_m \sum_n h(k-m,l-n) \cdot f(i,j)} \cdot f^{n-1}(i,j)$$

Or:

$$f^n(i,j) = W^{n-1}(i,j) \cdot f^{n-1}(i,j)$$

where $W^n(i,j)$ is the weighting function given by the previous equation. This expression for iteratively finding $f(i,j)$ can be modified in a variety of ways. $W^n(i,j)$ is dependent on n.

However, it probably does not change much from iteration to iteration, and a constant set of weights independent of n may be used. In this case $\{W^0(i,j)\}^p$ may be precalculated for p iterations, saving much computing.

Cormack [16] has used essentially the same equation, for nuclear medicine images, but on an event by event basis, rather than considering g(i,j) events in the image at i,j to lead to an estimate of f(i,j) events in the object. A number of other authors have reported the use of various non-linear smoothing and resolution recovery techniques which will not be developed here [17-21]. There is little evidence as to whether such non-linear processing techniques are better than linear operations or are in fact of clinical value, (but see however [9,10]). As for linear processing, it is suggested that display is also a very important factor in the quality of such medical images. Likewise, the availability of array processors could prove very significant.

4. QUANTITATION OF MEDICAL IMAGES

Quantitation of medical images can give intrinsic or derived information. Volume, or area, can be considered as the former, for example the sizing of stenoses in a digitized angiogram. Quantitation of cardiac wall motion from an angiogram or from a radioisotope study can be considered as the latter. Rate of change can be estimated intrinsically; compartment size after fitting a model is 'derived'.

As another example, CT scans can give, with reasonable precision, the radiological density at a point, or within a region of interest. Such quantitative information is intrinsic. If a question is asked of the form, what is the fat content of the muscle in a given CT slice, this must be derived from a knowledge of the expected density of fat and muscle. Such an estimation may be very simple. For example a CT scan of a patient with muscular dystrophy is shown in Fig 1, with a region of interest defined by the superimposed contour. Fig 2 shows a histogram of frequency of occurance of CT values obtained within that region. This should be compared with a similar image as shown in Fig 3 , for a 'normal' patient and the corresponding histogram as shown in Fig 4. Two main peaks may be observed, corresponding to 'fat'- and 'muscle'. Integrating each peak within appropriate limits gives the total number of 'fat' pixels and the total number of 'muscle' pixels, and thereby the relative fat content. The problem of course is how to define the limits of integration. Likewise a rigid classification has been supposed: a pixel is either 'fat' or 'muscle' but not a combination. Nevertheless, such a technique seems to give quite reasonable estimates of fat to muscle ratios.

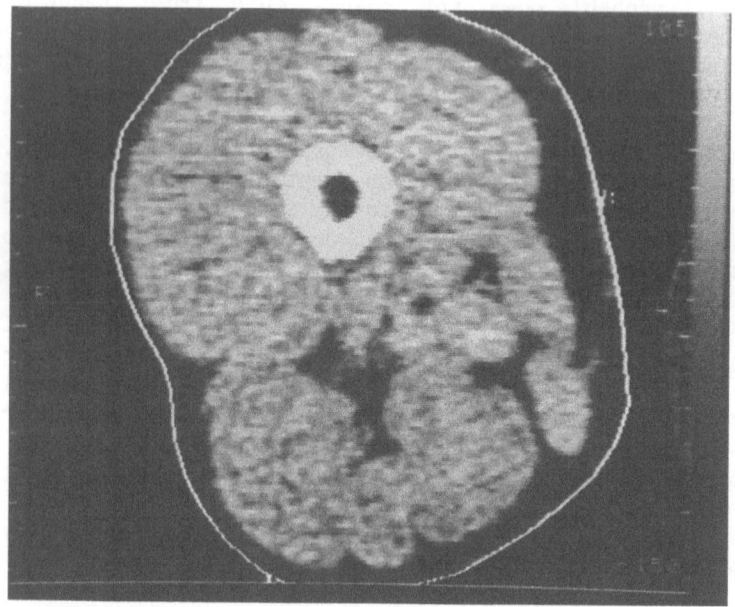

Fig 1. CT image of normal section through thigh.
The contour outside defines a region of interest.

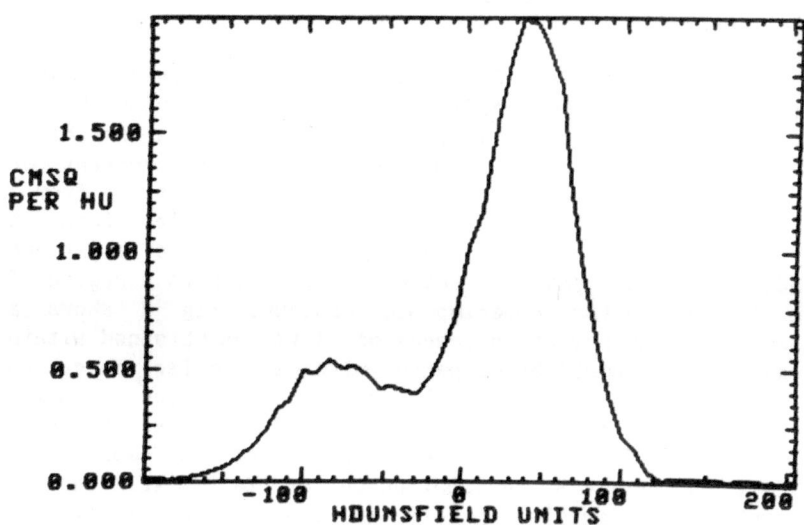

Fig 2. Histogram of CT values within the above region
of interest. The large peak corresponds to muscle, the
small peak to fat. Bone is off scale.

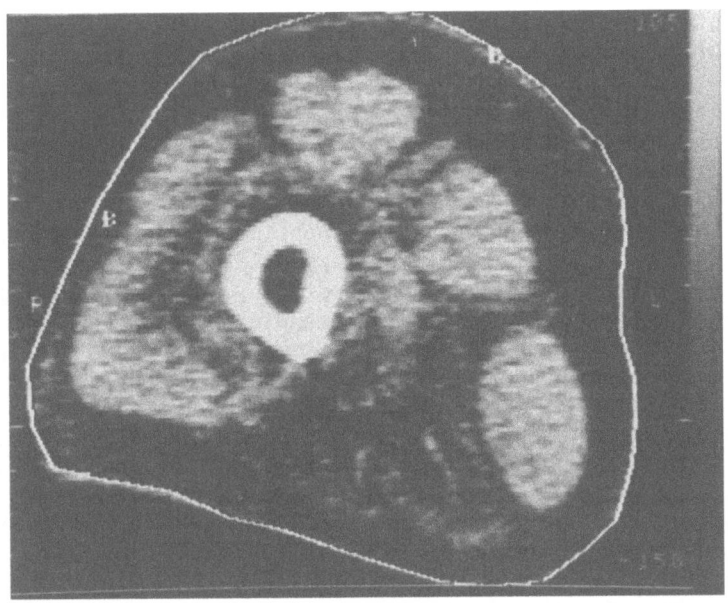

Fig 3. CT image of a similar slice through a patient with muscular dystrophy.

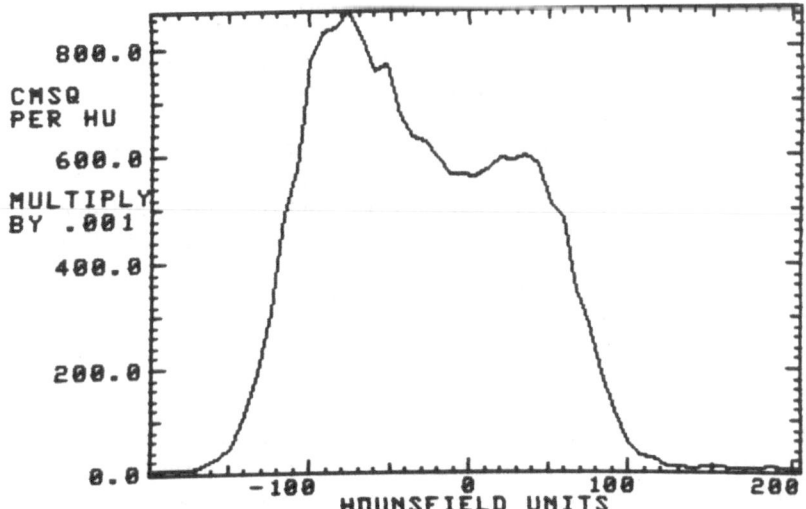

Fig 4. Histogram of CT value from above region of interest. Note the increase in height of the fat peak. The problem is to define suitable limits of integration.

Ejection fraction in nuclear cardiology is another interesting example. Ejection fraction is defined simply as (Max-Min)/Max volumes of a heart chamber, for example, the Left Ventricle (LV). Thus having obtained images of the heart synchronised with its 'beating' i.e. gated by the R-wave, then, if the activity per unit volume of blood is supposed constant, then the number of photons detected in a given region is proportional to the volume of blood in that region. Thus, ignoring background, scatter and attenuation, if a chamber can be isolated (in computer terms - segmented), then estimates of volume at different phases of the cardiac cycle can be determined to derive the ejection fraction. An example of one segmentation algorithm applied to an isotopic cardiac image is shown in Fig 5. The calculation of ejection fraction is not a direct measurement of the image, but is derived from such measurements. In comparison, if a gated tomogram (3-D synchronised data) is obtained, then, if the chamber can be isolated (segmented) volume can be determined directly as can ejection fraction. However, it is important to intercompare the two techniques suggested above to find out which is the more accurate.

Note that, for the planar image, attenuation is not taken into account; it is assumed to be constant. For the tomogram, the volume estimate is independent of attenuation. If, on the other hand, a quantitative estimate of 'activity' within a given volume is to be made, then both types of image need to be corrected for attenuation. Such corrections, while essentially trivial for positron systems (apart from problems associated with the signal to noise ratio), are difficult for single photon tomographic systems, and the subject of current research.

Similar problems exist in CT, for example as a result of beam hardening. Quantitation of ultrasound images, for example volume estimates of scanned objects, is routine, but estimate of derived parameters such as spectral reflection as a function of angle have proved to be tricky, for similar reasons. Physically such effects are 'poorly conditioned'. They are usually non-stationary, and often anisotropic. Suitable techniques for handling such situations are the subject of much current research.

Texture analysis has been used with a variety of medical images. Nuclear medicine images seem to have too much noise and too little data to be amenable to such analysis. CT images are likewise not very interesting since the dominant influence on texture is that of the noise character. However, ultrasound texture analysis for tissue characterization appears promising, and texture analysis of radiographic data is also quite common. However, the texture parameters used so far have been largely empirical (e.g. run length) and cannot as yet be called truely

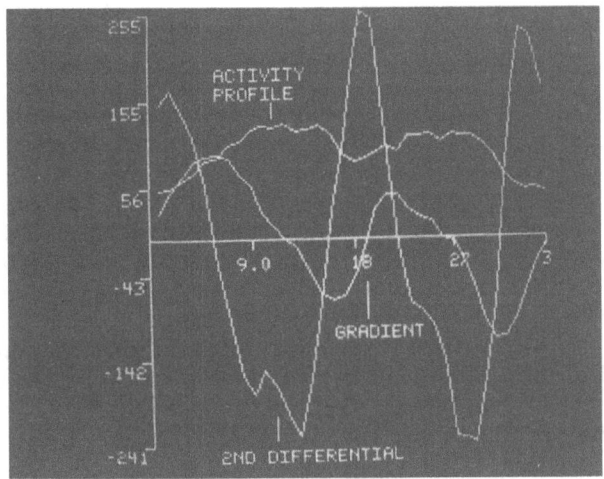

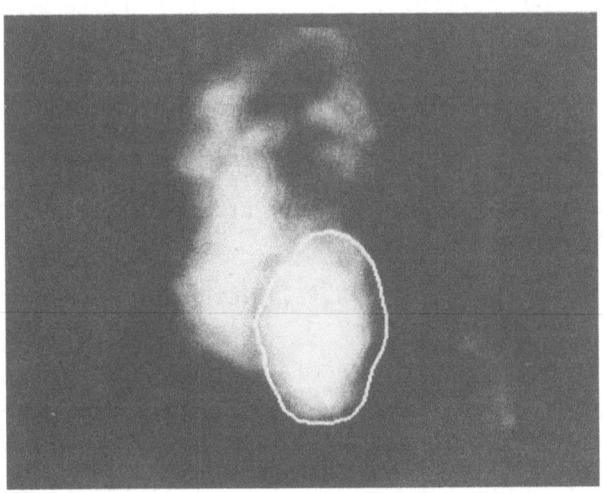

Fig 5. After selecting the centre of gravity of the LV,
a series of radial profiles are obtained, one example
being shown, above, labelled activity profile. The
first and second differentials are then obtained and
turning points detected, for all profiles at all angles
These turning points are combined to form a contour as
shown below. The problem is to define satisfactorily
and reliably the interventricular septum.

quantitative.

5. MATHEMATICAL TECHNIQUES FOR GENERATING FUNCTIONAL IMAGES AND ASSOCIATED NOISE CHARACTERISTICS

Much data in medicine (for example in nuclear medicine), and certainly most functional (physiological) data are essentially 3-D, being images spaced in time, (or space). While the use of regions of interest (ROIs) serve to extract curves, some form of data compression, reducing the 3-D array to a 2-D image, is potentially very powerful. Such a data compression is the generation of functional (or parametric) images. Two fundamentally different approaches exist. Either a model is supposed, and, using this a priori information, the model fitted as a function of position, the parameters of the fit being the values in the functional image. Alternatively, some technique based on diagonalizing the covariance matrix, such a factorial analysis, may be used to generate 'factor images', as has been widely used in general image processing and described under the title of 'compression' or 'coding', (amongst others [22,23]). Firstly, methods of generating functional images will be considered, and secondly, the question of noise generation and propagation will be examined.

5.1 Simple Functional Images - Washout

One common example of a functional image is that of washout, for example of ^{133}Xe in lungs or brain. The model supposed is that, at some time t_o the activity at a point i,j is $C_t(i,j)$ may be expressed as:

$$C_t D(i,j) = C_o(i,j) . \{ N_1(i,j).exp^{-A(i,j).t}$$

$$+N_2(i,j).exp^{-B(i,j).t}\}$$

where $A(i,j)$ and $B(i,j)$ are the fast and slow washout components, and $N_1(i,j)$ and $N_2(i,j)$ are the 'sizes' of each compartment. The simplification of assuming $B(i,j)$ to be large or $N_2(i,j)$ to be zero, a single compartment model, is normally used. The first and oldest method of calculating $A(i,j)$ is to look at the slope $R(i,j)=\{C_{t1}(i,j)-C_{t2}(i,j)\}/(t2-t1)$ from which an estimate of $A(i,j)$ can be made. However the numerator has very poor noise properties, as explained below. Note that to obtain $A(i,j)$ from the ratio given above a non-linear mapping function must be generated e.g. a look-up table giving value of $A(i,j)=f[R(i,j)]$. A second better technique [24] is to use the ratio of moments:

$$R(i,j) = \frac{\int C_t(i,j) \cdot t \quad dt}{\int C_t(i.j) \, dt}$$

The two integrals have much better noise properties than in the previous form. All events in the time series are used in the calculation. Note also that the integrals can be replaced by summations with little loss of precision and the result is independent of sampling. A mapping function is still required. A third method, as described by Budinger [25], is based on the maximum likelihood estimator:

$$\hat{A}(i,j) = \frac{\sum C(t) \cdot t \cdot \sum [C(t) \cdot \ln(C(t))] - \sum t \cdot C(t) \cdot \ln(C(t)) \cdot \sum C(t)}{\sum C(t) \cdot \sum [t^2 \cdot C(t)] - [\sum t \cdot C(t)]^2}$$

where C(t) represents $C_t(i,j)$. A fourth form for the same calculation is as follows. Replace $C_t(i,j)$ by $\ln[C_t(i,j)]$. The calculation of A(i,j) is then a simple linear regression:

$$\hat{A}(i,j) = \frac{\sum t \cdot \ln(C(t)) - N \cdot \sum t \cdot \ln(C(t))}{N \cdot \sum t^2 - [\sum t]^2}$$

The only difference between the last two forms is that of the weighting function used which is uniform in the latter case (which is incorrect), and equal to the square root of the observed values in the former, which reduces bias being introduced from low values of C(i,j) and thus reduces noise. These 4 different types of expression are very representative of the different ways of calculating functional images in general.

5.2 Washin

Washin or rise time supposes a model of form:

$$C_t(i,j) = N_0(i,j) \cdot \{ 1 - N_c(i,j) \cdot \exp^{-A(i,j) \cdot t} \}$$

For which one solution has been given in a previous paper [26] being:

$$\hat{g} = \frac{S_1^{1,N} - S_0^{1,N} \cdot (N+1)/2}{S_1^{0,N-1} - S_0^{0,N-1} \cdot (N-1)/2}$$

where

$$S_1^{p,q} = \sum C_t(i,j) \cdot t$$

$$S_0^{p,q} = \sum C_t(i,j)$$

for the limits given as superscripts p,q. $1-\hat{\beta}$ is an estimate of $exp(-A(i,j).T)$ where T is the sampling rate. An alternative technique is to apply an appropriate transformation, taking logs, and then perform a regression. Also, if $N_c(i,j)$ is supposed to be equal to unity, slopes may be determined and used as estimators of $A(i,j)$.

5.3 Time to Peak

Time to peak has been used for many organs, for example brain and kidney. An appropriate algorithm is:

IF [MAX(i,j) < C_t(i,j)] THEN
{ MAX(i,j)=C_t(i,j) ; TIME(i,j)=t }

where MAX(i,j) has an initial value of 0. This is easily calculated and requires storage only of current maximum and time for each pixel. As always, sampling is of great importance. Such a technique may then be combined with washin and washout estimators defining the time before which washin is to be determined, and after which washout to be estimated.

5.4 Phase

Phase images in cardiac studies are probably the most commonly used functional images (in nuclear medicine) at the present time [27-29]. They are really fits of sinusoids to the gated cardiac data, and are usually calculated as follows:

$$S(i,j) = \sum_t C_t(i,j).Sin(k.t)$$
$$C(i,j) = \sum_t C_t(i,j).Cos(k.t)$$
$$AMP(i,j) = [C(i,j)^2 + S(i,j)^2]^{1/2}$$
$$PHASE(i,j) = Tan^{-1}[S(i,j)/C(i,j)]$$

where $C(i,j)$ is the cosine images, AMP(i,j) is the amplitude image and PHASE(i,j) is the phase image. Note that the Fourier transform as proposed above can be replaced with little loss of 'accuracy' by a Hadamard transfrom and with a considerable gain in computation time such that, if Tan^{-1} is generated using a look-up table, a PHASE image could be generated in real time.

An alternative approach to fitting a sine (or square) wave is to try to fit a function more closely resembling the LV volume curve, by adding in higher order sine functions, or using some statistical technique such as factor analysis or the Karhunen-Loeve transform. It is not yet known whether this is clinically helpful.

5.5 Transit Time

Transit time images, e.g. in brain or kidney, are essentially deconvolutions, being solutions of:

$$g(i,j) = \sum_l \sum_k h(l-i,k-j).f(l,k)$$

to find h() the transfer function, given f() the input function and g() the output function. Practical implementations are by use of the Fourier transform F{ }, since F{h(i,j)}=F{g(i,j)}/F{f(i,j)}, or by (constrained) matrix invertion.

5.6 Factor images

Factor images have been considered in slightly more detail in a previous publications e.g [2]. In general eigenfunctions may be derived such that the original data G and its transpose G' can be expressed as:

$$[G] [G]' = [U] [L] [V]'$$

where [U] and [V] are sets of eigenfunctions, for example sinusoids for an operator such as the Fourier transform, and [L] a diagonal matrix of eigenvalues, being the weight associated with each eigenfunction, in the case of the Fourier transform, the weight of each sinusoidal component. However, there are many such decompositions. It is of interest to find one which minimises the correlation between different eigenfunctions. Such a transform is given by:

$$E[G\ G'] = [U_r] [L_r] [U_r]'$$

where $[U_r]$ is a (row) transform such as the Hotelling or Karhunen-Loeve, and E[G G'] is the expected value of G G', or in other words the covariance matrix. The approach called 'Principal Component Analysis' is essentially similar. Thus each eigenfactor is the weight associated with an eigenfunction or 'factor', where the 'factors' have minimal correlation. The eigenvalues are ordered such that the first is associated with the most variance in the image, etc, in decreasing order. In fact, in general, the importance of the eigenfunctions decreases very rapidly, and only a very few serve to 'capture' all the signal information contained in the image. These factor weights may be used to classify the image (as in discriminant function analysis). Alternatively, the eigenvalues and corresponding factors can be isolated and used in reverse to generate the corresponding factor image, corresponding to a single isolated factor. In general such images do not correspond to any physiological reality and a transformation must be used to combine factors with appropriate weights giving so-called oblique factor images. The use of such techniques applied to medical images is currently of considerable interest (see for example [22,23]) but cannot be considered in greater detail here.

5.7 Parameters to be Optimized

The following questions are important:
1. What spatial sampling is optimal?
2. What temporal sampling is optimal?
3. What is the expected error?
4. How much intermediate storage space is required?
5. What is the computation time?

Clearly, the maximum likelihood operator for determining washout is expensive since it requires 6 separate summations each of which must be stored for every pixel. The unweighted regression requires 4 summations, while the ratio of moments and the phase image require only 2. If a functional image is generated for every point of a 64x64 matrix, then each intermediate value may require 8K words of storage (since they almost certainly require greater precision than the original data), e.g. 48K words for the maximum likelihood operators.

5.8 Noise Propagation

Three types of error must be considered.
1. Absolute error (difference between estimate and true value)
2. Relative error, i.e. absolute error divided by true value
3. The expected error, effectively, the S.D. of the result

The following basic rules may be derived. After addition or subtraction, absolute error adds. After multiplication or division, relative error adds. The error $e_{f(x)}$ after an operation $f(x)$ is equal to $e_x.f'(x)$, i.e. the error is multiplied by the slope of the function. The error after an operation $f(x_1,x_2....)$ is amplified by the sum of the partial derivatives with respect to $x_1,x_2....$. With two random variables x,y then the expected error of x+y is:

$$var_{x+y} = (var_x + var_y)^{1/2}$$

where var_x is the variance of x. From this rule, the expected error after application of a filter $[a_i]$ is amplified by Σa_i^2.

The use of the above, plus their incorporation in recurrence relationships and their solution via linear difference equations, permits a reasonable analytic assessment to be made of the noise propagated by most functional imaging techniques [30]. However, note that the absolute error after subtraction of two nearly equal numbers x and y may be small, but the relative error

$(e_x+e_y)/(x-y)$ may be very large. For this sort of reason, relative error often seems more appropriate to characterize the error properties of processes than absolute error. The expected error (of uncorrelated values) defines a lower limit for the propagated error. When input noise is correlated, which is often the case after image manipulation, the absolute or relative error defines an upper limit. Some results can be derived directly, for example, the error propagation for a cosine image is simply the sum of the cosine weights squared (e.g. 8 for 16 images). The error is then passed to the phase image after multiplication by $1/(1+x^2)$. The error after deconvolution can be investigated by looking at the value of the determinant, etc. An alternative and often simpler technique than analytic assessment of error is to use a (Monte Carlo) simulation.

5.9 Guide Lines

The two general problems encountered are:
1. How can a reasonable signal to noise ratio be achieved?
2. How can noise be masked (or how should the image be segmented)?

Both by simulation (for example [31]) and by manipulation and resampling of real clinical data, it has been possible to compare 4 methods:
1. Smoothing the original data
2. Smoothing the functional images
3. Sampling more coarsely in time
4. Sampling more coarsely in space

The following general observations can be made. There is little difference between 1 and 2, although computationally 2 is cheaper. In both cases, some distortion of the functional image results. In many cases, sampling more coarsely in time is beneficial, or at least, not harmful. Both washout and washin rate are little changed by the temporal sampling rate (as can be expected from sampling theory which suggests that for such models, four time sample points are adequate). Phase images can be constructed similarily with very few points. As coarser spatial sampling is used, so the images become more and more difficult to interpret.

However it should be noted that in functional images:

Relative error is approximately proportional to resolution.

The final compromise has to be determined on clinical grounds, although figures of merit can be determined from simulations or ROC studies.

5.10 Masking

Masking or elimination of noise regions is essential. Some criterion has to be used since, in general, in regions where there is no signal, any numeric value can result in a functional image. As an example, in akinetic cardiac regions, the phase is undefined. Frequently, a simple threshold may be applied such that the functional image at a point is set to zero (or out of range) if the maximum counts, or total counts, or counts at some time t do not exceed this threshold. It is sometimes difficult then to get completely contiguous defined regions. Note also that smoothing of such segmented images is dangerous in that the data from defined regions is being mixed with data from undefined regions which can create serious edge effects. Fig 6 shows the effect of masking in the calculation of time to maximum for a dynamic brain study.

In conclusion, the mathematical methods available seem sufficient, even with the very noisy data encountered in nuclear medicine, to generate satisfactory functional images provided that the underlying models, (with either basic approach), are well defined. Care needs to be taken over spatial and temporal sampling to optimise the clinical value of such techniques.

6. DISPLAY IN TWO DIMENSIONS

The display of medical images is very dominated by technological details. However, although accepting that such considerations are very important in deciding what hardware system should be used to display images, the main area of interest, here, is to decide 'how' they should be displayed, or rather, what display algorithms might be of value. For example, while displays with a resolution of 256x256 or 512x512 or 1024x1024 or greater and with 16 -> 1024 grey levels exist, which is most appropriate and how should such a display be used? What kind of interpolation is is needed? How should pixel value be mapped onto grey values, and what is the value of colour? Indeed, what are the requirements of a display system for medical images?

6.1 Mapping

By 'mapping' is meant the relationship between input pixel values and output display level values. While the most obvious method of mapping a matrix onto a display is linear, there may be much better mapping functions. Let $d(i,j)$ be the display brightness at a point, and $m(i,j)$ be the value in the matrix at a corresponding point then linear mapping is given by:

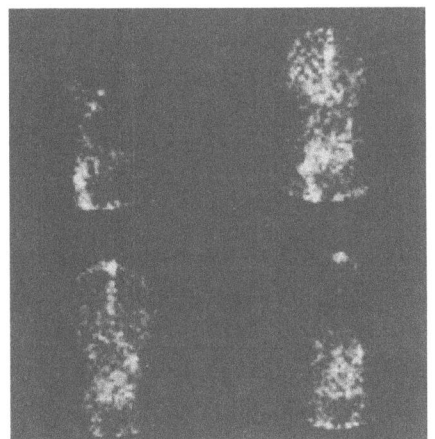

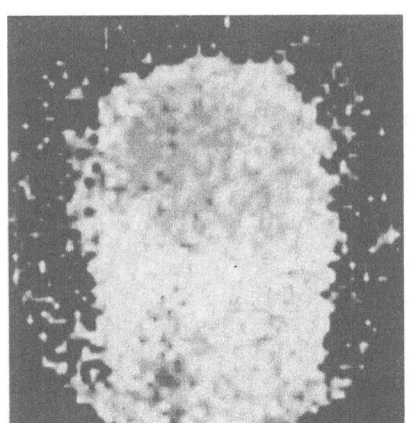
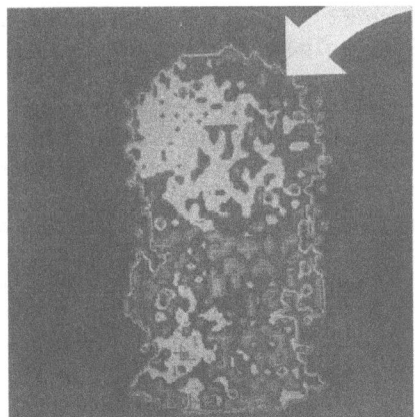

Fig 6. Four views, top, from a radioisotope cerebral
angiogram, showing clear differences in time of arrival
between left and right hemispheres. Below, left, is
shown the raw functional image for time-to-peak. Note
the presence of considerable quantities of noise outside
the brain. A partially processed, and 'masked' functional image is shown, right, with, arrowed, the site
of a subdural haematoma. Further processing of the
image tends to reduce the information content.

```
d(i,j) =  a.[ m(i,j) - b ]
                    while d(i,j) < dmax
```

where a and b are two constants. Background subtraction is
controlled by b and 'contrast' by a. This in fact defines a
window and many displays allow interactive control of a and b or
alternatively of b and dmax. However, many other functions are
possible, for example multiple windows such that areas in m
having very different values may be displayed simultaneously.
Likewise, logarithmic or other functions may be used such that,
for example:

```
d(i,j) =  a.[ log(m(i,j)-b) ]
                    while d(i,j) satisfies some constraint
```

or in general:

```
d(i,j) =  MAP[ f( m(i,j) ]
```

where f() is some function and MAP[] is an operator mapping input
pixel values into output intensities.

The first helpful concept in terms of such mapping is to
consider the process of linearisation, i.e. creating a set of
linearly spaced grey intensities perceptually, that is, to the
user [32]. Displays are normally very unlinear such that the
difference between equal increments in brightness of the display
appear to be very different to an observer. For example Weber's
law [33] suggests that the minimal detectible increment of
brightness (Δd) should be proportional to brightness d itself.
In reality more complex relationships seem to be found with real
displays. However, it may be hypothesised that Δd is a smooth
function of d. Thus it suffices to find Δd for a few values of d
from which by interpolation Δd can be defined for all values of
d. Using this information, a suitable table of values can be
generated for the mapping function MAP to generate an apparently
linear display scale such that equal increments of the scale are
equally perceptually different. This process is constrained by
the limited number of grey scales available, for example if only
16 grey levels exist on the display there is no point in trying
to linearize it. Some appropriate compromise must be adopted. The
question of defining a value for Δd the minimal perceptible
difference is well handled using ROC techniques, and the
interested reader is recommended Pizer [34] for further
information. It must be pointed out that linearisation needs to
be performed for each display, including each different colour
lookup table. A display linearised from the point of view of a
human observer, will not be linearised in term of photographic
hardcopy.

6. 2 Histogram Equalization

A commonly employed technique in display is called histogram equalization. Here the number of pixels with any given grey output level is to be made equal. Thus if VAL(m) is a function such that VAL has a value equal to the number of input pixels of value m, then the histogram equalization process is given by:

$$MAP[m] = k. \sum_{i=1}^{m} VAL(i)$$

Normally this procedure is carried out by calculating VAL over the whole image. However, it is possible to consider a region within the image of some size R. Now, a histogram VAL and a mapping function MAP can be determined for the region R, for every region R. If R=1, one pixel, the operation produces a uniform grey image. Some value of R intermediate between 1 and N the total number of pizels would seem to be appropriate. Pizer [35] has suggesting using values of N/4 and N/16. In order to spead up the algorithm, he has suggested caluulating VAL and MAP for each disjoint region of size R (for example for each quadrant when R=N/4) and than at a point i,j interpolating between the precalculated surrounding MAP functions. Fig 7 shows the result of using such a histogram equalisation procedure. Cormack [36] has suggested a procedure which is essentially similar.

6. 3 Interpolation

It should be stressed that, while data have presumably been collected correctly sampled according to the sampling theorem, there is no guarantee that if displayed with a single data pixel mapping on to a single display pixel that the image will be optimal from the point of view of an observer. The eye has greatest (contrast) sensitivity at certain spatial frequencies, and is less sensitive for both higher and lower frequencies. However, the spatial frequency content of an image is dependent not only on the number of pixels, but also their size (angle subtended at the eye) and such things as noise as generated by edges in the image. Thus while, if the image is minified, a one-to-one mapping from data to display may be adequate, if large images are desired, interpolation is normally helpful. (Note the vagueness of this last sentence: such assertions need to be tested [37].)

Ideally, if the data points in the matrix are supposed to be delta function samples of a continuous distribution, in order to obtain the continuous function (which is after all the aim of interpolation) the delta functions should be replaced by Sinc functions with their first zero crossing point equal to the pixel

340

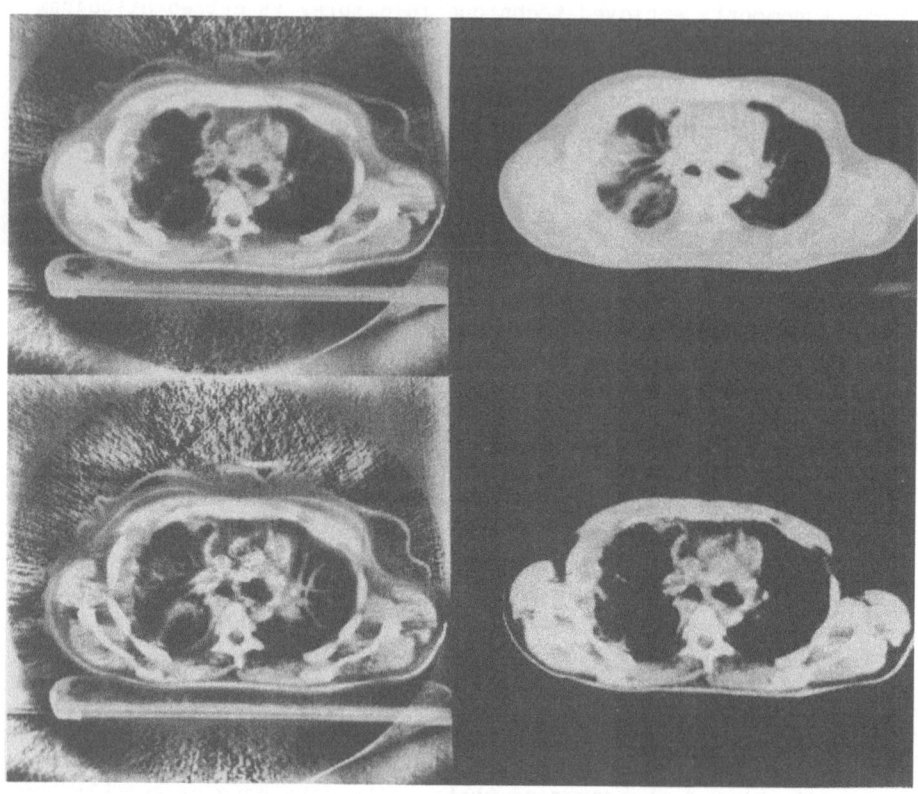

Fig 7. Four displays of a CT image of the chest. Two
windows were selected by clinicians as being optimal
for displaying 'lung', shown above right, and 'bone',
shown below right. Above left is the image obtained
by variable histogram equalization, without lineariza-
tion, while, below left, is the same display, with
linearizarion. Although the noise outside the patient
should be masked, most observers agree that the variable
histogram equalization images contain as much information as the two fixed window images. The above figure
is by permission of Steve Pizer.

size. By inspection, it may be seen that such a process is not very different to linear interpolation, the error being of the order of a few percent. For this reason, bilinear interpolation, being much faster to compute has been used almost exclusively.

7. DISPLAY IN THREE DIMENSIONS

Since so much data, and in particular tomographic data, is essentially three dimensional, it would be helpful if a simple and convenient 3-D display device existed. Many attempts have been made using 2-D displays to present an impression of the third dimension. Thus where surfaces are meaningful, a shaded surface (with perspective) may be portrayed [38]. Stereo pairs have been generated etc. However, the commonly used display technique of looking at series of transverse or coronal or saggital slices leaves much to be desired since it is up to the observer to perform the computation required to imagine an object in 3-D, which is not trivial. Many systems help the observer by paging different slices under interactive control such that the observer can in some manner move a 'bug' in 3-D and obtain the three orthogonal projection passing through the point indicated. However, it is important to realise that current 2-D display systems are intrisically limited in trying to display 3-D images. If the 3-D data are considered to be in a matrix of size 256x256x256 where each point is coded into 8bits (one byte), then, if each point is to be displayed, the corresponding information must be stored somewhere. A simple calculation indicates that the 2-D display must be of size 4096x4096 to contain all the data, essentially whatever display algorithm is used. Likewise, if a manipulation is to be performed, the data transfer rates are correspondingly very high (e.g. >16Mbytes/sec). Current technology can handle 3-D surfaces where the total data content is much less, but the problems of display of 3-D medical images are much more difficult.

However, several true 3-D displays have been developed, for example, the vibrating mirror ([39] amongst others). The principle of the vibrating mirror display is that, using a concave mirror driven in such a way that its radius of curvature changes at some relatively high frequency, for example 60Hz, a display is generated on a device such as a fast phosphor oscilliscope, which is sychronized with repect to the vibration of the mirror. Thus for one given radius of curvature, corresponding to an observer to some distance in 'depth' of the image of the 'scope, a given picture for that 'depth' is generated. Thus, if this is performed for all (useful) distances, a true 3 dimensional image is generated, which may be inspected simultaneously by several observers, and exhibits parallax motion. Perspective, if required, has to be computed in addition and is not computationally simple. For line drawings, for example molecular models, and certain visual scenes, such as aircraft flying over an airport, the 3 dimensional effect of such a display is remarkable.

For medical images, a problem remains, that of displaying 'translucent' objects. It is required to see inside an object (for example a brain). Thus one must be able to see simultaneously both data in front of, and data behind the object of interest. Such data must not be opaque as in conventional surface generating techniques. New display algorithms seem to be needed, for example, highlighting a depth or 3-D contour surface of interest. It should be pointed out again that one drawback of this display system is that of the very high data rates required when displaying complex data such as found in medical images.

Attempting to eliminate this data rate problem, other special purpose display devices have been developed. For example a clever rotating mirror system synchronized with a film projector [40] is commercially available, but the use of some intermediate medium (film) between computer and display seems undesirable since it prohibits interactive use of the display, which is probably essential for medical purposes (viz the opacity problem).

The use of time information for example by continuously rotating the object displayed is a powerful visual clue. A number of workers have used simple systems displaying for example the raw projection data without reconstruction which, for certain types of objects, is remarkably effective (and artefact free). Barber [41] has gone one stage further by incorporating stereo pairs of images such that the rotation of the data can be 'frozen' at some point in time and the stereo clue remains to assist the 3-D interpretation of the data.

Providing a satisfactory 3-D display system is a high priority in current medical imaging, for potential use in nuclear medicine, ultrasound, CT, and, certainly, NMR.

8. DIGITAL RADIOGRAPHY: A POSTSCRIPT

Radiography is evidently one of the areas of considerable interest with respect to the application of digital image processing techniques in medicine [42]. However, essentially, the major technique used in Digital Radiography at present is the subtraction of pairs of images either at different times or at different energies for the purpose of enhancing contrast, or both. While some attempt has been made to use functional imaging methods (as developed in nuclear medicine but apparently unknown

to authors in the radiographic field [43]), it does not appear
that any attempt to use deconvolution methods has been
implemented. An explanation of this is required. It could be
that, in fact, such radiographic data is still very photon
limited. An alternative hypothesis is that the amount of data
(matrix size) computation time, and display facilities are still
too limited. It may be expected that there will be an upsurge of
interest in this area in the near future when a small advance in
technology has taken place. Image processing is useful when the
raw data is of good quality. Handling large matrices with
appropriate operators requires the use of array processors. As
stated previously, the increasing availability of such devices is
likely to change dramatically the use of image processing
operations, in particular, of digital radiographs. Many of the
image processing techniques developed for other applications,
especially those for the creation of functional images, could be
applied directly.

Acknowledgement

The author would like to thank various colleagues for their
help and advice, notably Robert Di Paola with respect to image
processing, Steve Pizer for long discussions about display (and
for permission to use his material on variable histogram
equalization) and Sue Grinrod for helpful comments on CT image
processing and for providing the histograms given as Figs 1-4.
(The author would also like to thank A. T-P for typing the
manuscript.)

BIBLIOGRAPHY

[1] Budinger, T.F., G.T. Gullberg, and RH. Huesman. "Emission
     computed tomography." Topics in applied physics, Image
     Reconstruction from Projections 32 (Springer-Verlag,
     Berlin, 1979) 147.
[2] Di Paola, R. and A.E. Todd-Pokropek. "New developments in
     techniques for information processing in radionuclide
     imaging." Proc. Symp Medical Radionuclide imaging, (IAEA,
     Vienna, 1981) 1 287-312.
[3] Pratt, W.K. Digital image processing, (John Wiley, New
     York, 1978)
[4] Iinuma, T.A. and T. Nagai. "Image restoration of
     radioisotope imaging systems." Phys. Med. Biol. 12 (1967)
     501.
[5] Brown, D.W., D.L. Kirch, T.W. Ryerson et al. "Computer
     processing of scans using Fourier and other

344

transformations." J. Nucl. Med. 12 (1971) 287.

[6] Andrews, H.C. and B.R. Hunt. Digital image restoration, (Prentice Hall, Eaglewood Cliffs New Jersey 1977).

[7] Anscome, F.J. "The transformation of poisson binomial and negative data." Biometrica 35 (1948) 246.

[8] Boardman, A.K. "Constrained optimisation and its application to scintigraphy." Phys. Med. Biol. 24 (1979) 363.

[9] IAEA. "Co-ordinated research programe on the intercomparison of computer assisted scintigraphic techniques, 2nd progress report." Proc. Symp. Medical Radionuclide Imaging (IAEA, Vienna, 1977) 1 571.

[10] IAEA. "3rd progress report." ibid 1 585.

[11] Rai, G.S., J.W. Haggith, J.D. Fenwick and O. James. "Clinical evaluation of computer processing of liver gamma camera scans." Br. J. Radiol. 52 (1979) 116.

[12] Cordier, S., Y. Biraud, A. Champailler and M. Voutay. "A study of the application of a deconvolution method to scintigraphy." Phys. Med. Biol. 24 (1979) 577.

[13] Frieden, B.R. "Image enhacement and restoration." in Picture processing and digital filtering, (Springer Verlag, Berlin, 1975), 177.

[14] Kemp, M.C. "Maximum entropy reconstructions in emission tomography." Proc. Symp Medical Radionuclide imaging, (IAEA, Vienna, 1981). 1 313-323

[15] Ortendahl, D., L. Kaufman, D. Shosa, R. Herfkens, W. Rowan and S. Williams. "Resolution recovery in planar nuclear images." Phys. Med. Biol. in press.

[16] Cormack, J. and B.F. Hutton. "Incremental deconvolution." Phys. Med. Biol. 25 (1980) 339.

[17] Gustafsson, T. and A.E. Todd-Pokropek. "Design and application of filters with variable shape." 2nd Conf. on Data handling and Image Processing Hannover, unpublished (preprint available).

[18] Pizer, S.M., J.A. Correia, D.A. Chesler and C.E. Metz. "Results of nonlinear and nonstationary image processing." Information Processing in Scintigraphy Oak Ridge (1973) USERDA CONF-730687 93.

[19] Bell, P.R. and R.S. Dillion. "Comparison of some non-linear smoothing methods." Information Processing in Medical Imaging ORNL BCTIC-2 (1977) 596.

[20] Gustafsson, T. and S.M. Pizer. "Non-Stationary metz filtering" Information Processing in Scintigraphy (CEA, Orsay, 1975) 56.

[21] Tukey, J.W. "Nonlinear (nonsuperposable) methods for smoothing data." The congressional record EASCON (1974) 673.

[22] Barber, D.C. "The use of prinicipal components in the quantitative analysis of gamma camera dynamic studies." Phys. Med. Biol. 25 (1980) 283.

[23] Bazin, J.P., R. Di Paola and M. Tubiana. "Factor analysis of dynamic scintigraphic data as a modelling method." Information Processing in Medical Imaging, Les Colloques de l'INSERM 88 (1980) 345-366.

[24] Alpert, N.M., B. Hoop, D.A. Chesler, et al. "Dynamic studies with a multiprogrammed computer system." Proc. Symp. Dynamic studies with radioisotopes in Medicine (IAEA, Vienna, 1975) 1 27-43

[25] Budinger, T.F. "Clinical and research quantitative nuclear medicine system." Proc. Symp. Medical Radioisotope Scintigraphy, (IAEA, Vienna, 1972) 1 501-554

[26] Raynaud, C., A.E. Todd-Pokropek, D. Comar, et al. "A method for investigating regional variations of the cerebral uptake rate of ^{11}C-labelled psychotropic drugs in man." Proc. Symp. Dynamic studies with radioisotopes in Medicine, (IAEA, Vienna, 1975) 1 45-57

[27] Geffers, H., W.E. Adam, F. Bitter, H. Sigel, and H. Kampmann. "Data processing and functional imaging in radionuclide ventriculography." Information Processing in Medical Imaging ORNL-BCTIC-2 1977 322.

[28] Verba, J.W., I. Bornstein, N.P. Alazraki, et al. "Onset and progression of mechanical systole derived from gated radionuclide techniques and displayed in cine format." abstract, J. Nucl. Med. 20 (1979) 625.

[29] Bossuyt, A., F. Deconinck, R. Lepoudre and M. Jonckheer. "The temporal Fourier transform applied to functional isotopic imaging." Information Processing in Medical Imaging (Les Colloques de l'INSERM, 88 Paris, 1980) 88.

[30] Pizer, S.M. Numerical computing and mathematical analysis, (SRA, Chicago, 1975)

[31] Pizer, S.M. and A.E. Todd-Pokropek. "Processing of noisy functional images" Proc. 1st World Congress Nucl. Med., Tokyo, (1974) 161-163.

[32] Todd-Pokropek, A.E. and S.M. Pizer. "Displays in Scintigraphy." Proc. Symp. Medical Radionuclide Imaging (IAEA, Vienna, 1977) 1 505.

[33] Cornsweet, T.N. Visual perception. (Acamedic Press, New York, 1970).

[34] Pizer, S.M. "Intensity mappings to linearize display devices." Comp. Graphics and Imag. Proc. 17 (1981) 262-268.

[35] Pizer, S.M. "An automatic intensity mapping for CT display." in press.

[36] Cormack, J. and B.F. Hutton. "Minimisation of data transfer losses in the display of digitised scintigraphic images." Phys. Med. Biol. 25 (1980) 271.

[37] Sharp, P., R. Chesser and P. Dendy. "Pixel size and the quality of clinical radionuclide images." Proc. Symp 2nd Int. Conf. on Visual Pysychophysics and medical imaging, IEEE Special Issue, in press.

[38] Robb, R.A., E.L. Ritman, J.F. Greenleaf, R.E. Strum, G.T.

Herman, P.A. Chevalier, H.K. Liu and E.H. Wood. "Quantitative imaging of dynamic structure and function of the heart, lungs and circulation by computerized reconstruction and subtraction techniques." Proc. 3rd Anual Conf. Computer Graphics, Interactive Techniques and Image Processing (SIGGRAPH '76, Philadelphia, Pa, 1976) 246-256.

[39] Baxter, B.S. "Application of three dimensional display systems in diagnostic imaging." Proc. 3rd World Cong. of Nuclear Medicine, (Pergamon, Paris 1982).

[40] Zyntronics Corporation N.Y., exhibition 1980.

[41] Barber D.C. and I.S. Skellas. "Three dimensional display of radionuclide tomograms." Proc. Symp. 3rd World Congress of Nuclear Medicine Pergamon, Paris, 1982).

[42] Kruger, R.P. "A survey of computer processing of chest radiographs." Information Processing in Medical Imaging (ORNL-BCTIC-2 1977) 13.

[43] Hoehne, K.H., M. Boehm and G.C. Nicolae. "The processing of X-ray image sequences." Proc. Int. Symp. Bad Neuenahr, Advances in digital image processing, (Plenum Press, New York, 1979), 149.

FILM ANALYSIS SYSTEMS AND APPLICATIONS

Y. Yonekura and A. B. Brill

Brookhaven National Laboratory
Upton, N.Y. 11973, U.S.A.

1 INTRODUCTION

Quantitative film analysis systems are being used successfully in high technology applications, including earth's surface
mapping, aerial reconnaissance, and high energy physics particle
tracking. The intense interest in these types of images has led
to the development of sophisticated techniques for recording and
extracting high quality information from local and remote sensing
systems. The transfer of this technology to medicine awaited the
development of lower cost simpler systems. Such devices are now
available, and being utilized for radiological image analysis.

During the past 20 years, there has been a revolution in electronic technology so that high quality image analysis systems are
now widely used in hospital practice. Film analysis systems can
be classified as analog or digital. Section 2 of this manuscript
presents a brief review of the different systems elements that can
be used, including experience obtained with a system we are using.
Section 3 presents examples of medical applications to indicate
the potential utility of these techniques for the development of
new knowledge and for routine applications, as well.

Biomedical applications of autoradiography (ARG) have been
employed since Becquerel's discovery of natural radioactivity.
Heightened interest in ARG now exists in response to several recent developments. The thalidomide toxicity experience focused attention on the need to screen new drugs prior to use in humans for
unsuspected focal accumulations in animals. With the rapid increase in frequency and types of nuclear medicine procedures, information on radiation dosimetry of new compounds is needed, along
with dose ranges within organs. Rapid developments in positron

emission tomography (PET) technology include the synthesis of new radiolabelled compounds whose distribution, and metabolism in normal and disease states need to be evaluated. The use of in vitro ARG provides the high resolution needed to determine biodistribution in small animals, in regions which are far smaller than can be resolved by current PET technology.

For these reasons, and others that will be discussed in Section 3 of this report, we believe that these systems will be of increasing use in medical research and medical practice.

2 FILM ANALYSIS SYSTEMS

2.1 Components

2.1.1 Film. Many sizes and types of film are available commercially and the choice depends on the application. Key factors that determine the proper film are the spectral sensitivity, and resolution required. For radiographic studies, single and double-sided emulsions are available, and these are used with and without special intensifying screens depending on radiation dose and image resolution requirements. For example, when final detail is needed industrial grade film can be used without intensifying screens. Dose is of no concern in industrial radiography, and hence such small, fine grain, one-sided emulsion, high resolution films are useful for nondestructive materials testing using high energy gamma ray sources (^{60}Co). Alternatively, there is the need for high sensitivity film which can be used to image low energy radiation, for example beta rays (β^-) from tritium for ARG visualization. In this case, special films are now used in which the silver is on one side and there is no emulsion coating which would attenuate the low energy beta rays (1). Special films, and intensifying screens are used for mammography studies, to reduce patient dose. Since geometrical factors play a major role in determining the resolution (sharpness) of ARG images, close apposition between the imaged sample (radioactive tissue section) and the film is required.

When sensitivity is marginal, long contact times are needed. The time required for a given film can be reduced in several ways:

(1) Increasing the amount of nuclide given to the animal,

(2) Pre-irradiating the film to eliminate the low intensity heel of the curve, so that you start to work on the linear portion of the H(intensity x time) and D(density) curve, or

(3) By use of an intensifying screen and double-coated film
so that radiations that penetrate the emulsion and which ordinarily would be lost, can elicit additional light from the screen,
adding to the film exposure.

(4) Lastly, exposure in the cold will reduce fading of the
latent image during long exposures.

2.1.2 Sensing systems

2.1.2a Densitometers. Manual densitometers have been used in
sensitometry for many years. These are the typical systems used
for quality control of film processing systems, including
radiographic instrumentation. Measurement of the attenuation of
light transmitted through a film in comparison to calibration step
wedges is the standard method. Accurate quantitative data are
obtained for points in the image sampled with such equipment. The
light source sampling aperture, and sensitivity of the sensor are
uniform (positionally invariant) and permit accurate comparisons
from the few points one ordinarily samples. If it is necessary to
make many such measurements over large areas, to preserve spatial
as well as intensity resolution, then more automated methods are
used.

2.1.2b Flying spot scanners. These devices typically utilize a
scanning light beam which moves over the image, and intensity of
transmitted light is recorded over sequentially sampled regions.
High cost, high performance electromechanical systems of this type
were developed for physics application, i.e. nuclear track analysis (2). Simpler electro-optical systems now are available commercially and are used for most applications (3).

2.1.2c Television camera-based systems. Vidicon
(videoconverter) television pick-up tubes are the most commonly
used means of transducing 2-D images into electrical signals which
will drive a TV display. Vidicon tubes originally employed SbS_3
as the photosensitive material. The Plumbicon contained PbO
rather than SbS_3, and more recently Chalnicon tubes are used,
which contain $CdSe-As_2S_3$ (4). These changes in tube design have
resulted in increased sensitivity (wide dynamic range), improved
spectral response (covering IR through the UV) and diminished lag,
which provides a more faithful representation of the scene.

The TV camera records and displays a 2-D image from 2 or 3-D
objects and hence can be used for real time inspection, and measurement of moving as well as stationary objects. The output of
such devices is displayed on TV monitors with between 525 and 1024
lines/frames, depending on spatial resolution requirements. Typically TV systems operated at 30 frames (60 interlaced fields) per

second and provide a flicker-free display on black and white or color cathode ray tube (CRT) monitors. The major problems with TV recording and display systems are noise sensitivity, and differing resolution along X and Y directions due to the scan raster pattern.

2.1.2d Mosaic-array sensors. Linear arrays of photodiodes or charge storage devices - charge-coupled devices (CCDs) and charge injection devices (CIDs) - are used for imaging transmitted or reflected light from stationary objects (5,6). The linear arrays view an object (positive or negative film) mounted on a rotating drum. Alternatively, linear translation of the film (or transducer) can be used to acquire data from a 2-D scene. Such devices are available as components or as assembled systems whose output can be displayd directly as TV images, or can be digitized for subsequent analysis. Blemishes, i.e., non-uniformities in the response characteristics of different elements in these arrays, are always present and require either digital normalization or analog masks for correction. These systems have the advantage of better spatial sampling properties than TV pick-up tubes. These devices have further advantages in that they can perform real time analog signal processing operations, as well as lending themselves readily to digitization for computer analysis. Two dimensional CCD and CID cameras are also available as complete systems. Increasing use of such devices is occurring and more sophisticated processing options are emerging. Commercially available CCD camera systems have gone from 32 x 32 (1976) to 488 x 380 (1980) and arrays up 1024 x 1024 are expected in the next year or two. Linear arrays are now available at reasonable prices in 2048 x 1 assemblies, which are used for high quality digitization of images for facsimile transmission and for film image analysis. By utilizing scanning translations of film or the linear array, 2048 by arbitrary size images can be acquired, displayed, digitized, and processed. Sensor materials will become available in the near future that will yield an improved spectral response compared to silicon. Materials, such as GaAs, are now being developed for CCD devices. Hitachi Corp., for example, is offering a 512 x 512, fully compatible with U.S. Television Standards (NTSC), and larger arrays are anticipated.

2.1.3 Digitizers. The spatial and intensity resolution that can be achieved in a particular study is limited by factors inherent in the scene and the film recording system. Analog to digital converters (ADC) are used to transduce voltage levels from analog sensors to digitized values.

Spatial resolution for TV imaging systems is determined by the number of samples taken across the image, and the size of the field of view. By optical magnification, one can vary the size of the region represented by a given pixel. The sampling mesh can be adjusted by varying the number of bins into which the data are distributed. This is determined by the number of TV lines (y axis) and the number of samples taken along each line. Intensity resolution is limited by the number of levels into which the signal is divided. Digitizers with 8-12 bits resolution are commonly used which permit the construction of array sizes, or intensity levels, with 256-4096 different intervals.

TV frame digitizers are typically of two types. The first type is slow, but low in cost, while the second is fast, operating in real time and more expensive. The slow digitizer takes advantage of the fact that each of the 525 horizontal lines in a TV image has a 62.5 microsecond retrace time. Thus, if one samples and digitizes the signal level in one picture element at the beginning of each horizontal line, in sequence, and then advances through the image column-by-column it will take n(1/30) seconds to digitize the whole image, where n is the sampling mesh size chosen. Thus, an image can be digitized into a 256 x 525 mesh (actually only 480 horizontal lines are seen on a 525 line system) in 256/30 or approximately 8 seconds. This slow data rate permits easy acquisition and storage of the digitized image from stationary objects using low cost micro or minicomputer systems without special purpose components, besides the computer-based digitizer itself.

The second type of digitizer operates in real time. If one divides an image into 256 x 480 elements and samples it in 1/30 second, the system must digitize, and acquire more than 4 million 8 bit bytes/second. This requires fast data buffers in addition to fast ADCs and the usual computer hardware for imaging applications. This is the type of system that is used ordinarily for digitization of the output of CCDs and for real-time radiographic applications.

2.1.4 Processors. Image processing and enhancement can be achieved with analog, digital, and hybrid systems. Analog systems are usually fast and can handle large array sizes. Digital systems tend to be slower and more costly, but have greater flexibility. Actually, most systems have both analog and digital components and are best categorized as hybrids.

Simple optical data processing can be achieved very cheaply using TV cameras. The image from a single film viewed by a TV camera can be processed using contrast enhancement, background erase, and windowing with the resulting image displayed in black and white, or color. By the use of calibration step wedges in the field, intensity levels can be coded into pseudo-color intervals for visual "quantitative" comparisons within as well as between

352

films. Two different films taken at successive intervals can be
viewed by 2 different cameras, whose outputs can be subtracted to
display differences. In this fashion, images before and after contrast injection are used to display perfused structures without
background common to both films. Similarly, ARG images taken with
different labelled compounds can be displayed to reveal differences in metabolism of two compounds in the same tissue section.

More sophisticated optical data processing can also be accomplished using coherent light sources (lasers) and optical paths
which permit spatial and frequency filtering of images (7). Optical filters designed in digital systems can perform mathematically
prescribed operations and the results of these operations can be
recorded on film. To avoid delays and problems in film
processing, the "processed" images can be viewed in real time on
TV monitors when the optical path is projected onto a TV camera,
instead of film. Further, the ability to project video images
into a coherent optical path for optical data processing is under
development and such systems could have a significant impact on
real time image processing of digital as well as analog (film)
images (8).

Analog processing can also be achieved with CCD and CID
systems. By varying the weighting factors between adjacent elements attractive for use in modern image storage and processing
achieved; by varying weighting factors between adjacent rows and
columns in 2-D arrays, real time fourier transform operations can
be performed (9). The ability to use CCD, and CID buffers for
data collection, storage, and real time processing makes these element attractive for use in modern image storage and processing
systems.

The development of fast, high performance, low cost
microprocessors has revolutionized modern instrumentation. Because of the low cost involved in the cost of computer components,
it is now economically feasible to construct dedicated systems for
single applications, such as film analysis. The costs of software
development at present greatly exceed the costs of hardware.
Hence, until well-engineered commercial dedicated systems become
available at low cost, many users will find it preferable to share
the use of a larger computer developed for general purpose image
processing applications. Specialized biomedical image analysis
systems are now available in many institutions. A typical
hospital-based nuclear medicine laboratory contains one or more
general purpose digital computers which are used for image collection and processing and which can be used for film analysis. The
film analysis system we are using is basically a nuclear medicine
computer, and is described in Section 2.2.

The recent development and growth of digital radiography systems suggests that in the near future many hospitals will be equipped with high quality TV analysis and display systems for the conduct of routine radiographic studies. Since these systems, in general, digitize the output of a TV camera coupled to the back end of an x-ray image converter (image intensifier tube), it is clear that provision could be made easily to switch a second TV camera viewing a film into the data path when the x-ray system is not being used, to utilize the real time digitization, analysis, and display capability of the digital radiography equipment. The availability of such equipment should greatly expand the range of applications and use of film processing in radiological and allied studies.

2.1.5 Storage. Storage of large numbers of images is a difficult problem. Film itself, is the most commonly used high quality image storage medium. With the high cost of silver, logistic, and cost problems in storage, accessioning and distribution of films, alternative media are being sought for medical diagnostic and research purposes.

Analog images can also be stored on video tape (reels or cartridges), or on video discs. The former have large capacities, and are most useful for acquiring and storing cinematic images. This is due to the fact that the noise content of a single image (still frame) is often too high for direct viewing. Once recorded on video disc or tape the noise is a permanent part of the study. Since the noise from the TV system is random, this source of artifact can be removed from TV camera/film analysis systems by summing together and signal averaging multiple digitized images from a single high quality film record. In this way, TV-film analysis systems can produce relatively noise-free images.

Video discs permit rapid random access to single images in large files, whereas it takes a much longer time to move from the first to the last recorded image on a typical tape file. Further, the ability to stop-frame and digitize an image, and do subtraction studies, for example, is far simpler and more accurate when high performance video discs are used for video image recording. Such capabilities are useful for ARG and other imaging applications.

Higher fidelity can be retained by storing the data directly in digital form. Temporary storage in semiconductor or core memories is useful, prior to storage on a permanent archival media. Such archival materials include floppy discs (cheap, and can be used for individual patient files), or various types of disc cartridge systems. These can contain many studies and pro-

vide the capability of random access and permit retrival of large
numbers of images stored in compact form.

Permanent, non-reuseable laser-encoded files have been used
as an archival media for very large systems. Simpler systems used
mylar tape, and a laser written hole pattern encoding the digital
data. Currently, similar systems are being developed using multiple layer disc packs in which the laser-induced hole pattern determines the image element values. In one such system under development (Phillips), the information is digitized and recorded on a
disc, from which it can be displayed in video format or can be
retrieved in digital form for further numerical analyses. Several
such discs could be on-line simultaneously. The capacity of each
disc is of the order of 1,000 megabytes, equivalent in storage capacity to fifty 1200 foot magnetic tapes and the cost/disc should
be less than $200. Thus, such systems could provide the capacity,
and quality needed for archival purposes for clinical and research
purposes at reasonable costs.

2.1.6 Displays. The development and wide dissemination of high
quality x-ray computed tomography systems has brought state of the
art display systems into medical use for the first time.
Interactive systems which permit the operator to carry out different display processing options and to recover quantitative information from user-defined regions of interest now are a standard part
of radiological image analysis systems, including low cost nuclear
medicine data acquisition systems. These provide black and white
and color displays, and with specialized peripheral devices and
interfaces can be used to acquire and display images from various
sensors, including film analysis systems. Modern computer architectures often include general or special purpose array processors
which enhance the speed and complexity of operations that may be
performed in the display processing systems, with little or no dependence on the main frame computer itself. Such systems will be
of importance in correlative imaging situations, where images from
different devices are registered so as to display concordant and
discordant features.

2.2 Description and Characterization of a TV-Sensor Based System.

2.2.1 System Description. The Brookhaven National Laboratory,
Medical Department TV-film analysis system is illustrated in Figure 1.

2.2.1a Hardware. The TV camera is a Chalnicon (Hamamatsu Model
C1000-01) 1), coupled via a camera control unit (Hamamatsu Model
M999-05) to a Digital Equipment Corp. PDP 11/34 via a DMA

_____
1, Hamamatsu Systems Inc., 332 Second Ave., Waltham, Mass. 02154.

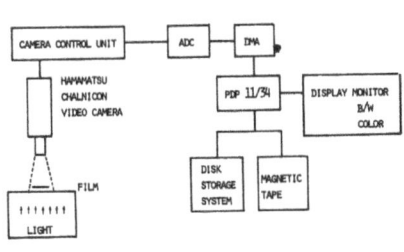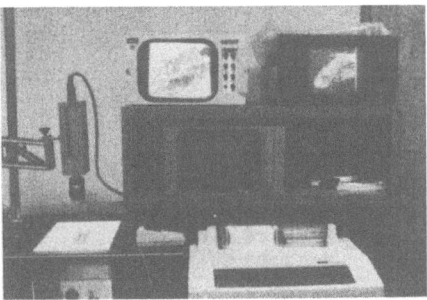

Fig. 1. Schematic diagram (left) and picture (right) of TV-film analysis system in Brookhaven National Laboratory, Medical Department.

interface (DR11B). An adapter ring permits the camera to be used with standard 35mm photographic lenses. By proper choice of lens and distance, the size of the field viewed can be adjusted for all film sizes one is likely to encounter. The camera control unit provides focus and gain controls for the TV camera, low level bias adjustment and variable digitizer mesh sizes (256^2, 512^2, and 1024^2).

The light box constructed for this application consists of eight tungsten filament light bulbs controlled by a variable autotransformer in a box covered with ground glass.

The display system used is a Unibus device which buffers 256 x 256 x 18 bits of data, and displays images up to 256 x 256 x 16 or 512 x 512 x 4, with 2 overlay planes (Computer Design and Applications - CD&A - Model MDP-3) 2). The display system is coupled to an array processor (CD&A Model MSP-3) for enhancing display system performance. Images are displayed on black and white and color TV monitors simultaneously. The color-coded images reveal more levels than can be perceived on the black and white, while the black and white displays provide an immediately recognized intensity scale that complements the color display.

2.2.1b Software. An RT-11 operating systems is used with Gamma-11 (DEC) and more recently Delta-11 (CD&A) has been added. The options used for film analysis procedures are:

---

2. Computer Design and Applications, Inc., 375 Elliot Street, Newton Upper Falls, Mass. 02164.

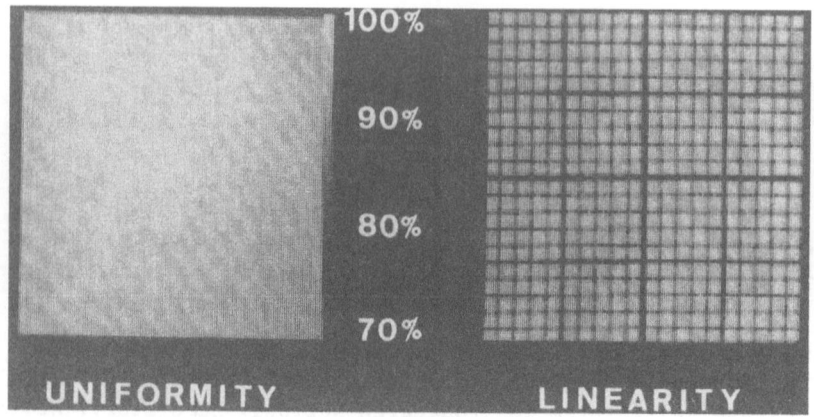

Fig. 2. Uniformity and linearity of TV-film analysis system.

(1) Variable array size digitization.

(2) Signal averaging by multiple integration (to improve signal to noise ratio).

(3) Display of the magnified image obtained from a small region with high resolution (1024 x 1024 sampling).

(4) Imaging system distortion corrections (uniformity, linearity, blurring).

(5) Registration of two images to compare and manipulate these images pixel-by-pixel. For double-isotope ARG analysis, blurring or resolution recovery of the digitized film image is done to permit spatially-congruent assessment of tracer content. This is important for example, when a blurred F-18 image is compared to a sharper C-14 image.

(6) Quantification of film density in each pixel, using a standard curve with linear interpolation between adjacent values.

(7) Histogram equalization displays are used to present images with wide variations in gray scale, while quantitative displays use linearized scales.

These utility programs operate under the RT-11 system, but some data analyses which need larger memory are performed on a 32 bit computer, VAX 11/780, to which the data are transferred via magnetic tape.

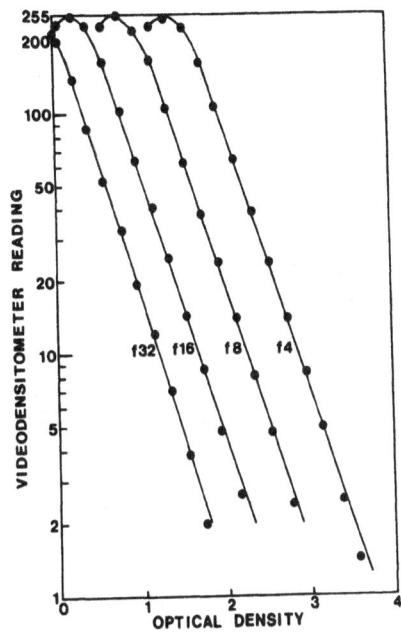

Fig. 3. Relation between optical density and digitized light intensity.

2.2.2 Performance characteristics.

2.2.2a Uniformity and linearity. The uniformity and the linearity of this system are illustrated in Figure 2. The coefficient of variation of the digitized number using a uniform intensity source (light box) is less than 2% when signal averaging is used (16 to 32 integrations). Intensity distortion is characteristic of the sensor response, and to a lesser extent non-uniformity in the illumination system. These need to be adjusted computationally to provide a flat field response. The maximum intensity distortion is approximately three times the coefficient of variation and the major distortion in our system is seen as a decreased mean response level in the lower right side of the field. Spatial linearity was measured using linear graph paper with reflected light. Measured spatial linearity distortion is less than 1% with a standard photographic close-up lens, and manufacturer specifications quote linearity as better than 0.2%.

2.2.2b Spatial resolution. The spatial resolution of the system depends on the focal length of the lens, the lens to film distance, and the array size used. The maximum spatial resolution of this system obtained by digitizing a 1 x 1 cm field into a 1024 x 1024 array, provides a 10 x 10 micron pixel size, which exceeds the resolution needed for ARG studies. Studies with TV test patterns show that the system can resolve between 8 and 16 lines per mm.

2.2.2c Light intensity response. Figure 3 shows the relation between optical density and digitized light intensity measured from a calibrated intensity step wedge. The response is linear for a broad range of optical densities when different lens openings are used. The response characteristics of the system rarely require digitization with more than a single lens opening.

2.2.2d Stability. A usual procedure involves 16 integrations to reduce noise from the video camera system. This requires 70 seconds for acquiring and signal averaging a 128 x 128 image array. The stability of the system was assessed by repeatedly digitizing the output of the light box for many hours. After initially turning on the system, it took approximately 10 minutes for a stable mean and standard deviation to be recorded (density recorded in the center of the field of view). Short term transients were not seen. Long term drifts, which ranged up to 2%, were observed over several hours. Since the procedure involves reference to calibration data with each image processed, these slow drifts do not interfere with the accuracy or precision of the study analyses.

3 METHODS AND APPLICATIONS

3.1 Film Enhancement

There are many ways to enhance films if one has the option of taking additional exposures. When one is dealing with unique images, this option is not available and it may be important to recover information by various tricks. The problem may arise because of under/over exposures, from sources of distortion which are inherent in the imaging system, or from subject related artifacts, such as motion. Each of these can be corrected, at least in part, by appropriate methods.

It is possible to extract additional information by methods which enhance the film image per se. Thus, neutron activation will render the developed silver grains radioactive, and then contact ARG (the activated film is used instead of a tissue section to produce the ARG) may reveal additional detail not perceived in the original negatives themselves (10). This method requires the availability of thermal neutron sources and is time and labor intensive in terms of the processing requirements. In addition, if other elements in the film are activated, high background levels will limit the enhancement achieved.

Autoradiography has also been performed on films using ^{35}S-labelled compounds which react with the developed silver grains in the film (11). Contact ARGs reveal detail in the second film exposed to the low energy beta rays from ^{35}S which could not be perceived in the original images. Figure 4 shows that a low contrast (low dose) X-ray can be contrast-enhanced chemically (ARG) to provide a xerograph-like image, without added radiation exposure to the patient. The method is time consuming and requires the use of radioactive chemicals and hasn't yet found wide application although very good results have been obtained with underexposed satellite photographs, and medical images (mammograms, and angiography studies) (11-14).

Another very promising method avoids the need for radioactive solutions, and does not require the ARG processing step. This involves the reaction of a fluorescent dye with the silver remaining on the film. By exposing the processed film to UV light, the fluorescent distribution can be imaged on film, or can be viewed with a high resolution lens-coupled video camera for real time processing and viewing of the image (15). In this system, processing time and complexity is small and as such could be useful for recovery of useful information from under-exposed images. It has been shown that the method can be useful if background fog levels are low, and care is taken in processing the original films, to avoid artifacts.

If one analyzes film without physical or chemical enhancements, there are analog and digital techniques which may be used to improve contrast and resolution. These include:

(1) Optical data processing - By using different band pass filters in the optical path, filtering operations can be accomplished which:

    (a) Remove characteristic artifacts, (such as scan lines)

    (b) Compensate for blurring due to imaging system distortions, and

    (c) Recognize patterns for which characteristic masks have been created.

(2) Contrast enhancement and background erase.

These operations can be carried out using analog or digital techniques. By adjustment of background cut-off, one may eliminate background fog or intensity levels below a threshold value.

360

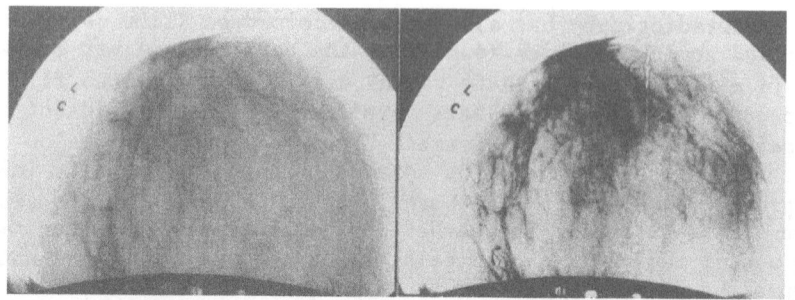

Fig. 4. Low contrast X-ray mammogram (left) and radiochemically-
enhanced image (right).

One may display all the intensity levels that can be viewed on the
display media (TV or film) for selected intensity bands through
the image where additional structural detail is desired. Similarly, one can recover information at the lowest or highest levels
where the film process is least efficient (the tails of the H&D
curve).

3.2 Autoradiography (ARG)

The autoradiographic method has been used widely for many
years, and a large literature exists on methods and applications
(16-20).

The ARG method enjoys new popularity because it provides data
not easily obtained otherwise. Small accumulations in parts of
organs cannot easily go unnoticed in studies using these
techniques. Further, improved sample preparation equipment for
whole body sectioning, now makes it simpler to conduct such
studies. Further impetus comes from the need to evaluate
biodistribution (including dosimetry) and to assess the potential
utility of new compounds developed for use in clinical nuclear medicine. The fact that nuclear medicine scientists skilled in these
procedures are actively involved in these studies should assist in
promulgating these mehtods for use in a growing number of
applications. Previously, most tracers used in diagnostic nuclear
medical imaging studies emitted low energy (100-200 KeV) gamma
rays which did not lend themselves readily to ARG. The development of new positron-emitting short radioactive half-life agents
has revived interest in ARG for various reasons.

Information on biodistribution at multiple times is needed
for:

(1) High resolution biodistribution data,

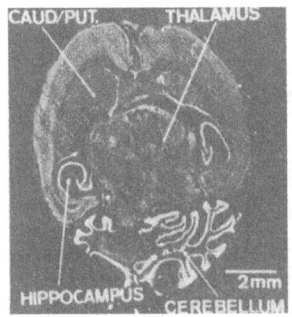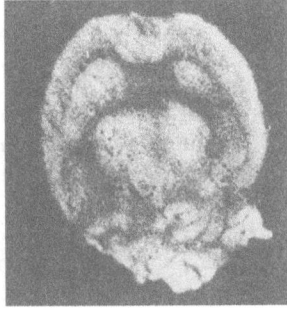

Fig. 5. Anatomical picture (left) and ^{14}C-2-deoxyglucose
autoradiogram (right) of transverse section (mouse
brain).

(2) Dosimetry,

(3) Improved understanding of normal physiological, and
biochemical mechanisms,

(4) Effects of drugs/disease on distribution and metabolism,
and

(5) Correlations between blood flow and metabolism.

Some examples of ARG studies which provide these types of
data are illustrated from our work and from the literature. The
ability to localize different compounds, one at a time, in the
body requires no new techniques. The ability to map two or more
processes, simultaneously, is now being explored in several
laboratories (21-26). Quantitative densitomety systems (26-28)
make it possible to quantitate the relative distributions of two
(or more) tracers simultaneously, and to assess the effects of various perturbations on metabolism (29). In addition, methods now
exist for doing ARG on samples containing stable isotopes which
make it possible to do new types of studies in human patients. Examples of different approaches will be presented for single, dual,
and multitracer studies. Variation in physiological state and
difficulties in cutting exactly comparable sections through experimental and control animals, contribute to the error in such
studies. In Section 3.2.2, the use of dual tracer techniques will
be shown to be a means of minimizing these errors.

3.2.1 Studies using a single tracer

3.2.1a Metabolic studies. ARG studies involve the production of
a film record of radioactive emissions from a thin tissue section
(typically 10-30 μ thick). Som et al. (28) in our lab have
developed procedures for whole body ARG in collaboration with Fand
and McNally (30). The images are a 1:1 mapping and hence visual
inspection reveals major correspondences. Figure 5 shows images
of ^{14}C-2 deoxyglucose (^{14}C-2DG) in mouse brain, next to a photograph of the anatomical section from which it was derived. The
histological section provides information on the anatomical structures which are spatially congruent with the ARG image of the
radioactivity distribution. Given

(1) that fiducials can be identified in both sets of images,
and corresponding locations in the two representations overlaid,
and

(2) that calibration data permit density to be transformed
into μCi content, and

(3) blood glucose levels and clearance of the injected ^{14}C-
2DG are measured, then it follow that regional glucose metabolic
rates can be computed for different body regions. Sokoloff and
his colleagues pioneered in the development of this method. Wolf
and his colleagues at BNL developed the ^{18}F labelled 2-fluoro-2-
deoxyglucose compound (^{18}F-2DG) which permits the use of this
method in patients (using PET) as well as for ARG in animals.
When data for different brain regions are calculated from such
studies and then summed, the results are in close agreement with
independent estimates from global measurements of total brain glucose metabolism.

From studies, such as these, regional cerebral glucose metabolism (RCGM) has been quantitated for different brain structures in
normal animals. Changes from these values are assessed by
studying groups of animals, each exposed to either mock procedures
or experimental agents, and differences between RCGM assessed
based on statistical tests of differences between means of different groups of experimental subjects. Additional data can be
extracted from studies such as the above. These include:

(1) 3-D anatomical mapping of organs, and/or organelles
established from a series of slices taken at multiple levels.

(2) Histochemical procedures can be used to localize and possibly to quantitate the distribution of metabolites in the various
organs (for example, glucose content may be mapped following glucose oxidase treatment of sections) (31). Such analyses would be

fostered by the use of color sensitive TV camera systems, since
stained regions have characteristic colors. Alternatively, color
filters could be used which increase contrast selectively for
particluar colors viewed by a black and white camera.

(3) The effect of different drugs, treatments, or disease,
can be studied in animals and analyses based on pattern changes.

(4) Radiation dose distributions in selected organs can be
assessed from sequential slices taken at different times following
injection into different animals. This will provide information
on mean dose as well as the range of doses in normal and abnormal
circumstances.

(5) By chemically analyzing tissue plugs sampled from regions of interest in particular sections, the chemical form of the
label can be assessed.

The analysis of chemical form of the injected tracer is
clearly a factor of major concern for understanding the biology underlying the observed images. For volatile compounds, such as
^{14}C-labelled chloroform (^{14}CHCl$_3$) it is possible to distinguish
metabolite distribution from the parent compound (^{14}CHCl$_3$) by the
use of two temperatures in the processing of the materials. The
initial AGR sections are made with tissues kept at low temperatures throughout the processing. This records the location of the
volatile parent compound, plus non-volatile metabolites. By
letting the specimens warm up and degass a second ARG image reveals only the fixed metabolites. Thus, one can separately analyze the distribution of ^{14}CHCl$_3$ plus metabolites, and metabolites
alone, and by difference determine the distribution of
unmetabloized ^{14}CHCl$_3$ that was present at the time the animal was
sacrificed (32).

3.2.1b Blood flow. Since metabolism is a convolution of
blood flow with subsequent metabolic pathways (transport and
change) it is necessary to assess blood flow and metabolism
independently if the two processes are to be separated (20,21).
Such studies can be accomplished readily by the use of labelled
10-15 micron diameter microspheres, which are trapped in perfused
capillaries. Gallium-68 is a very useful agent for such studies
since it is a short-lived positron-emitter, which can be obtained
readily from a long-lived generator system. For assessment of regional pulmonary perfusion, peripheral vein injections are made.
For systemic distribution, intracardiac injections of microspheres
are necessary. For the latter purposes, studies in rats (or animals larger than mice) may be needed where left heart injections
are more easily made.

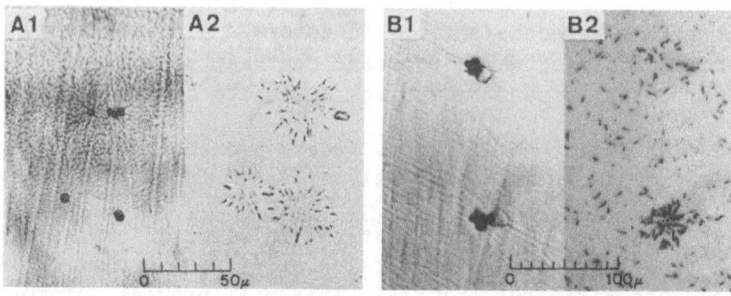

Fig. 6. Microautoradiographic images of deuterium (A2 and B2) in
human erythrocytes (A1) and transformed human lymphocytes
(B1).

With the development of increasing public concern about radiation exposures, potential benefits can be derived from the use of
non-radioactive tracers. Various stable tracers can be used for
tissue distribution studies. Tissue distribution studies can be
done in animals using sample counting (neutron activation analysis
or x-ray fluorescence) or ARG techniques. Some such studies can
be done in patients in easily sampled tissues (e.g. blood, and
urine) as well as in tissues from which biopsy samples are to be
collected for medically-justified reasons. Examples of stable
tracer studies with labelled compunds that could be conducted include the ARG assessment of the distribution of deuterium-labelled
compounds in blood cells and boron-labelled compounds in tumors.

Deuterium ARG takes advantage of a $D(T,n)^4He$ reaction. At
BNL, the uptake of deuterated thymidine into human lymphocytes in
vitro, during DNA synthesis was confirmed using 200 KeV tritons
from a Van de Graaf accelerator (33). The alpha particle emitted
from the triton activated deuterium nucleus has a maximum energy
of 4.7 MeV. A 6 μ teflon absorber which intervenes between the
sample and the alpha particle detector (cellulose nitrate plastic)
absorbs part of the alpha particle energy, and all of the tritons.
Thus, the radial pattern of tracks etched in the plastic around individual cells reflects the deuterium content of the cell. Figure
6 shows results achieved with this method. The method is complex
and requires relatively high concentrations of deuterium, but
could be useful when unique data are needed and when radiation
dose needs to be minimized or avoided.

A useful analog to these techniques for mapping alpha particles in tissue, has been developed at Harwell (34). Their
interest was to be able to assay and localize the dose from
alpha-emitters in bone (^{235}U and ^{239}Pu). The technique involves

alpha-particle "shadowing" of dewaxed specimens (also necessary
for neutron activation images). Shadow images (tissue "thickness"
images) are obtained by exposing the LEXAN plastic film to alpha-
radiations transmitted through the specimen from a high intensity
alpha-source (^{239}Pu). They then expose the samples to a thermal
neutron beam. The fissions induced in the ^{239}Pu and ^{235}U nuclei
produce densely ionizing fragments whose tracks are easily
identified in the ARG images. The long exposures needed for standard ARG of the spontaneous alpha radiations from the low levels
of ^{235}U, or ^{239}Pu encountered, was so long that fading of the latent images made direct ARG too insensitive. The method developed
using LEXAN plastic track etching provides higher sensitivity and
is able to measure high normal and elevated levels in human tissue
samples (34).

3.2.1c Tumor metabolism studies. The distribution of radiolabelled tracers can be assessed in animals using ARG. Packer et
al. of our group at Brookhaven National Laboratory have studied
the biodistribution of over 30 radiopharmaceuticals thought to be
tumor-seeking agents (35). Several animal models have been used.
Initially their work was with the Greene melanoma in hamsters and
more recently with the Harding-Passey melanoma (36) in mice. The
biodistribution studies were often erratic and it was not until
they started using autoradiography and obtaining melanin analyses,
that they learned that pigment-affinic radiopharmaceuticals were
distributed unevenly within the Greene melanoma. The distribution
in the Harding-Passey melanoma was quite uniform; therefore, we
now use autoradiography in the Harding-Passey melanoma for screening new radiopharmaceuticals. The results of these
biodistribution studies, and autoradiography, Fand (30), have been
published (37).

    Neutron capture therapy (NCT) involves the administration of
compounds which can be labelled with an element which has a high
cross-section for neutron capture followed by prompt emission of
an alpha particle - ^{10}B(N,α)^{7}Li - and relies upon the availability
of compounds which are concentrated heavily in tumors. If the
range of the alpha particle is sufficient, i.e., the site of attachment is within range of the radiosensitive tumor cell nucleus,
then such therapy can be clinically useful. It is important to
have compounds which localize in the tumor, and not in normal
radiosensitive structures which are present in the neutron-
irradiated field. Early trials with NCT of human glioblastoma
multiforme brain tumors failed due in large part to the poorly-
localizing compounds used. A significant effort is being made in
many laboratories to develop ^{10}B (and to a lesser extent Li and
Gd) compounds which have suitable properties for similar
applications. Fairchild et al. at Brookhaven National Laboratory
have been attempting to label melanoma seeking agents with boron.

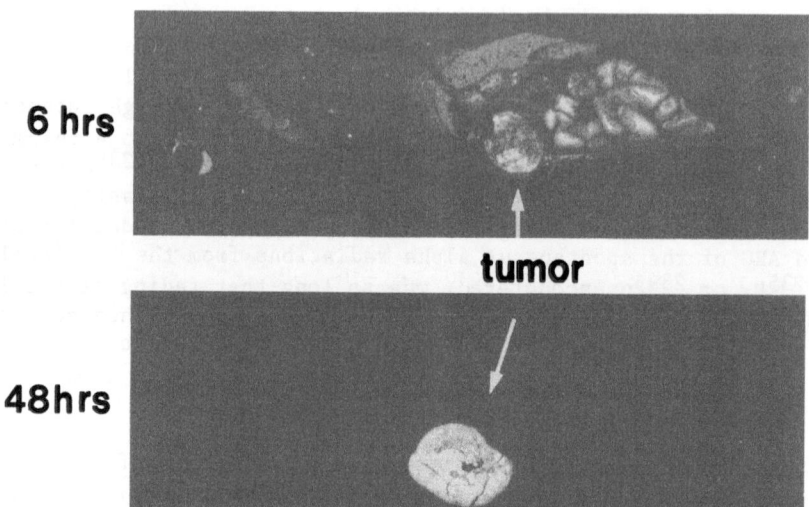

Fig. 7. ^{35}S-chlorpromazine ARG in Harding-Passey melanoma (mice).

The assessment of biodistribution of several of these compounds, including chlorpromazine is being accomplished with ARG in our laboratory in support of this effort. In the absence of ^{10}B-labelled compound, we have assessed the distribution of ^{35}S-labelled chlorpromazine in mice with a transplanted melanoma. The result is illustrated in Figure 7. The uptake of the ^{35}S-labelled chlorpromazine is more than 10 times higher than other agents studied, and if the borated compound behaves similarly, the prospects for its utility in tumor therapy would be significant. When the ^{10}B-labelled compound is available ARG studies will be carried out using techniques developed in Japan (38).

3.2.2 Studies using multiple tracers. It is possible to image multiple radioactive tracers in the same sample if either energy or their radioactive half-lives differ significantly. The short-lived positron-emitters can be studied in combination with longer-lived ^{14}C labelled compounds by taking advantage of $t\frac{1}{2}$ differences. Thus, a sample containing ^{68}Ga ($t\frac{1}{2}$ = 68 min) and ^{14}C ($t\frac{1}{2}$ = 5730 yrs) when imaged for 8 hours immediately after sample preparation will reveal the distribution of the ^{68}Ga with very little contribution form the longer-lived ^{14}C. A second film imaged for 2-4 weeks thereafter, will reveal the distribution of the smaller amount of ^{14}C given to the animals.

Alternatively, different penetrations of the radiations can be used to separate different radiations. Thus, low energy beta rays from ^{3}H-labelled compounds can be separated from higher energy beta radiations by use of differential absorbers. Thus,

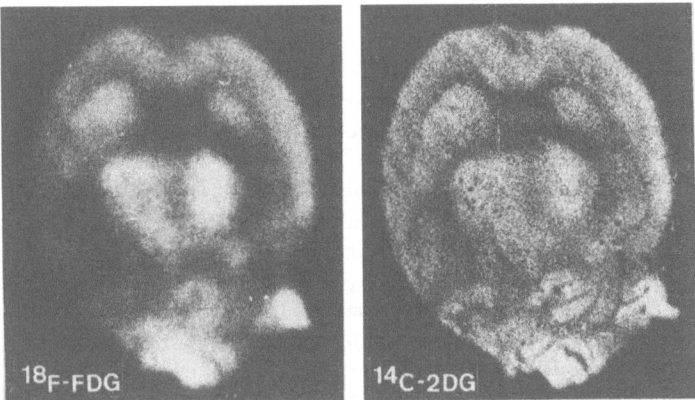

Fig. 8. Dual isotope ARG (mouse brain). Separate images of ^{18}F-
2DG and ^{14}C-2DG distributing in single mouse.

^{14}C and ^{3}H can be imaged simultaneously on 1 film. A second exposure using an intervening plastic film whose thickness is sufficient to attenuate the ^{3}H beta ray, images only the ^{14}C, and the
difference images then can be ascribed to the ^{3}H (39). A combination of ^{14}C, ^{3}H, and a short-lived β^{+} emitter could also be imaged
for 3-isotope ARG studies.

3.2.3 Simultaneous injection of two tracers. ARG studies have
been conducted in our laboratories with ^{18}F-2DG (^{18}F has a 110 min
half-life) and ^{14}C-2DG in the same animal (Fig. 8). The study reveals a close correspondence between the biodistribution of these
two compounds. An even more critical comparison would have been
to compare the biodistribution of stable fluorine-labelled ^{14}C-2DG
to show whether and to what extent the fluorine label is responsible for changes in biodistribution. Studies involving organ sampling of such a compound have been reported which show no major
differences (40), but we have not verified these with ARG.

The separate measurement of blood flow and metabolism in relative terms in the same animal can be accomplished using 2 tracers,
simultaneously. Absolute quantification will be more difficult,
but possible in principle. The simultaneous injection of ^{68}Ga-
labelled microspheres and ^{14}C-2DG injected into the left atrium
(or ventricle), provides systemic biodistribution data which permits assessment of the degree of coupling of blood flow and metabolism in normal animals. Such an experiment permits analysis of
changing patterns in animals exposed to stress, with different diseases and following different treatments.

The analysis of distribution and metabolism of vasoactive amines in the lung can be assessed with ^{14}C-labelled compounds, along with intravenously injected ^{68}Ga microspheres to study pulmonary pathophysiology correlates. Cardiac studies using ^{125}I labelled fatty acids could be correlated with regional metabolism of ^{18}F-2DG in the same tissue samples, and distribution patterns compared to other animals with disease, different treatments, etc.

The biological behavior of tumor localizing agents used in nuclear medicine can be assessed by studying the biodistribution of ^{67}Ga-citrate, for example, in tumor models where a second agent is also given. In such an experiment, for the second tracer, some animals would receive ^{18}F-2DG (for metabolic correlations) others would get ^{68}Ga microspheres (as a blood flow control) while others could receive ^{125}I IUdR or ^3H-thymidine (for cell replication rate comparisons). Additional studies can be readily performed on treated tumors (radiation, chemotherapy, etc.) to assess metabolic effects.

3.2.4 Sequential injection of two tracers. Most of the dual tracer studies described above were designed to identify differences in two processes in normal and disease states by analysis of the major biological variables simultaneously, i.e. blood flow and metabolism. If one finds that the difference appears to involve blood flow changes primarily, then a second set of experiments could be carried out to verify the results. An animal injected with a long-lived flow tracer (for example, ^{131}I-microspheres) could be exposed to the stress, drug, or disease, and a second microsphere tracer (Ga-68 for example) given to determine in the same animal if the previously-observed pattern could be substantiated with each animal serving as his own control. This information could help document the vascular effects in radiation therapy about which much debate exists. It should be noted a large number of microspheres would have to be given into the arterial supply of the irradiated field.

The use of film analysis systems makes it possible to quantitate these changes with reasonable precision. An example of such a study, which we have performed, involved the effect of the tranquilizer, chlorpromazine on the metabolism of glucose in mice. Control mice were given ^{14}C-2DG followed by a saline infusion and then ^{18}F-2DG. Experimental animals received ^{14}C-2DG and then chlorpromazine was administered (dose = 12 mgm/kgm) and 60 minutes later ^{18}F-2DG was injected. The animal was sacrificed 60 minutes thereafter and the relative distribution of the two labelled deoxyglucose tracers studied. The ARGs for two animals are shown in Figure 9 along with the quantitative assessment of the results. The quantitation was achieved by digitizing standards for the ^{14}C and ^{18}F studies from which a calibration curve is created relating

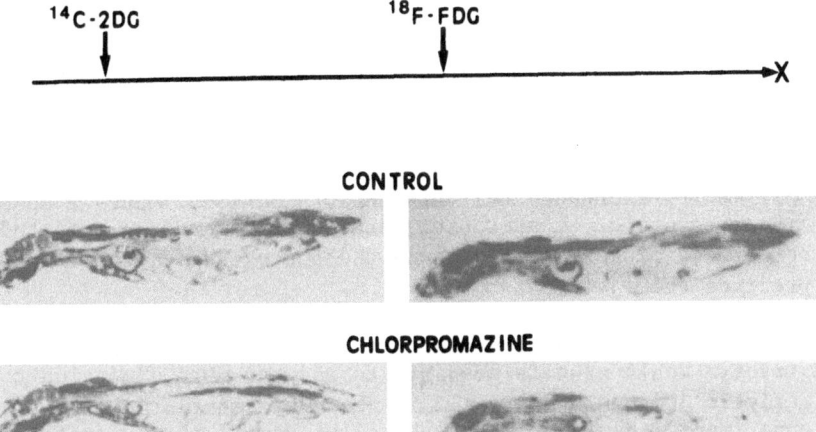

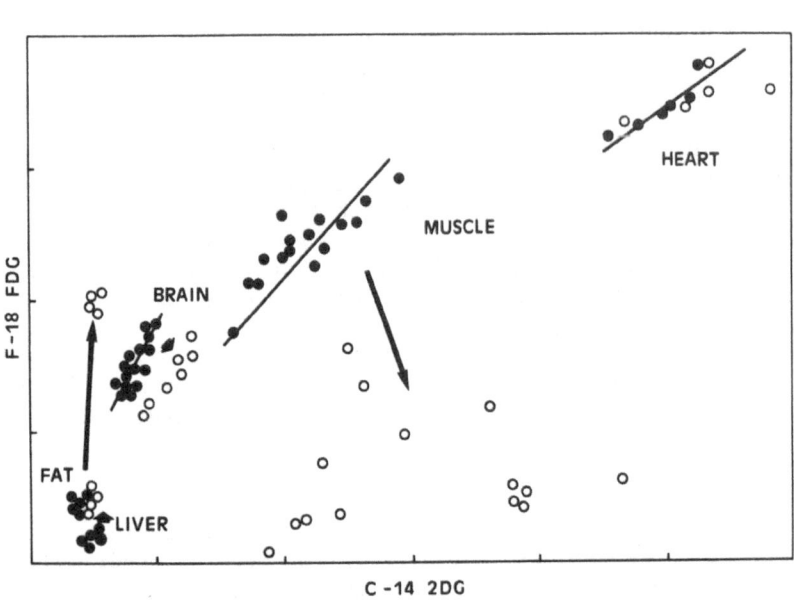

Fig. 9. Dual isotope ARG. Effect of chlorpromazine (CPZ) on glucose metabolism in mice. Upper: ARGs of control and CPZ treated mice. Lower: Quantification comparing ^{14}C-2DG and ^{18}F-FDG disribution in control (solid circle) and CPZ treated (open circle) mice.

optical density and μCi content of a pixel. The images of the animal recorded on the ^{14}C and ^{18}F films are analyzed and the activities in selected regions of interest in the image of these two nuclides are recorded and plotted (Fig. 9). It is clearly seen from the ARG and from the graph relating the change in tissue isotope content that the chlorpromazine had a profound depressing effect on metabolism in voluntary muscles, but not the heart, and that while the distribution decreased in skeletal muscles, the fat content of ^{18}F-2DG increased following chlorpromazine. Such a conclusion requires use of quantitative data to determine the magnitude of the effect, since differences in the photographic process, per se, preclude such judgments.

3.2.5 Studies involving 3 or more tracers. Extending ARG methods to 3 tracers would make it possible to add one more dimension to the analytic judgments and would increase the statistical power of the experimental design. Thus, a smaller number of observations would be needed to reach a given conclusion, since interanimal variations would be reduced. The problem is to ensure that experimental accuracy is not compromised and that the occasional loss of samples that occurs does not equal or exceed the efficiency gain. We have not yet carried out 3 isotope studies but plan to do so. An example of such a study could be to assess the effects of fast neutron therapy (14 MeV) on early changes in pulmonary blood flow. Thus, ^{125}I labelled microspheres could be injected prior to neutron hemithorax irradiation, followed one hour thereafter by ^{131}I-labelled microspheres, followed in six hours by ^{68}Ga-labelled microspheres. The evolution of changing patterns could be seen on the irradiated side and controlled with respect to the distribution to the unirradiated side. The time spans over which such studies can be carried out are limited by the tracer half-life, and by the in-vivo stability of the injected compounds.

3.2.6 Other applications of film analysis systems. The prime impetus for this review was to indicate the techniques and potential role of ARG for nuclear medical applications. However, it is clear that there are a wide variety of other medical applications for such systems.

Film imaging and analysis techniques are most useful when signals come at rates that are too high or too low for other modes of acquisition. For light photography, the photon fluxes are too high for other recording media, without loss of spatial and contrast resolution. Until recently, when higher performance measurement systems were developed, the same could be said for radiographic studies. The data rates in nuclear medicine imaging procedures are sufficiently slow that image data can be collected digitally. Hence, film analysis rarely is needed for nucler medical patient studies. For ARG studies, film is an ideal measurement media since a separate "system" (film) can be committed to a single patient (slide) for weeks or months without interruption or undue cost.

There are significant applications for film analysis systems which have been used for radiological research and which could be useful for patient diagnosis. Examples include the following:

(1) Enhancement of low contrast films. Where dose reduction is sought, films could be deliberately underexposed to minimize radiation dose (if subsequent enhancement would permit retrieval of needed data). It could also be used to enhance an archived low contrast film which did not reveal a lesion, whereas a current film is read as positive. The judgement as to whether the lesion was present at the earlier time might be assisted by enhancing the earlier film (41).

(2) Low pass filtering could be used to assist the radiologist in screening films, particularly when looking for low contrast large objects, such as lung nodules in chest films (42,43). If systems were readily available and easy to use, such techniques would be used routinely.

(3) Measurements of dimensions can be useful in classification of disease based on organ size/shape, structural anomalies, and temporal changes chronicled. Successful classification of valvular heart disease has been accomplished based on cardiac size/shape (44). Temporal changes in cardiac chamber size and wall motion are useful in the classification of coronary artery disease. Irregularities in the caliber, dimensions, and pulsatile character of coronary artery blood flow can be assessed from contrast dye injected into the arteries per se. Attempts are now being made to extract similar data from intravenous contrast injections, which if successful would be of great clinical value. (Such studies, however, will probably require digital radiography systems, and will not rely upon film analyses.)

(4) Measurements of textural features in chest x-rays have been useful for the classification of pneumoconioses using objective criteria (45). Similar methods are being used to diagnose osteoporosis from spine x-ray films (46).

(5) Progression of arthritic involvement of joints has been quantitated using sequential x-rays. Color coding of density levels in reproduced films (using a calibrated step wedge) is a sensitive means of displaying quantifiable changes without loss in spatial resolution. Thus, the spatial distribution of these changes can be perceived readily. Quantitative methods of assessing bone mineral changes from x-ray films are well estab-

lished. These procedures measure bone mineral content globally
and do not preserve high resolution spatial information (47).

(6) Blood flow to organs can be assessed from cine recorded
contrast angiography studies. Differential renal blood flow has
been measured as an average value (48) and as a pulsatile time
varying flow profile (49). The temporal variations in flow, and
the changes in vascular dimensions at different phases of the cardiac cycle provide additional information of pathophysiologic importance not available from the average flow values per se.

Microscopic analyses offer a wide range of options for quantification, many of which have been extensively explored. Representative examples of application areas include the following:

(1) Cell size/shape characterizations, and counting,

(2) 3-D structural reconstructions from sequential sections,

(3) Histochemical/structural correlations (multispectral
     analyses),

(4) Chromosome karyotyping and anomaly scoring,

(5) Sperm counting, and motility studies, and

(6) Cytological screening.

4 CONCLUSIONS

The different components that can be used in modern film analysis systems have been reviewed. TV camera and charge-coupled device sensors coupled to computers provide low cost systems for applications such as those described in this review. The increasing
availability of digital radiography systems can be used for film
analysis if they are available after hours for such applications.

There is a generally recognized need for the development of
unified viewing stations where the results of different procedures
can be compared. Until digital systems are developed in each center, film can be used to permit comparisons between analog and digital images from comparable structures provided by different
imaging modalities.

The ARG method provides an important tool for medical research and is especially useful for the development of new radiopharmaceutical compounds. Biodistribution information is needed
for estimation of radiation dose, and for interpretation of the

significance of observed patterns. The need for such precise information is heightened when one seeks to elucidate physiological principles/factors in normal and experimental models of disease. The poor spatial resolution achieved with current PET-imaging systems limits the information on radioreceptor mapping, neurotransmitter, and neuroleptic drug distribution that can be achieved from patient studies. The artful use of ARG in carefully-controlled animal studies will be required to provide the additional information needed to fully understand results obtained with this new important research tool.

The submitted manuscript has been authored under Contract No. DE-AC02-76CH00016 with the U.S. Dept. of Energy.

REFERENCES

1. Larsson, B. and Ullberg, S., A rapid film for gross autoradiography with tritium. Acta Pharmacol. et Toxicol. 41 (Suppl. I), 48-49, 1977.

2. Hough, P.V. and Powell, B.W., A method for faster analysis of bubble chamber photographs. Nuovo Cimento Ser. 10, XVIII, 1184-1191, 1960.

3. Gonzales, R.C. and Wintz, P., Digital Image Processing. Addison-Wesley Publishing Co., Mass., 1977, pp 7-9.

4. Yoshida, O., Recent chalnicon developments. In: Advances in Electronics and Electron Physics, Vol. 52. Academic Press, 1979, pp 39-50.

5. Borsuk, G.M., Photodetectors for acousto-optic signal processors. Proc. IEEE 69, 100-118, 1981.

6. Melen, R. and Buss, D., Charge-Coupled Devices: Technology and Applications. IEEE Press, 1977.

7. Casasent, D., Optical signal processing. In: Electro-Optical Systems Design, June 1981, pp 39-46.

8. Turpin, T.M., Real time input transducer for coherent optical processing. Proc. International Optical Computing Conf. Zurich, Switz., April 9, 1974, pp 34-37, 1974.

9. Special section on acousto-optic signal processing. Proc. IEEE 69, 48-118, 1981.

10. Ostroff, E., Early fox talbot photographs and restoration by neutron irradiation. J. Photoscience 13, 213, 1965.

11. Askins, B.S., Photographic image intensification by autoradiography. Appl. Optics 15, 2860, 1976.

12. Askins, B.S., Autoradiographic image intensification: Applications in medical radiography. Science 199, 684, 1978.

13. Askins, B.S., Brill, A.B., Rao, G.U.V., and Novak, G.R., Autoradiographic enhancement of mammograms. Radiol. 130, 103, 1979.

14. Brill, A.B., et al., Dose reduction in mammography-preliminary studies utilizing computer enhancement and autoradiographic image intensification. Space Sciences Laboratory, NASA, MSFC. Preprint Series No. 77-119, Nov. 1977.

15. Pettijohn, R.R., Photographic image enhancement using fluorescent light emission techniques. Proc. S.P.I.E. 175, 105, 1979.

16. Rogers, A.W. Techniques of Autoradiography. 3rd Ed. Elsevier, Amsterdam, 1979.

17. Graham, P.B., ed., Autoradiography for Biologists. Academic Press, New York, 1972.

18. Practical Autoradiography. Review 20, The Radiochemical Center Ltd., Amersham, Bucks, England, 1979.

19. Roth, L.J. and Stumpf, W.E. Eds., Autoradiography of Diffusable Substances. Academic Press, N.Y., 1979.

20. Ullberg, S., The technique of whole body autoradiography. In: Science Tools, The LKB Instrument Journal, Special Issue on Whole-Body Autoradiography, Sweden, 1977, pp 2-29.

21. Ericsson, Y. and L. Hammarström, The distribution in the mammal body of ^{18}F and ^{32}P from double-labelled Na_2PO_3F. Acta Physiol. Scand. 65, 126-137, 1965.

22. Lear, J., Reivich, M., Jones, S., Fedora, T. and Greenberg, J., An autoradiographic technique for the simultaneous measurement or local cerebral blood flow (LCBF) and local cerebral metabolism. In Chapter 2, Tenth International Symposium on Cerebral Blood Flow and Metabolism, June 20-23, 1981, St. Louis, Mo.

23. Diemer N.H. and Rosenørn J., Determination of local cerebral blood flow and glucose metabolism or transfer by means of a double

autoradiographic method. In Chapter 2, Tenth International Symposium on Cerebral Blood Flow and Metabolism, June 20-23, 1981, St. Louis, Mo.

24. Rooijen, N. Van, Double isotope autoradiography. Acta. Pharmacol. et Toxicol. 41, (Suppl. I), 72-73, 1977.

25. Miles, G. and Hossman, K.A., Double tracer autoradiographic investigation of regional blood flow and glucose metabolism during spreading depression. In Chapter 3, Tenth International Symposium on Cerebral Blood Flow and Metabolism, June 20-23, 1981, St. Louis, Mo.

26. Yonekura, Y., Meyer, M., Brill, A.B., et al., Quantitative digital autoradiography by videodensitometry. J. Nucl. Med. 22, p14, 1981.

27. Goochee, C., Rasband, W., Sokoloff, L., Computerized densitometry and color coding of (^{14}C) deoxyglucose autoradiographs. Ann. Neurol. 7, 359-370, 1980.

28. Som, P., Meyer, M., Brill, A.B., et al., Quantitative autoradiography with radiopharmaceuticals. J. Nucl. Med. 22, p66, 1981.

29. Sokoloff, L., Reivich, M., Kennedy, C. et al., The (^{14}C) deoxyglucose method for the measurement of local cerebral glucose utilization: theory, procedure, and normal values in the conscious and anesthetized albino rat. J. Neurochem. 28, 897-916, 1977.

30. Fand, I., and McNally W.P., The Technique of whole body autoradiography. Vol. 2. In: Current Trends in Morphological Techniques. Johnson J.E., Jr., Edit., CRC Press Inc., Boca Raton, Fla., 1981.

31. Meyer, M.A., Functional mapping of the brain with a histochemical method for the localization of glucose. Medical Hypotheses 7, 931-935, 1981.

32. Bergman, K. and Tjälve, H., Three-step autoradiography of organic solvents and plastic monomers to register total radioactivity, non-volatile metabolites, and non-extractable metabolites. Acta Pharmacol. et Toxicol. 41 (Suppl. I), 22-23, 1977.

33. Geisler, F.H., Jones, K.W., Fowler, J.S. et al., Deuterium micromapping of biological samples by using the $D(T,n)^4He$ Reaction and plastic track detectors. Science 186, 361-363, 1974.

34. Green, D., Howell, G.R., Thorne, M.C. and Watts, R.H., Imaging of tissue sections on lexan by alpha-particles and thermal neutrons: An aid in fissionable radionuclide distribution studies. Int. J. Appl. Rad. and Isotopes 29, 285-295, 1978.

35. Packer, S., Lambrecht, R.M., Fairchild, R.G., et al., Non-invasive nuclear detection of choroidal melanoma. Proc. of Int. Symposium in Intraocular Tumors, Schwern, East Germany, May 17-21, 1981.

36. Watts, K.P., Fairchild, R.G., Slatkin, D., et al., Melanin content of hamster tissues, human tissues and various melanomas. Cancer Res. 41, 467-472, 1981.

37. Packer, S., Lambrecht, R.M., Christman, D.R. et al., Metal isotopes used as radioactive indicators of ocular melanoma. Am. J. Opth. 83, 80-94, 1977.

38. Matsuoka, O., Hatenaka, H., and Miyamoto, M., Neutron capture whole body autoradiography of ^{10}B compounds. Acta. Pharmacol. et Toxicol. 41 (Suppl. I), 56-57, 1977.

39. Blomquist, L., Double isotope technique for simultaneous autoradiographic demonstration of protein-incorporable and protein-nonincorporable substances. Acta. Pharmacol. et Toxicol. 41 (Suppl. I), 26-27, 1977.

40. Reivich, M., Kuhl, D., Wolf A., et al., The ^{18}F-fluoro-deoxyglucose method for the measurement of local cerebral glucose utilization in man. Circ. Res. 44, 127-137, 1979.

41. Trussell, H.J. Processing of x-ray images. Proc. IEEE 69, 615-627, 1981.

42. Kruger, R.P., Hall, E.L. and Turner, A.F., Hybrid optical digital radiography based system for lung disease detection. Appl. Optics 16(10), 1977.

43. Hall, E.L., Kruger, R.P., and Turner, A.R., An optical-digital system for automatic processing of chest x-rays. Optical Engineering 13, 250-257, 1974.

44. Hall, E.J., Dwyer, S.J., Harlow, C.A., and Lodwick, G.S., A review of computers in diagnostic radiology. 2(4), 467-494, 1971.

45. Kruger, R.P., Thompson, W.B., and Turner, A.R., Computer diagnosis of pneumoconiosis. IEEE Trans. Systems. Man. and Cyb. 4, 40, 1974.

46. Personal communication. Cahill P., Nuclear Medicine Division, New York Hospital.

47. Colbert C., Fels microdensitometer/computer for bone mineral determinations from roentgenograms. Critical Rev. in Radiol. Sci. 1(3), 459-471, 1970.

48. Link, D.P., Lantz, B.M.T., Foerster, J.M., et al., New videodensitometric method for measuring renal artery blood flow at routine arteriorgraphy: Validation in the canine model. Invest. Radiol. 14, 465-470, 1979.

49. Kedem, D., Kedem, Dr., Smith, C.W., et al., Velocity distribution and blood flow measurements using videodensitometric methods. Invest. Radiol. 13, 46-56, 1978.

Part VI: Results of Clinical Evaluation: State-of-the-Art
Performance of New Radiographic Transmission Techniques

DIGITAL RADIOGRAPHY: DEVELOPMENTS, LIMITATIONS, CLINICAL RESULTS

J.Werner Ludwig and Pierre H.C. Engels

Department of Cardiovascular Radiology, Sint Antonius Hospital,
Utrecht, The Netherlands.

Angiocardiography has developed to a high degree of perfection
during the last years. Images with much diagnostic information
can be obtained of practically every vascular area. Disadvantages
are the intricacy of the examination and the chance of complications. Moreover, angiocardiography gives little information about
the circulation itself.
Angiocardiography as a so-called indirect method of investigation
(for instance to show displacement of vessels by pathological
processes) has been largely superceded by other techniques in
recent years. Next to function investigations new imaging techniques have come into existence that have partly superceded angiocardiography as an indirect method of investigation, for example:
computerized tomography, nuclear medicine, ultra sound, endoscopic retrograde cholangiopancreaticography.

For the angiocardiography, the so-called direct method, which
means investigation of heart and blood vessels with regard to
anomalies of the vessels themselves, a number of additional methods of investigation have been developed. Nearly all these methods refer only to the investigation of the function of the
blood vessels, for instance Doppler investigation, ocular pneumo-
plethysmography etc. The conventional angiocardiography as an intrinsic method of investigation can now partially be substituted
by digital vascular imaging technique.

This technique, the d.v.i., has been in use in the St. Antonius
Hospital, Utrecht, The Netherlands, sinice October 1980. The
technique is a mdified form of the subtraction technique, introduced in radiology in 1934 by Ziedzes des Plantes. (1).

D.v.i. was first developed by Mistretta (2) and Nudelman (3).
With this method the X-ray transmission data from the image intensifier are digitized and stored in a memory. This information
is used as a mask for subtraction from the next image which is
integrated in digital form in a second memory. After subtraction,
multiplication and conversion from digital to analogue the images are visible in real time on a monitor and stored on an analogue disk. (See fig. 1). After an intravenous injection of contrast material heart and vessel structures can be made visible
and documented on a disk. In most cases the images give excellent
information.

See figure 1.

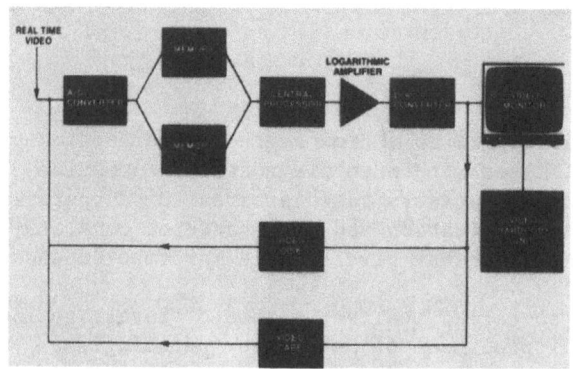

Schematic representations of the Philips system for digital vascular imaging.

Robb and Steinberg (4) have described the intravenous angiography
as early as 1939, but the quality of the images obtained
through their method was restricted by the amount of contrast material that had to be injected and the relative insensitivity of
the X-ray film to small differences in contrast between tissue
and the strongly diluted contrast material.
The recently developed, less toxic contrast materials are still
being used for intravenous angiography in combination with photographic subtraction. The large quantity of contrast material that
has to be injected (@ 150 ml.) to obtain a diagnostically usable
image does not make this a very attractive method and image quality is worse than that of d.v.i.
D.v.i. consists in general of two methods: the so-called mask
method (M-mode) and the time interval difference method (t.i.d.).

With the M-mode the image is stored on the first memory before
intravenous injection and used as a mask for all following
images. This method is used for investigation of non-moving objects, especially for vessel examinations.
The t.i.d.-method operates in the same way with two memories but
with this method each image is being subtracted from the previous
one. With a high frequency of 50 images per second this system
can also be applied to moving parts, and is thus usable for examination of the heart.
A disadvantage of this method is the much smaller contrast difference in the images after injection of contrast material in
comparison with the contrast obtained with the M-mode.

With M-mode an image either consists of one videosignal or it is
built up by integration of a number of videosignals. In our system one image is being built up by integration of four videosignals. Advantage of this integration is less noise. A videosignal is generated in 20m.sec. so that an image is built up in
80m.sec, short enough to give a sharp image of the vessels.
By altering the number of videosignals to be integrated a third
method is possible which is derived from the M-mode.
With this method a large number (e.g. 80) of videosignals is
being integrated, and this image serves as a mask for all following images that are in their turn being built up from one to
more videosignals. With this method a blurred mask is obtained.
This so-called continuous mask mode is also applicable for moving
structures i.e. for heart investigation.
In practice this method appears to give more information about
the heart cavities. The t.i.d. gives more information about the
outlines of the heart cavities and wall motion.

The pulsations of the aorta, especially the aorta ascendens and
the first part of the descendens cause less satisfactory subtraction images because of this movement. Sometimes the same difficulty presents itself with larger branches such as carotid arteries and renal arteries. Also the pulmonary arteries show a
rather strong motion when pulsating. To eliminate these subtraction disturbing movements we developed the possibility of ECG-
gating. Herewith the first image (mask) and all other images are
triggered on the ECG, preferably late in the diastolic phase. As
a result considerably better subtraction images are obtained.
The frequency of the images is therefore the same as the heart
rate.

METHOD, MATERIAL AND EQUIPMENT.

1. Injection of contrast material.

The contrast material can be injected intravenously or intra-arterially.

a. Intravenous injection: With the M-mode as well as t.i.d. the contrast material is injected preferably in the v.basilica. We use a conventional contrast material (Telebrix 38). An amount of 20-40 ml. of contrast material is injected with a flow of 12-14 ml. per second, administered with a high-pressure injector. The amount of contrast material depends on the region that will be visualized, for example the pulmonary arteries 20 ml.; for the intracranial arteries 40 ml. (adult patients). After the contrast material has been injected 15-20 ml. of a glucose solution 5% is subsequently administered. This is done by filling the syringe first with glucose solution and with the syringe in an upright position (with the filling point down) subsequently carefully sucking up the desired quantity of contrast material without the two solutions mixing.
To puncture the vein a needle with a plastic sheath (gauge 18) is used. The length of the sheath is 4,5 cm. During the injection the arm is held high. If it is not possible to puncture an arm vein, a canula is introduced into the femoral vein.

b. Intra-arterial injection: If contrast material is injected selectively in the aorta, through a catheter in an artery, this must be done after the first image has been stored in the memory.
With a minimal quantity of contrast material very good images can be obtained. When applying digitized subtraction with the selective injections sometimes more information can be obtained compared to conventional arteriography.
The quantity of the contrast material to be injected depends on the vessels to be studied. I.e.: for visualizing the abdominal aorta 8 ml. of contrast material is sufficient, either a.p. or lateral projection. For visualizing a carotid artery 1 ml. suffices. Arteriography with small quantities of contrast material is very attractive and is very important in patients with severe renal failure.

2. Conditions to obtain good images:

a. Especially with the M-mode prevention of motion is essential. There are different possibilities to prevent motion or to eliminate this afterwards. These are:
a1. Postprocessing. In the d.v.i. system the possibility of postprocessing is built-in. If the patient has moved in the interval between tha mask and the images to be subtracted motion artefacts occur. Chosing another mask more closely to the moment in which the contrast material is visible in the

vessels these artefacts can be partly or total eleminated.
Postprocessing is applied frequently and provides much more
information in many cases.
a2: During the interval of investigation, about 15 to 25 seconds, it is very important that patients refrain from breathing. Explicit instructions are necessary.With patients who
cannot prevent motions, e.g., strong dyspnoea or M. Parkinson,
poor images are obtained.
A3: In investigation of carotid arteries swallowing movements
are impediment to get good images. With the intravenous injections of contrast material many patients tend to swallow
as soon as they feel a sensation of heat. Helpful in suppres-
sing this tendency is positioning a wedge between the teeth
with which the mouth should be opened as far as possible.
A4: In order to obtain maximum immobility a supine relaxed
position is of utmost importance. For the different projections the equipment has to be turned around the patient.
A5: When investigating the abdominal vessels eliminating the
peristalsis is important. An intravenous injection of 1 mg.
glucagon 30 sec. before the contrast material is injected
results in a considerable decrease of the peristaltic movements of the intestines.

b. In case of a bad cardiac output slow circulation exists with
    a strong dilution of contrast material. To improve the quali-
    ty of the images in these cases a large amount of contrast
    material is helpful.
    The circulation is being affected unfavourably also by a Val-
    salva manoeuvre. To prevent this as much as possible the in-
    vestigation will not be done during deep inspiration.

3. Digital vascular imaging system.

a. Generator: X-ray generating part consists of an Optimus M 200
    generator, delivering 200 KW. Mostly used 60-95 KV.

b. X-ray tube: bifocal tube with 0.3 and 0.6 mm. focus, water-
    cooled with an anode capacity of 280 KW sec. or 380.000 heat
    units. During the d.v.i. examinations the 0.6 mm. of the two
    focal spots is used.

c. The image intensifier has an entrance screen with a 14" dia-
    meter and is switchable to either 10" and 6" field, resulting
    in magnification of resp. 1.4 and 2.3 times.
    Moreover the large field of view proves to be advantageous,
    i.e., in visualizing two kidneys or a considerable part of
    both the abdominal aorta and the renal artery. Both lung
    fields can almost be visualized completely.
    The t.v. camera contains a plumbicon.

d. Memories: we are using a 256 x 256 pixel matrix. The pixel
    sizes in the 6", 10" and 14" mode of the image intensifier are
    then resp. 0.64 mm., 1.1 mm. and 1.5 mm.

e. Exposure: the X-ray factors KV and mA are automatically set
    and locked in by the optimus generator which features auto-
    matic measuring shots during preparation time.
    The voltage used is dependent upon the area to be examined,
    the girth of the patient and the chosen image intensifier
    size. As a rule the voltage is between 60 and 90 KV. The cur-
    rent is also dependent upon the type of examination and the
    field size of the image intensifier.
    For example: when examining the carotid arteries we generally
    use the 6" field with a current of 300-400 milli amps. and a
    voltage of 60-65 KV. To examine the renal arteries we use the
    6" field with 75 KV and a current of 500 milli amps. To exa-
    mine the heart with time interval difference mode, we gene-
    rally use the 10" field in 30 degree R.A.O. with a voltage
    of 70 KV and a current of 250-275 milli amps.
    Dose levels:
    The dose by using 14" field by the mask mode is approximately
    70 micro R per exposure. By using the 10" field 150 and by
    the 6" field 355 micro R per exposure.
    By the time interval difference mode these values are respec-
    tively 11.6, 15 and 27.8 micro R per exposures on the 14",
    10" and 6" field size.

f. Exposure rate. A choice can be made from 1 exposure per 8 se-
    conds to 4 exposures per second. The chosen exposure rate cor-
    responds more or less with that of the conventional arterio-
    graphy. For examination of the carotid bifurcation a rate of
    2 exposures per second is used. When using a low frequency in
    this region there is a distinct possibility that the moment
    of maximum concentration of the contrast material in the ar-
    tery is not recorded. With the t.i.d. 25 or 50 exposures per
    second can be made.

g. Suspending system for image intensifier and X-ray tube.
    The image intensifiers and the X-ray tube are mounted on an
    U-arch (Polydiagnost). The X-ray stand makes it possible to
    choose all projections perpendicular to the head-to-toe axis
    without turning the patient. It is also possible to choose
    the cardiocranial and cardiocardial projections by utilizing
    the scissor-movement of both arms of the U-arch. The distance
    between the focus of the X-ray tube and the image intensifier
    can be altered by adjusting the height of the image intensi-
    fier over a distance of 40 cm. The examination table has a
    movable top which can be moved over a distance of 140 cm.

The end of the table top does not contain any metal parts.

See figure 2:

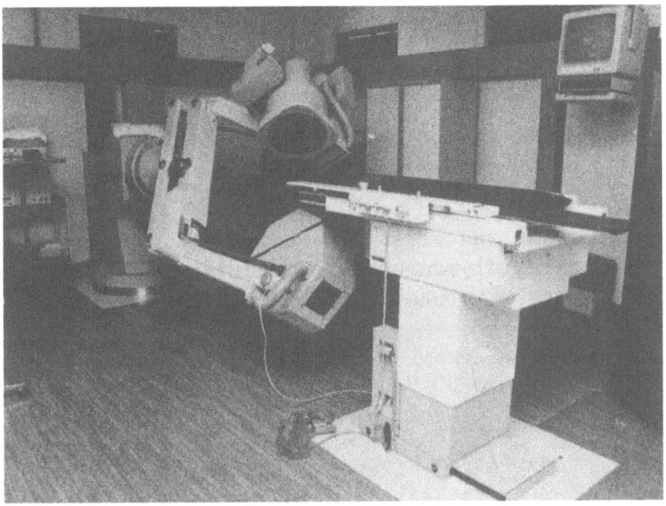

Suspending system for I.I. and X-ray tube. All projections can be made without pursuing the patient (a.p., lateral, r.a.v., l.a.v., caudocranial and cranio-caudal).

h. Disc. The subtracted images are stored on an analogue disc with 500 tracks. The disc is connected to a magnetic tape recorder, a cinefilm installation (16 mm), (Kinasope) tape recorder and a multiformat camera (8 x 10" film, divided into either 1, 4 or 9 images per film sheet).

Application.

The d.v.i. has been applied for the examination of various arterial areas as well as for the examination of the left ventricle. Until now we studied about 600 patients for vessel diseases and 60 patients for heart disease, especially the left ventricle ejection fraction and wall motion. In the next paragraphs the different areas of examination are described.

THE INTRACRANIAL ARTERIES.

The examination of the intracranial arteries is done with an intravenous injection of 40 ml. of contrast material. By mistake an injection of 20 ml. contrast material was given to one patient for basilar insufficiency; the basilar artery showed up very well

and did not show any lesion confirming the conventional angiogram
which was made the next day.
The exposures are made a.p. as well as lateral. If sufficient information is not available, sometimes additional L.A.O. and R.A.O.
projections are made.
For the investigation of these arteries we use generally the 10"
field. A frequency of two exposures per second is used.
Lower spatial resolution and the simultaneous filling of all the
intracranial arteries are disadvantages especially in this area.

The indications are:

a. Suspicion of aneurysms and arterial-venous malformations.
    In 4 patients an arterial-venous malformation was found, com-
    pletely in accordance with the conventional angiographies.

    See figure 3

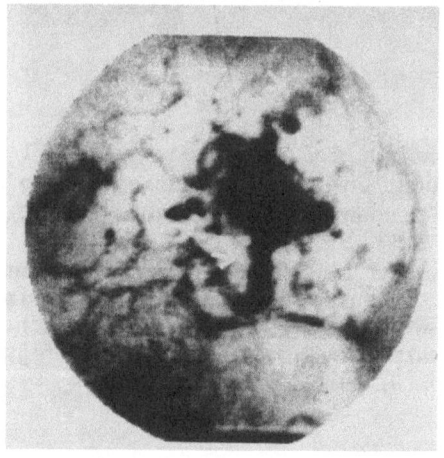

Patient with an a.-v. malformation in the left hemisphere. Feeding results are branches of the middle cerebral artery. Note
the veins. Exposure made on 6" field 60 KV 200 mA i.v. injection
of 40 ml. of contrast material.

    5 Patients were examined with suspected aneurysm. None of
    these patients was found to have an aneurysm; with 3 patients
    a conventional angiogram was made as well also showing no
    aneurysm.

b. Lesions of the siphon. In some patients we found irregulari-
    ties of the siphon and where a conventional angiogram was also
    obtained, similar findings were seen.

c. Suspicion of an insufficient vertebral basilar artery.
    10 Patients were examined for this indication. The findings
    were completely in accordance with the conventional angio-
    graphy. In one patient we found an occluded basilar artery,
    in all the other patients no lesions from the basilar artery
    or the vertebral arteries were found.

d. Post-operative results of an extra-intracranial anastomosis.
    In 3 patients we did a post-operative study and in all these
    we saw the anastomosis between a temporal artery and the
    middle cerebral artery.

    See figure 4.

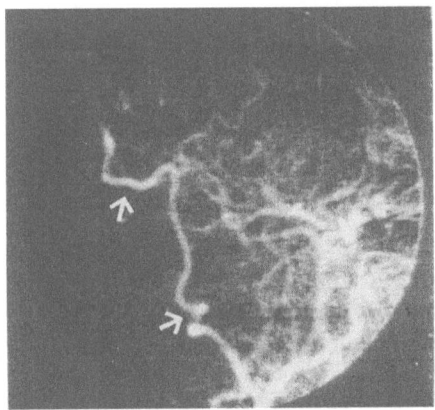

Figure 4: Study of a patient with total occlusion of middle cerebral artery. Patient has had surgery-anastomosis between temporal
artery and a distal branch of the middle cerebral artery.

ARTERIES IN THE NECK.

The examination was at the onset started by injection of 40 ml.
of contrast material. More recently we have injected 20 ml. of
contrast material only, also obtaining images which could very
well be used for diagnostic purposes. Exposures were made in 30°
R.A.O. and L.A.O. sometimes supplemented by a.p. projections.
When making exposures of the right arterial carotid bifurcation
the head was turned to the left over about 45° in R.A.O. projection and to the right over 45° in L.A.O. projection. For the left
carotid bifurcation the same projections were used. All exposures
were made with the 6" field.

We choose a frequency of two exposures per second in accordance with the frequency used for conventional angiography.

See figure 5

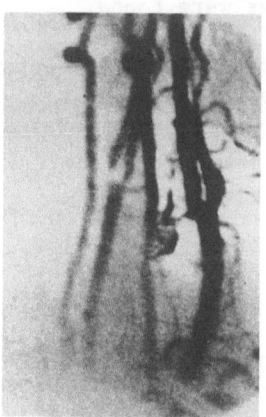

Figure 5: Investigations of left and right carotid bifurcation. The right internal carotid artery is nearly total occluded at the bifurcation; there is still a good filling of the artery. The left carotid artery shows no lesions.

The indications are the following:

a. T.I.A.'s (transient ischaemic attack)

b. A-symptomatic bruits

c. Suspected obstructions of an internal carotid artery.

d. Post-operative. Two groups of patients: the first group of patients who have had a surgical correction and to examine the operation-results; the second group of patients who have been operated and whose stenotic symptoms return.

e. To show arteriomalformations in the skull or neck area. In patients who have had a non invasive examination of the circulation of the brains; i.e. the o.p.g. (ocular pneumople-thysmosgraphy) and in which no significant results can be obtained. In these cases the intravenous angiography is a good method to determine whether a stenosis of the carotid artery is present. If the o.p.g. points to a haemodynamic significant

stenosis, it is important to look for lesions in accordance with the o.p.g. The patient described below makes this clear: During a routine physical examination of a patient an a-symptomatic carotid bruit was found both on the left and the right side. A bloodpressure difference between the left and the right arm was found as well. (right 140/80; left 120/70). An o.p.g. was done, showing a significant haemodynamic lesion on the left side. Because of the o.p.g. results, a d.v.i. was done of the carotid bifurcation. This showed a stenosis of the left internal carotid artery of approximately 40% and of the right internal carotid artery of about 95%. These lesions did not explain the findings of the o.p.g. Therefore an additional d.v.i. was made of the aortic arch. This examination showed a stenosis at the origin of the left common carotid artery of 95% and an obstruction of 70% of the left subclavian artery.
These findings explained the results of the o.p.g. completely. Two days later a conventional angiography was done in this patient pointing to deviations which are identical with those of the d.v.i.

Results:

A comparative study of d.v.i. and conventional angiography was done in 35 patients for lesions of the carotid bifurcation. We found an accuracy of 93%, a sensitivity of 90% and a specificity of 95%. (6)

AORTA.

a. Aortic arch: Before we did e.c.g.-gatings we did not obtain good images of the aortic arch. The exposures are preferably made at 80 KV. The exposures are made with the 10" field at an rate of 2 per second. We injected 40 ml. of contrast material.

    See figure 6.

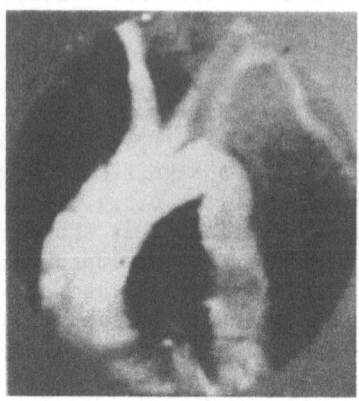

Figure 6: Study of an aortic arch in a patient with a small
shadow in the left hilus. We found a small coarctation just distal to the left subclavian artery.

The exposures are mostly made in L.A.O. projections. The indications are:
- Suspected aneurysm of the aorta. Two patients were examined
having a suspected aneurysm of the aortic arch. The d.v.i.
showed that the shadow seen on the thorax X-ray was in fact
an irregular contour of the aorta caused by a little coarctation.
- Suspected obstructions or stenoses of the large arteries.
One patient we examined was found to have a subclavian steal-
syndrome caused by occlusion of the left subclavian artery.
This concurred completely with the results of the conventional angiography.
A d.v.i. was done in one patient where we suspected an aneurysm of the anonymus artery, a complete normal anonymus was
found, the large shadow in the upper mediastinum on the right
side was found to be a large abberant thyroid gland.

b. The abdominal aorta: For the abdominal aorta the examinations
are mostly done in AP projection or lateral projection.
The indications are the following:
- Aneurysm. In several patients the aneurysm was clearly visible. In two patients the aneurysm was not visible as the
dissection did not fill with contrast material.
- Occlusions of the abdominal aorta. After translumbal aorta-
graphy of a patient a large dissection appeared. It was not
clear however to what degree the aorta was obstructed. The
d.v.i. showed an impression of the abdominal aorta, but the

aorta was found to be quite open (7). Complete stenosis of
the abdominal aorta was found with a second patient, situated some cm's below the renal arteries. Some arteries were
seen which took care of collateral filling of the blood supply
to the legs. A second injection was made to visualize the femoral arteries on both sides. This worked very well and adequate information was obtained about both the deep and the
superficial femoral arteries. Exposures of the right femoral
arteries were overexposed, making subtractions of this area
not of adequate quality.
- Stenoses of the renal arteries.

See figure 7.

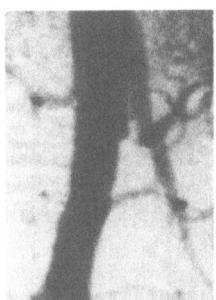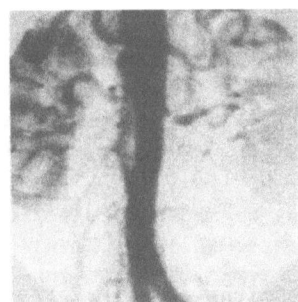

Figure 7: Abdominal aorta: left renal artery nearly occluded.

A comparative study of d.v.i. and conventional arteriography
of the renal arteries in patients with hypertension is in progress.   There seems to be a good correlation with conventional
arteriography.

THE ILIAC ARTERIES AND THE FEMORAL ARTERIES.

This study is also done with intravenous injections of 40 ml.
of a normal contrast material (Tlebrix 38). The exposures are
mostly made in AP projection. The indications are:
- In some patients with dysmasia. In several patients one of
the iliac arteries was occluded. In these patients we did
one more injection to get images of the more peripheral arteries. In all these patients it was possible to get an image
of the femoral arteries. We did a comparison of conventional
and d.v.i. in the follow-up of femoral crural bypass operation in 18 consecutive patients. These patients had a femoral

crural bypass graft inserted between 1971 and 1980. This study was undertaken to determine the value of intravenous angiography for the documentation of femoral crural bypass surgery, concerning the graft patency. No differences were found between both methods, given a diagnostic accurancy of 100%. The results of this study indicates that it is possible to determine the graft patency by d.v.i. Referring to the graft quality two stenoses were not seen by d.v.i.
A relative large disadvantage of the d.v.i. is that it is not possible to move the patient, so that only one area can be studied by one contrast material injection. If one wants to see the whole traject of femoral artery or a femoral crural bypass it is necessary to do many contrast material injections.

PULMONARY ARTERIES.

For the study of the pulmonary arteries we inject 20 ml. of contrast material intravenously. The images are made with E.C.G.-gating. After the first injection we made an overview on the 14" field in AP projection. For more details of the left lung projections of about 30° L.A.O., on the 10" or 6" field were made. For the right lung we made a projection of about 10° R.A.O. Indications:

  - Suspicion of lung embolism. A comparative study of nuclear medicine examination, conventional angiography and d.v.i. is now in study.
  - Arterio-venous malformations. We studied some patients and by these we got very good images of the malformations, concurring with conventional angiography.
  - Examinations of pathologic hili of the lungs.

LEFT VENTRICLE ANGIOGRAPHY BY DIGITAL VASCULAR IMAGING.

We did a study with the time interval difference method. We did a comparative study, on the one hand we measured the ejection fraction and wall motion pattern of the left ventricle by means of conventional left ventricle angiography. On the other hand the two parameters were measured with the t.i.d.-technique. Each patient was studied on two consecutive days. The t.i.d.-images were stored on an analogue disc and thereafter transferred to 60 mm. cinefilm at 50 frames per second.
The same projections were used in both examinations. The patient material we studied was divided over two equally large groups. A learning population and a testing population. In the testing population of 20 patients one observer analized the left ventricle angiograms, the other independently looked at the t.i.d.-images. The films were studied with the help of a computer.

End-diastole and end-systole were indentified and the contours
outlined by hand. The data were then processed by a mini computer, that produced ejection fraction and regional wall shorte-
nings, according to Leighton's method. The ejection fraction had
a correlation coefficient of 0.82.
For the wall shortening we found for the anterior wall and apex
a correlation coefficient of 0.94 and for the inferior wall a
correlation coefficient of 0.69.

DIGITAL VASCULAR IMAGING WITH INTRA-ARTERIAL INJECTION.

Up until now we did only a few examinations. In one patient with
a very poor kidney-function we made an aortogram. We inject twice
7 ml. of contrast material just proximal to the renal arteries
and images of the aorta in AP and lateral projection are made.
We got a very good image of the abdominal aorta and we made a
correct diagnosis. After that we injected 5 ml. of contrast material just above the bifurcation of the aorta. With this injection we had a very good picture of the bifurcation and the iliac
arteries.
In a second patient we did an intra-arterial injection in a femoral artery to demonstrate the lower leg arteries. The day before an arteriogram of femoral arteries was made and it was not
possible to show any of the three arteries of the lower leg because of an occlusion of the superficial femoral artery. With
d.v.i. we inject 5 ml. of contrast material in the iliac artery
and got a picture of the arteries in the lower leg.

Complications:

Until now we studied about 600 patients. Three times there was
an extravasation of contrast material in the arm.
This was painful for about half an hour and after that none of
these patients had any complains.
In one patient we had a severe allergic reaction.
On examining patients with a poor output of the left ventricle
one might see the contrast material appear retrograde in several
neck vessels. This however does not cause any complications for
the patient, but gives some interference in the interpretation.

Discussion:

The examinations we did until now have shown a wide area of applications. The information in a rather large number of patients
compared with the information obtained through conventional angiography, surgery and/or the pathologist reports gave a good
correlation. It is now always possible to determine the correct
diagnosis with intravenous angiography.

There are however many advantages to these methods, such as low
level of patient discomfort and physical taxation. The easy and
quick determination of diagnosis for a number of patients with
arterial problems, the small material costs and the possibility
of doing an examination on an out-patient basis.
This makes it extremely attractive. Moreover we can be certain
that the technique will be improved, thus increasing the number
of indications for the d.v.i.

The whole area of indications of conventional angiography has decreased the last few years because of the new non-invasive techniques, as already mentioned in the beginning. There will however remain an area particularly suitable for conventional angiography.
It is therefore desirable the d.v.i. will be administered in the
future to a large and varied number of institutions and to cen-
tralize the relatively small area of indications that remains
for conventional angiography in clinics that also contain the
possibility of arterial surgery on a large scale.

Literature:

1. Ziedses des Plantes, B., Planigraphy and Subtraction, Roent-
    genographic Differentation Methods, Thesis, Keunink en Zn.
    N.V., Utrecht.

2. Mistretta, Ch.A., Ort, M.G., Cameron, J.R. et al., Multiple
    Images Subtraction Technique for Enhancing Low Contrast Pe-
    riodic Objects, Invest. Radiol. 8: 43-44 (1973).

3. Ovitt, T.W., Nudelman, S.N., Fisher, D. et al, Computer-
    Assisted Video Subtraction for Intravenous Angiography, Pre-
    sented at Work in Progress at RSNA, Chicago, Ill, Nov. 27-
    Dec. 2, 1977.

4. Robb, G.P., Steinberg, I., Visualization of the chambers of
    the heart, the pulmonary circulation and the great blood ves-
    sels in man, Summary of method and results, JAMA 114: 474-
    480, 10 feb. 1940.

5. Ludwig, J.W., Engels, P.H.C., Eikelboom, B.C., Vorläufiger
    Bericht über Digital Vascular Imaging (DVI) bzw. intravenöse
    Angiographie,H. Karobath, M. Redtenbacher, Wien Nov. 1980,
    Witzstrock Verlag, Baden-Baden, Köln, New York.

6. Engels, P.H.C., Eikelboom, B.C., de Vries, A.R., Ludwig, J.W.
    Digital Vascular Imaging (DVI) in the evaluation of cerebro-
    vascular disease, Proceedings of the Symposium on cerebro-
    vascular disease, Bern, Sept. 1981, Witzstrock Verlag, Baden-
    Banden, Köln, New York, in Press.

7. Ludwig, J.W., Engels, P.H.C., Digital Vascular Imaging, een
    nieuwe angiografische techniek, Ned. Tijdschrift voor Genees-
    kunde 125, nr. 34, 1981.

- WORKSHOP IN CLINICAL APPLICATIONS OF TRANSMISSION TOMOGRAPHY

- J. VIGNAUD -

FONDATION OPHTALMOLOGIQUE A. de ROTHSCHILD - PARIS - FRANCE

In the field of X-Ray diagnosis, the advent of transmission tomography (C.T.) seems to be the most important discovery since that of X-Rays.

This non-invasive radiological technique allowing the spontaneous visualization of the brain and its cavities as well as any space-occupying lesions, is considered to be a miracle, especially by those who formerly practiced the painful invasive technique of pneumo encephalography.

The discovery of C.T. has opened an entirely new era in radiology within the last ten years, its development has been tremendous.

VISUALIZATION OF ANATOMICAL STRUCTURES

Up until now, there were many organs which were never spontaneously visualized by conventional techniques. Amongst these are organs of the brain such as : the white and grey matter, the ventricles, and the subarachnoid spaces.

Those of the orbits : the globe, lens, optic nerves, muscles
and vessels.

In addition, with scans of the abdomen, the pancreas is now
visualized. Fresh blood and fatty tissue has become possible
to distinguish.

For a better visualization of the vessels, an intra venous
injection or an iodized contrast media is administrated.

With this, even vessels of 0.5 mm such as the orbital ciliary
arteries can be detected.

This intravenous injection aids in determining modifications
in the blood brain barrier by the absorption and various
densities of the contrast media trapped within the extracellular space of the brain.

Such modifications are commonly found in cases of malignant
tumors or recent infarcts.

Intrathecal injection of a water soluble
contrast media increases the visualization of the subarchnoid
spaces and their contents ; i.e. : the nerves, vessels and
any existing tumors.

This technique also delineates the brain from adjacent cisterns
and is able to define such organs as the chiasma in the
chiasmatic cistern and the acoustic nerve in the cerebello
pontine angle cistern.

With scans of the spine, the spinal
cord is outlined by the contrast media. The exact location
of a tumor with regards to the cord is now easily diagnosed
as well as an enhanced intramedullary cyst in cases of
syringomyelia.

For example, the nerve roots in the
opacified subarachnoid spaces are sharply delineated whereas
in the epidural spaces, they may be spontaneously (without the

use of contrast media) visible thanks to the surrounding fatty
tissue.

An intrathecal injection introducing
a small amount of air directed towards the internal auditory
canal, will enable the visualization of the nerves and any tumor
within the canal.

The sharpness of the contour of the
structures is becoming more and more precise due to the
technical evolution of the matrix : with the first generation
of scanners, the size of the pixel was 3.2 X 3.2 mm, which
has now been decreased to 0.25 X 0.25 mm.
The same progress has been made with the thickness of the
slice, reducing it from 12 mm to 1 mm, thus diminishing the
partial volume effect and allowing a precise analysis of the
morphology and density of a structure.

With these technical advances, a precise
and accurate study of complex structures such as the sella and
para sellar region ; the petrous pyramids ; the inter vertebral
spaces including the disc, the spinal canal with its cord and
roots can be made.

The scanner has greatly contributed
to the facility in obtaining a basal view of the skull.

To date, with conventional radiology,
the axial basal view required the patient to remain in an
uncomfortable position with radiographic results being of
minimal quality.

For an accurate diagnosis as for
conventional radiographs, two orthogonal positions at

right angle are required. Coronal sections are applicable
for head C.T. scanning, and with some machines they are possible
for the body C.T.

The multiplanar computed reformation
is indispensable when scanning complex structures and gives
additional information when coronal sectioning is not
possible.
Even oblique reconstruction (reformation) is possible.
These are performed with thin joining slices.
The reformated images have a rather good spatial resolution
which accurately demonstrates organs such as the ossicles of
the ear and the ophthalmic vein.

A precise target on a structure can
be determined due to the numerical display of each voxel.
Therefore, it is possible with given plane references, to
determine the exact direction of a needle for a biopsy puncture
or a radioactive implant.
Moreover, the trajectory of the needle can be precisely
calculated and even automatically guided.
For any subsequent radiotherapy, axial scans and precise
measurements enable a detailed mapping of the lesion with
regards to surrounding tissue so that the dose is administered
directly and precisely to the lesion.

The biopsy technique is primarly utilized
for the brain but is as interesting for the visceral organs.
In these cases, the results are often comparable to those
obtained with ultrasound.

With the same plane references, superim-
position of digitalized angiography permit the calculation
of needle trajectory avoiding major vessels. Up till now,

stereogrammetry seems the most adequate technique.

ANALYSIS OF TISSUE CHARACTERISTICS

Densitometry is the basis of
such an analysis.
With thick slices, the partial volume effect becomes too
prominent and therefore decreases the optimum requisites
for an accurate interpretation.
With thinner slices of 1 mm, the partial volume effect is
avoided enabling a precise microdensitometry recorded
by a numerical density profile or a histogram. For example,
the demineralized or sclerotic part of the cochlea in otoscle-
rosis is well demonstrated by this technique.
Due to their densities, lesions with fatty components can be
identified, such as lipomas or dermoid cysts. This is also
the case for diagnosing fresh blood.

However, on the basis of densitometry
it is often difficult to differentiate with certainty lesions
of various natures, such as a glioma, a meningioma, a recent
infarct, an abscess or a metastasis.
The morphology of the lesion can be helpful but it is not
specific enough.
Correlations with clinical data and other procedures such
as isotopic nuclear exams, angiographies and body ultrasound
are often required.

ANGIO SCAN

Often referred to as rapid sequential C.T.,
angio scan is performed to study the dynamics of blood flow. An
intravenous bolus injection of contrast media is introduced

while a graph plotting the density levels with the time
of passage is diagrammed. This enables the study of the time
of circulation and the concentration of the opacified blood
in the region of interest.
Sequential images are obtained and subtraction films will
clearly demonstrate the modification of enhancement between
the serial images.
With the aid of the angio scan, we can differentiate an
aneurysm from a tumor.
In cases of transient vascular insufficiency, the angio scan
reveals its upmost efficiency by detecting a lack of opacifi-
cation in comparison with contra lateral region.

C.T. of the heart has not yet totally
evolved even linked with the E.C.G.
However, angio scan can evaluate the patency of a coronary
graft.

DOSES

The dose varies from 1 to 20 rads,
depending on the amount of photons used. With more photons,
the image becomes sharper but the dose is increased.
This is why high resolution images must be restricted to
the region of interest.
The lens of the orbit must be avoided by tilting the gantry
thus changing the section plane.

REVIEW MODE (OR SCOUT VIEW)

Most of the new C.T. scans offer a
spatial and density resolution equivalent to the quality
of a standard radiograph. Since the image is digitalized

various window settings allow the visualization of bone or
soft tissue.

Due to the axial translation, the
computed measures are precise and may be depended upon,
in particular, when the size of intervertebral spaces is
being calculated. This holds true for all measurements
determined on each slice, whereby allowing for an exact
diagnosis.

Today, the primary application of the
review mode is for exact slice positioning and accurate gantry
angulation in order to obtain precise sections of the area
in question. For example, the intervertebral space, the optic
nerve or the sella turcica.

VALIDITY OF A SCAN IN REGARDS TO OTHER AVAILABLE EXAMS

Aside from the fact of its high cost
and the problems of legal authorization, the C.T.scan should
replace conventional radiography, in many domaines.

In regards to polytomography : the bony
spatial resolution is equivalent and occasionally superior
to the polytomographic images thanks to certain high resolution
programs. The density resolution has proven to be superior.

The quality of the soft tissue visualiza-
tion found in C.T. is incomparable. Exploration of intricate
structures is to our advantage; such is the case with the
exploration of the middle or inner ear.
Up until now, polytomography offered concise and detailed

information but it was necessary to obtain several projections.
High resolution C.T. scanning in axial position, using
consecutive overlapping thin slices and multiplanar reformation may completely replace conventional tomography.
Moreover, the C.T. technique can decrease the radiation dose
while completely avoiding the orbital lens.

APPLICATIONS OF CT IN NEURORADIOLOGY

In regards to conventional neuro
radiological procedures, pneumoencephalography and diagnostic
angiography has become extinct. However, follow up angiographies
after scanning are often performed in order to obtain precise
information on the nature of a lesion and in pre operative
cases to be aware of arterial pedicles feeding the lesion.

Therapeutic angiographies are increasing.

Gas myelography is no longer used but
water soluble myelography still exists being complemented
by a C.T. scan.
But now, with the "review mode", myelographies may be performed
uniquely with C.T.

For Pediatric cases echography must replace CT as long
as the fontanels are opened, in order to avoid irradiating
the immature brain.

When exploring the thorax and mediastinum regions,
CT offers a large spectrum of densities in addition to axial
projections thereby allowing a precise morphological and
densitometric study far superior to those obtained in

conventional standard and tomographic radiography.

For abdominal exams especially the digestive tract,
conventional radiography is challenged by fibroscopy.
CT may provide additional information concerning surrounding
soft tissue in regards to a detected lesion such as tumors
of the rectum and oesophagus.

Concerning diagnosis of other visceral organs
echography and CT are in competition with each other.
In many cases, the two procedures are used as complement.
CT scanning provides the morphology of a lesion whereas
echography offers a better tissue characterisation.

In the oto-rhino-laryngology domaine the scanner may
eventually replace all other procedures.

PROSPECTIVE

Theoretically, digitalized radiology
might in most cases replace conventional techniques due
to the aforementioned advantages.
At the present time, the evolution of computerized transmission
tomography seems to have reached its climax.

Density and spatial resolution are
optimum with regards to the radiation dose.
Technological advances in these two domaines should not be
able to improve the ability to diagnose a lesion.

However, some further developments appear
to be required in regards to the microdensitometry of thin
slices to improve the visualization of pathological anatomy

and improvements concerning cardio and angio scans.

IN CONCLUSION

We would like to insist upon the
interesting capabilities of the "review mode". This technique
performed with an intravenous injection of contrast media
and the ability to apply subtraction quality films may
seriously challenge the future of digitalized angiography.

We must keep in mind that as long as
there is irradiation to the patient and a contrast media
injection, no technique can be considered entirely harmless.

Part VII: The Results of Clinical Evaluation: Studies of the Central Nervous System

THE INTERRELATIONSHIPS OF CEREBRAL BLOOD FLOW AND
CEREBRAL METABOLISM AND ITS STUDY WITH POSITRON
EMISSION TOMOGRAPHY IN MAN

J.C. BARON, M.D.

Service Hospitalier Frédéric Joliot, 91406 Orsay, France

Considerable interest has recently arisen into the study
of the local interrelationships of cerebral blood flow and
cerebral metabolism. This situation stems from two main factors.
One is that it has been realized that only partial or even
incorrect understanding of the mechanism by which drugs or
disease may affect brain homeostasis are derived if only flow
- or metabolism - is studied. The second factor relates to the
recent development of two powerful techniques for studying such
local relationships, namely quantitative autoradiography in the
experimental animal, and quantitative positron emission tomography
in man.

That the assessment of the primary target action, whether
circulatory or metabolic, of drugs appears necessary is self-
explanatory. Similarly, it would seem of the utmost importance
to define whether the local cerebral dysfunction seen in disease
states results from pathophysiological mechanisms affecting primarily either flow or metabolic rate, or even is the consequence
of disproportionate changes in these two parameters. Such studies
would help define whether therapy should be directed toward altering either flow or metabolism, or both, and in which direction,
as well as provide a direct quantitative estimation of the local
effects of therapy on these parameters.

Although important for all organs, the study of the flow-to-
metabolism relationship is especially crucial for brain, because
it has very little energy reserves, and its high metabolic rate
consequently depends on a constant supply of energetic substrates
by the blood circulation.

This paper briefly reviews, in the light of previous animal and human studies, the already large body of new information on this relationship provided by positron emission tomography (PET) in the normal and diseased brain of man.

First, a brief account of the previous knowledge on this relationship will be given. The data are derived from human and animal studies that have used various global and regional techniques for measuring cerebral blood flow (CBF), cerebral metabolic rate of oxygen ($CMRO_2$) or cerebral metabolic rate of glucose (CMRClc), either globally (e.g. the Kety-Schmidt technique, venous outflow, etc...) or regionally (e.g. the ^{133}Xe clearance technique, quantitative autoradiography, brain sampling, etc...). For a more detailed account, the reader may refer to excellent textbooks (Purves 1972, Siesjö 1978) or reviews (Lassen 1959, Ingvar and Lassen 1970, Olesen 1974, Sokoloff 1981).

1. RELATIONSHIP BETWEEN FUNCTION AND $CMRO_2$

The brain has to carry out an energetically costly work to maintain its ionic and structural homeostasis, even at rest. The energy, derived from ATP, results from the respiration which consumes glucose, in the presence of oxygen, to yield water and carbon dioxide. In the normal conditions, glucose is the only substrate for brain, and, since glycogen stores are relatively small, brain homeostasis depends on a minute-to-minute basis upon a constant supply of both glucose and oxygen. After circulatory arrest, unconsciousness occurs within seconds and irreversible brain death after only a few minutes. The deleterious effects of hypoxia or hypoglycemia on brain function, even though circulation is maintained, are well known.

That $CMRO_2$ is directly related to function is demonstrated by various facts : increased function (e.g. seizures, in vitro electrical stimulation) increases $CMRO_2$, whereas decreased function (e.g., hypothermia barbiturates) does the reverse. The mediating agent is probably ADP whose accumulation, immediately following the onset of increased function, stimulates the mitochondrial respiratory chain.

The in vitro measurements of oxygen consumption of brain slices has demonstrated that white matter (which contains only glial cells) consumes about 3-4 times less oxygen than grey matter (where both neurons and glia are found). It has been estimated that the neuronal cell consumes at least 10 times more oxygen than the gial cell, indicating that more than 75 % of whole brain $CMRO_2$ is due to neuronal work.

2. RELATIONSHIP BETWEEN THE DEMAND AND THE SUPPLY OF OXYGEN

It is obvious that, in any given situation, the oxygen uptake of the brain is equal to its supply times the fractional extraction of oxygen, that is $CMRO_2 = CBF.Ca.E$, where E is the fractional extraction of oxygen (OEF), CBF is the volumetric blood flow (ml/100 g/mn) and Ca is the arterial oxygen content (ml O_2/ml). This equation is a restatement of the classical Fick equation $CMRO_2 = CBF (Ca - Cv)$. Since, in steady state conditions, both CBF (to a given region) and Ca are constants, it follows that the ratio $CMRO_2/CBF.Ca$, i.e. the balance between oxygen demand and supply, is constant and equal to E, the OEF.

When primary changes in function occur in the structurally intact brain, the $CMRO_2$ changes are attended by parallel changes in CBF, so that the OEF remains constant. This phenomenon whereby supply is adjusted to meet the metabolic demand was first observed for the whole brain in various states of increased (e.g. seizures) or decreased (e.g. hypothermia, coma) function. More recently, this couple has been shown to hold even at the regional level, whereby the heterogenous distribution of metabolic rate in brain is associated with a similar pattern of regional CBF. This local coupling between flow and metabolism was first documented in man by regional measurement of CBF and $CMRO_2$ using the $H_2{}^{15}O-IIb{}^{15}O_2$ intra-carotid injection technique (Raichle et al. 1976), and later confirmed in minute structures of the rat brain by CBF and CMRGlc autoradiographic studies (Sokoloff 1981, Mies et al. 1981, Lear et al 1981). It is therefore clear that in normal brain CBF can be regarded as a reliable index of the metabolic rate.

The mechanisms by which CBF is adjusted to meet the metabolic demand have not been fully elucidated. One widely held hypothesis implicates that brain resistant vessels are submitted to the vasogenic influence of the extracellular pH. A shift to lower pH triggered by increased CO_2 production (and possibly of anaerobically produced lactate), itself secondary to increased metabolic rate, would thus induce local vasodilation and hence increased blood flow. Although supported by a number of studies, this hypothesis has been challenged on the basis of various experimental facts (see Siesjö 1978). Other vasoactive candidates have been proposed as the link between metabolism and flow such as extracellular potassium ion (K_e^+) or adenosine concentrations, both of which being vasodilating agents that could build up in metabolically hyperactive tissue. However, some studies would tend to minimize their role in the CBF-metabolism coupling mechanisms (see Siesjö 1978, Kuschinsky 1978). Recently, three other potential linkers have been suggested, namely prostaglandin derivatives, local oxygen tension, and central innervation of brain parenchymal vessels, but more data are needed to seriously implicate them (Kontos et al. 1978, Pickard et al. 1981, Tsubokawa et al. 1980).

Let us now consider the radically opposite situation where oxygen supply is primarily altered, without primary alterations in the metabolic rate. Obviously, this can result from primary changes in either CBF or Ca, but although the consequences are different in each of these two situations, in both cases the brain will tend, within certain limits, to maintain its function, i.e. $CMRO_2$ will tend to remain constant. In the case of changes in Ca (i.e. arterial hypoxia or hyperoxia), inversely proportionate changes in CBF occur so that oxygen supply remains constant (see Jones et al. 1981) and the OEF is not altered. Thus, although CBF values may seem uncoupled from $CMRO_2$, the oxygen supply infact remains adjusted to the metabolic demand. On the contrary, if primary changes in CBF occurs, the oxygen supply will change in parallel since Ca remains constant. Hence, uncoupling between supply and demand occurs and the OEF establishes at a new value either decreased (CBF increases) or increased (CBF decreases). A decreased OEF indicates lessened fractional O_2 extraction, i.e. decreased oxygen arterio-venous difference and "arteriolized" cerebral venous blood, whilst an increased OEF is witnessed by a darkened cerebral venous blood. Clearly, in these situations, CBF would be an extremely unreliable index of the existing metabolic rate.

3. PRIMARY CHANGES IN FUNCTION

As emphasized earlier, primary changes in neuronal function induce matched and proportionate changes in $CMRO_2$ and CBF.

States of globally increased function are observed during immobilization stress in unanesthetized animals and probably occur also in man in anxiety and painful situations, although indisputable evidence here is lacking. During generalized seizures, both in man and in animals, $CMRO_2$ increases are associated with CBF increases, but the latter frequently exceeds the former for reasons not quite understood yet.

Regional increases in cerebral function in the appropriate cortical areas in response to various stimulations, first described with CBF studies in man during visual, intellectual and sensory-motor tasks (Cooper et al. 1965, Ingvar and Risberg 1967, Olesen 1971), have since been amply confirmed and extended to animal studies. Matched increases is CBF and $CMRO_2$ occur in the sensory-motor cortex of man contralateral to vigorous hand exercise (Raichle et al. 1976). The fine ^{133}Xe intra-carotid injection CBF studies of the Scandinavian group in man have produced a wealth of fascinating data on the functional connections between various cortical areas in various activated conditions (see Larsen et al. 1978, Roland et al. 1976, Orgogozo et al. 1979). More recently, the quantitative CBF and CMRGlc autoradiographic techniques in the animal have provided high resolution 3D mapping of the highly focal functional changes that occur in the brain during various physiological conditions (for review, see Sokoloff 1981).

Conditions of decreased neuronal function are found in nonphysiological states such as coma (e.g. induced by barbiturates) and hypothermia. In senile or Alzheimer dementia, most investigators have found a coupled decrease in CBF and $CMRO_2$ (Lassen et al. 1960, Grubb et al. 1977). Normal human aging, on the other hand, has been the matter of controversial reports. However, present evidence suggests that normal aging is attended by matched decreases in CBF, $CMRO2$ and CMRGlc, but that considerable interindividual variations are present (Gottstein 1979, Kety 1956, Scheinberg et al. 1953) ; the subgroup consisting of elderly people with neither cognitive deficit nor systemic vascular risk factors have preserved $CMRO2$ and CBF (Dastur et al. 1963). Autoradiographic CMRGlc studies in senescent rats have provided somewhat discrepant data, but on the whole suggest that aging is accompanied by moderate decreases of glucose utilization (Smith et al. 1980, London et al., 1981).

Schizophrenic patients have been studied with the global Kety-Schmidt technique, and have been found to have normal CBF and $CMRO2$ values (Kety et al. 1947). However, clinical subgrouping has suggested that "productive" schizophrenics have quite high CBF and $CMRO2$ values, whereas hebephrenics show decreased values (Hoyer et al. 1975).

Many anesthetic agents (chloralose, althesin, barbiturates) as well as CNS depressants (benzodiazepines, phenotazins) induce coupled decreases in CBF and $CMRO_2$ (Smith and Wollman, 1972). Natural putative neuromediators, when given access to brain tissue, show either coupled CBF-$CMRO_2$ decreases (serotonin, GABA, phenylethylamine) or increases (noradrenaline) ; dopamine agonists also induce coupled CBF-$CMRO2$ increases (e.g. apomorphine, peribedil). Adenosin-tri-phosphate (ATP) also results in similar increases.

4. PRIMARY CHANGES IN CBF

As discussed above, primary changes in CBF induce uncoupling of the supply to demand relationship, witnessed by changes in the OEF. This can occur either at a generalized or at a regional level.

Global cerebral decreases in CBF may occur secondary to decreases of the cerebral perfusion pressure (CPP) below the lower limit of the autoregulation range if either systemic arterial pressure is decreased or intracranial pressure is increased. In these situations, although ischemia is global, it predominates in the borderzones between territories of the various terminal cerebral arteries, as is seen pathologically in circulatory arrest or in multiple occlusions of proximal cerebral arteries. Primary decreases in CBF are also induced by arterial hypocapnia (i.e. hyperventilation) and by various vaso-constrictive drugs (i.e. aminophylline, indomethacin). More circumscribed decreases in CBF follow arterial occlusion either at the proximal level (i.e. spontaneous or surgical occlusion of the internal carotid artery in the neck) or at the distal level (i.e. spontaneous or experimental occlusions of the middle cerebral artery). Whatever the cause of the primary CBF decrease, $CMRO_2$ tends to be maintained at its normal level as CBF falls within certain limits, i.e.the OEF increases and the cerebral venous oxygen content decreases. Various studies suggest that $CMRO_2$ and function are essentially preserved until CBF is reduced two-fold, i.e. the OEF has almost doubled its value (Bruce et al. 1972, Grubb et al, 1975). If CBF is further reduced, $CMRO_2$ then declines but at a slower rate than CBF, i.e. the OEF further increases to maximal values of about 70-80 %. Thereafter $CMRO_2$ falls precipitously as damage to the intrinsic metabolic pathways occurs. Rather well-defined thresholds for cerebral tolerance to ischemia have resulted from numerous experimental studies, and seem to hold even in man. Thus, electrical failure with *reversible* functional deficit occurs at CBF values below $\sim$ 20 ml/100 g/min (compared to normal ranges of $\sim$ 50-60 ml/100 g/min), and pump failure (release of intercellular potassium) with time-dependant potentially *irreversible* structural damage occurs below CBF values of about 10-12 ml/100 g/min (Branston et al. 1974, Astrup et al, 1977, Morawetz et al. 1978, Jones et al. 1981).

Primary increases in CBF result from induced vasodilatation in the face of unchanged metabolic demand. This is seen in arterial hypercapnia, but also when CPP is increased above the upper limit of the autoregulatory mechanisms, or when vasodila-ting pharmaceuticals are administered (e.g. papaverine, adeno-sine, nimodipine, dipyrridamole, prostacyclin, nicotine), including some analgesic compounds which may have, in addition, specific effects on $CMRO_2$ (e.g. halothane, protamine, gamma-hydroxybutyrate). In all the above situations, CBF is uncoupled from $CMRO_2$ and the OEF is decreased. Two special circumstances need be mentioned here. One is the seizure state, where, for unknown reasons, the CBF increases often largely exceed the metabolic increases ; another one is the hyperemic state that follows short-lasting ischemia, be it global or focal. The latter condition of "reactive hyperemia" may be regarded as a physiological compensatory mechanism. However, its long-lasting occurence, its values largely exceeding the post-ischemic metabolic rate, and finally its frequent linear dependence on CPP (loss of autoregulation) and poor or inverted reactivity to changes in arterial pCO_2 (i.e. a state "vasoparalysis") all indicate an abnormal vasodilation far in excess to the metabolic demand. Lassen (1966) speculated that such hyperemia was due to focal ischemic acidosis, and coined the term "luxury perfusion syndrome" to define this state where CBF is overabundant relative to the oxygen needs of the tissue, the corollary being that the oxygen A-V difference is lower than normal, cerebral venous blood is red, and the OEF is low. He indicated that CBF values could be either higher than normal (absolute hyperemia), or normal, or even lower than normal, but still in excess of metabolism.

5. RELATIONSHIP BETWEEN OXYGEN AND GLUCOSE CONSUMPTIONS

In normal brain, the pathways of glucose utilization differ from those of many organs, in that the glycogen storage is of little quantitative importance and is relatively fixed, and that the pentose pathway utilizes small amounts of glucose. Thus, in steady state conditions, the glucose uptake is equal to the glucose consumed in the anaerobic and aerobic glycolysis. Since the anaerobic glycolysis amounts to only 5-10 % of glucose consumption in normal conditions, it follows that $CMRO_2$ and CMRGlc are linked in a predictable fashion, the $CMRO_2$ being slightly less than 6 times the CMRGlc (in molar quantities), i.e. the value predicted stoichiometrically if anaerobic glycolysis were not existing. Thus, in most of the above mentioned situations where primary variations in function occur (e.g. normal regional heterogeneities, focal activation, aging, drug effects, etc...), $CMRO_2$ and CMRGlc remain coupled to each other as well as to CBF. Quantitative autoradiography in animals has demonstrated the highly focal coupling that exists between flow and CMRGlc (see Sokoloff 1981).

However, in abnormal conditions CMRGlc may become uncoupled from function and $CMRO_2$. When anaerobic glycolysis is enhanced by cellular hypoxia (e.g. arterial hypoxia, ischemia) or seizure states, CMRGlc overestimates the real cerebral energy requirements. On the other hand, some conditions are associated with the use of other substrates than exogenous glucose (e.g. ketone bodies in starvation, amino acids in hypercapnia), and CMRGlc may underestimate the metabolic rate. As Siesjö (1978) puts it, "in disease, $CMRO_2$ provides the reference to the true energy requirements of the brain".

6. UNCOUPLING BETWEEN CMRO$_2$ AND FUNCTION

However true the last statement may appear, CMRO$_2$ may not always be a reliable index of the functional state of the tissue. It is particularly true in various conditions where CMRO$_2$ may be preserved in the face of obvious functional failure (both clinical and electrical), e.g. in hypoglycemia and in arterial hypoxia. In the post-ischemic state, CMRO$_2$ may even be increased although function has not returned (Hossmann et al. 1976). Although it is possible that in the above situations energy is required for other tasks than neuronal transmission, or that the latter is impeded by an unknown "toxic" compound, a more likely (but not mutually exclusive) hypothesis suggests that mitochondrial respiration is in an uncoupled state, i.e. oxygen is consumed but little ATP is produced. This state may result from free-radical production induced by tissue hyperoxygenation (Kogure et al. 1980), possibly in the presence of arachidonic acid prostaglandin derivatives (Flamm et al. 1978).

Positron Emission Tomography (PET) studies of the interrelationships of CBF and metabolism

With the recent development of PET, a new era in the study of the local CBF-metabolism relationships in man has been opened. An original model has been designed for the measurement of local CBF and CMRO$_2$, and the deoxyglucose technique of Sokoloff has been adapted to PET for measuring local CMRGlc in man.

The principles of PET will not be described here (see Ter Pogossian et al 1975, Phelps 1977, Ter Pogossian et al. 1980). Briefly, it consists of 1) non-invasive administration to the patient of a suitable molecule labeled with a short-lived, cyclotron produced, positron-emitting radionuclide ; 2) external detection of the annihilation photons by NaI detectors that view a slice of the patient's head and are connected two by two by means of a coincidence circuit ("electronic collimation") ; and 3) reconstruction of the slice radioactivity distribution by a filtered back-projection algorithm.

Its advantages are numerous : 1) availability of radiochemicals well-adapted to the study of brain metabolism ; 2) non-invasive, repeatable, and simultaneously bilateral studies; 3) 3-D, tomographic imaging of high spatial resolution ; 4) accurate local absolute quantitation of radioactive concentrations provided stringent technological precautions are taken.

Numerous elegant models have been proposed, but, at the present time, only two have been thoroughly investigated and validated and have consequently gained wide use, namely the ^{18}F-fluoro-2-deoxy-D-glucose ([18]FDG) technique for measuring local

CMRGlc, and the $^{15}O_2$-$C^{15}O_2$ continuous inhalation technique for measuring local CBF and CMRO2. The former is an adaptation to PET of the Sokoloff autoradiographic model ; it is based on the same principle, i.e. that of using a labelled glucose analog which competes with glucose for the same carrier at the blood-brain-barrier as well as for the phosphorylation step, but remains trapped in the tissue at this step. It therefore accumulates in the tissue, and if its transport and phosphorylation rate constants are known, as well as the arterial input function and the local tissue radioactive concentration at a given time after I.V. injection, it becomes possible to measure the local phosphorylation rate of the analog ; knowing the arterial plasma glucose concentration and the analog-glucose coupling factor (the "lumped constant"), the rate of glucose phosphorylation can be derived. The latter is equated to the glycolytic rate since other metabolic routes for glucose-6-phosphate are normally negligible in brain (for details of the model and its assumptions, see Sokoloff et al. 1977). The use of the fluorine derivative of deoxyglucose does not modify the approach (Miller et al. 1981), but its use with PET offers the additional opportunity of measuring locally the rate constants of ^{18}FDG since repeated measurement of ^{18}F concentration in brain tissue can be obtained after the I.V. injection (Phelps et al. 1979, Huang et al. 1980). Although quite reliable in normal tissue (Maziotta et al. 1981) the CMRGlc measurements should be interpreted with more caution in abnormal states because of the uncertainties in both the rate constants and the "lumped" constant (Kuhl et al. 1980a, 1980b).

Inhalation of $C^{15}O_2$ labels in vivo the arterial blood water, and the $H_2^{15}O$ so produced will diffuse in brain tissue in proportion to blood flow (Jones et al. 1976). Because of the short half-life of ^{15}O (123 sec.), an equilibrium is reached after a few minutes of continuous inhalation whereby the $H_2^{15}O$ input in tissue is balanced by disappearance of the tracer from physical decay and tissue outflow. During continuous inhalation of $^{15}O_2$, the tracer is transported to brain by the oxyhemoglobin, and is taken up and converted to $H_2^{15}O$ in the tissue in proportion to $CMRO_2$. The $H_2^{15}O$ so produced in situ is constantly cleared by blood flow and recirculates. Thus, at $C^{15}O_2$ equilibrium, the $H_2^{15}O$ tissue concentration is a non-linear function of CBF, whereas that at $^{15}O_2$ equilibrium is a complex function of both CBF and CMRO2. However this difficulty can be overcome by dividing the $^{15}O_2$ quantitative image by the $C^{15}O_2$ corresponding image, a procedure which obtains a "ratio" image now linearly proportional to the OEF (Jones et al. 1976, Subramanyam et al. 1978). The $C^{15}O_2$ and ratio images can then be transformed into CBF and OEF images, respectively, if the $H_2^{15}O$ and $Hb^{15}O_2$ arterial concentrations have been measured. Multiplying one by the other and by the arterial oxygen content provides a $CMRO_2$ quantitative image. The validity of this model has been confirmed by experimental studies (Baron et al. 1980c, 1981c, Rhodes et al. 1981) although it does have some theoretical limitations (Lammertsmaa et al. 1981, Baron et al. 1981c). The regional values for CBF, OEF and $CMRO_2$ obtained in control subjects have been satisfactory (Frackowiak et al. 1980, Baron et al. 1981c).

1 - Results in normal brain

The above mentioned studies have provided indisputable evidence that local CBF matches exactly local $CMRO_2$ in normal brain. The heterogeneous features of the CBF image are exactly identical to those of the $CMRO_2$ image (Fig. 1). The constant relationship between oxygen supply and demand is well demonstrated by the plainliness of the OEF image (Fig. 1), i.e., the OEF is a constant thoughout brain (Baron et al. 1978, 1979, 1981c, Frackowiak et al. 1980). This is also well demonstrated by the plot of CBF versus $CMRO_2$ in 131 various brain regions in 19 subjects which provide a highly significant correlation and an intercept not very different from zero (Fig. 2). Recent studies combining the ^{15}O and ^{18}FDG studies have also confirmed that local CBF and CMRGlc are closely coupled (a fact already suggested by the combined $^{13}NH_3$ and ^{18}FDG studies of Kuhl et al. 1980), and that $CMRO_2$ and CMRGlc are also tightly matched in various brain regions (Fig. 3) (Baron et al., 1981e). Although the ^{18}FDG studies during activated states have clearly demonstrated the appropriate focal increases in CMRGlc (Phelps et al. 1981, Greenberg et al. 1981), parallel local increases in CBF, although highly probable (Roland et al, 1981), have not yet been documented in the same subject.

2 - Pathophysiological states where coupling is preserved

As documented by PET studies, the coupling of CBF and metabolism holds true on a *regional* basis in a number of situations where function is primarily altered. Thus, in normal aging, CBF and $CMRO_2$ decrease significantly in grey matter but not in white matter (Frackowiak et al. 1980) ; in all grey structures, the OEF was found unchanged when young (< 50 years old) were compared to older (> 50 years old) volunteers, whereas CBF and $CMRO_2$ values in the latter group were 28 % below those of the former (Lenzi et al, 1981a). However, some brain regions (e.g. parietal) did not show such age related changes. In patients with senile dementia (i.e., Alzheimer's disease), CBF and $CMRO_2$ showed a 30% decrease when compared to age matched controls, and the decrease correlated with the severity of dementia (Frackowiak et al, 1981). The depression in CBF and metabolism occurred for all brain regions studied, including white matter, but was more

CBF   **OEF**   **CMR O$_2$**

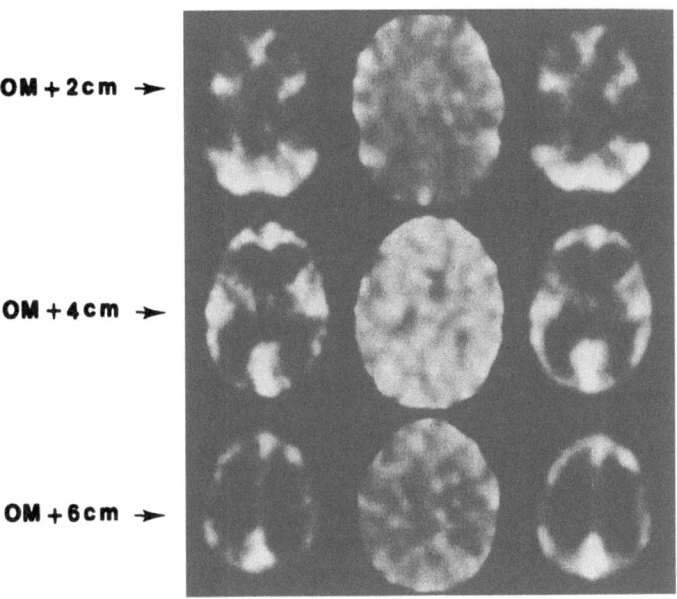

OM + 2cm →

OM + 4cm →

OM + 6cm →

Fig. 1 – Functional images representing CBF (left-hand row), OEF (middle row) and CMRO$_2$ (right-hand row) in a normal subject, at three different brain levels. The higher the activity, the whiter it appears on the images. Areas consisting essentially of grey matter are clearly delineated from white matter areas, and several physio-anatomic structures are identifiable. In this normally functioning brain, the normal regional couple between flow and metabolism is demonstrated by the close similarity of the corresponding CBF and CMRO$_2$ images and by the plainliness of the OEF images (Baron et al., SHFJ, Orsay, France).

418

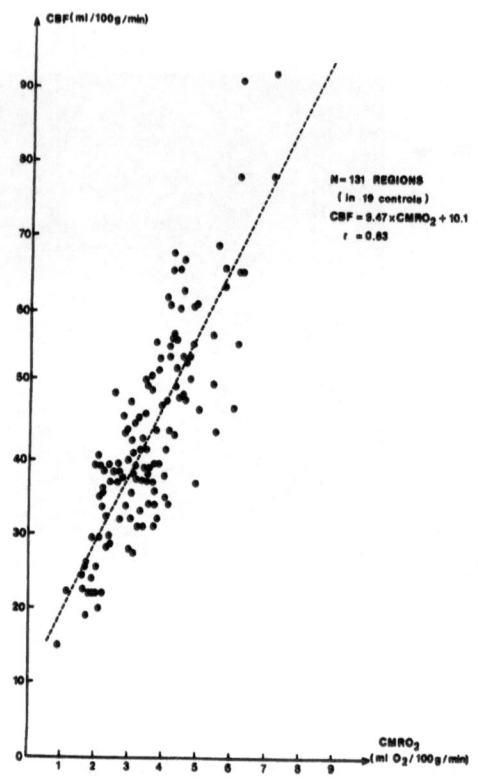

Fig. 2 – Plot of regional CBF versus CMRO$_2$ in 131 brain regions in 19 control studies, showing the constant relationship between CBF and CMRO$_2$ across a wide range of values (Baron et al., SHFJ, Orsay, France).

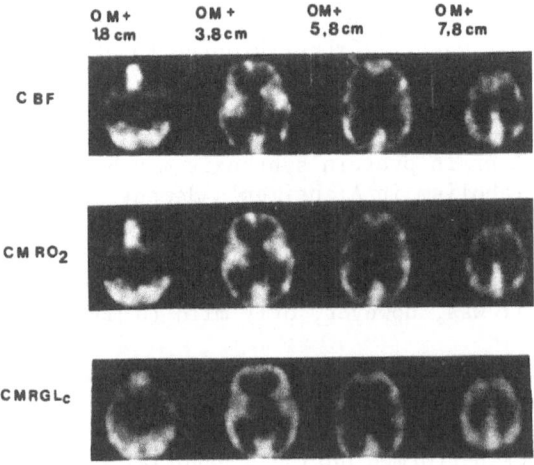

OM+ 1.8 cm   OM+ 3.8cm   OM+ 5,8cm   OM+ 7,8cm

C BF

CM RO$_2$

CMRGL$_c$

S.H.F.J   ORSAY

Fig. 3 - Functional CBF, CMRO$_2$ and CMRGlc images at 4 different brains levels in a control subject. The close coupling between CBF, CMRO$_2$ and CMRGlc is demonstrated by the corresponding regional variations in all three parameters (Baron et al., SHFJ, Orsay, France).

marked over the frontal lobes. In a preliminary study of senile dementia patients using ^{11}C-L-Methionine to assess the regional protein synthesis rate with PET, protein synthesis showed a 42 % decrease in mild dementia and 70% decrease in severe dementia when compared to age matched controls (Bustany et al, 1981), suggesting that brain protein synthesis may be more affected than energy metabolism in Alzheimer's dementia. In support of this hypothesis, a preliminary study of CMRGlc in senile dementia reported a 33 to 37 % decrease in glucose utilization in all examined structures (Ferris et al. 1981) ; the severity of the clinical deficit was, however, only mild to moderately severe.

Kuhl et al. (1980b) studied 17 patients with medically resistant focal epilepsy using the coupled $^{13}NH_3$-^{18}FDG PET technique to estimate local perfusion and glucose utilization. In three studies performed during behaviorial seizure activity, massive local increases in ^{13}N and ^{18}F substrates occurred in clinically corresponding areas ; although CBF was not quantitated, the tentative conclusion was that increases in metabolism were matched by similar increases in CBF. In the 15 studies carried out interictally in patients with unilateral EEG localization, 12 studies showed regional decreases in CMRGlc that were concomittant with presumably parallel decreases in CBF. These hypometabolic zones were found on repeated studies in the same patient irrelevant of the degree of interictal EEG abnormalities, and were located in morphologically intact (as seen on C.T. scans in 10 patients) but microscopically gliotic areas (as seen on temporal lobetomy specimens in 5 of 6 operated patients, including 5 patients with normal C.T. scans). This important study therefore suggested that focal areas of interictally diminished function (but without C.T. scan counterparts) correlated with the area identified both electrically and pathologically as responsible for the seizure condition. In both ictal and interictal states, primary changes in function were attended by apparently matched changes in CBF.

In schizophrenic syndromes, three preliminary studies of local CMRGlc have suggested a moderate metabolic decrease in the frontal lobes (Buchsbaum et al. 1981, Widen et al. 1981, Farkas et al. 1981), reminiscent of the earlier work of Ingvar and Franzen (1975) who reported CBF decreases in the frontal lobe of schizophenics. Paired studies of CBF and metabolism in schizophrenia, though, have not been performed to date. This comment would also apply to a recent ^{18}FDG study on patients with Huntington's chorea, showing metabolic depression in the caudate nuclei very early in the course of the disease (Kuhl et al. 1981).

The advent of PET allows one to map in detail the secondary metabolic depressions that occur remote from the site of focal brain injury, particularly in stroke. A better understanding of the clinical correlates in completed stroke, as well as of the mechanisms of the long term partial clinical recovery, may now be at hand. Thus, parallel decreases of CBF and glucose metabolism over the cortical mantle and/or the thalamus ipsilateral to circumscribed supratentorial infarction have been reported (Kuhl et al. 1980a). Although the mechanism underlying these phenomena remains controversal, a likely hypothesis incriminates transneural depression (i.e. deactivation) from interruption of the connecting neural pathways, a phenomenon known as "diaschisis". Similarly, the disputed occurence of metabolic depression over the contralateral cerebral hemisphere has received some support from PET studies (Kuhl et al. 1980a). In addition, a matched decrease in CBF and $CMRO_2$ over the *cerebellar* hemisphere *contralateral* to supratentorial infarction in the internal carotid artery distribution has recently been reported (Baron et al. 1980b). This transient phenomenon, called "crossed cerebellar diaschsis" suggests a transneural deactivation of the cerebro-cerebellar loop (i.e. the neural pathways connecting the sensori-motor cortex to the contralateral cerebellar cortex). It would thus stand as the most undisputable *in vivo* demonstration of transneural depression (Fig. 4).

3 - Pathophysiological states with flow-metabolism uncoupling

A number of PET studies on cerebral ischemic disorders have appeared lately. They have demonstrated the importance of studying the local CBF-metabolism relationship in spontaneously occurring human cerebral ischemia for an improved pathophysiological understanding. The main findings will be briefly summarized here.

Within the core of recent cerebral ischemia, in completed stroke patients studied less than 15 to 30 days after clinical onset, a state of focal mismatch between CBF and $CMRO_2$, evidenced by a focal OEF abnormality, has been an almost constant finding. In two studies, this was true in 20/20 studies (Lenzi et al. 1981b) and in 43/45 studies (Baron et al. 1981b), respectively. Two different types of uncoupling, both already discussed in the first section of this paper, have been encountered. In one, the OEF is focally decreased, i.e. indicating the "luxury-perfusion syndrome" (Lassen, 1966), whereas in the other, the OEF is focally increased. The latter state has been jocularly termed the "misery-perfusion syndrome" (Baron et al. 1980a, 1981a). The former, encountered in 37/45 studies (Baron et al. 1981a), could be associated with focally increased flow (i.e. absolute hyperemia), normal flow or decreased flow in respecti-

422

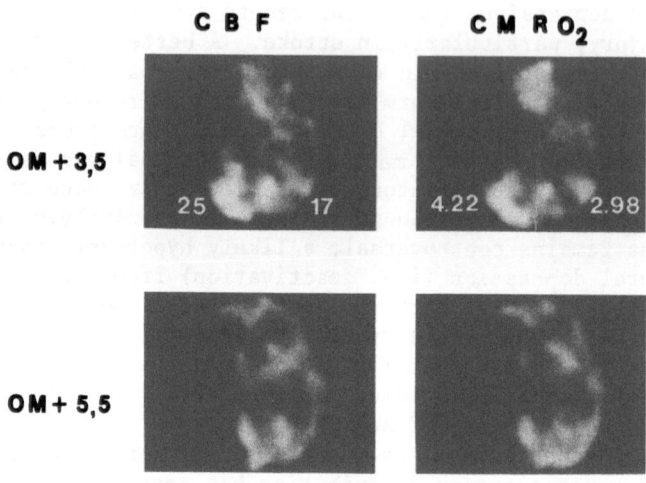

Fig. 4 - Crossed cerebellar diaschisis : tomographic maps of CBF
and CMRO$_2$ at two adjacent brain levels in a patient with a 4
day old infarction in the left middle cerebral artery territory. The ischemic region is clearly seen at both brain levels
as an area of greatly reduced CBF and CMRO$_2$. In addition, there
is a striking cerebellar asymmetry of CBF and CMRO$_2$, the right
side showing reduced values (indicated here in ml/100 g/min)
relative to the left side (OM + 0.5 cm). This functional asymmetry had no C.T. Scan counterpart (Baron et al., SHFJ, Orsay,
France).

vely 14 %, 34 % and 52 % of the times (Baron et al. 1981a), but
in all instances indicating that CBF was overabundant relative
to the metabolic needs. Misery-perfusion was observed in 9/45
patients, in all instances associated with decreased CBF (Baron
et al. 1981a). These results indicate that CBF cannot be regarded
as a reliable index of function in a brain region that has
recently suffered from ischemia. Moreover, in a given ischemic
core, CBF undergoes spontaneous changes with time, but does so
in a rather predictable manner. Thus, Baron et al. (1980a, 1981a)
showed that, with reference to the contralateral homologous zone,
CBF consistently went through a phase of near-normal or even
increased values between the 5th and 20th day after onset, together with profoundly depressed OEF, a finding confirmed by
Ackerman et al. (1981b). Earlier than the 5th day, CBF was most
often decreased, while the OEF was increased, although in some
cases the reverse was true.

The prognostic significance of these two types of flow-
metabolism uncoupling, namely luxury and misery-perfusion, have
been assessed by clinical and C.T. scan correlations. Semiquantitative studies have suggested that ischemic core areas
showing the luxury-perfusion syndrome, either early or during the
2-3rd week after onset, are undergoing ischemic necrosis. Conversely, when misery-perfusion is present, tissue prognosis is
often good (Baron et al. 1980a, 1981a, Ackerman et al. 1979,
1981b) unless CBF is at extremely low levels (Baron et al.
1981a). Preliminary quantitative studies indicate that prognosis
is poor if local $CMRO_2$ falls below 1.25 ml/100 g/min or if
CBF falls below 20 ml/100 g/min (Lenzi et al, 1981b). Further
quantitative studies will hopefully refine these prognostic
correlations and define quantitatively the $CBF-CMRO_2$ patterns
and thresholds that are indicative of spontaneous tissue outcome,
whether irreversible necrosis or functional reversible ischemia.
This information would be of paramount importance in trying to
select patients· in whom therapeutic manoeuvres aimed at salvaging
threatened but potentially viable areas (the "nenumbra" of
Symon and Astup, 1979) may be contemplated. Similarly, PET
studies would help quantitate the local effects of such therapy
on CBF and $CMRO_2$.

Tissue immediately surrounding the ischemic core may show
any or all of the four following patterns of $CBF-CMRO_2$ relationships : 1) increased CBF with a *moderately* decreased OEF
(luxury perfusion) ; 2) *moderately* decreased CBF with increased
OEF (misery perfusion) ; 3) *matched* increase in CBF and $CMRO_2$;
and 4) *matched* decrease in CBF and $CMRO_2$. Since the terms
"neighbouring tissue" imply that it is located outside the area
of ischemic necrosis defined on follow up C.T. scans, the inference is that the above-mentioned $CBF-CMRO_2$ patterns are

functional abnormalities that take place in morphologically essentially normal tissue, i.e. they indicate viable tissue.

The mechanisms responsible for such CBF-CMRO2 abnormalities in recent completed stroke are only partially understood to date. Within the necrotic core, late luxury-perfusion presumably indicates macrophage-laden softening. Early misery-perfusion in the ischemic core indicates continuing occlusion at the level of either the main feeding artery or the capillary bed (i.e. the "no-reflow" phenomenon of Ames et al. 1968). The latter hypothesis may also explain the experimental findings of delayed hypoperfusion with relatively maintained CMRO2 observed in the ischemic zones after circulation has been reestablished (Levy et al. 1979). Early luxury-perfusion in the ischemic core, on the other hand, would indicate that perfusion pressure has been partially (e.g. through collateral channels) or completely (i.e. after post-embolic recanalization) restored in a tissue with low metabolic demand and lost autoregulation (i.e. vaso-paralysis). In neighbouring tissues, similar phenomenons may explain the uncoupled states observed ; especially vasopara-lysis secondary to spreading acidosis could induce neighbouring hyperemia, whereas persistent occlusion of the main feeding vessel (e.g. the internal carotid artery) could be responsible for neighboring misery-perfusion (see below). Matched increases in CBF and CMRO2, on the other hand, implies post-ischemic hyper-metabolism, a condition already observed in experimental ischemia (Hossmann et al. 1976) but with ill-defined prognostic and pathophysiologic significance. Conversely, matched decreases in CBF and CMRO2 suggest functional depression secondary to either post-ischemic inhibition (toxic ?) or transneural deactivation, or both.

Obviously, the situation in ischemic completed stroke is made very complex by the spatially and temporally changing pattern of circulatory and functional states (see Fig. 5), thus making any oversimplification unrealistic. However the 3D simultaneous assessment of CBF and CMRO2 by PET allows such patterns to be studied, thereby clearly showing the superiority of this approach over conventional 2D CBF techniques.

Even more relevant pathophysiologic information may come from the coupled study of local CBF, CMRO2 and CMRGlc in stroke. This is feasible if ^{15}O and ^{18}FDG studies are done in sequence, and such studies are now underway in a number of research centers although none has been published to date. Kuhl et al. (1980a) carried out a study of 10 completed stroke patients using $^{13}NH_3$ and ^{18}FDG as essentially qualitative perfusion and glucose utilization tracers, respectively. These authors reported findings very similar to those described above for CBF-

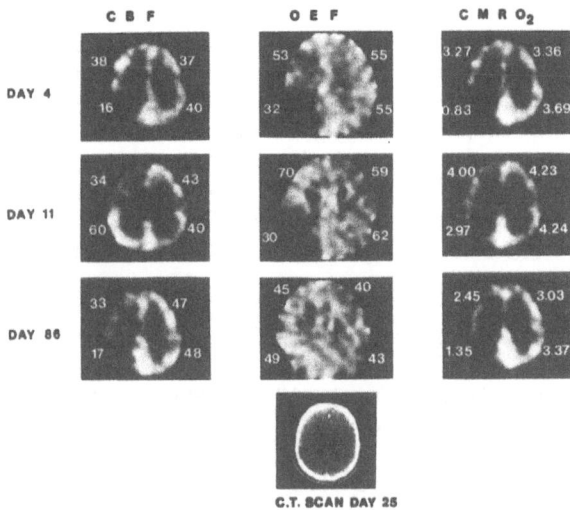

C.T. SCAN DAY 25

Fig. 5 - Ischemic completed stroke : CBF, OEF and CMRO2 at the level OM + 5.8 cm in the same patient on 3 different occasions. The patient suffered an extensive infarct in the left middle cerebral artery territory and distal to an occlusion of the ipsilateral internal carotid artery. The values shown indicate regional CBF (ml/100 g/min), OEF (percent value) and CMRO2 (ml O2/100 g/min). Unenhanced C.T. scan performed at day 25 at level OM + 6.0 cm shows that the necrotic area was essentially restricted to the left parietal region. *Within this area,* CBF was very low on day 4 but CMRO2 was even more depressed as evidenced by the lower OEF value relative to the remainder of the brain ("luxury perfusion" type of uncoupling) ; on day 11, there was focal hyperemia with continuing "luxury perfusion" - the OEF being about half the contralateral value - and CMRO2, although improved, was still reduced ; on day 86, both CBF and CMRO2 had returned to very low values in the infarcted area, and were at that time essentially coupled. In the cortical mantle *anterior to the infarct,* no changes were noted on day 4, but CBF was decreased at day 11 whereas CMRO2 was close to normal - the OEF value was therefore increased relative to the contralateral side ("misery perfusion" type of uncoupling) ; on day 86, CBF and CMRO2 were both lower than on the contralateral side, but the OEF relative increase was then only marginally significant compared to ranges in normal controls. These chronic changes in morphologically intact tissue may have been related to the persistent occlusion of the left internal carotid artery (Baron et al., SHFJ, Orsay, France).

$CMRO_2$ studies. For example, perfusion was more depressed than CMRGlc within the infarct in the first 2 days, whereas the reverse was observed during the second week. In surrounding tissue without evidence of structural damage on C.T. scans, matched decreases in both parameters were observed. The authors however stressed that caution was required in interpreting their results since : 1) tracer behavior of both ^{13}N and ^{18}F in ischemic tissue remained unexplored (Hawkins et al. 1981) ; and 2) anaerobic glucose metabolism may have been at play in some cases.

When several months-old infarcts are investigated, coupling of CBF and metabolism is consistently found in the remaining infarcted tissue (Baron et al. 1979, 1980a, 1981a, Kuhl et al. 1980a), presumably as a result of complete removal of necrotic tissue. In some instances however matched decreases in CBF and metabolism are found remote from the infarct per se , e.g. in the thalamus and cortical mantle ipsilaterally or in the cerebellar hemisphere contralaterally, presumably from trans-neural deactivation (Baron et al. 1980a, Kuhl et al. 1980a). Rarely, in some cases with persistent occlusion of the ipsila-teral internal carotid artery, widerspread "misery-perfusion" may be observed, suggesting a state of long-standing hemodynamic insufficiency.

In a few patients clinically selected for extra-intra-cranial by pass surgery because of continuing neurological events occurring distal to a previously demonstrated occlusion of the internal carotid artery (ICA), PET studies have disclosed two patterns of CBF-OEF relationships. In all patient, CBF was decreased over the appropriate cerebral hemisphere, and the area showing CBF decrease was much larger than the C.T. Scan abnor-malities. Two patients showed concomittant OEF increase (i.e. misery perfusion), and two did not (i.e. matched flow-metabolism depression), but in all cases the functional changes were maxi-mum at the cortical arterial boundary zones between the anterior, middle and posterior cerebral arteries. The PET features thus suggested a state of chronic hemodynamic failure distal to ICA occlusion, a finding in accordance with the clinical presenta-tion of hemodynamic, not embolic, cerebral ischemia in 3 of the 4 patients. Following surgery, all patients clinically improved and all showed disappearance of the previously demonstrated physiologic abnormalities (Baron et al. 1981b, 1981d). This study (Fig. 6), which is consonant with previous PET investiga-tions showing improvement of CBF after extra-intracranial anastomosis (Yamamoto et al. 1979), strongly suggested that, in selected patients, surgical revascularization may be of physiological benefit. Both CBF-OEF patterns thus appeared potentially reversible, but it remained unclear why uncoupling

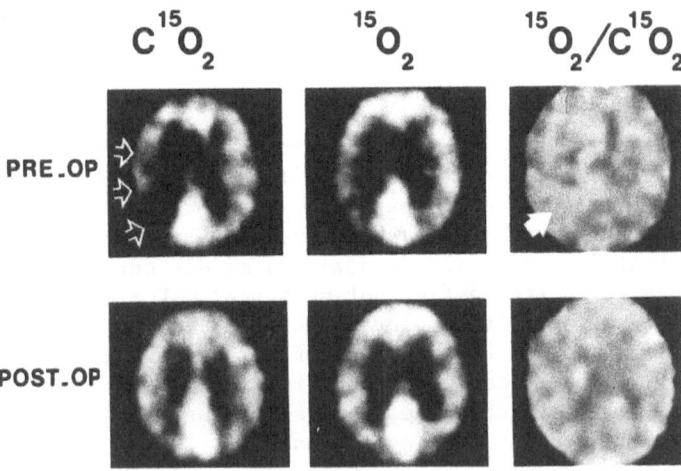

$$C^{15}O_2 \qquad {}^{15}O_2 \qquad {}^{15}O_2/C^{15}O_2$$

PRE.OP

POST.OP

Fig. 6 - Pre- and post-operative studies performed at level OM + 6 cm in a patient who presented with repeated transient ischemic episodes involving the left cerebral hemisphere, which led to the discovery of a left internal carotid artery (ICA) occlusion. Despite anticoagulation, the attacks continued and were triggered by diabetic orthostatic hypotention. He had two severe episodes of right hemiplegia and aphasia, resolving almost entirely within a few days. Repeat angiogram showed that the middle cerebral artery filled solely from the left ophthalmic artery. A left extra-intracranial arterial bypass (EIAB) was performed in 1979. The attacks stopped immediately and had not recurred as of 1981. A post-operative C.T. Scan showed only moderate cortical atrophy over the left watershed, and a control angiogram revealed a patent and functional anastomosis. The images shown are equilibrium $C^{15}O_2$, $^{15}O_2$ and $^{15}O_2/C^{15}O_2$ ratio images, which are representations of CBF, both CMRO2 and CBF, and OEF, respectively. Pre-operatively, there was a marked decrease in CBF over the left cortical mantle (hollow arrows) associated with an increased OEF (filled arrow), both abnormalities predominating over the posterior wasterhed. All post-operative images were normal.

could be found in some cases and not in others. However, both patterns of abnormalities may constitute rational indications for surgery. Earlier studies using intra-carotid ^{15}O injections had reached similar conclusions (Grubb et al. 1979).

One report of PET study in a case of left occipital migrainous infarction has appeared (Bousser et al. 1980). The study at day 14 showed a decreased CBF with decreased OEF within the infarct, i.e. a luxury-perfusion syndrome not different from that seen in common stroke. However, distant functional changes were detected in : 1) the ipsilateral middle cerebral artery territory as increased flow but unchanged OEF ; and 2) the contralateral occipital pole as decreased flow and increased OEF, i.e. misery-perfusion. These findings suggested an involvement latent clinically, of arterial territories distinct from the clinically affected one, thus stressing the unusual nature and extent of the underlying process.

Only very preliminary results on brain tumor studies with PET have appeared. From these abstracts, it appears that, although tumor flow may vary from high to low values, tumor $CMRO_2$ is consistently decreased ; the tumor OEF thus may be either normal or decreased relative to surrounding brain (Lammerstsmaa et al. 1981, Ackerman et al. 1981a). An interesting report of ^{18}FDG uptake in human glioma has revealed high uptake in 6 cases and low uptake in 7 cases but the former were correlated with higher grades of malignancy (Di Chiro et al. 1981). It would thus seem that in high grade gliomas, glucose utilization may be elevated whilst $CMRO_2$ is decreased, suggesting a shift to anaerobic glycolysis possibly correlated with the degree of malignancy. Combined quantitative studies with ^{15}O and ^{18}FDG, ans possibly ^{11}C-Methionine, may provide direct in vivo insight into the circulatory and metabolic features of brain tumor, and their correlation with histologic grades, prognosis and therapeutic effects. The distant effects of tumor over the ipsilateral and contralateral cerebral hemisphere and their pathophysiological importance are now also open to study.

REFERENCES

1. Ackerman, R.H., Alpert, N.M., Correia, J.A., Grotta, J.C., Fallick, J.T., Chang, J.Y., Brownell, G.L., Taveras, J.M. Correlations of positron emission scans with TCT scans and clinical course. In Gotoh F., Nagai H., Tazaki Y. (eds). Cerebral blood flow and metabolism. Copenhague, Munksgaard, Acta Neurol Scand. 60, 1979 (Suppl. 72), 230-231.

2. Ackerman, R.H., Davis, S.M., Correia, J.A., et al. Positron imaging of CBF and metabolism in patients with cerebral neoplasms. J. CBF Metabol.,1981a, 1, Suppl. 1, 575-576.

3. Ackerman, R.H., Correia, J.A., Alpert, N.M. et al. Positron imaging in ischemic stoke disease using compounds labeled with oxygen 15. Arch. Neurol., 1981b, 38, 537-543.

4. Ames, A., III, Wright, R.L., Kowada, M. et al. Cerebral ischemia II. The no-reflow phenomenon. Am. J. Pathol., 1968, 52, 437-453.

5. Astrup, J., Symon, L., Branston, N.M., Lassen, N.A. Thresholds of cerebral ischemia, in "Microsurgery for stroke" Springer, New York, 1976, p. 16-21.

6. Baron, J.C., Comar, D., Bousser, M.G., Soussaline, F., Crouzel, C., Plummer, D., Kellershohn, C., Castaigne, P. Etude tomographique chez l'homme, du débit sanguin et de la consommation d'oxygène du cerveau par inhalation continue d'oxygène 15. Revue Neurol., 1978, 134, 545-556.

7. Baron, J.C., Comar, D., Bousser, M.G., Plummer, D., Loc'h, C., Kellershohn, C., Castaigne, P. Patterns of CBF and oxygen extraction fraction (EO2) in hemispheric infarcts : a tomographic study with the ^{15}O inhalation technique. Acta Neurol. Scand., 1979, 60 (Suppl. 72), 324-325.

8. Baron, J.C., Bousser, M.G., Comar, D. et Kellershohn, C. Human hemispheric infarction studied by positron emission tomography and the ^{15}O inhalation technique, in "Computerized tomography", J.M. Caillé and G. Salamon, eds., Springer-Verlag, Berlin, p. 231-237, 1980a.

9. Baron, J.C., Bousser, M.G., Comar, D. et Castaigne, P. "Crossed cerebellar diaschisis" in human supratentorial brain infarction. Ann. Neurol., 1980b, 8, 128.

10. Baron, J.C., Naquet R., Steinling, M., Loc'h C. et Soussaline, F. Tomographic measurement of cerebral blood flow with the $C^{15}O_2$ continuous inhalation technique : experimental evidence. Ann. Neurol., 1980c, 8, 99-100.

11. Baron, J.C., Bousser, M.G., Comar, D., Soussaline F. and Castaigne, P. Non invasive tomographic study of cerebral blood flow and oxygen metabolism in vivo : potentials, limitations and clinical applications in cerebral ischemic disorders. Eur. Neurol., 1981a, 20, 273-284.

12. Baron, J.C., Rey, A., Guillard, A., Bousser, M.G., Comar, D., Castaigne, P. Non-invasive tomographic imaging of cerebral blood flow and oxygen extraction fraction in superficial temporal artery to middle cerebral artery anastomosis, in "Cerebral Vascular Disease", Vol. 3, J.S. Meyer, H. Lechner and M. Reivich eds., Excerpta Medica, Amsterdam, 1981b, p. 58-64.

13. Baron, J.C., Steinling, M., Tanaka, T., Cavalheiro, E., Soussaline, F. and Collard, P. Quantitative measurement of CBF, oxygen extraction fraction (OEF) and CMRO2 with the ^{15}O continuous inhalation technique and positron emission tomography (PET) experimental evidence and normal values in man. J. Cereb. Blood Flow Metabol., 1, Suppl. 1, 5-6, 1981 b, c.

430

14. Baron, J.C., Bousser, M.G., Rey, A., Guillard, A., Comar, D. et Castaigne, P. Reversal of focal "misery-perfusion syndrôme" by extra-intracranial arterial by-pass in hemodynamic cerebral ischemia : a case study with I50 positron tomography. Stroke, 1981d, 12, 454-459.

15. Baron, J.C., Lebrun-Grandie, P., Collard, P. et al. Non-invasive measurement of blood flow, oxygen consumption and glucose utilization in the same brain locus in man by positron emission tomography, 1981e (in press).

16. Bousser, M.G., Baron, J.C., Iba-Zizen, M.T., Comar, D., Cabanis, E., Castaigne, P. Migrainous cerebral infarction : a tomographic study of cerebral blood flow and oxygen extraction fraction with the Oxygen-15 inhalation technique. Stroke, 1980, 11 : 145-148.

17. Branston, N.M., Symon, L., Crockard, H.A., Pasztor, E. Relationship between the cortical evoked potential and local cortical blood flow following acute middle cerebral artery occlusion in the baboon. Esp. Neurol., 1974, 45, 195-208.

18. Bruce, D.A., Schutz, H., Vapalahti, M., Gunby, N., Langfitt, T.W. Interactions between cerebral blood flow and cerebral metabolism. Neurol. Surg., 1972, 23, 417-419.

19. Buchsbaum, M.S., Kessler, R., Bunney, W.E. et al. Simultaneous electroencephalography and cerebral glucography with positron emission tomography in normals and patients with schizophrenia. J. CBF Metabol., 1981, 1, Suppl. 1, 457-458.

20. Bustany, P., Sargent, T., Saudubray, J.M., Henry, J.F. et Comar, D. Regional brain uptake and protein incorporation of ^{11}C-L-Methionine studied in vivo with PET. J. CBF Metabol., 1981, 1, Suppl. 1, 17-18.

21. Cooper, R., Crow, H.J., Walter, W.G., Winter, A.L. Variations of occipital blood flow, oxygen availability and the EEG during reading and flicker in man. Electroenceph. Clin. Neurophysiol., 1965, 19, 315.

22. Dastur, D.K. et al. Effects of aging on cerebral circulation and metabolism in man, in "U.S. Public Health Service publication, 986", 1963, 59-76.

23. DiChiro, G., Delapaz, R., Smith, B. et al. ^{18}F-2-Fluroro-2-Deoxyglucose positron emission tomography of human cerebral gliomas. J. CBF Metabol., 1981, 1, Suppl. 1, 11-12.

24. Farkas, T., Wolf, A.P., Fowler, J., et al. Regional brain glucose metabolism in schizophrenia. J. CBF Metabol., 1981, 1, Suppl. 1, 496-497.

25. Ferris, S.H., Leon, M.J., Wolf, A.P. et al. Positron emission tomography in the study of aging and senile dementia. Neurobiol. Aging, 1981, 1, 127-131.

26. Flamm, E.S., Demopoulos, H.B., Seligman, M.L., Poser, R.G., Ransohoff, J. Free radicals in cerebral ischemia. Stroke, 1978, 9, 445-447.

27. Frackowiak, R.S.J., Lenzi, G.L., Jones, T., Heather, J.D. Quantitative measurement of cerebral blood flow and oxygen metabolism in man using ^{15}O and positron emission tomography : theory, procedure and normal values. J. Comp. Ass. Tomog., 1980, 4, 727-736.

28. Frackowiak, R.S., Pozzili, C., Legg, N.J., Duboulay, G.H., Marshall, J., Lenzi, G.L., Jones, T. A prospective study of regional cerebral blood flow and oxygen utilization in dementia using positron emission tomography and oxygen-15. J. CBF Metabol. 1981, 1, Suppl. 1, 453-454.

29. Gottstein, U. Cerebral blood flow, $CMRO_2$ and CMR of glucose in patients with hypo-, and hyperchronic anemia and polycythemia. The effect of hemodilution on CBF, CMR and hematocrit, in "Cerebral Vascular Diseases", Vol. 2, J.S. Meyer, H. Lechner and Reivich, eds. Excerpta Medica, Amsterdam, 1979, 225-229.

30. Greenberg, J.H., Reivich, M., Alavi, A., et al. Metabolic mapping of functional activity in human subjects with the ^{18}F-fluorodeoxyglucose technique. Science, 1981, 212, 678-680.

31. Grubb, R.L., Raichle, M.E., Phelps, M.E., Ratcheson, R.A. Effects of increased intracranial pressure on cerebral blood volume, blood flow, and oxygen utilization in monkey. J. Neurosurg., 1975, 43, 385-398.

32. Grubb, R.L., Raichle, M.E., Gado, M.H., Eichling, J.O., Hughes, C.P. Cerebral blood flow, oxygen utilization and blood volume in dementia. Neurology, 1977, 27, 905-910.

33. Grubb, R.L., Ratcheson, R.A., Raichle, M.E., Kliefoth, A., Gado, M.H. Regional cerebral blood flow and oxygen utilization in superficial temporal-middle cerebral artery anastomosis patients. J. Neurosurg., 1979, 50, 733-741.

34. Hawkins, R.A., Phelps, M.E., Huang, S.L., Kuhl, D.E. Effect of ischemia on quantification of local cerebral glucose metabolic rate in man. J. CBF Metabol., 1981, 1, 37-51.

35. Hossmann, K.A., Sakaki, S., Kimoto, K. Cerebral uptake of glucose and oxygen in the cat brain after prolonged ischemia. Stroke, 1976, 7, 301-305.

36. Hoyers, S., Oesterreich, K. Blood flow and oxidative metabolism of the brain in patients with schizophrenia. Psychiat. Clin., 1975, 8, 304-313.

37. Huang, S.C., Phelps, M.E., Hoffman, E.J. et al. Non invasive determination of local cerebral metabolic rate of glucose in man. Am. J. Physiol., 1980, 238, E69-E82.

38. Ingvar, D.H., Risberg, J. Increase of regional cerebral blood flow during mental effort in normals and in patients with focal brain disorders. Exp. Brain Res., 1967, 3, 195-211.

39. Ingvar, D.H., Lassen, N.A. Cerebral blood flow and cerebral metabolism. Triangle Sandoz, 1970, 9, 234-243.

40. Ingvar, D.H., Franzen, G. Abnormalities of cerebral blood flow distribution in patients with chronic schizophrenia. Acta Psychiat. Scand., 1974, 50, 425-462.

432

41. Jones, M.D., Traystman, R.J., Simmons, M.A., Molteni, R.A. Effects of changes in arterial O_2 content on cerebral blood flow in the lamb. Am. J. Physiol., 1981, 240, H209-215.

42. Jones, T., Chesler, D.A., Ter Pogossian, M.M. The continuous inhalation of oxygen 15 for assessing regional oxygen extraction in the brain of man. Brit. J. Radiol., 1976, 49, 339-343.

43. Jones, T.H., Morawetz, R.B., Crowell, R.M. et al. Thresholds of focal cerebral ischemia in awake monkeys. J. Neurosurg., 1981, 54, 773-782.

44. Kety, S.S., Woodford, R.B., Harmel, M.H. et al. Cerebral blood flow and metabolism in schizophrenia. The effects of barbiturate semi-narcosis, insulin coma and electroshock. Am. J. Psychiat., 1947, 104, 765-770.

45. Kety, S.S. Human cerebral blood flow and oxygen consumption as related to aging. J. Chron. Dis., 1956, 3, 478-486.

46. Kogure, K., Busto, R., Schwartzman, R.J., Scheinberg, P. The dissociation of cerebral blood flow, metabolism and function in the early stage of developing cerebral infarction. Ann. Neurol., 1980, 8, 278-290.

47. Kontos, H.A., Wei, E.P., Raper, A.J., Rosenblum, W.I., Navari, R.M., Patterson, J.L. Role of tissue hypoxia in local regulation of cerebral microcirculation. Am. J. Physiol., 1978, 234, H582-591.

48. Kuhl, D.E., Phelps, M.E., Kowell, A.P., Metter, E.J., Selin, C., Winter, J. Effects of stroke on local cerebral metabolism and perfusion mapping by emission computed tomography of [18]FDG and [13]NH$_3$. Ann. Neurol., 1980a, 8, 47-60.

49. Kuhl, D.E., Engel, J., Phelps, M.E., Selin, C. Epileptic patterns of local cerebral metabolism and perfusion in humans determined by emission computed tomography of ^{18}F-DG and [13]NH$_3$. Ann. Neurol., 1980b, 8, 348-360.

50. Kuhl, D., Phelps, M., Markham, C. et al. Local cerebral glucose metabolism in Huntington's disease determined by emission computed tomography of ^{18}F-fluorodeoxyglucose. J. CBF Metabol., 1981, 1, Suppl. 1, 459-460.

51. Kuschinsky, W., Wahl, M. Local chemical and neurogenic regulation of cerebral vascular resistance. Phys. Rev., 1978, 58, 656-689.

52. Lammertsmaa, A.A., Itoh, M., McKenzie, C.G., Jones, T., Frackowiak, R.S. Quantitative tomographic measurements of regional cerebral blood flow and oxygen utilization in patients with brain tumors using oxygen 15 and positron emission tomography. J. CBF Metabol., 1981, 1, Suppl. 1, 567-568.

53. Lassen, N.A. Cerebral blood flow and oxygen consumption in man. Phys. Rev., 1959, 39, 183-238.

54. Lassen, N.A., Feinberg, I., Lane, M.H. Bilateral studies of cerebral oxygen uptake in young and aged normal subjects and in patients with organic dementia. J. Clin. Invest., 1960, 39, 491-500.

55. Lassen, N.A. The luxury perfusion syndrome and its possible relation to acute metabolic acidosis localized within the brain. Lancet, 1966, 2, 1113-1115.

56. Larsen, B., Skinhoj, E., Lassen, N.A. Variations in regional cortical blood flow in the right and left hemisphere during automatic speech. Brain, 1978, 101, 193-209.

57. Lear, J.L., Jones, S.C., Greenberg, J.H., Fedora, T.J., Reivich, M. Use of ^{123}I and ^{14}C in a double radionuclide autoradiographic technique for simultaneous measurement of lCBF and lCMRGlc. Theory and Method. Stroke, 1981, 12, 589-597.

58. Lenzi, G.L., Frackowiak, R.S.J., Jones, T., Heather, J.D., Lammertsma, A.A., Rhodes, C.G., Pozzilli, C. $CMRO_2$ and CBF by the oxygen 15 inhalation technique. Eur. Neurol., 1981a, 20, 285-290.

59. Lenzi, G.L., Frackowiak, R.S., Jones, T. Regional cerebral blood flow, oxygen utilization and oxygen extraction ratio in acute hemispheric stroke. J. CBF Metabol., 1981b, 1, Suppl. 1, 504-505.

60. Levy, D.E., Van Uitert, R.L., Pike, C.L. Delayed postischemic hypoperfusion : a potentially damaging consequence of stroke. Neurology, 1979, 29, 1245-1252.

61. London, E.D., Nespor, S.M., Ohata, M., Rapoport, S.I. Local cerebral glucose utilization during development and aging of the fisher-344 rat. J. Neurochem., 1981, 37, 217-221.

62. Mazziotta, J.C., Phelps, M.E., Miller, J., Kuhl, D.E. Tomographic mapping of human cerebral metabolism : Normal unstimulated state. Neurology, 1981, 31, 503-516.

63. Mies, G., Niebuhr, I., Hossmann, K.A. Simultaneous measurement of blood flow and glucose metabolism by autoradiographic techniques. Stroke, 1981, 12, 581-588.

64. Miller, A.L., Kiney, C. Metabolism of ^{14}C-fluorodeoxyglucose by rat brain in vivo. Life Sci., 1981, 28, 2071-2076.

65 - Morawetz, R.B., Degirolami, U., Ojemann, R.G. et al. Cerebral blood flow determined by hydrogen clearance during middle cerebral artery occlusion in unanesthetized monkeys. Stroke, 1978, 9, 143-149.

66 - Olesen, J. Contralateral focal increase of cerebral blood flow in man during aim work. Brain, 1971, 94, 635-646.

67 - Olesen, J. Cerebral blood flow : methods for measurement, regulation effects of drugs and changes in disease. 1974, Copenhagen, Fads Forlag.

68 - Orgogozo, J.M., Larsen, B., Roland, P.E., Lassen, N.A. Activation de l'aire motrice supplémentaire au cours des mouvements volontaires chez l'homme. Rev. Neurol., 1979, 135', 705-717.

69 - Phelps, M.E. Emission computed tomography. Sem. Nucl. Med., 1977, 7, 337-365.

434

70 - Phelps, M.E., Huang, S.C., Hoffman, E.J., Selin, C., Sokoloff, L., Kuhl, D.E. Tomographic measurement of local cerebral glucose metabolic rate in humans with (F. 18) 2-fluoro-2-deoxy-D. Glucose : validation of method. Ann. Neurol., 1979, 6, 371-388.

71 - Phelps, M.E., Mazziotta, J.C., Kuhl, D., Nuwer, M., Packwood, J., Metter, Engel, J. Tomographic mapping of human cerebral metabolism : visual stimulation and deprivation. Neurology, 1981, 31, 517-529.

72 - Pickard, J.D., Kelly, P.A., McCulloch, J. Prostaglandin mechanisms and the relationship between local cerebral glucose utilization and local blood flow. J. CBF Metabol., 1981, 1, Suppl. 1, 291-292.

73 - Purves, M.J. The physiology of the cerebral circulation, University Press, Cambrige, 1972.

74 - Raichle, M.E., Grubb, R.L., Gado, M.H., Eichling, J.O., Ter-Pogossian, M.M. Correlation between regional cerebral blood flow and oxidative metabolism. Arch. Neurol., 1976, 33, 523-526.

75 - Raichle, M.E. Quantitative in vivo autoradiography with positron emission tomography. Brain Res. Rev., 1979, 1, 47-68.

75 - Rhodes, C.G., Lenzi, G.L., Frackowiak, R.S., Jones, T., Pozzilli, C. Measurement of CBF and $CMRO_2$ using the continuous inhalation of $C^{15}O_2$ and $^{15}O_2$. J. Neurol. Sci., 1981, 50, 381-389.

76 - Roland, P.E., Larsen, B. Focal increase of cerebral blood flow during stereognostic testing in man. Arch. Neurol., 1976, 33, 551-558.

77 - Roland, P.E., Meyer, E., Yamamoto, Y.L., Thompson, C.T. Dynamic positron emission tomography as a tool in neuroscience : Functional brain-mapping in normal human volunteers. J. CBF Metabol., 1981, 1, Suppl. 1, 463-464.

78 - Scheinberg, P., Blackburn, I., Rich, M., Saslaw, M. Effects of aging on cerebral circulation and metabolism. Arch. Neurol. Psychiat., 1953, 70, 77-85.

79 - Siesjö, B.K. Brain energy metabolism, John Wiley, Chichester, 1978.

80 - Smith, A., Wollman, H. Cerebral blood flow and metabolism. Anesthesiology, 1972, 36, 378-400.

81 - Smith, C.B., Goochee, C., Rapoport, S.I., Sokoloff, L. Effects of aging on local rates of cerebral glucose utilisation in the rat. Brain, 1980, 103, 351-365.

82 - Sokoloff, L., Reivich, M., Kennedy, C. et al. The ^{14}C-Deoxyglucose method for the measurement of local cerebral glucose utilization : theory, procedure and normal values in the conscious and anesthetized albino rat. J. Neurochem., 1977, 28, 897-916.

83 - Sokoloff, L. Relationships among local functional activity, energy metabolism and blood flow in central nervous system. Federation Proc., 1981, 40, 2311-2316.

84 - Sokoloff, L. Localization of functional activity in the central nervous system by measurement of glucose utilization with radioactive deoxyglucose. J. CBF Metabol., 1981, 1, 7-36.

85 - Subramanyam, R., Alpert, N.M., Hoop, B., Brownell, G.L., Taveras, J.M. A model of regional cerebral oxygen distribution during continuous inhalation of $^{15}O_2$, $C^{15}O_2$ and $C^{15}O$. J. Nucl. Med., 1978, 19, 48-53.

86 - Symon, L., Astrup, J. Phenomena associated with focal ischemia in the central nervous system. Acta Neurochir., 1979, (Suppl. 28), 215-217.

87 - Ter-Pogossian, M.M., Phelps, M.E., Hoffman, E.J., Mullani, N.A. A positron-emission transaxial tomograph for nuclear imaging (PETT). Radiology, 1975, 114, 89-98.

88 - Ter-Pogossian, M.M., M. Raichle, M., Sobel, B. La tomographie par émission de positrons. Pour la Science, 1980, 38, 32-45.

89 - Tsubokawa, T., Katayama, Y., Kondo, T., Veno, Y., Hayashi, N., Moriyasu, N. Changes in local cerebral blood flow and neuronal activity during sensory stimulation in normal and sympathetectomized cats. Brain Res., 1980, 190, 51-65.

90 - Widen, L., Bergstrom, M., Blomquist, G. et al. Glucose metabolism in patients with schizophrenia : emission computed tomography measurements with ^{11}C-glucose. J. CBF Metabol., 1981, 1, Suppl. 1, 455-456.

91 - Yamamoto, Y.L., Little, J., Thompson, C., Meyer, E., Feindel, W. Positron tomography with krypton-77 for evaluation of topographical in CBF changes following EC-IC bypass surgery. Acta Neurol. Scand., 1979, 60, Suppl. 72, 522-523.

DYNAMIC EMISSION TOMOGRAPHY OF REGIONAL CEREBRAL BLOOD FLOW

Niels A. Lassen, M.D.

Department of Clinical Physiology, Bispebjerg Hospital, DK-2400 Copenhagen N.V., Denmark.

The diagnostic value of X-ray tomography ("CT scanning") is well recognized. It offers, however, only one rather gross parameter of the state of the regional tissue: its density. In relation to patients with brain ischemia this constitutes a limitation. X-ray tomography allows one to see frank infarction as hypodense areas. But, this image takes days to develop and it does not delineate areas of possibly reversible ischemia, viz. tissue that may be salvable. Hence, there is felt to be a great need for tomographic methods allowing to map regional cerebral blood flow. Such methods also allow to map areas of increased blood flow, hyperemia, as associated with increased neuronal function in the normal brain or in epilepsy, features not seen on X-ray tomography. In fact, tomography of blood flow or of metabolic parameters as currently being developed would, if all other factors were equal - resolution, costs, etc. - probably even replace the X-ray technique.

This paper reviews, however, only tomographic blood flow methods: this appears to be the field in which a wider clinical use can be foreseen in the next few years.

PRINCIPLE

The 3 methods are all based on computerized tomographic reconstruction of the tracer distribution. The principle is the conventional one of having a set of lateral projections of a slice of brain tissue, apply-

ing a filter to enhance contrast in each projection
and then project them back into the image field.

1. Single Photon Transmission Tomography Enhanced by

   Stable Xenon (1).

   This method is based on the conventional, single
photon absorption measurement technique using X-rays
transmitted through the head from a rotating external
source ("CT scans"). Inhalation of appr. 50% stable
Xenon is used, higher doses having a clearcut anesthetic effect. Because the maximal enhancement is small -
about 5 to 8 Hounsfield units above the initial value
of appr. 1000 units - the signal to noise ratio is
very unfavorable. Consequently the arrival and washout of the indicator is not easy to measure on the
series of CT scans. Integration over many pixels is
necessary to reduce random errors. Therefore the very
high spatial resolution of the X-ray technique cannot
be made use of. On the other hand, specific anatomical
structures may be outlined on the non-enhanced density maps and then used as areas of interest in the flow
calculation.

The mild anesthetic effect, and the high cost of stable Xenon are limiting factors. Another limitation lies
in only being able to study blood flow in one "slice"
of brain tissue per Xenon inhalation. This is a purely
technical problem, that could be overcome but at considerable cost.

2. Dual Photon Emission Tomography of Krypton-77 (2).

   This method is based on positron annihilation radiation detection, viz. on detecting simultaneously
the pair of photons emitted in coincidence at practically 180° from one another. The isotope is supplied
by inhalation and a series of 20 second scans is performed from 3 slices of brain simultaneously. Due to
the dynamic nature of the study - its brief duration -
and the dose of radioactivity used, the number of im-
pulses recorded is limited. Consequently the spatial
resolution achieved is not impressive, in the order of
1.5 to 2.0 cm to judge from the pictures published.
Other positron emitting tracers notably Oxygen-15 labelled CO_2 have been used to study regional blood flow
in the human brain. But this approach is not based on
inert gas clearance principles and does not readily
lend itself to quantification in terms of ml/100g/min.

The positron technology demanding access to an onsite
medically dedicated cyclotron and a costly detector

system is expensive and also cumbersome to run on a routine basis.

3. Single Photon Emission Tomography of Xenon-133 (3).

This method we have developed on the basis of a rotating gamma-ray detecting system as pioneered by Kuhl and coworkers (4). Commercially available Xenon-133 gas is inhaled a a concentration of 10 mCi/l for 1 minute. The brain uptake as wash-out is followed for 4 minutes using a 3-slice, rapidly rotating detector system essentially consisting of four gamma cameras. The spatial resolution is about 1.7 to 2.0 cm. Dynamic single photon emission tomography may yield maps of regional cerebral blood flow with other tracers as Xenon-127 or Iodine-123-Isopropyl-Amphetamine that may improve the resolution.

The technique, to be discussed in detail below, offers the advantage of a favorable signal to noise ratio. It is atraumatic and suited for routine clinical application because of the more moderate costs and of the ease of operation.

3.1. Blood flow imaging by Xenon-133 and dynamic emission tomography; methods.

The single photon tomograph we use was developed (3) with the specific aim of allowing dynamic studies of inhaled Xenon-133. It consists of 4 gamma cameras each having 16 sodium iodide crystals*. The instrument rotates at constant speed and collects data in brief intervals (1/8 of a second). Thus, in each interval one "view" or "projection" of the isotope distribution in a slice of brain tissue is recorded. Conventional filtering and back-projection techniques are used for reconstructing the isotope distribution in the slice; 3 slices of brain tissue are recorded simultaneously.

One half turn of the tomograph, allowing sampling of a complete set of projections, 40 in all, lasts 5 seconds. This rapid rotation is necessary because of the known speed of Xenon-133 arrival and wash-out from the brain: the tomograph must move so fast, that the Xenon-133 concentration is practically constant during collection of one complete set of projections. However, due to the low count rate a series of 5 second tomograms cannot be reconstructed with adequate resolution.

* Footnote: Tomomatic 64, Medimatic Inc., Gersonsvej 7, DK-2900 Hellerup, Denmark.

Text to Fig. 1

CBF tomograms in normal man. Example of brain activity induced CBF changes.
During rest with closed eyes the middle slice shows almost symmetrical flow pattern with a fairly high flow in the midline posteriorly (1,a). When copying a text writing with right hand and with open eyes CBF increases in left central cortex and in occipital cortex (1,b). The upper slice shows at rest highest flow anteriorly (1,c). During the hand movements with open eyes flow increases anteriorly in an area including the supplementary motor area bilaterally (1,d).

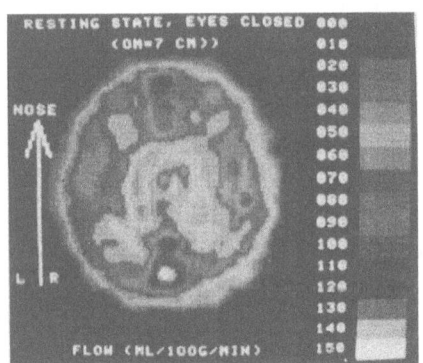
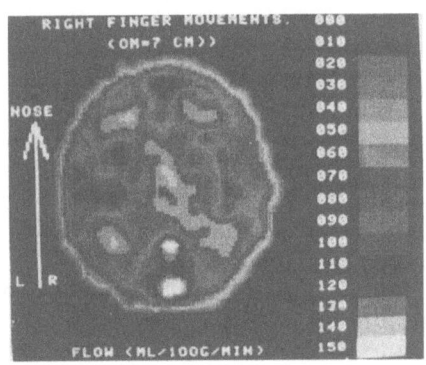
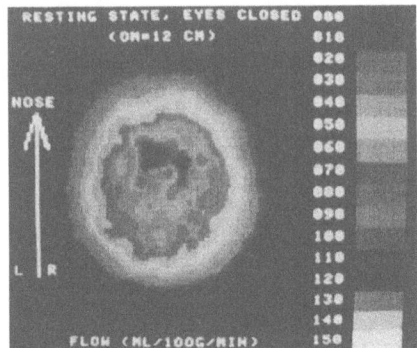
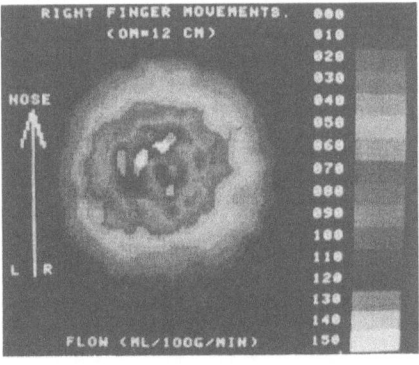

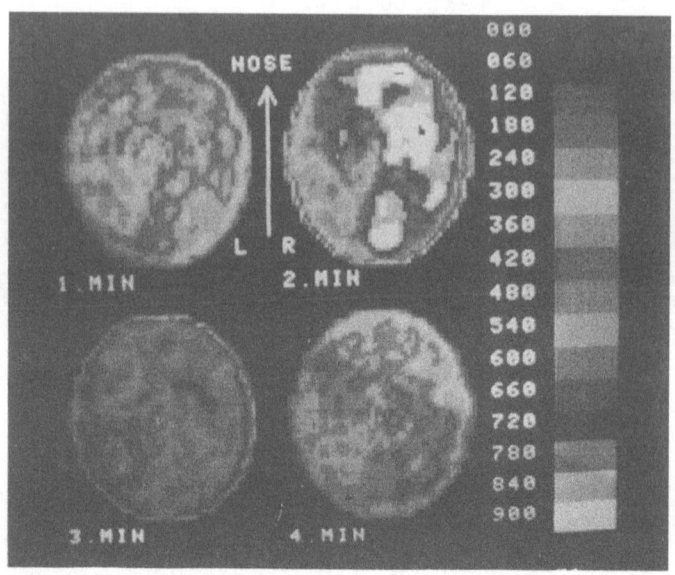

Text to Fig. 2
Xenon-133 tomograms of middle slice in a case of apoplexy. The images are the raw data; the four 1-minute
images used to calculate CBF. The asymmetry with low
Xenon uptake in infarct area is obvious. CT scan showed
a much smaller hypodense area.

Hence several sets of projections, typically 12, are added before reconstruction. As the raw data, the 12 sets added together, are the average count rates over one minute, the tomograms give the average isotope concentration in that minute. A series of four one-minute pictures is taken during and after the inhalation of Xenon-133 (10 millicuries/liter) for one minute.

3.1.1. Spatial resolution: With the collimators used the resolution is appr. 1.7 cm in the plane and 2.0 vertical to the plane. Resolution is here given in the conventional terms of the full width of the bell shaped curve at half its maximal (peak) height (Full-Width-Half-Maximum, FWHM).

This rather coarse resolution is related to the basic problem of accomplishing dynamic tomograms, viz. the trade off between sensitivity (getting many counts in a short time for a given amount of isotope) and resolution (getting a small FWHM). In the system used here high sensitivity - of appr. 60,000 cps for a 20 cm diameter phantom with an isotope concentration of 1 μCi/l for 1 minute gives an absorbed dose of ca. 0.4 rad in the critical organ - the lung(3). The gonadal dose is much lower, appr. 0.005 rad/study. It is considered preferable not to exceed the dose mentioned in order to be free to perform repeated studies in normal volunteers without undue radiation exposure.

As mentioned, each slice is 2 cm thick. However, the distance between the midline of adjacent planes is 4 cm; each slice is seen by 4 cm of crystal length in order to achieve a high resolution. Thus a "non-seen" interval, 2 cm wide, exists between the slices. This construction feature was considered necessary in order to achieve the sensitivity mentioned above. A series of continguous slices can only be obtained by repeating the measurements after shifting the position 2 cm.

3.1.2. Calculation of rCBF. For each slice the raw data consists of the series of four one minute average images of Xenon-133 concentration. In addition the shape of the input curve to the brain is available as the concentration curve over the right lung is recorded. Based on these data rCBF is calculated using the bolus distribution principle on the "early pictures" (5). This calculation is essentially the same as used by Kety in developing the autoradiographic method for calculating rCBF. However, as an individual scaling factor relating head counts to air curve is not available, the scaling is accomplished by using all four one-minute images.

This calculation has the advantage of exploiting the fair degree of isoefficiency in space and in time of the tomograph.

RESULTS

In normal man the CBF tomograms are symmetrical at rest with a flow level of about 60 ml/100g/min. Usually the three slices are positioned 0, 4, and 8 cm above the orbitomeatal plane. With this positioning, slice I (OM + 0) gives a good image of the cerebellum including the brain stem; slice II (OM + 4) cuts through the deep part of the hemispheres and shows the lateral (Sylvian) cortex, the midline cortex, and the deeper nuclei as high flow regions; slice III (OM + 8) shows the upper cortex with evidence of the subcortical white matter to a variable extent (it depends on the size of the head).

During visual stimulation an increase of appr. 30% in CBF in the striate occipital region - posteriorly in the midline - is seen (6). Movement of the hand results in a flow increase in the contralateral primary hand area and in the supplementary motor area on both sides (7).

In apoplexy the rCBF tomograms allow detection of the ischemic areas. In a series of 10 consecutive cases the flow maps showed low flow regions in the appropriate location in all cases (8). The defects tended to be larger than the hypodense areas on X-ray tomography. In one case studied several days after the onset of the stroke, the X-ray tomogram was even completely normal. Thus the CBF tomogram may reveal areas of borderline perfusion, a perfusion too low to sustain normal function and yet high enough to avoid frank tissue necrosis.

In transient ischemic attacks, TIA, a recently completed series of 12 cases showed asymmetry of the CBF maps in all cases (9). In 11 cases the low flow side corresponded to a severely stenosed or occluded internal carotid artery; the 12th case had CT proven brain atrophy probably explaining the flow asymmetry.

DISCUSSION

Single-photon emission tomography of Xenon-133 gives regional flow maps, that allow to detect areas of increased or decreased CBF. The technique avoids the

superposition of tissue layers and it is consequently
basically superior to the conventional methods based
on Xenon-133 inhalation and stationary detectors, a
technique often unable to identify the side affected
correctly in major stroke cases (10).

Many clinical problems suggest the usefulness of a
tomographic method for imaging CBF. Indeed in cases
where surgical interventions are indicated X-ray tomography (CT scanning) tends to be negative. This is
the case with focal cortical epilepsy, where only the
often associated atrophic lesions can be seen, not the
high flow region of an active focus. It is also the
case for borderline ischemia not evolving into frank
infarction.

We have in this article commented on patients with TIA.
But many other relevant patient groups exist, e.g. arterial spasms after a bleeding aneurism. In such cases
measurement of regional CBF should reveal the haemodynamic significance of the spasms. Repeated measurements
may readily be made. This might well influence the decision of when and how to operate?

Two other methods for obtaining CBF tomographically
are currently being explored. Their technical features
were summarized in the introduction. The choice between
the various tomographic CBF methods is not an easy one
and will depend on a multitude of considerations. The
clinical need for this type of measurement is a challenge and will prompt many to make a choice and get started.

REFERENCES

1. Drayer, B.P., Wolfson, S.K., Reinmuth, O.W., Dujov-
   ny, M., Boehnke, M. and Cook, E.E.. Stroke 9 (1978)
   123-126.

2. Yamamoto, Y.L., Thompson, C., Meyer, E., Nukui, H.,
   Matsunaga, M. and Feindel, W. Cerebral Blood Flow
   and Metabolism , Acta Neurol. Scand. suppl. 72,
   vol. 60 (1979) 186-187.

3. Stokely, E.M., Sveinsdottir, E., Lassen, N.A. and
   Rommer, P. J. Comput. Assist. Tomogr. 4 (1980) 230-
   240.

444

4. Kuhl, D.E., Edwards, R.Q., Ricci, A.R., Yacob, R.J., Mich, T.J. and Alavi, A. Radiology 121 (1976) 405-413.

5. Celsis, P., Goldman, T., Henriksen, L. and Lassen, N.A. J. Comput. Assist. Tomogr. (1981). In print.

6. Henriksen, L., Paulson, O.B. and Lassen, N.A. Eur. J. Nucl. Med. 6 (1981). In print.

7. Lauritzen, M., Henriksen, L. and Lassen, N.A. (sent to J. Cerebral Blood Flow & Metabolism).

8. Lassen, N.A., Henriksen, L. and Paulson, O.B. Stroke 12 (1981) 284-288.

9. Lassen, N.A., Henriksen, L., Hemmingsen, R. and Vorstrup, S. (unpublished observations).

10. Halsey, J. rCBF Bulletin 1 (1981) 5-6.

SPECT BRAIN PERFUSION STUDIES USING N-ISOPROPYL I-123 P-IODOAMPHETAMINE (IMP)

Thomas C. Hill, B. Leonard Holman, Richard Lovett,
Daniel H. O'Leary, Robert G. L. Lee, Philippe Magistretti, and
Melvin E. Clouse

From the Department of Radiology, New England Deaconess Hospital,
Brigham and Women's Hospital, Beth Israel Hospital and Harvard
Medical School, Boston, Massachusetts 02215 U.S.A.

Positron emission computed tomography has graphically demonstrated changes in regional brain physiology in patients whose transmission CT scans show normal anatomy. These results have stimulated interest in single-photon techniques that can have widespread distribution throughout the medical community (1). N-isopropyl I-123 p-iodoamphetamine (IMP), developed by Winchell and colleagues (2), is a single-photon radiopharmaceutical that penetrates the normal blood brain barrier due to its lipophilic form. Initial distribution of IMP has been correlated to the regional cerebral blood flow (3).

In this study we assessed the feasibility of evaluating regional cerebral perfusion in patients with neurologic diseases using single-photon emission computed tomography (SPECT) and IMP (4).

Imaging Technique

Over 100 patients have been studied to date using the Harvard scanning multidetector brain system. This single-photon system is a single slice, multidetector, circular array brain unit with a sensitivity of 14,000 counts/sec/uCi/cc in a 20 cm diameter phantom and a resolution of 10mm with FWHM. Its count rate is linearly related to the activity concentration, and both sensitivity and resolution are independent of the position with the slice (5). Thus, the system is able to obtain quantitative data from regional brain perfusion maps of the radiopharmaceutical.

446

Because the I-123 used for the radiolabel is produced by Te-124 (p,2n)^{23meV}I-123 reaction, 2.1-4.6% contamination with I-124 was present at the time of injection. The effects of scatter and lead "punch-through" by high energy photons from the I-124 contamination was minimized in the images by an approximate background subtraction applied to the raw data before reconstruction. The studies were all performed in dual channel mode with the low energy pulse-high window set at 135-185 keV (surrounding the I-123 peak) and the high-energy window set at 310-360 keV. Before scanning patients, three cylindrical phantoms were used to obtain a scatter mask. One of the cylinders was filled with 0.04 mCi of pure I-124 and placed in the gantry. The other two were filled with 0.08 mCi of I-124 and placed on the patient couch in the position approximating the patient's lung fields and lower torso. The two-dimensional projection intensity distribution recorded in the low energy window provided a close approximation to the shape of the distribution from the I-124 background when scanning the patient with I-123. This technique is not an exact compensation for punch-through and does not replace the requirement for very pure I-123.

Normal Distribution

When injected into the internal carotid artery, 65% of the radiopharmaceutical was extracted in the first pass without evidence of recirculation to the opposite hemisphere and independent of the carrier amphetamine (range 0.1 to 0.4mg) (Fig. 1).

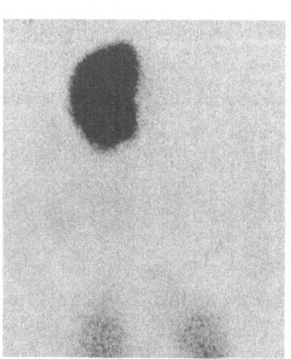 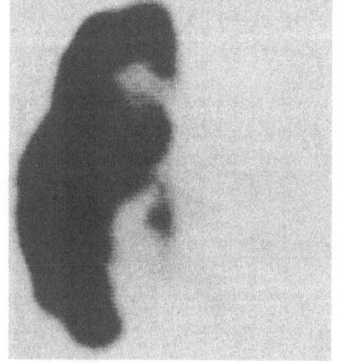

Fig. 1 Anterior Anger camera and SPECT image after right internal carotid artery injection.

After intravenous injection in patients, 50% of the brain activity was achieved at two minutes, 80% at ten minutes, and 100% at twenty minutes. The activity within the brain was constant from twenty minutes to at least two hours, allowing for tomographic images and quantification of the biodistribution. Therefore, the regional brain perfusion map reflects the perfusion during the first minutes after intravenous injection and is frozen for a substantial time to allow quantitative SPECT imaging.

Patient Studies

Eight patients served as normal controls. These patients had primary malignancies, but no evidence of brain metastasis by clinical examination or transmission CT scans. The average brain uptake after intravenous injection in this group of patients was 7.5% ± 0.9% of the injected dose. The activity was greatest in the strip of cortex along the convexities of the frontal, temporal, parietal, and occipital lobes, corresponding anatomically to the cortical brain matter. Activity was also high in the region corresponding to the basal ganglia. The region between the basal ganglia and convexity corresponding anatomically to cortical white matter has less IMP activity. Activity in the cortical grey matter was uniform in the temporal, parietal and occipital regions, but appeared patchy in the frontal regions.

The contours of this activity were undulating and reflected the gyral architecture observed on transmission CT examination. The impressions to the inner hemispheric and Sylvian fissures are also present (Fig. 2)

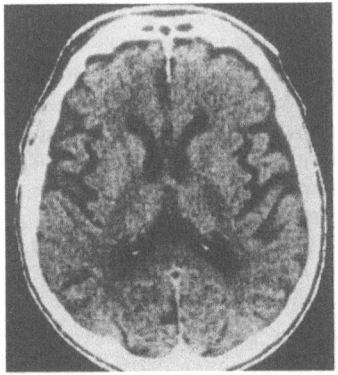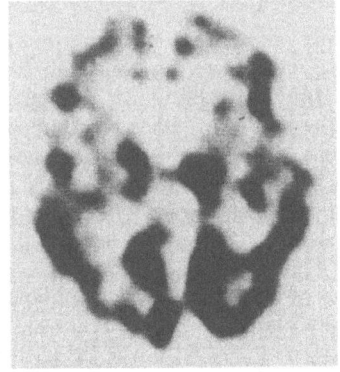

Fig. 2   SPECT-IMP brain scan of normal patient.

For patient studies, at least one tomographic image was obtained at 2cm above the orbitomeatal line. Additional images were obtained depending upon the clinical situation. The injected dose was 5 mCi, and imaging was performed between twenty and sixty minutes after the injection. To improve the statistical quality of the image, 4 to 6 slices (5 minutes each) from the same level were summed for presentation.

In patients with cerebral infarction, the abnormality on the IMP-SPECT image is visible immediately after the incident. This is far earlier than the defect on transmission CT, which does not usually appear until days after onset of symptoms (Fig. 3).

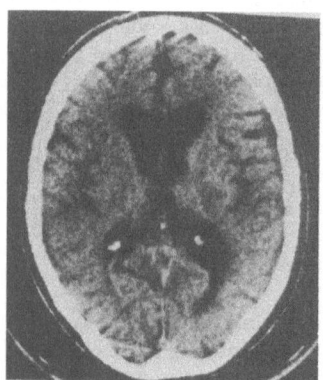 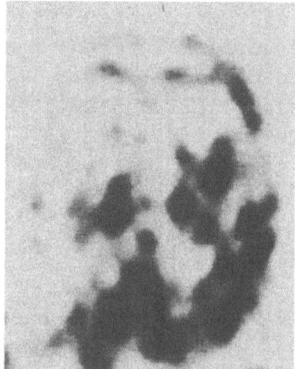

Fig. 3   SPECT-IMP scan 12 hours after onset of symptoms.

In our experience with cerebral infarctions, 21 of 22 patients with acute cerebral infarction had perfusion defects on their IMP study. Eight of these 21 patients had normal transmission CT studies at the time of hospital admission. When the IMP studies were compared to the infarcts that were eventually demonstrated on the transmission CT examination, 10 patients had IMP studies with larger perfusion defects than the abnormalities demonstrated on the transmission CT scan and 8 patients had perfusion abnormalities on the IMP that were equal to the size of the infarct on the x-ray CT scan. In the 19 patients with middle cerebral artery infarction, the perfusion deposits involve the grey and white matter of the temporal, parietal lobes with variable extension into the frontal and occipital lobes and the basal ganglia. In these patients there were sensory and motor deficits on the contralateral side to the perfusion defects. In the 3 patients with posterior cerebral infarction, there were corresponding perfusion defects involving the occipital lobes with involvement of the visual associated areas. In these 3 patients, there were corresponding visual field cuts. One patient had an abnormal transmission CT scan and a normal IMP study. Two patients had old cerebral infarctions.

In patients with epilepsy injected during seizure activity, there was markedly increased activity involving portions of the cerebral cortex corresponding to the epicenters of the seizure focus on electroencephalography examinations (Fig. 4).

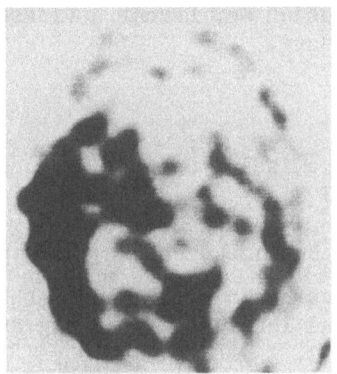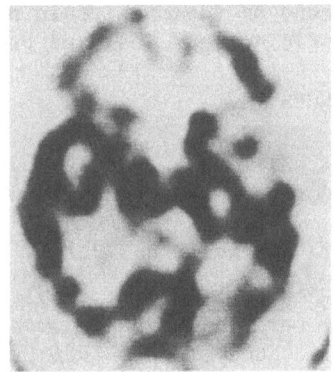

Fig. 4   SPECT-IMP scans; Right temporal lobe seizure before and after medical therapy.

Clinical Utility

It appears that single-photon emission computed tomography with N-isopropyl I-123 p-iodoamphetamine will be useful to assess regional brain perfusion in a number of neurologic situations:

1.   Acute cerebral infarction where a transmission CT scan may be normal for several days after onset of symptoms and where physiologic abnormalities may exceed the anatomic abnormality. The perfusion study with IMP may be used to evaluate the effectiveness of therapy or to obtain prognostic information.

2.   Before and after endarterectomy or superficial temporal artery bypass to document the effectiveness of surgical intervention.

3.   In patients with epilepsy for whom the extent and location of the hypermetabolic and, hence, hyperperfused focus may be important to medical and surgical management. Followup examination may be useful for documenting the effectiveness of medical therapy.

4. In patients presenting an ambiguous clinical pattern in which the transmission CT examination alone does not provide the diagnosis.

We anticipate that with additional increasing clinical experience the list of clinical indications for this procedure will increase substantially. Since quantitative data are the inherent advantage of tomography, regional measurements of cerebral blood flow are possible. With the potential for commercial distribution of IMP and availability of SPECT imaging systems, non-invasive assessment of regional brain perfusion may become a widespread diagnostic nuclear medicine procedure.

REFERENCES

1. Hill, TC. Single-photon emission computed tomography to study cerebral function in man. J Nucl Med 21; 1980:1197-1199.

2. Winchell, HS, Hirst, WD, Braun, L, et al: N-Isopropyl [123]I p-iodoamphetamine: Single pass brain uptake and washout; Binding for brain synaptosomes, and localization in dog and monkey brain. J Nucl Med 21; 1980:947-952.

3. Kuhl DE, Wu JL, Lin TH, et al: Mapping local cerebral blood flow by means of emission computed tomography of N-Isopropyl-p-I[123]Iodoamphetamine. J Nucl Med 22; 1981:16.

4. Hill TC, Holman BL, Lovett R, et al: Initial experience with SPECT of the brain using N-isopropyl I-123 p-iodoamphetamine (IMP). J Nucl Med 23; 1982:191-195.

5. Hill TC, Zimmerman RE. Single-photon ECT of the Brain: System Performance and Clinical Utility in Emission Computed Tomography: The Single-Photon Approach. Paras P, Eikman EA, eds. HHS Publication FD, 81-8177, pp 274-285.

*Part VIII: The Results of Clinical Evaluation: Studies of the
Heart and Lungs*

452

Utility of Imaging Techniques to Predict and Manage
Patients with Cardiovascular Abnormalities

W.E. Adam, H. Sigel, J.Zaorska-Rajca,F. Bitter

Department Radiology III (Nuclear Medicine) Ulm University, 7900 Ulm/Donau, FRG

1. INTRODUCTION

Newly developed technologies are going to revolutionize
the diagnostic procedure in cardiology. Recent progress
has been made in nuclear cardiology, sonography, transmission computer tomography and digital video-techni-
ques. Nuclear magnetic resonance seems to offer another
possibility for imaging of the heart. Besides the fact,
that these procedures are non-invasive and thus avoid
the risks of catheter techniques, special advantages of
the various techniques are obviously dependant on the
cardiac abnormalities under investigation. The information revealed by these various techniques may in some
ways even surpass the results obtained by catheter
techniques, whereas on some occasions the catheter is
obligatory. The history up to the present state of the
art of the various techniques has some highlights:
Nuclear cardiology started even before artificial
radioisotopes were available: In 1927 BLUMGART and
WEISS (1) investigated the pulmonary circulation time
with the help of radon. In 1948 PRINZMETAL et al. (2)
described radiocardiography as a new method for studying the blood flow through the human heart. NYLIN and
CELANDER 1950 (3) determined the heart stroke volume
with the help of radiophosphorus. DONATO, GIUNTINI et
al. (1964) (4) finally published their results on
quantitative radiocardiography largely based on the
concepts first developed by MEIER and ZIERLER (1954)
(5). The introduction of camera systems started a new
era of heart investigation (6,7,8).

Gated blood pool procedures started with systems
(HOFFMANN and KLEINE (9), WAGNER et al (10), and application of the procedure to the camera (11,12) resulted
in parametric scanning (13) for detection of regional
wall motion abnormalities (RWMA) in Europe. But the
breakthrough of nuclear cardiology in the USA finally
succeeded with the radionuclide ventriculography (14).
A further impetus for nuclear cardiology was provided
by the concomitant development of myocardial scintigraphy, based on experimental observations of SAPIR-
STEIN (15). BURCH (1955) (16) and CARR (1962) (17) who
applied potassium 43 and analogues of potassium.KAWANA
et al. (1970) (18) were the first to discuss the potential of Thallium, which marked the breakthrough in
myocardial scintigraphy after production of this radionuclide by BELGRAVE and LEBOWITZ (1973) (19). Imaging
of myocardial metabolism (20,21) finally completed the
spectrum of nuclear cardiology thus far, allowing
imaging of myocardial perfusion, metabolism and function. What about other non invasive imaging procedures?
As compared with nuclear cardiology and ultrasound
their history is short, their experiences in cardiology
limited and a final assessment of their clinical utility
seems not possible at present. Cardiovascular abnormalities cover a wide range of diseases. The next
chapter deals with the problem of how the spectrum of
methods available fits into the various cardiovascular
abnormalities.

2. DEFINITION OF CARDIAC ABNORMALITIES AND TECHNIQUES FOR THEIR IMAGING

Considering the heart as a pump enables a simplified
consideration of heart function and its abnormalities.
Anatomical abnormalities of the cardiovascular system
may reverse the blood flow (shunts, valvular insufficiency) or act as a barrier for flow (valvular stenoses
of large vessels). On the other hand flow impairment
may result from myocardial insufficiency. This might
be due to perfusion defects, metabolic failures or
regional motion abnormalities (scars, aneurysms). Finally abnormalities of the conduction system for steering and coordinating the pump function may be present
and may limit the pump function. Fundamentally all of
these abnormalities can be imaged by one or more than
one imaging procedure enumerated above.

2.1. Abnormalities of the Cardiovascular System which Influence Flow Direction or Serve as Barrier against flow

The valvular function is predominantly assessable by
ultrasound (US). It was in just this way that US
started out with its A,B and TM scans, before it
switched over to the more ambitious program of two
dimensional imaging of heart wall motion. Though first
pass investigations can be used to detect valvular
failure gated blood pool imaging can also contribute
significantly to the diagnosis and assessment of the
degree of valvular insufficiency. The method is based
on the fact, that the stroke volume of the left chamber
equals that of the right chamber in the normal heart,
unless there is valvular insufficiency or a shunt (22,
23). In terms of counts collected over the left and
right ventricle this means equal systolic-diastolic
count difference over both chambers. Due to geometrical
conditions and tissue absorption which favour the left
ventricle in LAO 30° direction, the left to right ratio
is 1.43 $\pm$ 0.27 (23).
Atrial septal defects have a similar effect on ventricular function as valvular insufficiency: A left-right
shunt leads to a volume overload of the right ventricle
with a decrease in the left to right ratio of systolic-
diastolic differences, and vice versa. The size of the
shunt can be assessed. The reliability of this assessment will be discussed later.
Ventricular septal defects are best investigated by
first pass techniques. The early, appearance of activity
in the left ventricle after intravenous injection of
the tracer is convincing proof of a right to left shunt.
A very interesting US technique is positive and negative contrast echocardiography to detect intracardiac
shunting. The echocardiographic contrast effect occurs, when the ultrasonic beam is reflected by microbubbles, produced by intravenous injection of fluid
into the circulation. Its arrival in the heart and its
transport through the heart chambers can be observed.
Heart structures and vessels can be identified. Abnormal flow direction as in the case of shunts becomes
apparent. This method is highly sensitive for right to
left atrial and ventricular shunts in a qualitative
manner (HUNTER 1980)   , unfortunately quantification
is not yet possible.

2.2. Abnormalities of Myocardial Perfusion and Meta-
bolism

One of the most surprising observations in nuclear
cardiology is the fact that, nearly simultaneously,
procedures have been developed which image the three
determinants of the myocardial state: myocardial per-

fusion, myocardial metabolism and myocardial function
(regional motion). The interrelationship between perfusion, metabolism and function becomes especially
clear in coronary artery disease (CAD). Decreased myocardial perfusion results in impaired metabolism and
restricted myocardial motility, which means impaired
pump function of the heart. Infarction results when
basic metabolic demands cannot be met. For complete
understanding of all nuclear procedures and their
meaning we need a more detailed interpretation of myocardial perfusion for substrate and oxygen delivery,
and myocardial metabolism or energy utilization for
myocardial function and cell maintenance. Oxygen and
metabolic substrates are delivered by the coronary
blood. Oxygen extraction in the myocardium reaches 75 %,
whereas in normal muscle the extraction rate is only
25 %. This is a very critical point because oxygen
delivery can not be effectively improved by a higher
extraction rate. An improvement is only possible by increasing the myocardial blood flow. This is normally
achieved by taking full advantage of the "coronary
reserve". Maximum dilatation of the coronary arterial
system causes an improvement in coronary flow by a
factor of 5 to 6. Coronary flow depends on the effective
perfusion pressure and the coronary resistance. Resistance is influenced by the cyclic compression of the
contracting myocardium. The coronary flow decreases
very fast, when isovolumetric contraction starts. Even
a reversal of the direction of flow is possible. Myocardial perfusion in the normal LV essentially occurs
during diastole. The influence of contraction on myocardial perfusion can be assessed during asystole: under
this condition perfusion increases by 50 %. It seems
obvious that the intraventricular pressure is especially effective on the inner (subendocardial) layer of the
myocardium. The subendocardial layers compensate for the
increased external pressure by decreasing the internal
resistance. This decreases the coronary reserve and will
exhaust it under stress conditions. For this reason
most non-transmural infarctions are subendocardial. It
is well established, that fatty acids, lactate and
glucose are the main sources of energy, whereas glucose
is used in only modest amounts. Glucose is transformed
into glucose -6-phosphate. This molecule may follow 3
pathways. The mainstream of carbohydrate metabolism is
that of anaerobic glycolysis. The latter way is the
prerequiste for entry into the most important energy
liberating process: the citric acid cycle (Krebs cycle).
This continuous cyclic process results in the breakdown
of the "acetyl" group by decarboxylation. The net result

of this process is the complete oxidation of 1 molecule of the 3-carbon pyruvate to 3 molecules of CO_2
and the associated release of the previously trapped
energy between the bonds. Glycolysis is of limited
value in energy production, representing a release of
only 9 % of the energy content of glucose. The net
output in breaking down glucose to pyruvate is 2 ATPs
by anaerobis glycolysis, whereas in the presence of
oxygen the break down of 2 pyruvate molecules in the
Krebs cycle yields another 30 ATP molecules. This
pinpoints the importance of oxygen supply to the myocardium. Decrease in oxygen consumption causes an increase of the glucose extraction coefficient, glucose
is taken up in great amount and glycogen is broken
down, so that the flux through the glycolytic chain is
markedly increased. Glycolytic production of ATP cannot compensate for loss of the more efficient oxidative
phosphorylating mechanism. The high energy phosphate
stores fall and electrial and mechanical functions become impaired. Anoxia causes an acute decline in creatine phosphate and in ATP to levels, which might continue to be sufficient for basal metabolic demands
of the myocardium, if maintained by the glycolytic
production of ATP. The high energy phosphates built
up in aerobic and anaerobic myocardial metabolism can
be stored as ATP or in a "reservoir" from creatine
phosphate. ATP is transported out of the mitochondria
to the cytoplasm where it is directly used for most
of the energy requiring reactions of the heart. These
reactions principally concern:

a) synthesis of cell proteins and nucleic acids for
cell maintenance and repair. This basal metabolism of
the noncontracting heart accounts for 15 to 20 % of
the energy generated by the heart. Cell necrosis results when these basal metabolic demands cannot be met.

b) The myocardial pumping function: this includes
ion "pumping" which results in electrical activity
and the interaction of contractile proteins. The energy
required for contractile work is approximately 80 %
of total cardiac energy consumption during rest conditions. During stress this share may increase to 95 %.
The energy required for electrical activity is less
than 1 %.

2.2.1. Imaging of myocardial perfusion defects: The indicator clinically most used for myocardial perfusion
imaging is Thallium 201. This substance bears some
resemblance to potassium. The uptake of both substances into the cell is similar, due to their comparable ionic radius, which is an important determinant

for the passive penetration of the cell membrane.There
is some evidence for the active transport of Thallium
into the cell by Na-K-ATPase. The role of the Na-K-
ATPase in the cellular uptake has been proven experimentally (24). Perfusion of the interventricular branch
of the left coronary artery with venous blood showed a
significant decrease of Thallium uptake in the corresponding region. Normalization of Thallium uptake was
observed after reperfusion with arterial blood. It is
now obvious, that the distribution of Thallium in the
myocardium is not only a function of perfusion, but
also to a significant extent a function of metabolism.
But fortunately for clinical reasons the metabolic
changes in hypoperfused regions reinforce the Thallium
defect. Decreased flow combined with decreased extraction means even a more significant Thallium defect in
the myocardial scan. This is indeed valid for most of
the myocardial radiopharmaceuticals. They are indicators
of both perfusion and metabolism. Even the radioactive
Xenon reveals a non-linearity to flow with underesti-
mation of higher flow rates. There is one procedure in
nuclear cardiology, which shows the true distribution
of coronary blood flow: The injection of microspheres
into the coronary artery. But even these results are
doubtful, when the main branch of the left coronary
artery is short and homogeneous mixing cannot be guar-
anteed. Besides the conventional scintillation camera
with high resolution and 7 pinhole collimator, nowadays
single photon emission computer tomography (SPECT) and
positron emission tomography (PET) is acquiring an increasing share in coronary heart disease investigations.

2.2.2. Imaging of failures of myocardial metabolism:
Radiopharmaceuticals for the visualization of myocardial
metabolism are in general physiological substrates, and
hence are assimilated into the metabolic pathways which
we have considered in the preceeding sections. The most
important substrates for myocardial metabolism are
glucose, fatty acids and lactate. Indeed, analogues of
two of these substrates have been successfully used,
Fluorine-18 2-deoxyglucose (FDG) as an analogue for
glucose, and, as an analogue for free fatty acids
Carbon-11 labelled palmitic acid (APA), or long chain
fatty acids labelled with Iodine-123. The turnover rate
of the radionuclide primarily reflects the hydrolysis
of triglycerides and subsequent β – oxidation of free
fatty acids. Under anaerobic conditions β – oxidation
is not possible and turnover rate decreases significantly, whereas glycolysis is the last reservoir for
energy liberation. For this reason glucose and glycogen

are essential for survival of the ischemic myocardium.
Fluorine-18 2-deoxyglucose behaves like glucose with
relation to its movement through the interstitium and
across the cell membrane. The initial metabolic steps
are comparable to glucose. It is initially phosphorylated by hexokinase to FDG-6 phosphate, but then becomes trapped. It does not enter glycolysis nor is it
stored in form of glycogen. Metabolically unbound FDG
subsequently leaves the myocradium. Images obtained by
positron emission tomography (PET) reflect the local
distribution of metabolic rates for glucose, when they
are obtained at equilibrium. We have to bear in mind,
that using these radiopharmaceuticals and a PET leads
to truly quantitative results. Cross sectional images
permit quantitative assessment of the local distribution of the radioindicator in μCi/g and thus resemble
"in-vivo autoradiographs". This makes possible physiologic modeling, e.g. mathematical formulation of a
multicompartment model. However, myocardial perfusion
abnormalities and failures of metabolism become apparent within short time: They cause motion abnormalities
in the hypoperfused region within seconds. Frequently,
the ischemic portion of the ventricle bulges outward
with systole, impairing the hearts pumping function.
Imaging of these subtle and frequently small regional
wall motion abnormalities (RWMA) with sufficient reliability is one of the most rewarding and challenging
tasks cardiology requires from imaging techniques.

2.3. Failures of Myocardial Function (Regional Wall
Motion Abnormalities) and Techniques for their
Imaging

The heart has been compared with a mechanical pump.
Heart function therefore has been described in terms
of volume and pressure and their time derivatives. But
determination of global volume of e.g. the left ventricle alone does not fulfill completely the requirements of cardiology. The heart is more complicated
than a mechanical pump and description of its function
by global parameters, like ejection fraction (EF) may
yield false negative results. Hyokinesis of one myocardial region may be compensated for by hyperkinesis
of another region preserving a normal stroke volume
and normal EF. The requirement for the exact definition
of RWMA by a non-invasive procedure has provoked increased developments in nuclear cardiology, US and
digital imaging, not to mention CT. The subsequent
sections will focus on the problem of how nuclear
cardiology can fulfill the strong requirements of

cardiology for imaging and quantitative evaluation of RWMA.

2.3.1. Approach of nuclear cardiology for imaging and quantitative evaluation of RWMA: Detailed description of RWMA requires the exact localisation (x,y,z) of each myocardial region (m$_i$) as a function of the heart cycle (t). The approach of nuclear cardiology is based on the assumption, that the cyclic motion of each myocardial region can be described as a set of time dependant count rates C (t), forming a representative time-activity-curve, which corresponds to the time-volume-curve of the respective region. We started with two heart regions, left and right ventricle (11,12). Finally, a set of regional curves was obtained (13,25, 26), each one representing the cardiac cycle of one small region corresponding to or smaller than the resolution of the camera computer system. The sum of the time-activity-curves of all regions of the heart contains all information concerning myocardial motion and therefore fulfills the fore-mentioned requirements (13). The resulting set of regional time-activity-curves and the LV global curve was extremely high. In more than 78% of the LV pixels, r was better than 0.9. activity-curves is reliability, which has been proven in the following way: The similarity of each pixel curve with the global left ventricular curve was evaluated by comparison of corresponding curve points. The resulting correlation coefficient (r) is a measure of the similarity of both curves. The plot of all correlation coefficients is termed the "correlation" scan. Investigation of more than 20 normokinetic subjects showed that the correlation between the pixel time-activity curves and the LV global curve was extremely high: In more than 78 % of the LV pixel r was better than 0.9. This shows that time-activity curves from single image points reflect very well the synchronous motion of the left ventricle and suggests that even small local deviations within the behaviour of time-activity curves may have statistical significance. Within infarcted regions the correlation coefficients may drop to low values of the order of zero and even may become negative in aneurysms. Thus, the correlation scan figures outline very clearly regions with wall motion abnormalities. But it does not indicate which kind of RWMA is present. For this reason we do not use the correlation scan in routine investigations. But we have learned and can prove by this special form of parametric scans, that the pixel time activity curves are reliable and can be used for further data processing providing careful

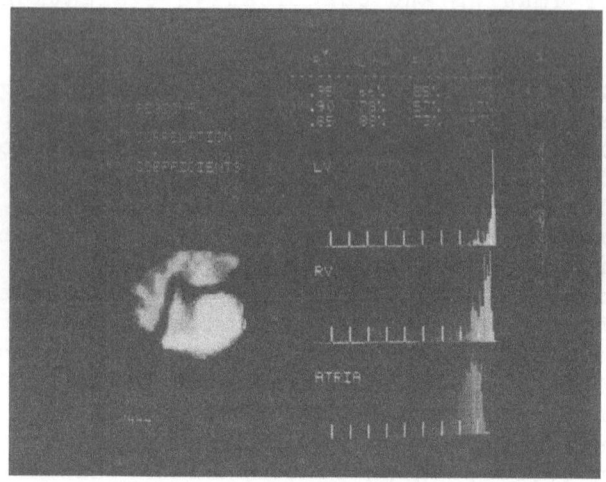

Figure 1: Correlation scan, showing the correlation of
the pixel curves to the global left ventricular curve.
78% of the LV pixels show correlation (r) better than
0.9. Normal heart with synchronous contraction.

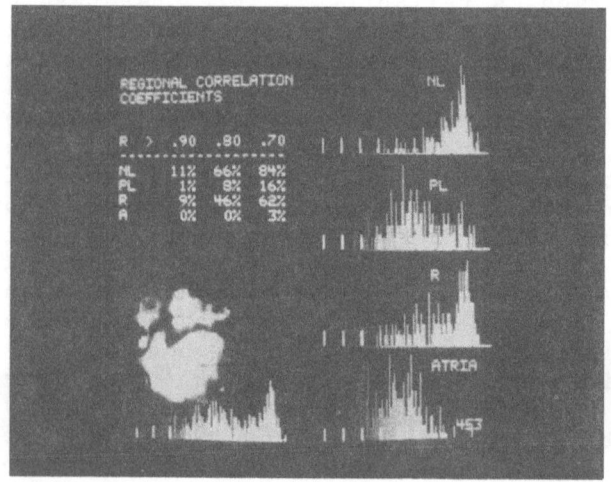

Figure 2: Decreased correlation in the antero-lateral
region of the LV. The correlation coefficient (r)
approaches zero in the infarcted area. Histograms:
NL = normal LV, PL = pathologic LV area, R = RV.

data accumulation and correction occur. Further data
processing in the analysis of myocardial motion requires the complete and valid time -activity-curves
for each of the heart pixels. Uncorrected curves obtained in frame mode often show a decrease of the
curve in end-diastole. This results from the variation
of cycle length, in the range of 10 % in normals and
to more than 50 % in patients with heart failure. In
our eyes it is not sufficient just to count and correct for the number of cycles which contribute to the
particular frame. In conclusion, the proper time correction is mandatory for exact parametric scanning.

2.3.2. Imaging of myocardial function abnormalities
(RWMA): The parametric scan mode. The complete assessment of heart function (wall motion) includes the
regional position as a function of time (x,y,z,t).
Imaging in nuclear cardiology results in a matrix of
regional time-activity-curves, which indeed fulfills
this requirement with sufficient exactness. The disadvantage of this matrix of regional curves is its
abstract presentation. It is impossible for the eye
to reveal the huge amount of information hidden in the
multitude of curves. Parametric scanning fundamentally
can solve the problem. Various essential features of
the regional curves are chosen as parameters. A parametric scan shows the regional distribution of one
parameter in the heart. The selection of parameters
should follow the criteria of clinical demands and
reliability. The parameters chosen should reveal abnormalities of myocardial motion and - if possible -
differentiate between functional or anatomical lesions
and conduction abnormalities. The cardiologist utilizes
the contrast angiogram to detect RWMA, differentiating
akinetic, hypokinetic and dyskinetic regions. Diagnosis of conduction abnormalities is based on the ECG.
Nuclear cardiology based on the concept of parametric
scanning facilitates the diagnosis of RWMA and conduction abnormalities. Hypo- and akinesis show decreased
or deleted systolic-diastolic differences and dyskinesis
is revealed as asynchronous motion, e.g. delayed end-
systole. Left bundle branch block (LBBB) shows delayed
contraction of the whole LV. This can be demonstrated
in a parametric scan utilizing the interval "R-wave-
endsystole" (IRE) as parameter (endsystolic time).
Similar results are possible by utilizing amplitude
and phase of the base frequency after Fourier analysis.
The amplitude corresponds to the systolic-diastolic
differences, the phase to the IRE. But beyond the scope
of conventional angiography parametric scanning yields

additional information (e.g. the "peak filling rate
(maximal relaxation velocity) scan"), which may prove
to be of importance in early stages of myocardial insufficiency. The reliability of each individual parameter has yet to be fully elucidated. Systolic-diastolic
count differences, commonly used in parametric scanning,
may show considerable statistical errors using the
original curves. Parameters derived from only two
points of a statistically "blurred" pixel curve, like
S-D differences and E.F. show a considerable degree
of uncertainty corresponding to the statistical uncertainty of the two points chosen. In contrast, parameters based on the total number of curve points should
reveal higher reliability. This could indeed be proven
by Fourier analysis of the pixel curves. The reliability
of the parameter "amplitude" as representative of the
entire pixel curve was clearly better than "difference"
parameters. A multiplicity of parameters has been
proposed and applied within the last few years (27,28,
29,30). Those parameters describing the "extent of myocardial contraction" (for detection of hypo- and akinetic regions), may be classified separately from those
describing the "coordination of myocardial motion"
(for detection of dyskinetic regions and conduction
abnormalities). Finally it is necessary to classify a
third group of parameters describing abnormalities of
wall motion which although genuine cannot usually be
displayed angiographically. The extent of myocardial
contraction frequently is assessed using the "two
points" parameter "diastolic-systolic differences"
(D-S) or (synonymous) "stroke volume" (D-S). This is
true also for the parameter "ejection fraction" (EF),
which is indeed the ratio of two "two points" D-S/D-B
(B=background) parameters. Besides statistical uncertainties mentioned previously another problem
arises with these parameters: Regions with normal
extent of contraction, but incoordinate motion show
up as hypokinetic areas. In contrast the parameter
"amplitude" of the basal frequency, of the pixel curve
after Fourier analysis (13,31,32) describes more exactly
the extent of regional motion. Fourier analysis and
its implication for parametric scanning will be discussed in the context of a later section.The coordination of myocardial motion is partly reflected by the
correlation scan, mentioned previously. At the moment
the phase scan is the simplest mode for visualization
of dyskinetic regions and conduction abnormalities.
Finally imaging of the negative values of (D-S) has
been used for paradoxical myocardial motion (30). In
conclusion, "amplitude" and "phase" scans provide both

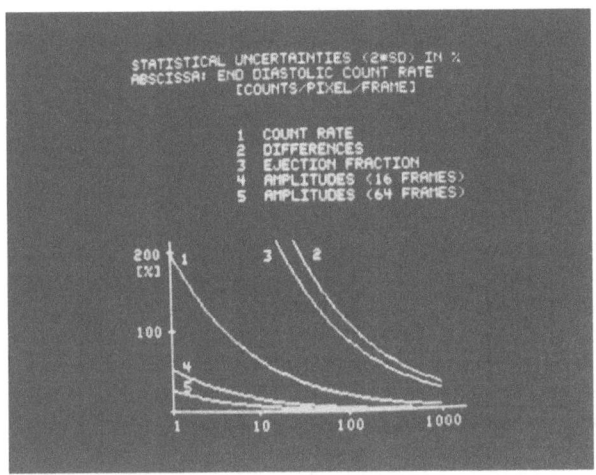

Figure 3: Statistical uncertainties (2 SD) of various
parameters as function of the enddiastolic count rate.
Assumed background 50%, assumed E.F. 50%.

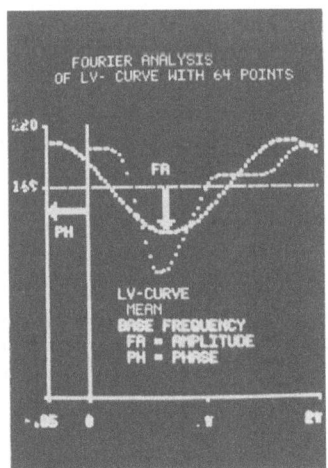

Figure 4: The amplitude (FA) corresponds to the extent
of contraction, the phase (PH) to the temporal sequence
FA reveals hypo- and akinetic,
PH dyskinetic regions.

requirements stated previously, clinical relevance and reliability. The "two points" scans "regional ejection fraction", "stroke volume" (diastolic-systolic difference) including "paradox imaging" are clinically relevant, but may lack reliability, unless the pixel curves are filtered prior to analysis.

2.3.3. Further data processing for complete quantitative evaluation of gated blood pool investigations: For quantitative evaluation of the extent and grade of RWMA further data processing is necessary. Complete quantification can be obtained in two ways:

a) Presentation of the distribution of one parameter within the heart as histogram and comparison with the histogram of a normal group. The set of all histograms then yields the complete information. Our results show a Gaussian distribution for the phases but an empirical distribution with negative skew for the amplitude and the "two points" parameters (ED-ES, reg. EF).

b) The enddiastolic LV area is divided into sectors. Comparison of the sector sum of the various parameters with a **group** of normals reveals pathologic areas. For intra-and interindividual comparison a normalization of the parametric scans is necessary. The distribution of the ventricular phase is arbitrarily normalised to $-\frac{1}{2}\pi$, provided a bundle branch block can be excluded. Normalization of the parameters FA, ED-ES and EF is based on the EF of the LV. Within the last years two dimensional US has made great progress in the recognition of RWMA. Best results are obtainable in children. Limitations exist for adults, because only approximately 60 to 70 % of the myocardial wall can be visualized sufficiently. Most difficult is assessment of the left ventricular apex. Comparison of 5 wall segments in 105 patients by angiography and 2 dimensional US agreement in 70%. This agreement could be improved to 80% after revision of the US results (33). However, radionuclide procedures are presently more useful in patients with CAD than US. Digital angiocardiography has a surprisingly high degree of similarity with radionuclide ventriculography:"Image subtraction" corresponds to background subtraction, "image integration" to gated imaging and "subtraction image enhancement" to contrast enhancement. Even the parametric scan mode finds its analogue in "functional imaging" of digital angiocardiography, extracting a single parameter from the "pixel densitogram" (34,35, 36). The data array obtained by applying this operation to the pixel densitogram can be rescaled and displayed as an image. This functional image may describe the

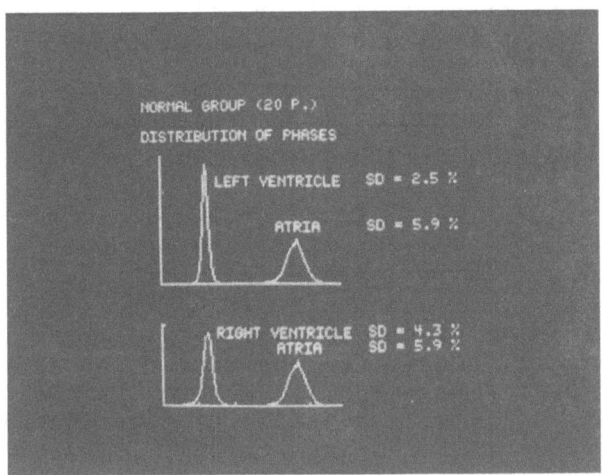

<u>Figure 7</u>: The phase histograms of 20 subjects without heart failure shows Gaussian distribution of the phases in the right and left ventricle with small standard deviations (SD).

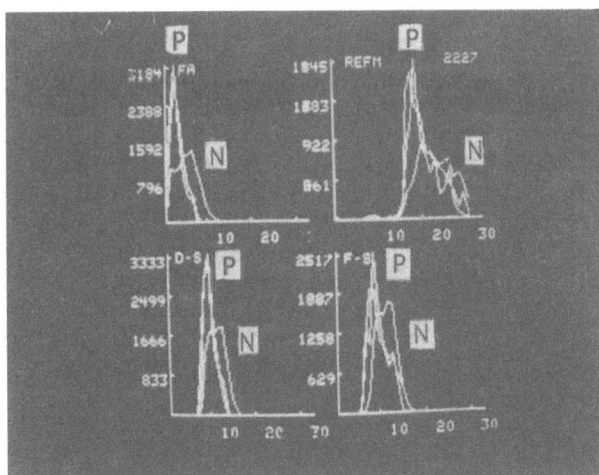

<u>Figure 8</u>: Histograms of amplitude (FA), regional ejection fraction (REFM), systolic-diastolic difference(D-S) and difference (fast filling-endsystole)(F-S) extracted from 20 normal subjects (N). All parameters show empirical distribution. Pat. with anterior wall infarction (P) before and after medication reveals partially impaired parameters (outside the distribution of N).

distribution of transit times or other parameters.
Their clinical utility has not been described up to
now.

2.4. Failures of the Conduction System of the Heart
     and Techniques for their Imaging.

Conduction abnormalities (CA) can be imaged with
sufficient exactness using the phase scan. This is due
to the conformity of the phase scan with the "enddiastolic time scan" and to the fact, that the electromechanical linkage of the myocardium preserves the
correspondence of mechanical contraction and electrical
activation. Differentiation between CA and regional
dyskinesia is clinically possible by the typical pattern
of CA. The present predominant role of Fourier analysis
in parametric scanning is based on the fact, that the
main diagnostic problems "localization and assessment
of the size of hypo- and akinetic myocardial regions"
by help of the Fourier amplitudes (FA) scan, "localization and assessment of the size of dyskinetic regions"
by the Phase (PH) scan, and finally "description and
analysis of conduction abnormalities" by the PH scan
can be solved very elegantly by only one algorithm.
Another reason is the fact, that the normal phase
histogram shows a Gaussian distribution with surprisingly small standard deviation (SD = 2,5 % in the LV
area), which simplifies recognition and even makes
possible exact definition of dyskinetic regions. Parametric scanning with the mono- or the multicrystal
camera translates heart motion into two dimensional
scans. Hence the requirements of exact localisation
of myocardial regions are not completely fulfilled.
PET further extends cardiac imaging and in combination
with the possibilities of imaging myocardial perfusion
and metabolism, yields a complete assessment of the
status of the heart.

3. UTILITY OF IMAGING TECHNIQUES FOR THE DIAGNOSIS AND
   PROGNOSIS OF CARDIOVASCULAR ABNORMALITIES

Discussion of clinical results of non-invasive imaging
techniques will follow the scheme used previously:
     a) Anatomical abnormalities of the cardiovascular
system (shunts, valvular failures).
     b) Myocardial insufficiency due to perfusion defects,
metabolic failures and/or wall motion abnormalities.
     c) Conduction system abnormalities.

3.1.Shunts and Valvular Failures

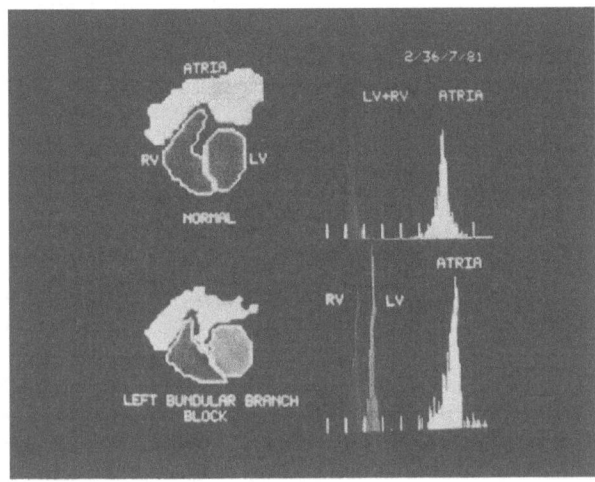

Figure 5: Phase scans and histograms.
Above: Normal heart, LV and RV show corresponding peaks.
Below: Left bundle branch block; delayed peak of the
LV.

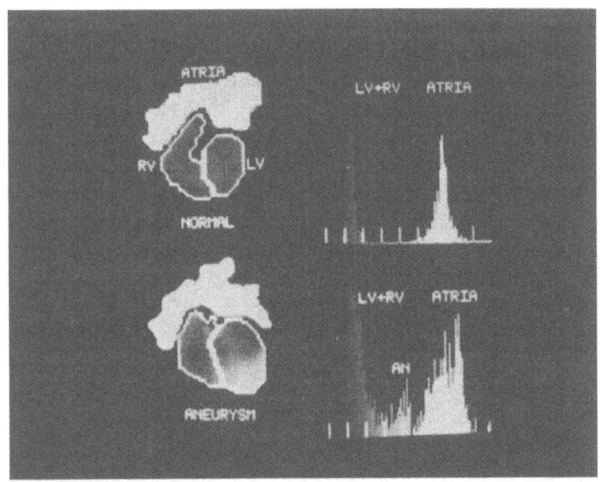

Figure 6: Phase scans and histograms.
Above: Normal heart.
Below: Aneurysm of the LV apical region. Myocardial
insufficiency.

The gated blood pool procedure and assessment of the
left to right ratio of count rates has been applied in
13 patients with a left to right shunt. The shunt size
was proven by oxymetry. The correlation was 0.77 (37).
The same method has been applied for assessment of
aortic and mitral valve regurgitation by RIGO and
WAGNER (38). The results were stated by KRESS (39) from
our group, who compared the results of the GBP study
with a hemodynamic ratio. The stroke volume of the
left ventricle was determined by angiography, the stroke
volume of the right ventricle by thermodilution. In 33
patients with aortic and mitral valve regurgitation
the correlation was 0,75. Due to a broad range of
normal values the sensitivity of the nuclear medicine
procedure is low, but the specifity high. In 64 patients
with all types of heart diseases false positive results
could not be observed. The value of US for detection of
valvular lesions goes without question. Valvular
stenoses with and without calcification can easily be
seen. Valvular incompetence can not be recognized
directly from the valve echogram except in papillary
muscle rupture. In all other cases only indirect signs
like diameter or volume increase of heart chambers and
valve fluttering or prolapse can be detected by conventional 1D or 2D- echocardiography. Contrast echocardiography has been shown to be useful for the detection of tricuspid insufficiency by observing the
to and fro motion of the ultrasound reflecting microcavitations across the tricuspid valve (40). Pulsed
Doppler echocardiography detects disturbances of intracardiac blood flow based on frequency shifts induced
by these disturbances in pulsed, reflected ultrasound
(41). It can be used to identify and estimate mitral
and aortic regurgitation and prosthetic valve dysfunction. Contrast 2D-echocardiography offers new aspects
to diagnose intracardiac shunting. Right to left
shunting is present if microcavitations are visible on
the left side of the heart after peripheral vein injection of fluid (e.g. saline or indocyanine green dye),
because in the lung capillaries these microbubbles are
dissolved. Left to right atrial shunting can be demonstrated by a negative contrast or wash-out effect of
the turbulences in the right atrium after peripheral
vein injection. Both methods are highly specific.

3.2. Myocardial Insufficiency due to Perfusion Defects,
     Metabolic Failures and/or Wall Motion Abnormalities

Coronary artery disease (CAD) is of primary interest
for this group of cardiovascular abnormalities. The

subsequent sections, therefore, will focus into this abnormality. Resting coronary flow and regional distribution are not affected by narrowing of up to 85 % of arterial diameter and therefore provide little insight into the effects of stenoses on coronary hemodynamics. However, maximal coronary flow and coronary flow reserve are markedly reduced by constrictions that do not affect resting flow. Coronary flow reserve begins to decrease with stenosis of 30 to 45 percent of arterial diameter (42). PROUDFIT, SHIREY and SONES (43) assumed that 50 % diameter stenosis in a coronary artery represents significant CAD. This was based on data from patients with angina and a positive ECG stress test. Those patients with a 5o % or greater reduction in luminal diameter in two or more coronary angiographic projections of one or more coronary arteries are considered having significant coronary artery disease. We are aware of the limitations of this definition, because it does not take into account site and length of the stenoses. A "coronary score" would better correspond to the real coronary state. However, for clinical purposes and listings of the literature, this seems roughly appropriate. "Subcritical stenoses" subsequently are defined by a 25 to 49 percent reduction in luminal diameter in two or more coronary angiographic projections of one or more coronary arteries. The group " significant stenoses" comprises stable angina and unstable angina. The subsequent sections deal with contributions of myocardial perfusion scintigraphy and myocardial motion scintigraphy (radionuclide ventriculography) to the diagnosis of CAD, ranging from subcritical stenoses to postinfarct state.

3.2.1. Contribution of nuclear cardiology to the diagnosis of subcritical stenoses: POHOST et al. (44) found, that 12 of 18 patients with subcritical CAD (20 to 49 % narrowing) had one or more defects on their initial postexercise Thallium imaging study. Only one of the patients had typical angina. These findings illustrate the special value of the perfusion scans. While angina pectoris and ECG changes are associated with functional ischemia, the Thallium 201 study depends only upon the presence of inhomogeneous flow and not on the presence of functional ischemia. However, a real estimate for the predictive value in diagnosing subcritical stenoses up to now is not possible.

3.2.2. Contribution of nuclear cardiology to the diagnosis of significant stenoses: The Thallium exercise test (TET) in patients with significant stenoses is

now accepted as being more reliable than the exercise
ECG (EECG). The sensitivity in various independent
groups ranges between 75 % and 99 % (as compared with
EECG 61 % to 79 %) and the specificity between 69 %
and 90 % (EECG 69 % and 82 %) (44,45,46,47,48). The
superiority of the TET becomes especially clear in
single vessel disease (SVD); the sensitivity was 73 %
versus 43 % (EECG). Stenosed coronary arteries with
angiographically proven collaterals yielded TET defects
in only 65 of 92 patients (48). Of paramount interest
is the "redistribution effect", which permits the
differentiation of ischemic, but viable myocardium from
infarcted myocardium. Variant or Prinzmetal's angina
(coronary artery spasm with transmural ischemia) shows
characteristic behaviour; during the occlusion phase,
Thallium 201 kinetics in the ischemic zone resembles
that of infarcted myocardium. After reflow slow accumulation can be observed in the previously ischemic
myocardium until it achieves a level equivalent to that
in the nonischemic myocardium. Although late imaging
may demonstrate total disappearance of defects (complete redistribution) after 2 hours, sometimes the
delay of redistribution may last up to 6 hours. Perfusion defects have an immediate impact on ventricular
function. BORER et al. (49) have shown a decrease of
left ventricular ejection fraction (E.F.) and motion
abnormality in the ischemic zone, whereas in normals
E.F. increased. By this way differentiation of a normal
and CAD group with sensitivity and specificity of more
than 90 % was possible. These fascinating results could
not be attained by other groups. CALDWELL and HAMILTON
(50) published results with a comparable sensitivity
of 93 %, but lower specificity of only 55 %. Our own
results revealed optimal sensitivity (100 %) with poor
specificity (54 %), when "normal behaviour" was defined
as "increase of E.F. more than 3 % ". In contrast, when
"normal" was defined as "E.F. unchanged or increasing",
specificity was increased to 85 %, combined with a
still good sensitivity of 84 %. These results are comparable to those attained by TET. However, at the
present state high sensitivity and lower specificity
should be taken into account for radionuclide ventriculography with respect to detection of CAD. This gives
high yield in detecting CAD in a population with high
prevalence of this disease. Best results of the RNV
exercise test (RNVET) were obtained by regional wall
motion analysis. Special interest deserves the publication of BODENHEIMER (51), who pinpoints that qualitative evaluation of regional wall motion failed in
detecting smaller abnormalities, which could be re-

vealed by the parametric scan procedure, the applied parameter
"regional E.F."

3.2.3. Contributions of nuclear cardiology to the
diagnosis of myocardial infarction (MI): Though most
acute myocardial infarctions offer no diagnostic
problems in the coronary care unit, still a substantial
group of patients remains with a questionable history
and a nondiagnostic ECG. In these cases perfusion
scintigraphy offers a highly valuable diagnostic tool.
WACKERS et al. (52) could demonstrate, that in the
period within 6 hours after onset all infarctions
could be detected, irrespectively of location, size and
their transmural or nontransmural quality. The sensitivity decreased to 78 % (transmural) and 52 % (nontransmural), respectively, after 24 hours. The sensitivity of Thallium 201 to detect acute MI was determined by WACKERS in 200 consecutive patients with proven
myocardial infarction. Overall, positive scans were
obtained in 82 %. Assessment of the infarction size
was based on the SGOT level in the serum. Large infarctions were characterized by a level more than 3,5
times upper limit of normal, and small infarctions by
a level below 3,5 times upper limit of normal. Large
MI showed positive scans in 94 % and small MI in only
57 %. Nontransmural MI revealed a lower sensitivity of
63 % as compared with the 88 % positive scans in transmural infarctions. It becomes evident, that the fast
decrease of sensitivity after 24 hours limits the value
of Thallium 201 in detection and assessment of older
myocardial infarctions. In our opinion starting with
the stage of infarction RNV should become the prevalent
diagnostic procedure for the subsequent reasons:
    a) sensitivity of RNV is comparable within the first
hours after infarction and seems to become superior
after 24 hours; 89 consecutive patients, who were
admitted to our ward with suspected acute or older infarction, were diagnosed by RNV. The correct diagnosis
was still unknown for the nuclear physician. 77 patients revealed wall motion abnormalities. All of them
finally were diagnosed as having infarction. This
corresponds to a sensitivity for detection of MI of
93 %, whereas in all subjects without wall motion abnormalities further observation could rule out MI.
    b) RNV allows assessment of myocardial function in
terms of global LV parameters (e.g. LVEF, EDV) and of
parametric scans with analysis of regional wall motion.
Assessment of resting myocardial function and follow
up of myocardial function are now of prior interest
for the prognosis of the individual patient.

Table 1:
Thallium 201 Exercise Tests: Significant Coronary Stenoses

	N	201 TL		E C G	
		Sensit.	Specific.	Sensit.	Specific.
1980 POHOST(44) (MULTIPLE CENTERS, USA)	1077	82 %	90 %	61 %	82 %
1980 SIMOONS HUGENHOLTZ(45)	118	75 %	86 %	59 %	76 %
1980 SAUER, SEBENING(46)	120	91 %	94 %		
1980 LÖSSE, LOOGEN(47)	169	99 %	69 %	79 %	69%
1981 HÖR(48) (MULTIPLE CENTERS)	3092	83 %	90 %		

Table 2:
Radionuclide Ventriculography Exercise Tests: Significant Stenosis

	Sensitivity	Specificity	
BORER et al.(49)	94 %	91 %	Global EF
BODENHEIMER et al.(51)	91 %	87 %	Reg.Wall.Mot. (PEF)Handgrip
CALDWELL, HAMILTON(50)	93 %	55 %	Global EF
NOLAN et al.(58)	89 %	88 %	Reg.Wall Mot.
SAUER, SEBENING(46)	83 %	100 %	Reg.Wall Mot.

Table 3:
Own Results of RNV in 89 Consecutive Patients with Suspected Infarction

	Motion Abnormality	No Motion Abnormality
Infarction clinically proven	77 (93%)	6
Infarction not clinically	0	6 (100%)

6 false negative

no false positive result

3.2.4. Contributions of nuclear cardiology to the post-infarction period: The ECG pattern of MI are not helpful in predicting prognosis of patients who have survived. Nontransmural infarctions may have a prognosis as poor as transmural infarctions. MI may be a marker of CAD, but not necessarily an indicator of its severity. TAYLOR et al. (53) could demonstrate, that low post infarction E.F. was associated with a high risk of sudden cardiac death. Multivariate analysis of 30 clinical and laboratory variables identified previous myocardial infarction and an E.F. less than 40 % as the best predictors of mortality. All patients who died were identified by these two variables. Once the information of these two variables were considered, neither three vessel disease nor complicated late hospital phase ventricular arrhythmias provided any additional information about mortality. E.F., which can easily be obtained by RNV, thus far plays a important role in the rehabilitation phase after infarction. But this shall remind us, that E.F. is only a byproduct of the much more informative imaging of regional myocardial motion, which can be assessed in a quantitative manner, or in a semiquantitative way by parametric scanning. In conclusion, nuclear cardiology may contribute considerably to all stages of CAD. Whereas the stages of infarction and the postinfarction area are domain of RNV, especially in the more sophisticated presentation of parametric scanning, Thallium scans are preferrably applied to the preinfarction stages of CAD.

3.3. Abnormalities of the Electrical Activation and
     Conduction System

The phase scan provides an accurate means of detecting and localizing abnormal foci of ventricular contraction. FRAIS et al. (54) observed foci of earliest contraction either in the anterior wall of the left ventricle or in the septum, in patients with WPW syndrome. This corresponded exactly to the sites of pre-excitation determined on electrophysiologic mapping. Similarly among 8 patients with pacemakers the site of earliest excitation was localised to the RV in 7 patients and to the left ventricle in 1 patient. Within each ventricle the site corresponded to the radiographic location of the pacemaker electrode, results also reported by PAVEL et al. (55). Typical pattern of left bundle branch block with characteristic changes in the phase histogram became apparent. Changes of the pacemaker from the upper to the lower septum showed corresponding pattern changes in the phase scan. In conclusion: With each

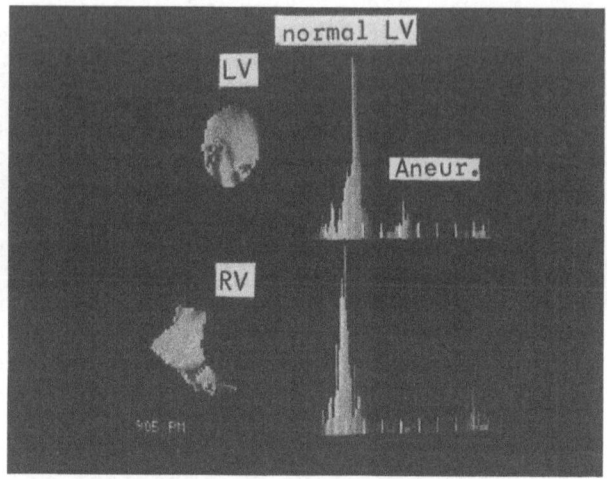

Figure 9: Phase scan and histogram of a patient with pacemaker (apex right ventricle).Excitation starts in this region. Contraction of the LV slightly delayed. Paradoxical motion of the aneurysm in the LV apical region.

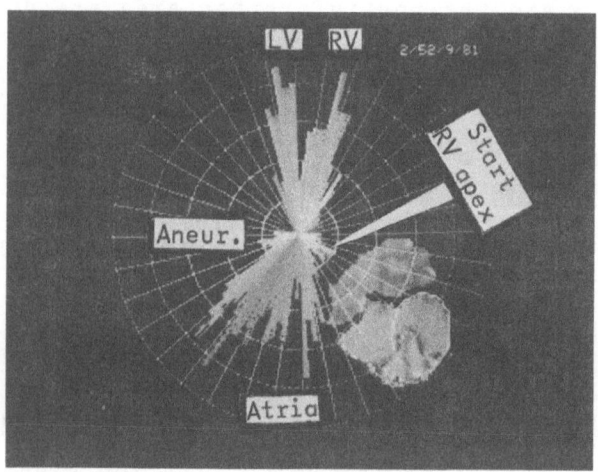

Figure 10: Phase scan and histogram in polar coordinate presentation. The cycle turns round counterclockwise, starting at about 4 o'clock.

case serving as its own control phase images showed
clearly the effect of different activation patterns.

4. FUTURE DEVELOPMENTS OF TECHNIQUES FOR IMAGING OF CARDIOVASCULAR ABNORMALITIES

Published images of nuclear magnetic resonance (NMR)
up to now have been proton images. That is, they depict
the distribution of mobile protons in the sample, and
thus far are able to yield tomographic images of the
heart. But the techniques of NMR imaging can possibly
be applied to any isotope having a nuclear magnetic
moment. FOSSEL, DELAYRE and INGWALL (56) have carried
out experiments which form the basis for a classification scheme whereby a high resolution P-31 spectrum
can be used to classify tissue as reversibly damaged,
potentially reversibly damaged or irreversibly damaged
based on the biochemical profile presented by the
spectrum. Whether clinical application of this classification sees the light of day in the form of spatial
images or high resolution spectra from surface coils
or topical magnetic resonance spectroscopy remains to
be seen. ^{31}P spectra of ischemic rabbit hearts show
little or no phosphocreatine and greatly enhanced
inorganic phosphate peaks. Thus far, NMR could greatly
enhance the information of myocardial metabolism
revealed by PET (57). Further software development
for gated blood pool scans should result in physiologic
data, which combined with other methods could yield
new and unexpected information, e.g., the vector ECG
reflects the spreading of electrical activation of the
heart muscle. A similar vectorlike mapping of the
mechanical contraction of the heart muscle could offer
an immediate assessment of the electro-mechanical
linkage of the heart. Finally, esophageal echocardiography could improve considerably the results of two
dimensional US and make possible flow studies in
combination with contrast media.

5. CONCLUSIONS

Newly developed non invasive imaging techniques at
present make possible a nearly complete description of
the state of the heart and for this reason help to
manage patients with cardiovascular diseases. The
selection of imaging techniques depends on the suspected abnormality:

Valvular stenoses are the domain of ultrasonography,
valvular insufficiency can be diagnosed by contrast

US and gated blood pool (GBP) scans. This procedure also yields reliable quantitative data. The same is true for atrial shunts, whereas ventricular shunts again are domain of first pass investigations or contrast US.

Myocardial insufficiency due to perfusion defects, metabolic failures or regional motion abnormalities is domain of nuclear cardiology up to now. Imaging of regional perfusion defects by Thallium has improved the diagnostic accuracy for CAD by about 20 per cent. A nearly 100 % sensitivity for the early detection of infarction within the most critical first hours after the event helps in the management of patients with masked infarction. For the management in the rehabilitation phase the radionuclide ventriculogram presently seems to be unsurpassable, because global parameters of LV function (volumes, EF) combined with exact definition of RWMA by parametric scans makes possible the early recognition of the development of an aneurysm.

Finally excitation and conduction abnormalities can be described precisely by the phase scan. Although the scientific utility of metabolic investigations with the PET up to now is superior to clinical applicability, further developments have to be taken into account. Nuclear magnetic resonance is of interest for its ability to detect the content of the energy store of the myo- cardium, phosphocreatine and its claim to differen- tiate between viable and non viable myocardial areas. Digital radiography makes possible imaging with high spatial distribution (as compared with nuclear cardio- logy).But a final assessment of the capabilities of this method for the prediction and management of patients with cardiovascular abnormalities seems to be premature.

REFERENCES

1. Blumgart, H.C., S. Weiss: Studies on the velocity of blood flow.VII. The pulmonary circulation time in normal resting individuals. J. Clin. Invest. 4 (1927) 399.

2. Prinzmetal, M., E. Corday, H.C. Bergman: Radio- cardiography: a new method for studying the blood flow through the heart in human beings. Science 198 (1948) 340.

3. Nylin, G., H. Celander: Determination of blood volume in heart and lungs and cardiac output through injection of radiophosphorus. Circulation 1 (1950) 76.

4. Donato, L., C. Giuntini, R. Bianchi, A. Maseri: Quantitative radiocardiography for the measurement of pulmonary blood volume. Dynamic Clinical Studies with Radioisotopes (R.M. Knisley, W.N. Tauxe, Eds.USAEC Washington (1964) 267.

5. Meier, P., K.L. Zierler: On the theory of the indicator dilution method for measurement of blood flow and volume. J. Appl. Physiol. 6 (1954) 731.

6. Bender, M.A., M. Blau: Evaluation of renal and cardiac dynamics with the autofluoroscope. J. Nucl. Med. 4 (1963) 186.

7. Scheer, K.E., E. Jahns, I. Kazem, P. Gelinsky: Klinische Untersuchungen mit der Szintillationskamera und 99m-Tc- Radioactive Isotope in Klinik und Forschung K. Fellinger, R. Höfer, Eds. Urban & Schwarzenberg, Verlag, München-Berlin-Wien (1967) 103.

8. Adam, W.E., W.J. Lorenz, K.E. Scheer: Quantitative radiokardiographische Untersuchungen mit der Szintillationskamera. 5. Jahrestagung der Gesellschaft für Nuklearmedizin, Wien (1967).

9. Hoffmann, C., N. Kleine: Eine neue Methode zur unblutigen Messung des Schlagvolumens am Menschen über viele Tage mit Hilfe von radioaktiven Isotopen. Verh. Dtsch. Kreislaufforschung 31 (1965) 93-96.

10. Wagner, H.N.jr., R. Wake, E. Nickoloff, T.K. Natarajan: The nuclear stethoscope: A simple device for generation of left ventricular volume curves. Am. J. Cardiol. 38 (1976) 747-750.

11. Adam, W.E., F. Bitter, W.J. Lorenz: Der Computer als Hilfsmittel zur Verbesserung der nuklear-medizinischen Funktionsdiagnostik. In: Computers in Radiology, edited by R.de Haene and A. Wambersie, Basel, Karger Verlag (1970) 459-464.

12. Bitter, F., W. Besch, N. Schäfer, E. Sigmund: Integrierte Herz-Kreislauf-Analyse mit Hilfe der quantitativen Funktionsszintigraphie. In: Frontiers of Nuclear Medicine, edited by W. Horst, Berlin-New York, Springer Verlag (1971) 250-261.

13. Geffers, H., G. Meyer, F. Bitter, W.E. Adam: Analysis of Heart Function by Gated Blood Pool Investigation Camera-Kinematography Int. Conference Orsay (1975) 462-465.

14. Zaret, B.L., H.W. Strauss, P.J. Hurley, T.K. Natarajan, B. Pitt: A noninvasive scintiphotographic method for detecting regional ventricular dysfunction in man. N. Eng. J.Med. 28 (1971) 1165-1170.

15. Sapirstein, L.A.: Fractionation of the cardiac output in rats with isotopic potassium. Circulation Res. 4 (1956) 689.

478

16. Burch, G.F., S.A. Threefoot, C. Ray: The rate of disapearance of Rubidium-86 from the plasma, the biologic decay rates of Rubidium-86 and the applicability of Rubidium-86 as a tracer of Potassium in man with and without chronic congestive heart failure. J. Lab. Clin. Med. 45 (1955) 371.

17. Carr, E.A.Jr., W.H. Beierwaltes, M.E. Patno, J. D. Jr. Bartlett, A.V. Wegst: The detection of experimental myocardial infarcts by photoscanning. Am. Heart. J. 64 (1962) 650.

18. Kawana, M., H. Krizek, J. Porter, K.A. Lathrop, D. Charleston, P.V. Harper: Use of 199-Tl as a potassium analog in scanning. J. Nucl. Med. 11 (1970) 333.

19. Lebowitz, E., M.W. Greene, P. Bradley-Moore, H. Atkins, A. Ansari, P. Richards, E. Belgrave: 201-Tl. for medical use. J. Nucl. Med. 14 (1973) 421.

20. Schelbert, H.E., M.E. Phelps: Physiologic tomography. A new means for the non-invasive measurement of myocardial metabolism, blood flow and function. Europ. Nucl. Med. 5 (1980) 209.

21. Freundlieb, C.H., A. Hoeck, K. Vyska, L.E. Feinendegen, H.J. Machulla, G. Stoecklin: Use of 17-C-123-I-labelled heptadecanoic acid for noninvasively measuring myocardiac metabolism. Proceed. 15th international annual meeting of the Society of Nuclear Medicine (1977) 216.

22. Rigo, P., P.O. Alderson, R.M. Robertson, L.C. Becker, H.N. Wagner: Measurement of aortic and mitral regurgitation by gated cardiac blood pool scans. Circulation 60 (1979) 306.

23. Geffers, H., M. Stauch: Assessment of regurgitation fraction by radionuclide ventriculography. Z. Kardiol. 68 (1979) 491.

24. Levenson, N.I., R.J. Adolph, D.W. Romhilt, M. Gabel, V.J. Sodd, L.S. August: Effects of myocardial hypoxia and ischemia on myocardial scintigraphy. Am. J. Cardiol. 35 (1975) 251.

25. Adam, W.E., H. Sigel, H. Geffers, H. Kampmann, F. Bitter, M. Stauch: Analyse der regionalen Wandbewegung des linken Ventrikels bei koronarer Herzerkrankung durch ein nichtinvasives Verfahren Radionuklid-Kinematographie. Z. Kardiol. 66 (1977) 445.

26. Adam, W.E., A. Tarkowska, F. Bitter, M. Stauch, H. Geffers: Equilibrium (gated) radionuclide ventriculography. Cardiovascular Radiology 2 (1979) 161.

27. Geffers. H., H. Sigel, F. Bitter, H. Kampmann, M. Stauch, W.E. Adam: Untersuchungen der segmentalen Wandbewegung des linken Ventrikels bei Herzgesunden und Myokardinfarktpatienten mit einer katheterlosen nuklearmedizinischen Methode (Kamera-Kinematographie

des Herzens). Z. Kardiol. 65 (1976) 680.

28. Noelpp, U., N. Schad, H. Rösler: Trendszinti-graphie. J. Nucl. Med. 16 (1977) 232.

29. Goris, M.L.: Non interactive identification of the left ventricular area. Proceed. Nuclear Cardiology, selected computer aspects, Published by SNM (1978) 139-145.

30. Holmann, B.L., J. Wynne, J. Idoine, J. Zielonka, J. Neill: The paradox image a noninvasive index of regional left-ventricular dyskinesis. J. Nucl. Med. 20 (1979) 1237.

31. Bossuyt, A., F. Deconinck, R.L. Lepoudre et al.: The temporal Fourier transform applied to functional isotopic imaging. Proceed. 6. Int. Conference on information processing in Medical Imaging, Paris (1979)

32. Verba, J.W., I. Bornstein, N.P. Alazraki, A. Taylor, V. Bhargava, R. Shabetai, M. Le Winter: A new computer program for the extraction of global and regional behaviour of all four cardiac chambers from gated radionuclide data. J. Nucl. Med. 20 (1979) 665.

33. Kisslo, J.A.: Nuklearmedizinische Methoden in der Kardiologie. Z. Kardiol. 67 (1978) 428-441.

34. Robb, R., E. Ritman, E. H. Wood: Cardiovascular imaging and image processing (D.C. Harrison, Ed.) SPIE, Palos Verdes Estates, California (1975) 183-194.

35. Brennecke, R., T.K. Brown, J. Bürsch, P.H. Heintzen: Digital processing of videoangiocardiography image series using a minicomputer. Computers in Cardiology, Long Beach, California: IEEE Computer Society (1976) 255.

36. Brennecke, R., H.J. Hahne, K. Moldenhauer, J.H. Bürsch, P.H. Heintzen: A special purpose processor for digital angiocardiography design and applications. Computers in Cardiology. (1979) 343-346.

37. Kress, P., F. Bitter, M. Stauch, N.W. Garvie, W. Nechwatal, H. Sigel, W.E. Adam: Radionuclide ventriculography: a noninvasive method for the detection and quantification of left-to right shunts in atrial septal defect. Shunt diagnosis by radionuclide ventriculography. Clin. Cardiol., in print.

38. Rigo, P., P.O. Alderson, R.M. Robertson, L.C. Becker, H.N. Wagner: Measurement of aortic and mitral regurgitation by gated cardiac blood pool scans. Circulation. 60 (1979) 306

39. Kress, P., H. Geffers, M. Stauch, W. Nechwatal, H. Sigel, F. Bitter, W.E. Adam: Evaluation of aortic and mitral valve regurgitation by radionuclide ventri--culography: comparison with the method of Sandler and Dodge. Clin. Cardiol. 4 (1981) 5-10.

480

40. Lieppe, W., R. Scallion, V.S. Behar, J.A.Kisslo: Detection of tricuspid regurgitation with 2-D echocardiography and peripheral vein injection. Circulation 57 (1978) 128.

41. Johnson, S.L., D.W. Backer, A.R. Lute, H.T. Dodge: Doppler echocardiography: The localization of cardiac murmurs. Circulation. 48 (1973) 810.

42. Gould, K.L., K. Lipscomb: Effects of coronary stenoses on coronary flow reserve and resistance. Am. J. Cardiol. 34 (1974) 48

43. Proudfit, W.L. L.K. Shirey, F.M. Sones: Selective cine coronary angiography: Correlation with clinical findings in 1000 patients. Circulation 33 (1966) 901.

44. Pohost, G.M. et al.: Thallium redistribution: Mechanisms and clinical utility. Sem. Nucl. Med. 10 (1980) 70.

45. Simoons, M.L., P.G. Hugenholtz: Value and limitations of exercise testing in coronary artery disease. Proceed. Int. Symposium Dubrovnik (1980).

46) Sauer, E., H. Sebening: Myokard- und Ventrikel-szintigraphie. Mannheim (1980).

47. Loogen, F., B. Lösse: Comparative study between thallium scintigraphy and coronary angiography. Proceed. Int. Symposion Dubrovnik (1980).

48. Hör, G., N. Kanemoto: 201 Tl scintigraphy: Curvent status in coronary artery disease. Nucl.Med. (in print).

49. Borer, J.S. et al.: Real time radionuclide cineangiography in the non invasive evaluation of global and regional left ventricular function at rest and during exercise in patients with coronary artery disease. N. Engl. J. Med. 296 (1977) 839.

50. Caldwell, J.H., G.W. Hamilton et al.: The detection of coronary artery disease by radionuclide techniques: A comparison of rest exercise thallium imaging and ejection fraction response. Circulation 61 (1980) 610.

51. Bodenheimer, M.M.et al.: Comparison of wall motion and regional ejection fraction at rest and during isometric exercise. J. Nucl. Med. 20 (1979) 724.

52. Wackers, F.J.: Myocardial imaging in the coronary care unit. The Hague, Boston, London (1980).

53. Taylor, G.J. et al.: Predictors of clinical course, coronary anatomy and left ventricular function after recovery from acute myocardial infarction. Circulation 62 (1980) 960.

54. Frais, M.A. E. Botvinick, J. O'Connel, D. Shosa, M. Scheinman, R. Hattner: The phase image: an accurate means of detecting and localizing abnormal foci of ventricular activation. Proceedings of the 28th annual

meeting of the Society of Nuclear Medicine (1981) 18.

55. Byrom, E., S. Swiryn, D. Pavel, C. Meyer-Pavel, B. Handler, K. Rosen: Correlation of phase image pattern with various cardiac activation patterns induced by pacing. Proceedings of the 28th annual meeting of the Society of Nuclear Medicine (1981) 18.

56. Fossel, E., J. DeLayre, J. Ingwal: P^{31} NMR measurements. Abstracts of Journal of Computer Assisted Tomography (1981).

57. Scott, K., H. Brooker, J. Fitzsimmons: Phosphorus nuclear magnetic resonance: potential application to diagnostic chemistry. Abstracts of Journal of Computer Assisted Tomography (1981).

58. Nolan, N.G., J. Lindsay: The radionuclide cardiac ventriculogram. Eur. J. Nucl. Med. (1980) 4o7-410.

UTILITY OF RADIONUCLIDE STUDIES IN PATIENTS WITH PULMONARY VASCULAR AND AIRWAYS DISEASES

Philip O. Alderson, M.D.

Professor of Radiology
College of Physicians and Surgeons
Columbia University
New York, NY
U.S.A.

Radionuclide studies aid the diagnosis of pulmonary diseases by providing information about regional pulmonary ventilation, perfusion and ventilation-perfusion (V-P) relationships which cannot be obtained by other methods. Ventilation-perfusion lung studies are used to evaluate regional lung function in patients prior to pulmonary surgery, to detect obstructive airways disease and to aid management of patients with suspected pulmonary embolism. The following sections will discuss each of these subjects in detail.

TECHNICAL FACTORS

Perfusion

Pulmonary perfusion is usually assessed following the intravenous injection of radiolabeled particles. The most commonly used radio-pharmaceuticals are Tc-99m labeled macroaggregates of albumin (MAA) or human albumin microspheres (HAM) (Table 1). These Tc-99m labeled particles lodge in the pulmonary arterioles or capillaries and allow the relative distribution of pulmonary perfusion to be assessed by radionuclide imaging. Nonparticulate perfusion lung imaging agents like Xe-133 in saline and Kr-81m in glucose have also been used.

Table 1

	Perfusion Lung Imaging Agents		
Agent	Physical Half-Life	Principal Photon Energy (keV)	Particle Size (microns)
Tc-99m MAA	6 hrs	140	10-60
Tc-99m HAM	8 hrs	140	10-30
Xe-133 in saline	5.2 days	80	-
Xe-127 in saline	36.4 days	203, 172 (375)	-
Kr-81m in glucose	13 sec	190	-

The standard perfusion lung imaging examination consists of anterior, posterior and both lateral views. Oblique perfusion images are a useful addition (1-3). Caride et al. (1) showed that significantly more perfusion defects were seen when the left and right posterior oblique views (LPO, RPO) were added to the four standard views. Nielson et al. (2) demonstrated similarly improved capabilities with posterior oblique views. In our laboratory the four standard views plus all four oblique views (LAO, RAO, RPO, LPO) are routinely obtained.

Ventilation

The predominant method for assessing pulmonary ventilation in the USA is Xe-133 imaging. This review will emphasize data obtained using Xe-133 in V-P studies. Recently, other inert gases like Kr-81m have also been used. The properties of these agents are shown in Table 2.

Table 2

	Radioactive Gases for Ventilation Imaging	
Agent	Physical Half-Life	Principal Photon Energy (keV)
Xe-133	5.2 days	80
Xe-127	36.4 days	203, 172 (375)
Kr-81m	13 sec	190

The relatively low energy of Xe-133 is disadvantageous, as emitted photons undergo scatter which degrades image quality. The 80 keV energy is also below that of the perfusion tracer, so there is down scatter from the photons present in the patient if the ventilation study follows the perfusion study. There are several different breathing maneuvers which may be used to administer Xe-133 gas to patients.

These include the single breath inhalation and tidal breathing to equilibrium. The single breath study is effort-dependent. The distribution of the tracer is greatly affected by the speed of inhalation and the volume of the lung at the beginning of the single breath (4). Clinically, patients are directed to initiate the single breath from functional residual capacity and take a slow and steady inhalation. The ability of the patient to cooperate is less important when using tidal breathing to equilibrium for delivery of the tracer. Most patients with obstructive pulmonary disease only approach equilibrium during this phase, but this approximation is used as the beginning point for the clearance phase. During the clearance phase (washout) the patient breathes room air and the exhaled Xe-133 is vented from the room or trapped in a lead-lined charcoal-filled container. Xenon-133 has a physical half-life that is long relative to pulmonary clearance times, so areas of abnormally slow washout, i.e., regions of obstructive airways disease, are detected as regions of retained activity. This retention is evidence of two of the hallmarks of obstructive lung disease, uneven ventilation and slow ventilation.

The physical properties of Kr-81m are compared with Xe-133 in Table 2. Its energy exceeds that of Tc-99m, so ventilation imaging can be performed after the perfusion study without fear of image degradation. Krypton-81m has only a 13 second half-life and is produced from a 4.5 hour half-life Rb-81 generator. The generator can be used for only one day. Krypton-81m decays to undetectable levels as the image of ventilation is being made. Thus, the image reflects the regional distribution of tidal breathing and does not show regions of retained activity during the clearance phase. Krypton-81m became commercially available in the USA late in 1980, but has been used in Europe for several years. It allows the acquisition of ventilation images in multiple projections at a substantially lower radiation dose to the patient than received from a standard Xe-133 study. The major disadvantages of Kr-81m at present are its expense and its lack of availability in certain areas.

Another approach to ventilation imaging is the use of radiolabeled aerosol particles. These particles are deposited by impaction or sedimentation on the bronchial mucosa (particles 1-10 microns in diameter), or by random contact with bronchial or alveolar walls during diffusion (particles less than one micron in diameter). The range of particle sizes in the inhaled aerosol is an important determinant of their regional distribution. The radioaerosols originally used in clinical nuclear medicine were produced in ultrasonic generators and had a wide range of particle sizes. Recently, the late George

Taplin and his colleagues (5) introduced a simple way for generating aerosols with relatively uniform particle size for clinical use. The system requires the interposition of a "settling bag" between the aerosol generator and the patient. First, the aerosol generator delivers the aerosol into the settling bag. In the settling chamber the larger particles stick to the sides of the bag. The generator portion of the system is then clamped shut, and the patient inhales the smaller particles from the settling bag. This type of aerosol shows good peripheral penetration and helps minimize the central hot spot deposition pattern which has been a frequent problem in clinical radioaerosol studies (5, 6). Taplin has recommended the use of Tc-99m DTPA for labeling these aerosol particles. This radiopharmaceutical is widely available and clears rapidly from the body. Indium-113m has been used for the same purpose in Europe (F. Fazio, personal communication). Aerosol systems may become more widely used for clinical lung imaging in hospitals where inert gases are unavailable.

Clinical ventilation-perfusion studies can be obtained in analog or digital formats. In either format, it is best to combine ventilation and perfusion imaging. The nonspecificity of defects seen in perfusion lung images has been recognized for several years (7). Perfusion defects are commonly seen secondary to pulmonary emboli, in areas of parenchymal lung consolidation or compression and in regions of obstructive pulmonary disease. The hypoperfusion in regions of airways disease occurs by reflex vasoconstriction of pulmonary vessels and can be considered an attempt by the lung to retain normal ventilation-perfusion balance. The appearance of a perfusion defect does not indicate whether it is caused by emboli, airways disease or some other pulmonary problem. Approximately 80% of emboli appear as defects conforming to known bronchial pulmonary segmental anatomy, but 20% are nonsegmental. Conversely, roughly 80% of defects secondary to airways disease are nonsegmental, with only 20% of defects appearing segmental (8). The latter defects usually occur in areas of moderate to severe obstructive airways disease. Because of this nonspecificity, combined V-P imaging is more specific for the diagnosis of pulmonary embolism than is perfusion imaging alone. This will be discussed later in the section on pulmonary embolism.

Widespread application of computer techniques to radionuclide studies has resulted in several approaches to quantitating regional lung function. These include the simple determination of the relative distribution of ventilation, determination of the Xe-133 clearance half-time, determination of the fractional exchange of air, or the analysis of Xe-133 clearance as a biexponential function (9). The fractional ex-

486

change of air is an index of the mean rate of change of the downslope of the pulmonary clearance time-activity curve. This approach takes into account both the early and late phases of clearance, thus including clearance of Xe-133 from the pulmonary "slow space" as well as that of the "fast space." In patients with obstructive lung disease the poorly ventilated "slow space" may comprise a large portion of the anatomic lung volume, though it contributes little to overall lung function. Thus, it is important to evaluate its contribution when quantitating regional ventilation.

Regional ventilation-perfusion ratios can also be calculated from radionuclide lung studies. There are two basic approaches to this calculation. The first is to compare the relative distribution of perfusion to the relative distribution of ventilation. The second is to compare some dynamic measure of regional ventilation, such as the fractional exchange of air, to the relative distribution of perfusion. These various parameters are usually normalized to regional lung volume so that all figures are presented as ventilation or perfusion per unit lung volume. Computers can then be used to produce analog images and quantitative maps of regional V-P ratios. Radionuclide lung studies are the only means for quantifying or visually displaying information about regional ventilation-perfusion balance. Clinical applications of quantitative lung studies will be discussed below.

CLINICAL APPLICATIONS

Surgical Lung Disease
Evaluation of pulmonary function is an important aspect of pre-operative care in patients who are to undergo many types of surgery. If the surgery involves resecting a portion of the lung, knowledge of regional pulmonary function becomes critical. In these patients quantitative radionuclide V-P studies provide important information. The value of differential radiospirometry in evaluating patients prior to pulmonary resection was pointed out by Svendberg (10) and later by Olson et al. (11, 12). Olson and his colleagues showed that accurate predictions of postoperative pulmonary function could be made by combining the results of routine preoperative spirometry and regional quantification of lung function by radionuclides. They showed a good correlation ($r = 0.72$, $p < .01$) between predicted postoperative and actual postoperative $FEV_{1.0}$ in 13 patients who had quantitative Tc-99m perfusion lung scanning and standard spirometry prior to operation. For example, if a patient had a forced expiratory volume in 1.0 sec (FEV) of 1.5 liter prior to surgery and was to undergo removal of his left lung, his post-

operative lung function could be predicted by multiplying his preoperative FEV by the percentage of total Tc-99m MAA activity located in his right lung. If this hypothetical patient had 80% of the Tc-99m MAA activity in his right lung, the predicted postoperative $FEV_{1.0}$ would be 1.2 liter (1.5 l x 0.8). Using the criteria that the overall pulmonary $FEV_{1.0}$ after surgery must be greater than 0.8 l, this patient could undergo resection. However, if this patient's right lung had contributed 50% or less of his overall function, he would have been unlikely to maintain adequate pulmonary function postoperatively. The ability of a ventilation-perfusion study to reveal regional V-P balance is also important. If the region being considered for resection shows V-P imbalance, the decision to operate is strengthened because the area is either contributing to systemic hypoxemia or wasted ventilation in the patient.

Some authors have suggested that V-P lung imaging has a role in the detection of early lung cancer. The recent work of Katz et al. (13) helps resolve this issue. They obtained V-P lung images in a series of patients who had been intensively screened for several years to detect lung cancer. Their results suggest that the lung scan has limited utility in the early detection of lung cancer. Perfusion and ventilation defects were often present in regions of surgically confirmed lung cancer, but no characteristic scintigraphic pattern was found. In addition, most patients had multiple regions of abnormal ventilation and perfusion remote from the lung cancer. This occurred because of the high prevalence of obstructive airways disease in the population. Another 27 patients underwent surgery for suspected lung cancer but were proven to have benign lung disease. The V-P abnormalities in this group could not be distinguished from those in the patients with lung cancer. Thirteen patients in the study had radiographically occult lung cancer. In one of these patients a segmental perfusion defect and abnormal ventilation were present distal to the tumor, and the rest of the lung was relatively normal. Thus, V-P lung imaging helped localize the radiographically occult lung cancer. However, in the other patients with radiographically occult lesions the lung scan added little. The results of this study suggest the role of V-P lung imaging in the patient with lung cancer should be reserved for preoperative quantification of regional pulmonary function.

Detection of Obstructive Airways Disease

Theoretically, the ability of radionuclide V-P studies to evaluate regional pulmonary function makes them well suited for early and sensitive detection of obstructive airways disease. Even the most sophisticated tests of overall lung function, such as flow-volume loops, closing volume, and frequency dependence of compliance do not allow

localization of regional airways disease. Xenon-133 ventilation studies
are more sensitive than radiographs in detecting and localizing obstructive airways disease. In one study (14), radiographs failed to reveal
obstructive airways disease in 40% of patients who had clearly abnormal
Xe-133 ventilation studies. Correlation with pulmonary function tests
in these patients confirmed that those with normal radiographs and abnormal Xe-133 studies had mild abnormalities on standard spirometry.
Patients who had abnormal radiographs and abnormal ventilation studies
had significantly more severe spirometric abnormalities (Table 3).

Table 3

Pulmonary Function* in Patients with Xe-133 Evidence of Obstructive
Lung Disease

Chest Radiograph	Vital Capacity	Forced Expiratory Volume(1.0 sec)	Maximum Mid-expiratory Flow (L/sec)
Normal (n=10)	69 ± 17	59 ± 18	42 ± 23
Obstructive lung disease (n=14)	49 ± 19	35 ± 14	18 ± 7

*Results expressed as mean percent of predicted normal value $\pm$ stan-
dard deviation. All values in group with abnormal radiographs
significantly ($p < 0.005$) worse than in those with normal x-rays.

These data suggest that Xe-133 imaging is able to detect mild airways disease which is undetected radiographically. This seems logical,
since severe airways disease is probably necessary to create morpho-
logic abnormalities which can be detected radiographically. Several
small studies have also assessed the relative sensitivity of Xe-133
imaging and spirometric tests like closing volume and frequency dependence of compliance. The results are inconclusive at this time, but
suggest that ventilation imaging with inert gases can detect airways
disease with a sensitivity comparable to or greater than these spirometric approaches.

The equilibrium phase of Xe-133 imaging is less likely to detect
regional airways abnormalities than the single breath inhalation or washout phase (15). The washout phase is the most sensitive portion of a
Xe-133 study for detecting regional abnormalities which match regional
perfusion defects. The washout phase has several advantages. First,
serial images over several minutes time can be obtained. Secondly,
washout is not effort-dependent. Third, it detects abnormal regions
as retained activity in a field of background activity. This ability to

detect abnormalities as a "hot spot in a cold field" aids sensitivity. However, all portions of the washout phase do not provide clear separation between normal areas and areas of obstructive airways disease. Retention of Xe-133 for the first two minutes of washout can be seen in normals. However, localized Xe-133 retention seen three minutes or later into the washout study is strong evidence of regional obstructive airways disease. In our laboratory, washout is continued for at least five minutes, and often seven minutes. Images are obtained for a fixed time of 60 seconds during this washout phase. This allows the regional Xe-133 retention time to be subjectively judged by inspecting the images and also provides good evidence for regional differences in clearance rate. Washout images are routinely obtained in three projections: posterior, RPO and LPO. The routine addition of oblique washout images allows better localization of sites of airways disease, especially when they are in the anterior portions of the lung (16, 17).

Pulmonary Embolism

The utility of V-P imaging in the evaluation of patients with suspected pulmonary embolism (PE) is controversial. The role of the lung scan in evaluating these patients was questioned by Robin (18). He stated that lung scans may be used to exclude pulmonary embolism, but suggested that angiography was required to diagnose the condition with a certainty that would allow therapy. The data base for Robin's assertions is quite tenuous. He cites his own clinical experience at Stanford, the urokinase-streptokinase pulmonary embolism study (USPES) and data on ventilation alterations which occur with acute pulmonary vascular occlusion. Robin's experience at Stanford is controversial. McDougall, Goris and Kriss (19) feel that the Stanford lung scan-angiographic data have been misinterpreted by Robin. The USPES data offer little support. None of the USPES patients had ventilation studies, most were scanned with I-131 macroaggregates, half of them had only anterior and posterior perfusion images and all were done on rectilinear scanners. These techniques are outdated and the scan results obtained cannot be compared to current clinical V-P imaging. In addition, the goal of the lung scan panelists in the USPES trial was not to diagnose pulmonary embolism. Each patient in the trial was known to have PE. Categorization of the scans as high, medium or low probability was done informally and was not an official part of the trial. Nevertheless, Robin relied to a large extent on this data base and continues to do so. He has recently stated (20) that ventilation imaging as an adjunct to perfusion scanning "leads to unacceptable errors," though he has no new data on which to base that statement. He has also stated (20) that 60% of patients with suspected PE need pulmonary angiography. This is a much higher number than the proportion (15-25%) that undergo angiography in most major institutions in the USA.

Recent data indicate that V-P lung imaging has excellent predictive
value in patients with suspected PE. Biello (21) found positive and
negative predictive values greater than 0.90 in a large series of patients
with angiographically confirmed diagnoses (Table 4).

Table 4
Ventilation-Perfusion Lung Imaging in Diagnosis
of Pulmonary Embolism

Scan Diagnosis	N	PE by Angio	%PE
High probability	26	24	92
Nondiagnostic	80	28	35
Low probability	40	1	2.5
TOTAL	146	53	36

Another series (22) evaluated the problem of coexistent airways disease
and PE. In the presence of widespread obstructive lung disease, it is
difficult to determine whether perfusion defects are caused by local reactive vasoconstriction secondary to alveolar hypoxia or whether they
are secondary to pulmonary emboli. Moderate to severe obstructive
lung disease can cause segmental perfusion defects simply due to this
reactive vasoconstriction. Because of the common coexistence of obstructive airways disease in pulmonary embolism, it is necessary to
assess V-P match and mismatch for each perfusion defect. Some
authors (23) have stated that patients showing areas of V-P match plus
areas of V-P mismatch should be placed in a nondiagnostic category.
However, this does not seem necessary (22). When two or more segmental or subsegmental areas of V-P mismatch are present in a patient
with clinically suspected pulmonary embolism, the case can be designated high probability even if other areas of V-P match are present.
When the obstructive airways disease (OPD) causes Xe-133 abnormalities
in 50% or less of the visible lung fields, V-P imaging is as accurate as if
no ventilation abnormalities existed (Table 5).

Table 5
V-P Imaging in Patients with Limited OPD*(n=67)

V-P Scan	Results of Angiography	
	PE+	PE-
High probability	19	3
Low probability	1	44

*Obstructive pulmonary disease

There are certain pitfalls to V-P imaging which must be remember-
ed. The first is the differential diagnosis of V-P mismatch. V-P mismatch is not synonymous with pulmonary thromboembolism. V-P mismatch can occur with other types of emboli, such as fat, air or foreign
body emboli. More importantly, V-P mismatch can occur secondary to
pulmonary vasculitis. This may occur in any of the rheumatoid variants,
such as systemic lupus, polyarteritis nodosa, or rheumatoid arthritis.
It can also occur in sarcoidosis and tuberculosis. Thus, one must be
particularly skeptical of a PE diagnosis when an isolated apical ventilation-perfusion mismatch is found in a patient who has a past history of
tuberculosis. Such a mismatch can occur even when the radiograph does
not reveal classical findings of tuberculosis. In addition, vasculitis is
probably in part responsible for the perfusion defects seen in chronic,
idiopathic pulmonary hypertension. The perfusion deficits in these
patients are usually associated with normal ventilation and can simulate
pulmonary emboli. Patients with mitral stenosis also have nonembolic
perfusion deficits which are associated with normal ventilation. Rare
congenital abnormalities such as peripheral coarctations of the pulmonary
arteries or other abnormalities secondary to congenital heart disease or
its surgical correction can also cause V-P mismatch. In addition, the
obliterative vasculitis which occurs following localized thoracic irradiation can cause a V-P mismatch. Thus, one must be constantly aware of
the clinical situation and not overextend a "high probability" reading in a
patient with these conditions.

Another theoretical pitfall of V-P imaging is reactive bronchocon-
striction following pulmonary embolism. This phenomenon clearly
occurs in experimental animals, but caused Xe-133 abnormalities in only
two of 136 (1.5%) regions containing experimentally-induced emboli in
dogs (3). When assessing the possibility of this phenomenon in patients,
it is important to distinguish matched ventilation and perfusion abnormalities from abnormal (but unmatched) ventilation-perfusion abnormalities which occur in the same region. For example, segmental perfusion
defects can occur secondary to moderate-severe obstructive airways
disease, but not secondary to mild airways disease. Thus, if a segmental perfusion defect is associated with mild Xe-133 retention (e.g., seen
only through a 3-minute washout image) this is V-P mismatch. In addition, it is useful to recall that bronchial constriction secondary to
emboli persists only several hours and seems to require large central
vascular occlusions. Since this phenomenon is infrequent and transient,
it is not likely to be a major clinical problem. However, it should be
considered when patients are studied shortly after the onset of symptoms
suggesting pulmonary embolism. In this regard, any patient who is
wheezing when referred to the lung scanning laboratory should not be

studied. Bronchospasm, whether on the basis of asthma, congestive failure, emboli, etc., can cause multiple segmental perfusion defects and a confusing scintigraphic picture. If a patient is wheezing, the lung scan should be delayed until the next day or until the wheezing has abated.

Since currently available data demonstrate that the sensitivity and specificity of V-P imaging for pulmonary embolism is on the order of 90%, one might wonder why a controversy exists about the utility of V-P imaging in patients with suspected pulmonary embolism. There is general agreement that the clinical diagnosis of pulmonary embolism is extremely difficult even with the help of laboratory tests and the chest radiograph. The pulmonary angiogram is a definitive diagnostic procedure, but should not be used indiscriminately. Arguments in favor of using the pulmonary angiogram to minimize uncertainty in the diagnosis of pulmonary embolism are based on arguments that heparin is responsible for a high rate of drug-related morbidity. However, angiography also has risks. Kelly and Elliot (24) cite a death rate during angiography of between 4 and 5 per 1,000. Indiscriminate use of angiography to replace indiscriminate use of heparin carries an increased risk of mortality and this may be increased further when angiography is performed without the expertise available in a major medical center. For these reasons, neither heparin nor the pulmonary angiogram should be used indiscriminately.

As indicated above, the lung scan occupies an important position in evaluation of the patient with suspected pulmonary emboli. Even though it is not a definitive test, it helps the clinician estimate the probability of PE. The V-P lung scan should be perceived as an aid to clinicians in making a management decision, rather than as a definitive diagnostic procedure. If a patient with suspected pulmonary embolism has a normal V-P lung scan, clinically significant emboli are excluded. If a lung scan is abnormal and shows regions of V-P mismatch which suggest emboli, the patient is categorized as having a high probability scan. When patients in this group are otherwise healthy, have no contraindications to anticoagulant therapy, do not have a history of past emboli, and are not being considered for surgical therapy of embolism, they are usually anticoagulated without corroboration of their disease by angiography.

If the patient has an abnormal lung scan with small, unimpressive defects, or larger perfusion defects demonstrating V-P match, he is considered to have a low probability for pulmonary embolism. In otherwise healthy patients with no obvious source for repeated emboli, no treatment is given and these patients do not undergo angiography. However, if these patients are at high risk for repeated emboli (e.g., active deep vein phlebitis is present), then angiography should be considered. In addition, these patients may undergo angiography if the clinical suspicion of PE is especially high.

If a patient has a nondiagnostic lung scan (e.g., perfusion defects and corresponding radiographic opacities of equal size or widespread airways disease), other studies are usually obtained. If emboli are strongly suspected, these patients go on to angiography. However, another alternative is to investigate the venous system. In our institution this usually means contrast venography, impedance plethysmography and/or Doppler ultrasound studies. Radionuclide venography and the fibrinogen uptake test are other suitable alternatives, but these are not commonly employed at our institution. If the study of the venous system is normal, the patient is followed without additional therapy. If venous disease is present, the patient will usually be anticoagulated and a repeat lung scan will be obtained 4-5 days to evaluate possible change in the perfusion pattern. Substantial resolution of perfusion defects during that time period increases the probability that they were caused by emboli.

SUMMARY

Quantitative V-P studies provide important regional lung function information in patients who are to undergo pulmonary surgery. However, V-P studies have limited utility in early detection of lung cancer and will probably not replace spirometry as screening procedures for early detection of airways disease. The major role of V-P imaging is in evaluating patients with suspected pulmonary embolism. Current data demonstrate that the predictive value of V-P imaging is excellent even when many types of coexistent lung disease are present. Thus, it can provide a useful aid to the clinician in making management decisions about patients suspected of having pulmonary embolism.

REFERENCES

1. Caride V. J., Puri S., Slaven J. D., et al. "The usefulness of the posterior oblique views in perfusion lung imaging." Radiology 121 (1976) 669-671.

2. Nielsen P. E., Kirchner P. T., Gerber F. H. "Oblique views in lung perfusion imaging and selective pulmonary angiography in animals with experimental pulmonary embolism." J Nucl Med 18 (1978) 967-973.

3. Alderson P. O., Doppman J. L., Diamond S. S. et al. "Ventilation-perfusion imaging and selective pulmonary angiography in animals with experimental pulmonary embolism." J Nucl Med 19 (1978) 164-171.

4. Bake B., Wood L., Murphy B. et al. "Effects of inspiratory flow rate on regional distribution of inspired gas." J Appl Physiol 37 (1974) 8-17.

5. Taplin G. V., Chopra S. K. : "Lung perfusion-inhalation scintigraphy in obstructive airway disease and pulmonary embolism." Radiol Clin N Amer 16 (1978) 491-513.

6. Greening A. P., Miniati M., Fazio F. "Regional deposition of aerosols in health and in airways obstruction: A comparison with Krypton-81m ventilation scanning." Bull Europ Physiopath Resp 16 (1980) 287-298.

7. Poulouse K. P., Reba R. C., Wagner H. N. Jr. "Characterization of the shape and location of perfusion defects in certain pulmonary diseases." N Engl J Med 279 (1968) 1020-1025.

8. Alderson P. O., Rujanavech N., Secker-Walker R. H. et al. "The role of Xe-133 ventilation studies in the scintigraphic detection of pulmonary embolism." Radiology 120 (1976) 633-640.

9. Alderson P. O. "The role of radionuclide studies in the diagnosis of pulmonary disease." In: Siegelman S., Ed., Multiple Imaging Procedures. Vol 1, Pulmonary System, Grune & Stratton, New York, 1979, 49-67.

10. Svendberg L. "Bronchospirometry in the study of regional lung function." Scand J Resp Dis 62 (Suppl) (1966) 91-102.

11. Olsen G. N., Block A. J., Tobias J. A. "Prediction of post pneumonectomy pulmonary function using quantitative macroaggregate lung scanning." Chest 66 (1974) 13-16.

12. Olsen G. N., Block A. J., Swenson E. W. et al. "Pulmonary function evaluation of the lung resection candidate: A prospective study." Am Rev Resp Dis 111 (1975) 379-387.

13. Katz R. D., Alderson P. O., Tochman M. S., et al. "Ventilation-perfusion lung imaging in early detection of lung cancer." Radiology, in press.

14. Alderson P. O. Secker-Walker R. H., Forrest J. V. "Detection of obstructive pulmonary disease. Relative sensitivity of ventilation-perfusion studies and chest radiography." Radiology 112 (1974) 643-648.

15. Alderson P. O., Lee H., Summer W. R. et al. "Comparison of Xe-133 washout and single-breath imaging for the detection of ventilation abnormalities." J Nucl Med 20 (1979) 917-922.

16. Alderson P. O., Line B. R. "Scintigraphic evaluation of regional pulmonary ventilation." Sem Nucl Med 10 (1980) 218-242.

17. Liehn J. C., Farrand O., Jouet I. B. et al. "Regional pulmonary ventilation studies with multiple view late xenon washout images." Int J Nucl Med Biol 7 (1980) 319-325.

18. Robin E. D. "Overdiagnosis and overtreatment of pulmonary embolism: The emperor may have no clothes." Ann Int Med 87 (1977) 775-781.

19. McDougall I. R., Goris M. L., Kriss J. P. "Letter to the editor." Ann Int Med 88 (1978) 711.

20. Robin E. D. "Diagnostic management of pulmonary embolism. Thrombos Hemostas 46 (1981) 250 (abstract).

21. Biello D. R., Mattar A. G., McKnight R. C., Siegel B. A. "Ventilation-perfusion studies in patients with suspected pulmonary embolism." Am J Roentgenol 133 (1979) 1033-1037.

22. Alderson P.O. , Biello D.R. , Sachariah K.G. , Siegel B.A. "Scintigraphic detection of pulmonary embolism in patients with obstructive pulmonary disease." Radiology 138 (1981) 661-666.

23. McNeil B.J. "Ventilation-perfusion studies and diagnosis of pulmonary embolism." J Nucl Med 21 (1980) 319-323.

24. Kelley M.J. , Elliot L.P. "The radiologic evaluation of the patient with suspected pulmonary thromboembolic disease." Med Clin North Am 59 (1975) 3-36.

Part IX: The Results of Clinical Evaluation: Studies of the Abdomen and Pelvis

CLINICAL STUDIES OF THE ABDOMEN:
Scintigraphic and Other Techniques in the
Management of Patients with Abdominal Disease

Leon S. Malmud, M.D.
Professor and Chairman,
Department of Nuclear Medicine
Temple University School of Medicine
Philadelphia, PA   19140 (U.S.A.)

INTRODUCTION

Abdominal diseases are among the most frequent ailments which specialists in diagnostic imaging must examine. Imaging procedures, in order to be used most effectively, should complement the history, physical examination, and other laboratory tests in order to achieve the most accurate, rapid, and cost efficient diagnosis. The choice of diagnostic procedures currently available is greater than ever before. The selection of appropriate studies and the order in which they are performed may have a profound effect on diagnostic accuracy and clinical success. This chapter will deal primarily with scintigraphy of the abdomen as it relates to esophageal disorders, liver-spleen scintigraphy, gastroesophageal reflux, gastric emptying studies, hepatobiliary scintigraphy, and gastrointestinal bleeding studies, including the detection of Meckel's diverticulum.

Quantitative scintigraphy of upper gastrointestinal motor function represents a major advance in our ability to diagnose and investigate gastrointestinal disease and physiology. Most alternative methods are limited in that they are somewhat indirect, insensitive, invasive, or have poor patient acceptance. For example, roentgenographic contrast studies employing barium are somewhat insensitive to many subtle motor disturbances of the upper gastrointestinal tract, and the radiation burden to the patient from fluoroscopy may be significant. While most non-scintigraphic techniques are either semi or non-quantitative, scintigraphy permits quantitation using available gamma camera imaging and computer data processing of each sequential gamma camera digital image.

The use of in vivo radionuclide procedures to quantitate upper gastrointestinal function began in 1966 when Griffith and his associates employed orally administered Cr-51 radiolabeled material in order to quantitate gastric emptying, using a scintillation detector (1). The advantage of Griffith's technique in comparison to previous methods, was that the tracer procedure was tubeless, quantitatable, and associated with a low radiation burden. But early radionuclide methods were limited in accuracy in that they relied upon blind placement of the detector probe over the stomach. This problem was resolved partially by the use of the rectilinear scanner. Subsequently, the rectilinear scanner was replaced by the combination of a gamma camera and digital computer, which permitted continuous quantitative imaging of the stomach, or any other organ, so that time-function curves could be generated for rapid determination of the rate of gastric emptying (2,3). The problem of overestimation of gastric emptying rate, which had been due to dissociation of the radiolabel from the food ingested (with more rapid emptying of the label than of the food) has been resolved by techniques which firmly bind radioisotopes to food, such as Tc-99m sulfur colloid chicken liver (4).

In addition, new radiopharmaceuticals have been introduced for the study of hepatocystic function (5); and new applications of older established radiopharmaceuticals, such as Tc-99m sulfur colloid have been introduced (6-11). Employing modern nuclear medicine instrumentation and radiopharmaceuticals, techniques have been developed for the quantitation of esophageal transit and clearance (10,11), the detection and quantitation of gastroesophageal reflux (6,12,8), the detection and quantitation of enterogastric reflux (9), the simultaneous quantitation of the rate of gastric emptying of each component of a mixed liquid-solid meal (7), quantitation of gallbladder function (13), and lower gastrointestinal bleeding detection. This chapter deals with each of these techniques, in addition to liver scintigraphy.

ESOPHAGEAL SCINTIGRAPHY

As food enters the esophagus, peristalsis and gravity transport it to the esophagogastric junction. The movement of a swallowed bolus over the length of the esophagus is defined as esophageal transit, as distinguished from esophageal clearance, which is the emptying from the esophagus of material which has refluxed from the stomach. Many disorders of the esophagus are characterized by abnormal motor function. Yet, until the development of esophageal scintigraphic techniques, there had been no non-invasive, quantitative method to evaluate esophageal transit and clearance.

The non-scintigraphic techniques employed to study esophageal motor function include the barium cine-esophagogram, double contrast esophagram (14), the acid clearance test and esophageal manometry. Each of these techniques has significant limitations and none is quantitative. Although cine-esophagography is non-invasive, the radiation burden to the patient is large. The acid clearance test requires intubation with and placement of a pH electrode and at best it is semiquantitative. Esophageal manometry records intraluminal pressures. Correlation of esophageal motor activity with transit has not been established.

The double-contrast esophagram has become the routine radiographic procedure in many departments for patients undergoing an upper gastrointestinal examination (14). A liquid effervescent agent such as a Seidlitz solution is often used to cause esophageal distension. Citric acid or sodium bicarbonate solutions are alternative solutions used by some radiologists for double-contrast upper gastrointestinal examinations. The goal is to create a greater dilitation of the esophagus, and any effervescent agent is considered preferable to a full barium column.

The esophagus is most easily studied radiographically with the patient in an upright position for anatomic abnormalities. When esophageal atresia, aspiration or a tracheo-esophageal fistula is suspected, a barium sulfate suspension rather than a water-soluble iodinated contrast medium is employed in order to avoid the serious complications which can result from aspiration of a water-soluble hyperosmolar contrast agent (15). When esophageal perforation beneath the diaphragm is suspected barium sulfate is contraindicated and the water-soluble agents are used. If a motility disorder is suspected, then the patient is usually studied in both the upright and recumbent positions since gravity may obscure abnormal motility, although scintigraphy is both a more sensitive and specific procedure.

METHOD

Esophageal scintigraphy was developed as a sensitive and non-invasive method to quantitate the rate of esophageal emptying of a liquid bolus in patients with a variety of esophageal disorders. Esophageal scintigraphy is useful in patients with motor disorders of the esophagus such as achalasia, diffuse esophageal spasm, scleroderma and symptomatic gastroesophageal reflux.

Initially, the procedure was also performed in normal controls in order to establish normal criteria. The primary motor disorders of the esophagus were identified by manometric criteria and symptomatic gastroesophageal reflux was defined as heartburn in patients with gastroesophageal reflux demonstrated by gastroesophageal scintigraphy. Patients with reflux disease were

subdivided based on manometric findings into two groups with
normal and abnormal esophageal motor function.

Following an overnight fast, subjects are positioned supine
under the diverging collimator of a standard size gamma camera
with the imaging window set at 140 Kev $\pm$ 30%. Three hundred
microcuries of Tc-99m sulfur colloid, diluted in 15 ml of water,
is ingested through a sipping straw in a single swallow. Following this, the subjects are instructed to perform dry swallows on
command, at 15 second intervals for 10 minutes. Data are stored
in and processed by a dedicated nuclear medicine computer. An
esophageal area of interest is designated for the esophagus in
each patient using a light pen (Figure 1).

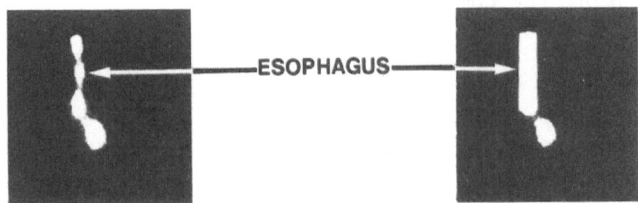

ESOPHAGEAL TRANSIT

**Counts per 15 second interval following serial swallows at
15 second intervals for 10 minutes.**

$$\frac{E_{max} - E_t}{E_{max}} \times 100$$

Figure 1

Esophageal scintigraph and esophageal area of interest for
quantitating esophageal clearance. Formula for calculating
esophageal clearance after either a single swallow or
multiple swallows is shown where E_{max} represents the maximal
count rate in the esophagus (immediately after the initial
swallow) and E_t the esophageal count rate at time t.

502

$$C_t = \frac{E_{max} - E_t}{E_{max}} \times 100$$

where C_t represents percent esophageal transit at time t;
E_{max}, represents the maximal count rate in the esophagus and
E_t, the esophageal count rate at time t. Esophageal emptying is determined by counting the esophageal activity for 15
seconds following successive swallows at 15-second intervals
for 10 minutes. The rate of esophageal emptying after a
single swallow is determined by counting esophageal activity
at one second intervals for 15 seconds after the initial
swallow.

In normal subjects, sequential esophageal activity decreases
rapidly. Within 4-10 seconds after the first swallow, the esophagus is usually not visualized on the gamma camera, but low
count rates were still detectable over the esophageal area of
interest using the computer (Figure 2).

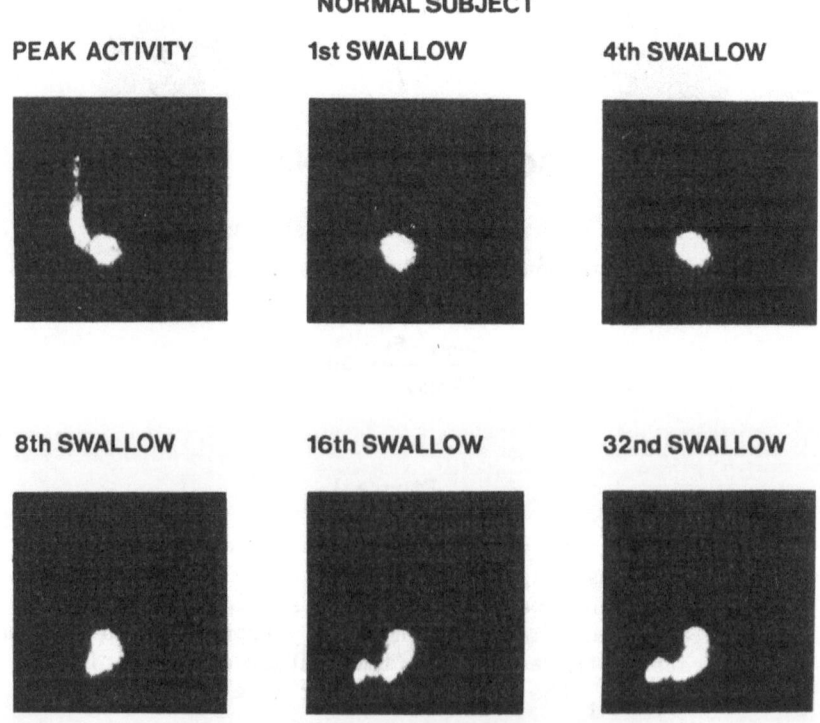

Figure 2
Esophageal transit after multiple swallows in a normal subject.

In marked contrast, patients with achalasia fail to clear activity from the esophagus for 10 minutes, despite continuous swallows at 15 second intervals (Figure 3).

ACHALASIA

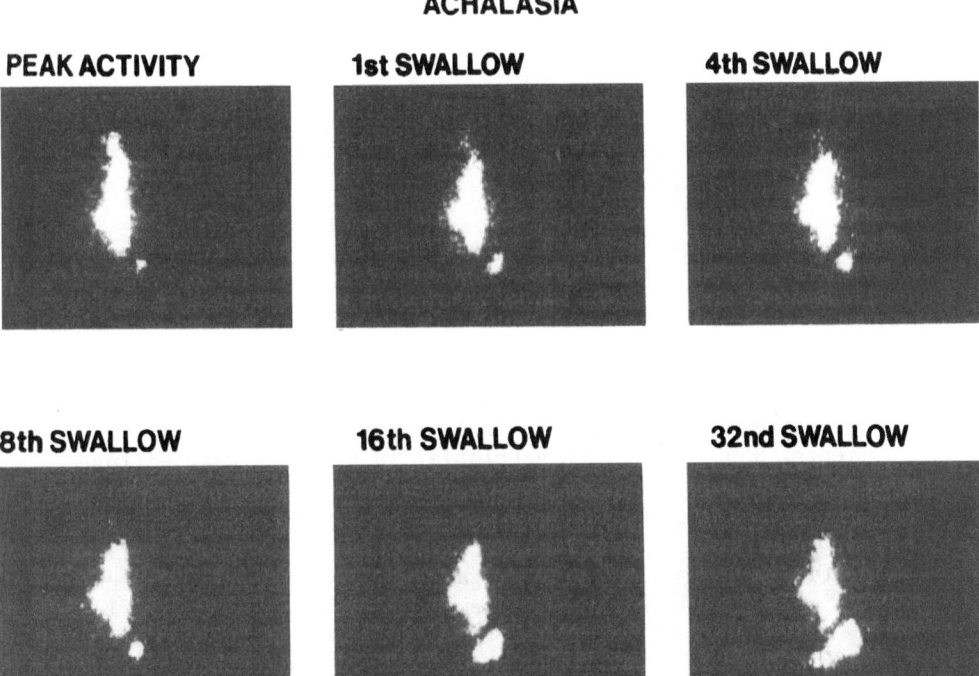

PEAK ACTIVITY   **1st SWALLOW**   **4th SWALLOW**

8th SWALLOW   **16th SWALLOW**   **32nd SWALLOW**

Figure 3
Esophageal transit scintigraphy in a patient with
achalasia. Note persistent esophageal activity
(delayed clearance) even after 32 swallows.

Esophageal emptying is diminished significantly throughout the study period in patients with both achalasia and scleroderma as compared to normal subjects (Figure 4). In the initial study, after 8 swallows, the emptying rates were $26.7 \pm 10.8\%$ in the achalasia patients ($P < 0.001$) and $23.6 \pm 14.6\%$ in patients with scleroderma ($P < .001$) compared with $92.8 \pm 1.2\%$ in normal subjects. After 40 swallows, esophageal emptying rates were $31.0 \pm 10.0\%$ ($P < .001$), $42.4 \pm 15.4\%$ ($P < .001$) and $95\% \pm 4.0\%$, respectively.

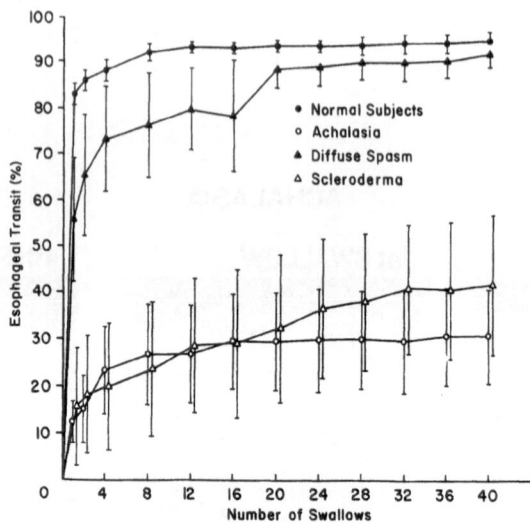

Figure 4
Esophageal transit after single swallow in 15 normal subjects, 8 patients with achalasia, 10 patients with diffuse
esophageal spasm and 5 patients with scleroderma. Each
point represents the mean ± SEM for esophageal transit.

Patients with diffuse esophageal spasm represent an intermediate group in whom esophageal emptying was reduced significantly during the first half of the study period but was normal
after 20 swallows. In patients with diffuse spasm, esophageal
emptying rates were 76.2 ± 11.4% (P < .05), 88.5 ± 3.8% (P > .05)
and 92.7 ± 3.0% (P > .05) after 8, 20, and 40 swallows respectively. The rates of esophageal emptying during the first 15
seconds following the initial swallow of the test bolus were
decreased significantly throughout the first 15 second test
period in all groups of patients with primary motor disorders of
the esophagus, including those with diffuse esophageal spasm
(Figure 5). In patients with symptomatic gastroesophageal
reflux, esophageal emptying rates after serial swallows are
diminished (Figure 6).

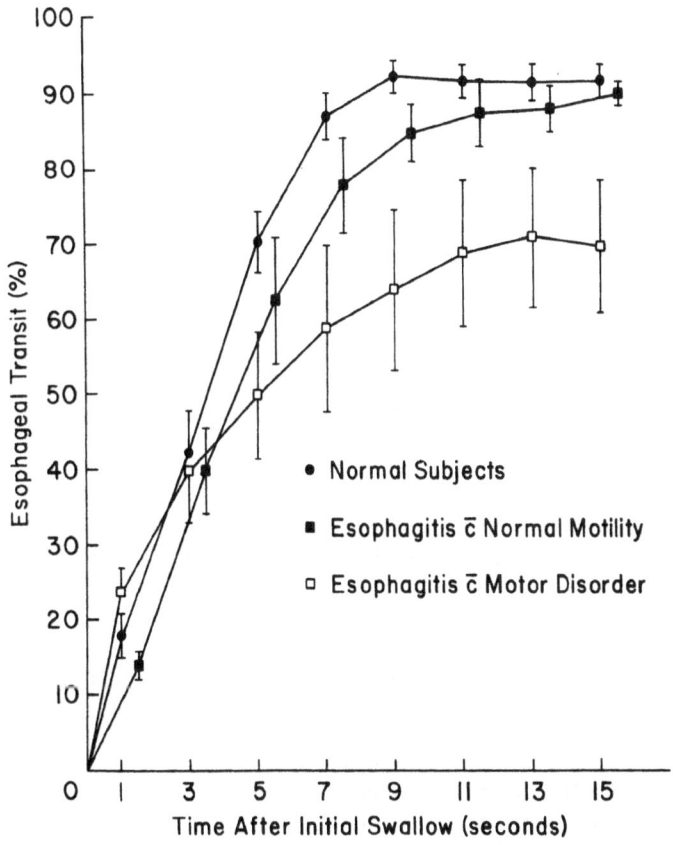

Figure 5
Esophageal transit after single swallow in 15 normal subjects, and patients with symptomatic gastroesophageal
reflux with and without a motor disorder of the esophagus.
Each point represents the mean ± SEM for esophageal transit.

506

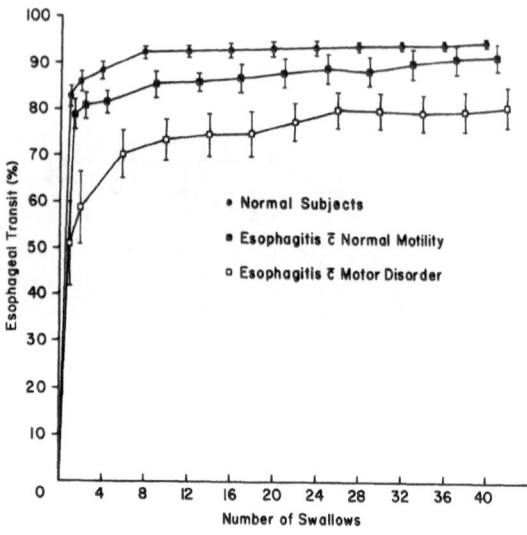

Figure 6

Esophageal transit after multiple swallows in 15 normal
subjects and patients with symptomatic gastroesophageal
reflux with and without a motor disorder of the esophagus.
Each point represents the mean ± SEM for esophageal transit.

The abnormality is more severe in those patients whose
reflux disease was accompanied by a manometric disorder of esophageal motor function. After 8 swallows, the esophageal emptying rates were 83.6 ± 4.2% (P < .05), 85.5 ± 2.7% (P < .05) and
92.8 ± 1.2% in patients with symptomatic reflux and a motor
disorder, patients with reflux without a motor disorder, and
normal subjects, respectively. After 40 swallows, emptying was
still reduced significantly in patients with reflux and motor
dysfunction (81.2 ± 4.3%, P < .05), but not in heartburn patients
with normal motility (92.3 ± 3.0%, P < .05) as compared to normal
subjects (95.0 ± 1.3%). During the first 15 seconds following
the initial wet swallow, emptying was diminished significantly
only in patients with reflux disease accompanied by a non-specific esophageal motor disorder.

Not only are disturbances in esophageal clearance demonstrable in patients who have obvious esophageal motor abnormalities on roentgen studies, but also subtle abnormalities can be
demonstrated in patients with normal radiographic studies.
Scintigraphy offers several advantages over barium cine-esophagography and acid clearance testing. In comparison to cineesopha-
gography, scintigraphy is quantitative, more sensitive, and has
a lower radiation burden. Previous studies have shown that the
density (specific gravity 1.5 to 2.0) and viscosity of barium
influence its behavior within the lumen of the gastrointestinal

tract (16). Acid clearance testing requires intubation with a
fragile pH electrode, gives only semiquantitative information and
is unphysiologic, in that the indwelling electrode could interfere with esophageal clearance. Further, acid must be ingested
or instilled into the stomach (17,18). In some normal individuals acidification of the esophagus may affect esophageal
motor function (19,20). On the other hand, esophageal scintigraphy can be adapted to study emptying not only of acid solutions, but also of any material which can be suitably labelled
with a gamma-emitting radionuclide.

The specificity of esophageal scintigraphy appears to be
high. All patient groups with abnormal esophageal motor function
manometric testing demonstrated decreased esophageal emptying by
scintigraphy. Patients with achalasia and scleroderma had similar abnormal patterns of esophageal clearance when studied in the
supine position. Patients with diffuse esophageal spasm demonstrated an intermediate defect. In these latter patients esophageal emptying was decreased significantly for the first 20
swallows, although they were able to achieve normal emptying with
additional repetitive swallows.

In recent years, it has been speculated that the contact
time between the gastric refluxate and the esophageal mucosa
might be an important determinant of the severity of mucosal
damage and/or symptoms in patients with gastroesophageal reflux
disease (21). Esophageal emptying as determined scintigraphically is decreased in patients with symptomatic gastroesophageal
reflux disease. As might be expected, emptying is impaired more
significantly in those patients who have a co-existing identifiable esophageal motor abnormality on manometry.

In summary, esophageal scintigraphy is a sensitive test for
evaluating esophageal emptying. Use of this test provides
useful information about esophageal function to both the clinician and the investigator (22). The method is more sensitive
than other techniques for subtle abnormalities of esophageal
transit, such as diffuse esophageal spasm or non-specific motor
abnormalities, and is the first quantitative test of esophageal
transit.

Barrett's Esophagus

In Barrett's esophagus, columnar epithelium resembling that
in the stomach is found in the distal portion of the esophagus,
in some cases possibly as the result of chronic gastroesophageal
reflux (23). Tc-99m pertechnetate is concentrated in the mucus-
producing glands of the stomach and may therefore be used to
identify the ectopic gastric mucosa found in Barrett's esophagus.
The technique employs approximately 5 mCi Tc-99m pertechnetate

administered intravenously (24). In order to eliminate Tc-99m
activity in the saliva from entering the esophagus, the patient is
instructed not to swallow or optimally may be assisted by oral
suction of the type used by dentists. A barium contrast study is
compared to the gamma camera image obtained 20-40 minutes following the radionuclide administration. Activity seen cephalad to
the gastroesophageal junction is indicative of the ectopic gastric mucosa of Barrett's esophagus. Although mucosal biopsy is
always essential to confirm the diagnosis, the scintigraphic
technique is a useful adjunct to contrast fluoroscopy and the
more invasive techniques which require intubation, such as manometry and the measurement of mucosal electric potentials.

Gastroesophageal Scintigraphy

Gastroesophageal scintigraphy is a technique which was
developed to detect and quantitate gastroesophageal (GE) reflux
(25,6,12,7,8,22). In the discussion of this technique, symptomatic gastroesophageal reflux was defined as heartburn with a
positive acid reflux test. Each of the other tests employed to
evaluate symptomatic GE reflux has some limitation. Barium eso-
phagography and barium cine-esophagography are able to detect
reflux directly, but are relatively insensitive (26,27). Esophageal endoscopy and mucosal biopsy findings may or may not be
attributable to reflux (28,29,11). Lower esophageal sphincter
and esophageal manometric findings may not necessarily be related
to symptomatic reflux (30,31). The acid perfusion test is a measure of mucosal sensitivity to acid, not a direct test of reflux
itself (18). The most sensitive and specific test of reflux, the
acid reflux test, requires endogastric intubation and accurate
placement of a pH electrode in the distal esophagus. Because each
of these tests for GE reflux is either non-specific, insensitive,
or 'invasive' in character, and because none of them is quantitative, GE scintigraphy was developed as a rapid, safe, sensitive,
non-invasive technique for the detection and quantitation of GE
reflux.

METHOD

Studies were initially performed in 10 normal subjects with
a double lumen tube assembly in place. An isotopic marker was
placed in the wall of the tube, midway between two pressure
recording orifices located 10 cm apart. Following manometric
placement of the marker at the LES, subjects were positioned
supine under a gamma camera, using a diverging medium energy
collimator, with a window setting of 140 keV $\pm$ 30%. Three hundred milliliters of isotonic saline containing 100 to 300 uCi Tc-
99m sulfur colloid were instilled into the stomach through the
tube, and 30 second timed gamma camera images were obtained, as
an externally placed inflatable abdominal binder was employed to

sequentially increase the gastroesophageal pressure gradient from 10 mmHg to 35 mmHg by 5 mmHg increments. Data from the gamma camera were stored on magnetic tapes for processing later using a computer.

PATIENT WITH REFLUX

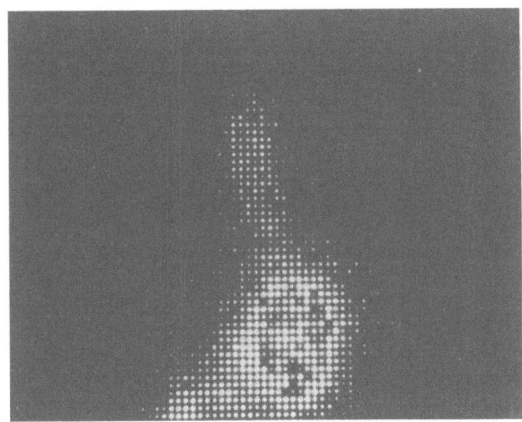

NORMAL SUBJECT

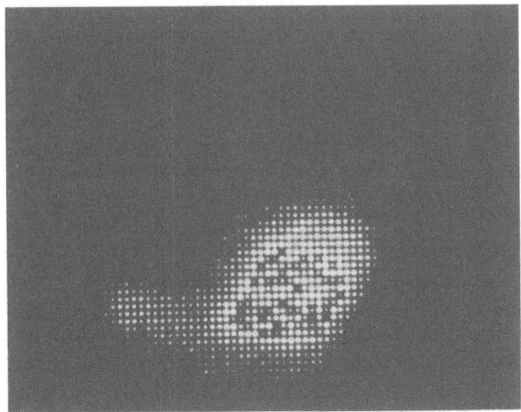

Figure 7
Gastroesophageal scintigraphy in a patient with reflux (above) and a patient with no gastroesophageal reflux (below).

In the interpretation of a typical gastroesophageal scintigraphy, any activity above the marker represented gastroesophageal reflux (Figure 7). Gastroesophageal reflux was detected in
27 of 30 symptomatic patients (90%). By comparison, none of the
other standard diagnostic techniques evaluated was as sensitive
(Table 1).

Table 1. Diagnostic Tests of Gastroesophageal Reflux

Diagnostic Test	Subject	Positive	Percent
Radiographic HH*	30	18	60.0
Fluoroscopic reflux	30	15	50.0
LES† pressure $\leq$ 10 mmHg	30	17	56.7
LES pressure $\leq$ 15 mmHg	30	23	76.7
Phenol red reflux test	30	14	46.7
Acid perfusion test	30	19	63.3
Endoscopic esophagitis	30	12	40.0
Histologic esophagitis	30	14	46.7
Gastroesophageal scintiscan	30	27	90.0

*HH, hiatal hernia

†LES, lower esophageal sphincter

Quantitation of GE scintigraphy was performed after recalling
the data which had been stored on magnetic tape, having used the
histogram mode for the collection of the data. Areas of interest
were identified, corresponding to the stomach activity, esophageal
activity, and background. The gastroesophageal reflux was determined. The mean reflux index for the test patients was 11.7 $\pm$
1.8% compared to 2.7 $\pm$ 0.3% for the controls (P < .001) (Figure 8).
Using quantitative criteria, the upper limit for reflux in normal
subjects was 4%, which coincided with the point at which gastroesophageal reflux became visible using the non-quantitative
technique. In the 2 of 20 normal subjects in whom gastroesopha-

geal reflux was observed, the quantity of reflux was minimal and occurred only at the highest gastroesophageal pressure gradient.

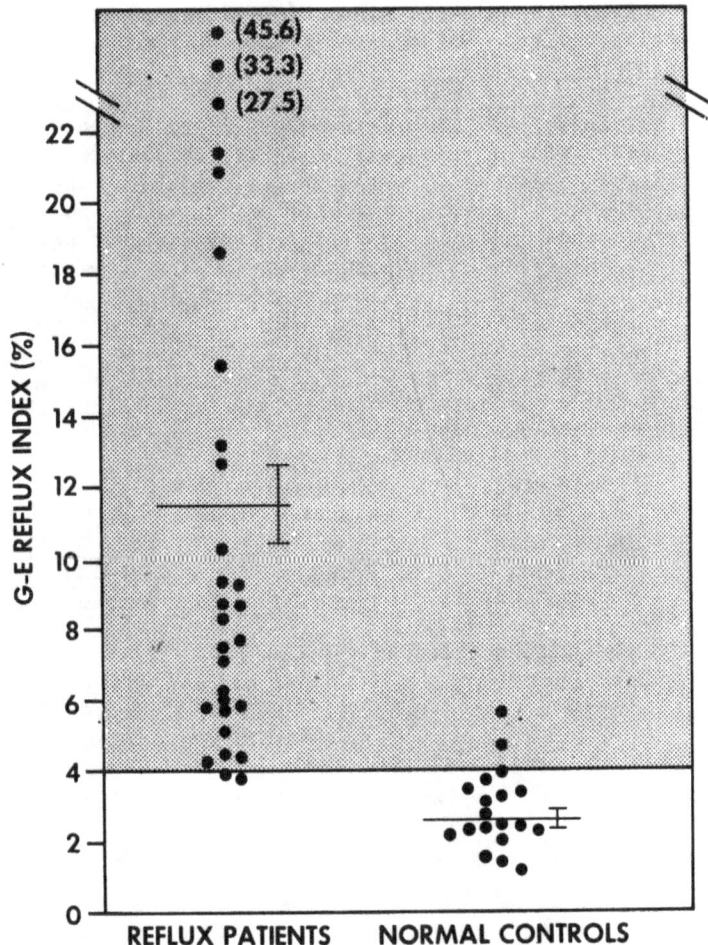

Figure 8

Gastroesophageal reflux index in all patients with reflux and normal subjects studied. Each point represents the maximal gastroesophageal reflux index of a single patient in percentage. Gastroesophageal reflux was visualized at a reflux index at or above 4%.

The gastroesophageal reflux index was computed, using the formula: $R = E_1 - E_B/G_0 \times 100$ where R represented the GE reflux index in percent, E_1, esophageal counts at t_1, E_B, esophageal background counts, and G_0, gastric counts at beginning of study. Since the Tc-99m binding was firm for the duration of the study, the background counts were negligible in each case. The amounts of activity in the esophagus, stomach, and background were determined by counting the scintillations within the outlined areas of interest, using a light pen on a 64 x 64 cell grid on the oscilloscope face.

The relationship of LES pressure and reflux has been studied following application of therapeutic modalities commonly used in the clinical management of gastroesophageal reflux. These included change in body position (upright vs. supine), administration of bethanechol, antacid, and an antacid-alginate preparation (Gaviscon), and Nissen fundoplication (Table 2). One of the findings was that the alginic acid-antacid compound reduced reflux from $9.1 \pm 1.3\%$ to $6.5 \pm 0.8\%$ (P < .01) as measured by the gastroesophageal scan. This was accomplished without significant alteration of resting LES pressure (Figures 9 and 10). Nissen fundoplication was the only therapeutic modality which returned reflux indices to normal values.

Table 2. Treatment of G-E Reflux

	Patients Studied	LES Pressure (mmHg)		G-E Reflux Index (%)	
		Before	After	Before	After
Supine to Erect	15	8.4 ± 0.8	6.0 ± 0.9**	14.8 ± 3.3	7.6 ± 1.7**
Bethanechol	15	8.9 ± 0.8	18.5 ± 1.9***	11.9 ± 2.4	6.0 ± 1.3***
Antacid	15	9.1 ± 0.9	17.3 ± 1.7***	11.2 ± 1.3	7.7 ± 1.0***
Alginic Acid + Antacids	15	10.1 ± 0.9	10.7 ± 0.8*	9.9 ± 1.3	6.5 ± 0.8***
Nissen Fundoplication	10	8.2 ± 1.3	12.0 ± 1.4***	17.4 ± 2.4	2.7 ± 1.1****

```
*    P > .05
**   P < .05
***  P < .01
**** P < .001
```

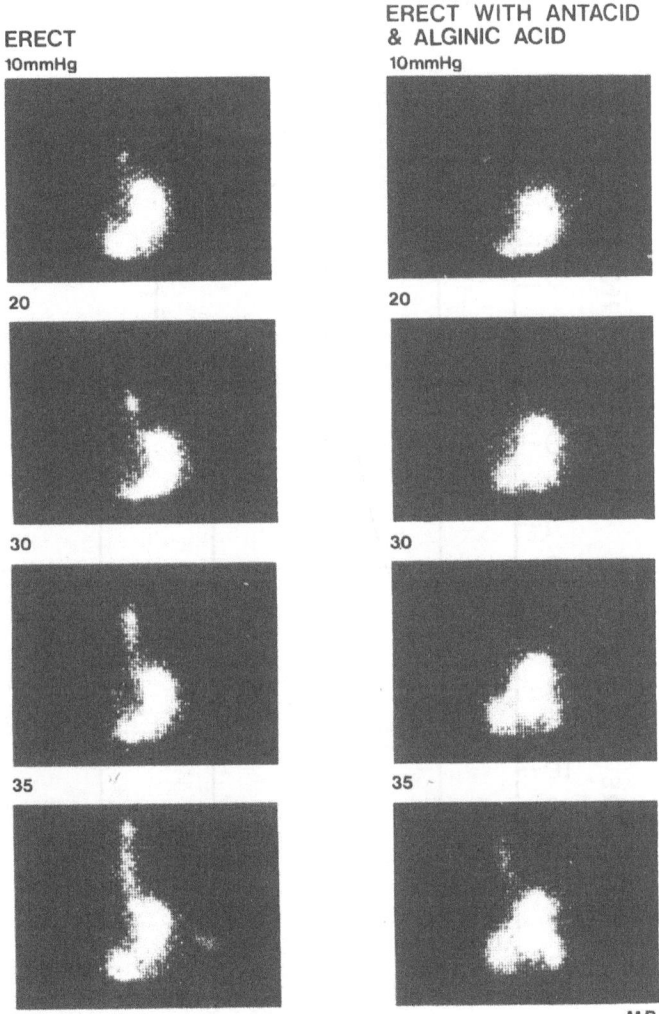

ERECT

ERECT WITH ANTACID
& ALGINIC ACID

Figure 9
Serial gastroesophageal scintigraphy in one patient with
gastroesophageal reflux before and 30 minutes after
administration of alginic acid antacid compound. Serial
scans are shown at gastroesophageal pressure gradients
of 10,20,30, and 35 mmHg.

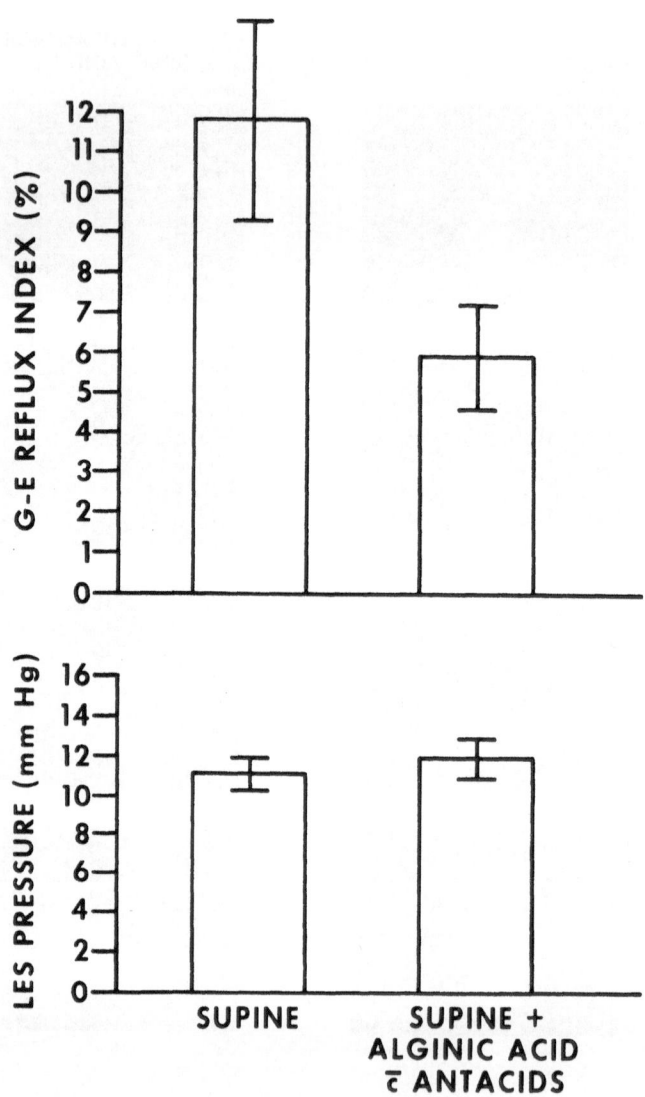

Figure 10
Gastroesophageal reflux indices and LES pressure gradients
before and after the use of alginic acid-antacid (Gaviscon).
Note reduction in reflux without alteration in LES pressure
gradient.

Gastroesophageal scintigraphy seems to be a safe, reliable non-invasive test for gastroesophageal reflux that can be performed rapidly with minimal patient discomfort. Reflux has been detected in 90% of approximately 300 symptomatic patients studied in our laboratory and on over 90% of 500 patients studied in Munich, Germany (Leisner, personal communication). None of the other diagnostic tests for reflux has been as sensitive. The scanning technique is also the first test which permits quantitation of gastroesophageal reflux. The equipment required for its performance is readily available in any nuclear medicine department. The procedure has now gained world wide acceptance and has been employed by pediatricians to identify reflux in children as a cause of recurrent pneumonia, recurrent vomiting, sleep apnea, and failure to thrive (32,33).

CHOLECYSTOGASTRIC SCINTIGRAPHY TO MEASURE ENTEROGASTRIC
REFLUX

Reflux of bile and digestive enzymes from the small bowel into the stomach has been observed in patients with a variety of gastrointestinal disorders including post-surgical alkaline gastritis (34-38), gastric ulcer (39-43), reflux esophagitis (44-47), gallstone dyspepsia (48) and functional dyspepsia (49). The role of enterogastric reflux in the pathogenesis of these disorders is poorly understood. This is in part, because a convenient non-invasive test for detection and quantitation of enterogastric reflux had not been available.

The scintigraphic technique for simultaneous measurement of gastric and gallbladder emptying was developed as a sensitive, quantitative non-invasive method which can be adopted to detect and quantitate enterogastric reflux. Normal values for gallbladder emptying and gastric emptying of a standardized meal and enterogastric reflux were established in normal, asymptomatic volunteers and then the method was employed to evaluate gastric and gallbladder emptying and enterogastric reflux in several groups of patients.

METHODS

The technique for simultaneous gastric-cholecystic imaging and quantitation requires that patients be studied following an overnight fast, at which time Tc-99m-HIDA N (2.6-Dimethylphenyl carbamoylmethyl) iminodiacetic acid (5 millicuries) was administered intravenously. Between 40 and 60 minutes later, a standardized liquid meal containing 300 ml Meritene and 20 ml Lipumol mixed with 250 microcuries In-111-DTPA (diethylenetriaminepentacetic acid) was ingested. At the time of administration of the meal, the liver and biliary tree were identified by imaging the Tc-99m-HIDA activity in the Tc-99m window of the gamma camera and

the stomach was identified by imaging the In-111-DTPA activity in
the In-111 window set at 170 Kev ± 5%. The activity of In-111
was separated from Tc-99m by setting the Tc-99m window to 140 Kev
± 5%. Both radionuclides were imaged simultaneously or separately
using these two windows on the gamma camera. The patients were
positioned supine under a gamma camera while 60 sec. images and
counts over gastric, gallbladder and hepatobiliary areas of
interest were obtained at 15 min. intervals for 2 hours. Data
were collected on disc and processed by a digital computer.

In the initial series, thirty-five subjects were studied
including 10 normal volunteers, 5 patients with gallstones, 7
patients with functional dyspepsia and 13 patients who had
previously been subjected to vagotomy, hemigastrectomy and Bilroth
II gastrojejunostomy. Functional dyspepsia was defined as epigastric or right upper quadrant pain, accompanied by abdominal
bloating or distention, nausea, vomiting or excess belching.
These patients all had normal upper gastrointestinal and gallbladder radiography, normal ultrasound studies of the biliary
tree and normal upper gastrointestinal endoscopic examinations.
All of the post surgical patients had been operated upon at least
6 months prior to participation in this study.

Quantitative cholecystogastric scintigraphy was performed
immediately after meal ingestion, defined as time zero, and at
one and two hours. In a typical normal subject, greater than 75%
of gallbladder activity had cleared by 60 minutes. Almost all
(more than 90%) had cleared by 2 hours (Figure 11). In patients
with gallstones, the gallbladder emptying was delayed and diminished both at one and two hours. In patients who had previously
undergone a vagotomy, hemigastrectomy and gastrojejunostomy,
gallbladder emptying was diminished and delayed at one and two
hours, respectively.

Gastric emptying was imaged in the Indium window. In normal
subjects, less than 40% of the standard meal emptied from the
stomach by 60 minutes, and between 50% and 75% of the activity
had emptied by 120 minutes. In patients with gallstones, gastric
emptying was not different from normal. In the post-operative
group, gastric pouch emptying was quite rapid initially, with
greater than 50% emptying by 30 minutes (Figure 12).

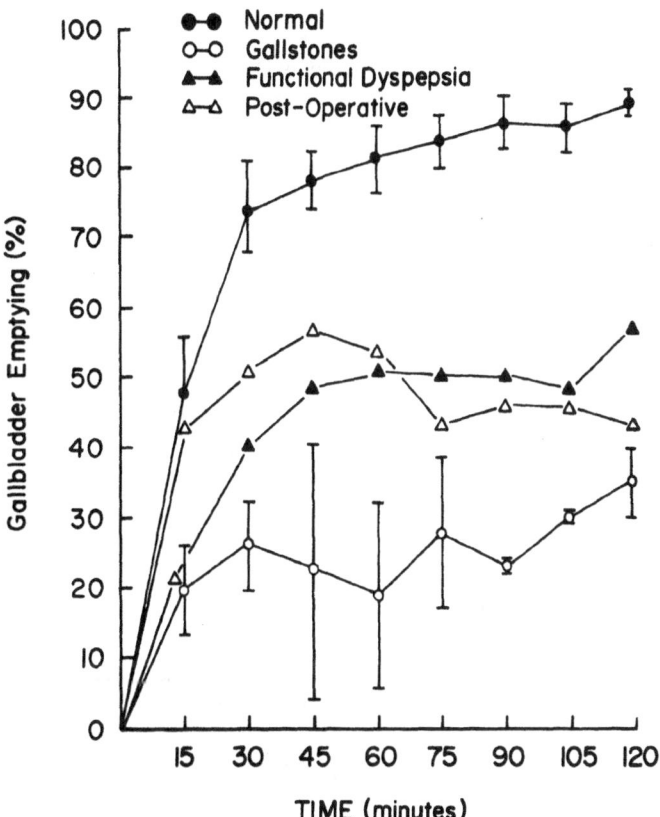

Figure 11
Rate of gallbladder emptying, expressed as percent gallbladder activity which has emptied versus time for two
hours. Note the clear separation of normals from patients
with gallstones, functional dyspepsia, and post-operative
patients.

518

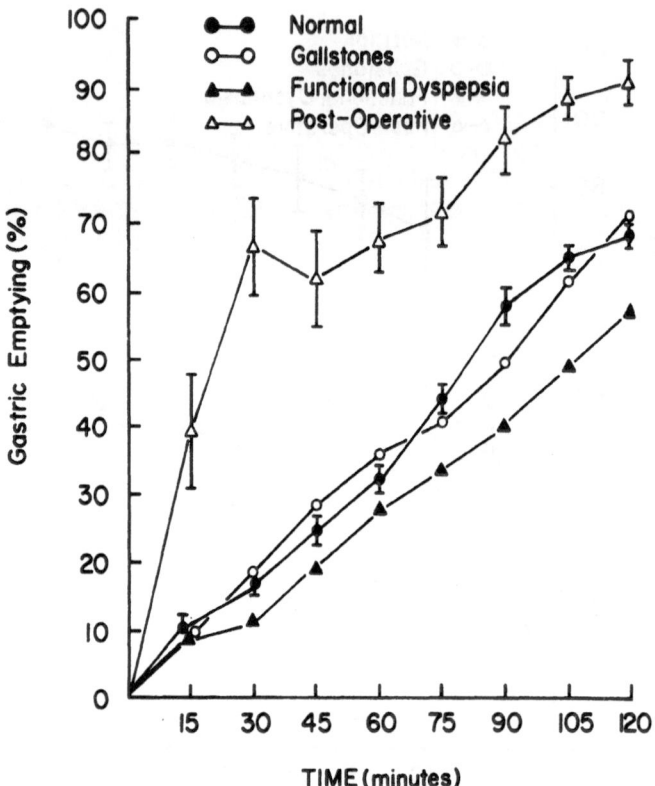

Figure 12

Rate of gastric emptying, expressed as percent gastric
activity which has cleared the stomach versus time for
two hours. Note that only the post-operative patients
had rapid emptying compared to normals and the other
two groups.

The enterogastric reflux index is a measure of bile reflux
from the small bowel into the stomach over a specified time
period $(0 \rightarrow t)$ and was defined as the increase in Tc-99m activity
in the gastric areas of interest divided by the decrease in Tc-
99m activity in the hepatobiliary tree. It was expressed by the
following formula:

$$EGRI_{(0 \rightarrow t)} = \frac{S_t - S_o}{HB_o - HB_t} \times 100$$

where $EGRI_{(0 \to t)}$ represented the enterogastric reflux index from time zero to time t expressed in percent; S_o, the Tc-99m activity in the stomach area of interest immediately after meal ingestion (time zero); S_t, the Tc-99m activity in the stomach area of interest at time t; HB_o, the Tc-99m activity in the hepatobiliary tract area of interest immediately after the meal (time zero); and HB_t, the Tc-99m activity in the hepatobiliary area of interest at time t. The denominator represented the amount of Tc-99m activity which left the hepatobiliary tree and therefore, was available for reflux into the stomach or gastric pouch.

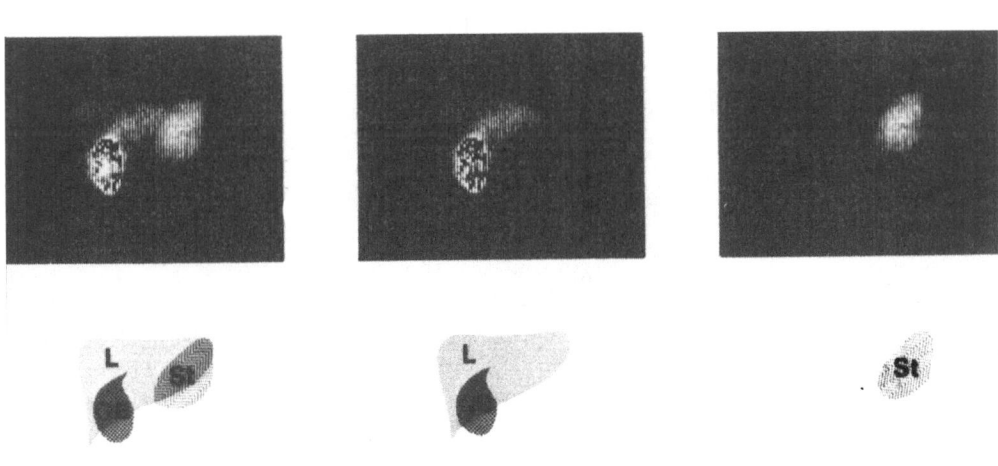

Figure 13
A combined gastric gallbladder study demonstrating areas of interest outlined.

In normal subjects, only a small amount of the cholecystic agent, Tc-99m-HIDA, was visualized over the gastric area of interest (Figure 13). In contrast, serial scans obtained from a post-surgical patient with the syndrome of clinical alkaline gastritis demonstrated that the majority of Tc-99m activity,

520

which emptied from the hepatobiliary tree, pooled in the gastric
pouch despite relatively rapid gastric emptying of In-111-DTPA.
Analysis of the composite results of enterogastric reflux studies
on 10 normal subjects and 13 post-surgical patients showed that
the reflux indices in asymptomatic post-surgical patients were
significantly higher than those in normal subjects and those in
patients with post surgical alkaline gastritis were the highest
of all (Figure 14).

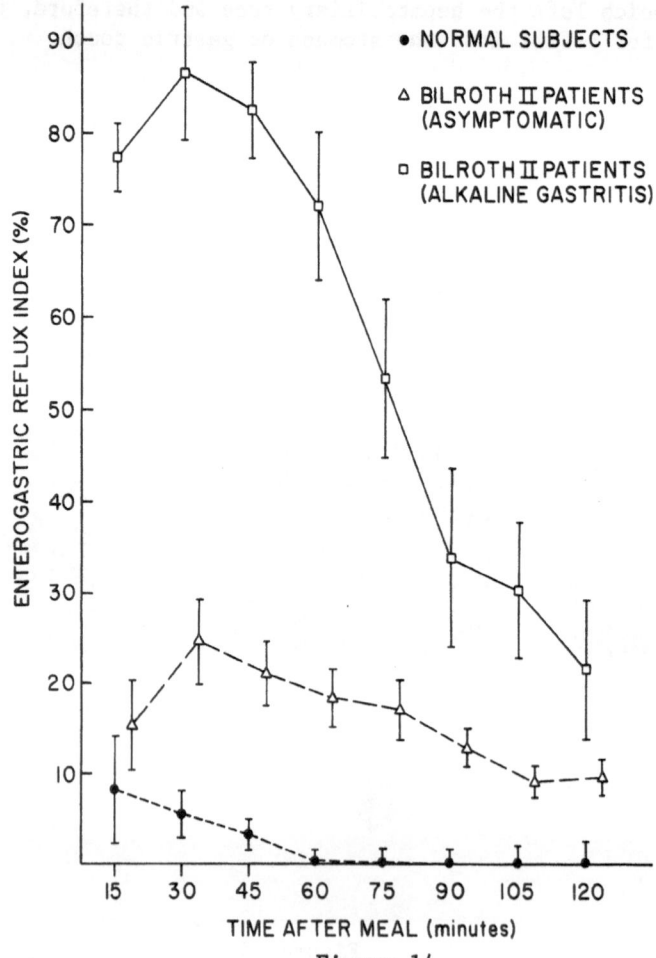

Figure 14

Enterogastric reflux indices in patients following Bilroth
II procedures and in normal subjects. The reflux indices
were significantly higher in all post-operative patients
as compared to normal. Amongst the post-operative group,
the reflux indices were highest in the symptomatic group.
Note that even normal subjects have minimal bile reflux,
i.e., less than 10% at 30 minutes.

The clinical criteria for alkaline gastritis (37,16,50,13,26) included recurrent post-prandial epigastric pain, nausea and bilious vomiting. Symptoms were partially or completely relieved by vomiting. Oral cholecystography, upper gastrointestinal roentgenography, gastroscopy and serum amylase measurements revealed no other cause for the symptoms.

Cholecystogastric scintigraphy is a safe, non-invasive, sensitive technique for the simultaneous quantitation of gastric emptying, gallbladder emptying and enterogastric reflux. No other technique has such broad capability.

GASTRIC EMPTYING

A wide range of techniques to measure gastric emptying has been introduced over the last 150 years, ranging from Beaumont's observations through a gastric fistula (51), to a variety of intubation tests (52-56), roentgenographic tests (57,58), radio-nuclide tests (21,1-4,59), and most recently, a ferro-magnetic technique (60).

The recent increased interest in gastric emptying studies has resulted from two stimuli: 1, inquiries into the role of gastric secretion and motor function in the etiology of peptic ulcer disease (61), and 2, the availability of new, reproducible quantitative techniques for measuring gastric emptying patterns and rates. Abnormalities in the rate of gastric emptying occur in diseases other than active peptic ulcer disease, and have been demonstrated following ulcer surgery, in patients with diabetes (62), and in gastric neoplasia (63). Several rather elegant techniques recently introduced (54,55,64), afford the gastro-intestinal physiologist information regarding both the rate of gastric emptying and gastric secretory patterns. While these techniques may become the standards for comparison, they are relatively cumbersome, require endogastric intubation, and may not meet either widespread acceptance by clinicians or their patients.

Radionuclide techniques for determining gastric emptying rates are by comparison, rather easily performed (21,65). They are non-invasive, safe, reproducible, accurate and increasingly available due to the ever-increasing presence of quantitative gamma camera imaging equipment.

Control and Regulation of Gastric Emptying

When food passes the lower esophageal sphincter and enters the stomach, it resides in the fundus and body, from where regu-lar slow contractions in the fundus and peristaltic waves in the

body propel it towards the antrum (66). As the food is carried
to the distal antrum and pylorus, the weaker waves fade, but the
stronger ones result in contractions of the antrum and coordinated duodenal muscular activity (67). Liquid and particulate
food passes in part into the duodenum. Solids, however, are
mostly retropulsed back to the gastric body and fundus, where
they are further broken up, mixed and emulsified with gastric
secretions. Gastric emptying, therefore, is a factor of pyloric
strength, and coordination between antral and duodenal muscular
activity. Gastric emptying of liquids is also dependant upon the
gastroduodenal pressure gradient (68). Because the fundus of the
stomach is able to relax considerably in response to increased
volume of food (69), there is not a rapid or direct relationship
between increased gastric volume and the rate of gastric emptying, although a definite relationship has been demonstrated (70).

Other factors which moderate gastric emptying include electrical activity, probably mediated by both autonomic and higher
neural activity; and hormones such as enterogastrone, gastrin and
secretin. Gastrin increases antral activity and delays gastric
emptying. Secretin decreases antral activity and delays gastric
emptying (71). The rate of gastric emptying also depends upon
the characteristics of the meal itself, including solid vs.
liquid (72), pH osmolarity (73), and volume (69).

Methods for Measuring Gastric Emptying Time

There are three methods which are in general use for describing gastric emptying time. The results can be expressed simply
as the amount of material remaining in (or passed through) the
stomach at any time, t_n, after a meal. This may be plotted on
either an arithmetic or logarithmic scale as a percent of the
administered volume vs. time and the half emptying time, $T_{1/2}$ calculated. This is a particularly convenient technique for radionuclide gastric emptying studies, where the gastric contents are
determined as a percent of the administered activity over a
period of time. Alternative approaches have also been employed,
such as, determining the square root of the remaining volume
(53). Presently, the $T_{1/2}$ technique and component method of
analysis appear to be most widely accepted (4,21,60,64,65). The
component method of analysis permits evaluation of the initial
rapid phase of emptying, as well as the slower components, which
primarily reflect emptying of the solid components (74).

Gastric Emptying Tests

Three types of gastric emptying studies are in use currently: 1. intubation tests, 2. roentgenographic tests, and, 3.
radionuclide tests (74). A fourth test, using a ferro-magnetic
tracer (60) was recently introduced, and may have potential

clinical use.

Intubation Tests

In the serial test meal, a non-absorbable marker is added to liquid meals of known volume, and the entire gastric contents are aspirated at different times, as the test is repeated on sequential days. By measuring the amount and concentration of the marker in each aspirate, the investigator is able to calculate the rate of gastric emptying and volume of gastric secretions (75). The test has served well in studies of normal gastric emptying, but has limited applicability in symptomatic patients who are unable or unwilling to be subjected to repeated endogastric intubation (74). The double sampling technique was introduced (76) in an effort to overcome the need for repetitive intubations and prolonged study time. Essentially, a liquid meal of known volume is administered, and small volumes of non-absorbable markers are introduced, as the stomach contents are sampled. The main limitation of the technique is that it is suitable only for liquid meals.

In 1973, Meeroff, et al. (77) introduced a variation of this technique, in which the duodenum is first perfused to a steady state, and then a test meal with a marker is placed in the stomach. As the duodenum is aspirated sequentially, the rate of gastric emptying is calculated from the concentration of the marker in the duodenal aspirate. The technique of Fordtran's group (61), is an improvement over that of Meeroff in that solid, physiologic meals are able to be employed. However, it requires perfusing the stomach to an intragastric pH of 5.5 by repeated titration of $NaHCO_3$, which is by no means a physiologic study.

Roentgenographic Techniques

Two general categories of roentgenographic tests exist: barium liquid and enteric coated barium granules. The barium liquid technique is not quantitative, and is unphysiologic as the barium may precipitate out and irritate the gastric mucosa (74). The enteric coated barium granules were developed in order to avoid the gastric irritation, but contrast radiography is simply not suited to quantitative studies (78), since the observer can only estimate what percent of the contrast remains in the stomach. Variations of these techniques, such as the acid barium test or the barium burger have similar limitations.

Nuclear Medicine Techniques

In 1966, Griffith (1) reported measuring the rate of gastric emptying using a Cr-51 labeled meal. No intubation is required and the meal could be either solid, liquid, or a mixture. As a result, a host of other nuclear medicine techniques has followed, using not only different meals (liquid and solid), but a variety of radionuclides, and equipment ranging from detectors and scanners to sophisticated gamma cameras on line to computers with data analysis.

Each subsequent radionuclide technique has attempted to correct, a deficiency in a preceding one. For example, Griffith employed Cr-51-sodium chromate as the radiochemical. This was replaced by a better imaging agent, I-131, attached to human serum albumin. Though the isotope I-131 had better imaging characteristics, the albumin is degraded in the duodenum, the I⁻ is reabsorbed, and then resecreted into the gastric juice. The gastric secretion volume could be calculated from the known concentrations and volumes. Other radionuclides have been employed, including In-111, In-113m, and Tc-99m. All of these gamma emitters are suitable for repetitive studies with low radiation burden to the patient. However, some degree of association between the solid marker and the food to be labeled was usually demonstrable. As a result, conflicting data were reported. Amongst all of the existing techniques, there were simply too many variables: first, the choice of meal: liquid or solid; second, if solid, then paper chips, porridge, beef stew, hamburger, chicken liver, or scrambled eggs; third, the isotope itself - I-131, C4-51, Cs-129, I-131, In-111, In-113m or Tc-99m; fourth, the kind of equipment - scintillation detector, rectilinear scanner or gamma camera.

Present technology suggests that the following technique is best: A gamma emitting radionuclide with no associated beta emissions and a relatively short half-life, such at Tc-99m or In-111. The equipment of choice is a gamma camera, preferably one suitable for simultaneously processing data from two isotopes of different energy peaks and on line to a digital computer capable of processing the scintigraphic data from either or both isotopes.

The problem of a tight bind between the isotope and the solid food appears to have been solved by a clever innovation reported by Meyer (4). He administered Tc-99m sulfur colloid to live chickens. Since Tc-99m sulfur colloid is phagocytized by Kupffer cells in the chicken's liver, the Tc-99m label becomes an intracellular one. The chicken is then killed, its liver removed, cooked, and fed to the patient along with additional solid food. More recently, Knight, et al. (79) have validated a number of Tc-99m labeled-egg preparations for measuring gastric emptying rates in man, and also compared labeled egg and liver preparations.

Using a dual isotope technique with a gamma camera, similar
to that reported by Heading, et al. (59) using a rectilinear
scanner, we have performed dual isotope studies in man using the
Tc-99m chicken liver or Tc-99m scrambled egg sandwich in a solid
meal with an In-111 DTPA (DiethyleneTriamine-Pentacetic Acid)
labeled liquid component. The use of two isotopes permits sequential visualization and quantitation of the movements of solid
and liquid components of meals simultaneously and permits us to
study the movement of meals of various types, i.e. meals of
varying volume, fat carbohydrate and protein content, specific
gravity, pH, fiber content, and osmolarity, in the same patients
repetitively.

Gastric Emptying Following Gastric Surgery

There has been considerable interest in gastric emptying
studies following surgery, and this has resulted in copious data
regarding gastric emptying following post-gastrectomy and vagotomy. There appears to be a concensus regarding faster emptying
of liquid meals following vagotomy and pyloroplasty (80-83).
When solid meals are used, the results are confusing. Here
again, new studies using a firm solid marker are needed.

In conclusion, a number of techniques have been used in the
past to quantitate gastric emptying. It is only in the last
decade, however, that quantitative techniques have become available which are suited to measuring gastric emptying of physiological solid meals in man. Of these, the radionuclide techniques
employing solid foods are the least invasive, most easily quantitative and most physiologic, since no intubation is required and
no alterations in intra-gastric pH by infusion are required
during the study.

HEPATIC SCINTIGRAPHY

Despite recent rapid advances in imaging modalities such as
ultrasound (US), digital radiography, and computerized tomography,
hepatic imaging with Tc-99m sulfur colloid remains the initial
study of choice in the search for focal disease of the liver.
Ultrasound and CT are recommended as complementary investigations
when the liver-spleen scan findings are questionable. In general,
ultrasound is the next study of choice. However, when suspected
abnormalities are found in the region of the portahepatis, CT may
prove to be the next most useful complementary technique.

The most frequent clinical situation in which a liver scan is
obtained is in the patient with possible metastasis. A discussion
of the relative merits of different imaging techniques is included
elsewhere (see McCready). We believe the most rational approach
to the investigation of a patient for possible hepatic metastasis

following a physical examination is to obtain liver function studies
followed by a liver scan in those patients with hepatomegaly or
with abnormalities in liver function tests. When an abnormality
is observed by liver scan, it should be further evaluated by either
US or CT. Since US costs less, does not involve the use of ionizing radiation, and can scan the liver in more than one plane, it
is preferable to CT scanning at the present time. Furthermore,
neither the sensitivity nor the specificity of CT scanning has
been demonstrated to be superior to US in the evaluation of hepatic
metastatic disease, and the use of CT scanning in this situation,
therefore, remains investigative (84).

HEPATOBILIARY IMAGING

The replacement of I-131 Rose Bengal with Tc-99m labeled
iminodiacetic acid (IDA) compounds has made possible the rapid
and accurate diagnosis of a variety of biliary tract disorders.
The low count rates and poor imaging characteristics of Rose
Bengal resulted from the I-131 label which permitted only micro-
curie doses to be employed. With the advent of Tc-99m labeled
compounds, the liver, biliary tree, and gallbladder could all be
imaged sequentially, resulting in anatomic, and more importantly,
functional information, not previously obtainable. In addition,
ultrasound and computerized tomography (CT) have provided morphological data regarding cystic duct and common duct size and
potency and the presence of stones, cysts or masses. Thus,
within the last 5 years, the traditional approach to gallbladder
and biliary tract disease - oral cholecystography and invasive
procedures - has undergone revolutionary changes, especially in
the diagnosis of acute cholecystitis.

Acute cholecystitis is initiated by obstruction of the cystic
duct. The Tc-99m-IDA imaging techniques rely upon detecting
cystic duct potency, so that the diagnosis of acute cholecystitis
can be made reliably by non-visualization of the gallbladder in
patients whose liver and intrahepatic ducts are visualized
scintigraphically. The technique requires that the patient be
fasted for a minimum of two hours prior to administration of 5 mCi
(3-15 mCi) Tc-99m-IDA agent, generally referred to as HIDA.
Images are obtained for 500,000 counts at 5 minute intervals for
30 minutes, and then at 30 minute intervals for up to 2 hours or
until the gallbladder is visualized. If no gallbladder activity
is seen by 4 hours in the presence of satisfactory liver and
intrahepatic bile duct activity, then a diagnosis of acute or
chronic cholecystitis is made. At our institution, we wait only
2 hours, then administer cholecystokinin (CCK) 20 ng/kg slowly
intravenously followed by a second 5 mCi Tc-99m-HIDA. Persistent
non-visualization 2 hours after CCK is interpreted as acute
cholecystitis in a patient with no history of cholecystectomy and
adequate hepatocystic activity to result in intrahepatic bile

duct visualization. An alternative approach, advocated by
Eikman (85) employs intravenous CCK (40-75 Ivy dog units over 5
minutes), followed by 3-15 mCi Tc-99mHIDA 30 minutes later.
Failure to visualize the gallbladder within 2 hours is a highly
sensitive and specific test for acute cholecystitis (cystic duct
obstruction) in acutely ill, fasting patients. The advantage of
the latter method is its speed (2 hours vs 4 or more without CCK
priming). However, CCK is not universally available and is,
therefore, not routinely employed. In the initial series of 90
patients reported by Weismann, et al. (86), the overall accuracy
of the procedure was greater than 95%, with a false positive rate
of zero and a false negative rate of 5%. Similar data have been
reproduced by other groups, including Rosenthal (87).

Chronic cholecystitis may present with a variety of scintigraphic findings ranging from normal (prompt gallbladder visualization) to markedly delayed gallbladder visualization even after
CCK.

The range of findings in acute cholecystitis may depend in
part upon the degree and location of stones or sludge. Other
applications of hepatobiliary scintigraphy include bile leaks due
to trauma or surgery (88) and in the differential diagnosis of
cholestasis, although this author finds most HIDA studies of
little use in cholestasis. The more recently available IDA
analogs, such as diisopropyl IDA may yet prove to have some
usefulness in this area.

Combined ultrasound and scintigraphic evaluation of the
gallbladder can now offer anatomic and functional information
including gallbladder wall thickness, presence of stones, duct
size and functional patency. In those instances where a mass
lesion is suspected in patients with cholestasis, CT may also
prove useful, though in acute cholecystitis, scintigraphy and
ultrasound combined usually are quite specific.

SCINTIGRAPHIC DETECTION OF ACUTE GASTROINTESTINAL
HEMORRHAGE

Recently, two new radionuclide techniques for detection of
lower gastrointestinal bleeding have been introduced (89,90).
These techniques represent a potential advance in the diagnosis
of lower gastrointestinal bleeding. Contrast radiography is able
to detect lower gastrointestinal hemorrhage only if the patient
is actively bleeding at the time of the study, and then only if
the rate of bleeding is at least 0.5 milliliters per minute. The
scintigraphic techniques appear to be technically superior to
contrast radiography in sensitivity, thus affording the clinician
a valuable technique in dealing with a difficult problem of the
acute lower gastrointestinal bleeder in whom a delay in diagnosis

or therapy might prove fatal. Lower gastrointestinal bleeding sites have not proven as amenable to rapid diagnosis with endoscopy as has upper gastrointestinal bleeding due to the inability to quickly and reliably prepare the colon for accurate fiber optic examination. Unfortunately, proctosigmoidoscopy permits evaluation only of a relatively small portion of the distal lower gastrointestinal tract. Due to the limitations of the radiographic and endoscopic techniques, the scintigraphic technique for detecting lower gastrointestinal bleeding has begun to assume increasing clinical significance.

Radiographic Studies

The diagnostic yield of emergency barium studies in the active lower gastrointestinal bleeding patient is limited. Usually, the lower colon contains fecal material as well as blood and conventional barium studies fail to demonstrate the source of gastrointestinal bleeding in a considerable portion of patients. Furthermore, the presence of barium in the bowel may interfere with later attempts at angiographic evaluation of the lower intestinal tract for acute gastrointestinal bleeding.

As stated above, angiography is generally accepted as being able to detect bleeding rates of 0.5 ml/minute, although even that figure may represent an overestimate of the sensitivity of angiography. The radiographic technique is further limited by an inability to detect venous bleeding, intermittent bleeding, failure to include all potential sites of blood loss in this study, and difficulty in detecting lower rectal hemorrhage.

Due to the limitations of the endoscopic and angiographic techniques, the introduction of the scintigraphic methods now offers the clinician a more sensitive, possibly superior technique in the detection and management of lower gastrointestinal bleeding.

The first of the two techniques employs Technetium-99m sulfur colloid. Approximately 15 mCi of the colloid is injected intravenously. The colloid is cleared rapidly by the liver during the first pass, so that very little vascular pool remains. A bleeding site would be an area of activity in an abdomen with very low blood pool, or extracellular fluid background. Thus, the bleeding site would be seen as a focus of activity, usually within the lumen of the bowel, in high contrast to the surrounding tissue activity. The requirement for the Technetium-99m-sulfur colloid technique to be successful is that the patient be hemorrhaging at the moment of injection. Using this technique in an animal preparation, bleeding rates of 0.1 ml/minute could be detected (89).

The other technique employs autologous red blood cells labeled _in vivo_ with stannous pyrophosphate and Technetium-99m. Several methods have been proposed for labeling the red cells, including an _in vitro_ technique in which the red cells are partially heat damaged, and in vivo technique in which the stannous pyrophosphate is first injected systemically, and the red blood cells labeled in vivo, and lastly a modification of the in vivo technique in which the patient is first administered stannous pyrophosphate intravenously and the red blood cells labeled in a slightly heparinized syringe (90,91). The Technetium 99m-labeled red blood cell technique permits the detection of bleeding sites, even when the blood loss is intermittent, as the red blood cells are constantly recirculating in the vascular compartment.

Both techniques appear to be of equal sensitivity in detecting slow rates of lower gastrointestinal bleeding. However, the two techniques differ quite a bit in their strengths and limitations. In the active lower gastrointestinal bleeder, the Technetium-99m sulfur colloid technique permits the rapid detection of the focus of blood loss within minutes of administration of the pharmaceutical. However, in patients with intermittent blood loss, probably the majority of all such patients, the colloid technique may miss the bleeding site. The red cell technique can be employed to detect an intermittent bleed by virtue of its ability to re-image the patient at regular intervals following administration of the radiopharmaceutical, while the colloid technique is further limited in its sensitivity in that the liver activity is so intense as to possibly obscure a bleeding site adjacent to the liver or in the hepatic flexure. The major limitation of the red cell technique is that imaging at infrequent intervals may result in inaccurate distal localization of the site of bleeding in patients with rapid bowel transit.

The approach which we use in our institution is to employ the Technetium-99m sulfur colloid method only in patients who are briskly and actively bleeding at the time of injection. In patients who are bleeding intermittently, we prefer to use the Technetium-99m labeled red blood cells. At the present time, our own experience, and that reported in the medical literature is not sufficient to recommend one technique in favor of the other. However, both appear to be considerably more sensitive for detection of lower gastrointestinal bleeding than is contrast angiography.

SUMMARY

In summary, gastrointestinal nuclear medicine procedures have progressed from the stage of anatomic imaging alone to their present applications which are in the study of gastrointestinal

530

function and pathophysiology. These tracer techniques have
several specific advantages over other procedures. Scintigraphy
require no intubation, has excellent patient acceptance, is
Quantitative, delivers lower radiation burdens to the patient
than does the average contrast radiographic study, and most
importantly, provides functional, rather than anatomic, information not obtainable from other imaging modalities.

REFERENCES

1.   Griffith, G.H., G.M. Owen, S. Kirkman, and R. Shields.
"Measurement of rate of gastric emptying using Chromium-51."
Lancet 1 (1966) 1244-1245.

2.   Harvey, R.F., N.J.G. Brown, D.B. Mackie, D.H. Keeling,
and W.T. Davies. "Measurement of gastric emptying time with a
gamma camera." Lancet 1 (1970) 16-18.

3.   Jones, T., J.C. Clark, N. Kocak, A.G. Cox and H.I. Glass.
"Measurement of gastric emptying using the scintillation camera
and Cs-129." Brit J Radiology 43 (1979) 537-541.

4.   Meyer, J.H., M.B. MacGregor, R. Gueller, P. Martin, and
R. Cavalieri. "Tc-99m-tagged chicken liver as a marker of solid
food in the human stomach." Digestive Dis 21 (1976) 296-304.

5.   Harvey, E., M. Loberg, and M. Cooper. "Tc-99m-HIDA. A
new radiopharmaceutical for hepatobiliary imaging." J Nucl Med
16 (1975) 533.

6.   Fisher, R.S. et al. "Gastroesophageal (GE) scintiscan-
a new method to detect and quantitate GE reflux." Gastroenterology 70 (1976) 301.

7.   Malmud, L.S. "Radionuclide studies of gastric emptying
and enterogastric reflux." In Peptic Ulcer Diseases -- An
Update. Third International Symposium on Gastroenterology (March
18-24, 1979), New York, Biomedical Information Corporation, 1979.

8.   Malmud, L.S., and R.S. Fisher. "Quantitation of gastroesophageal reflux before and after therapy using the gastroesophageal scintiscan." South Med J 71 Suppl 1 (1978) 10.

9.   Tolin, R.D., et al. "Enterogastric reflux in normal subjects and patients with Bilroth II gastroenterostomy" Gastroenterology 77 (1979) 1027.

10. Tolin, R.D., et al. "Esophageal scintigraphy to quantitate esophageal transit." Gastroenterology 76 (1979) 1402.

11. Weinstein, W.M., E.R. Bogach and K.L. Bowes. "The normal human esophageal mucosa: a histological reappraisal." Gastroenterology 68 (1975) 40-44.

12. Fisher, R.S. et al. "The lower esophageal sphincter as a barrier to gastroesophageal reflux." Gastroenterology 72 (1977) 19.

13. Stelzer, F., et al. "Abnormal gallbladder emptying in patients with gallstones or vagotomy and Bilroth II gastroenterostomy." Clin Res 27 (1979) 272.

14. Skucas, J., and W.W. Schrank. "The routine air-contrast examination of the esophagus." Radiology 115 (1975) 482-484.

15. Margulis, A.R. "Water-soluble radiographic contrast agents in the gastrointestinal tract." In Radiographic Contrast Agents. R.E. Miller and J. Skucas, Eds., (University Park Press, Baltimore, 1977) p. 188.

16. Sandmark, S. "Hiatal incompetence." Acta Radiol Supplement 219 (1963).

17. Bernstein, I.M., and I.A. Baker. "A clinical test for esophagitis." Gastroenterology 34 (1958) 760-781.

18. Battle, W.S., L.M. Nyhus and C.T. Bombeck. "Gastroesophageal reflux: diagnosis and treatment." Ann Surg 177 (1973) 560-564.

19. Donner, M.W., et al. "Acid barium swallows in the radiographic evaluation of clinical esophagitis." Radiology 87 (1966) 220.

20. Hookman, P., et al. "Acid induced esophageal motor abnormalities. A cine-manometric study." Gastroenterology 48 (1965) 822.

21. Calderon, M., R.E. Sonnemaker, T. Hersh, J.A. Burdine. "Tc-99m human albumin microspheres (HAM) for measuring the rate of gastric emptying." Radiology 101 (1971) 371-374.

22. Malmud, L.S., and R.S. Fisher. "Scintigraphic evaluation of disorders of the duodenum, esophagus and stomach." Med Clinics N Amer. (1981) in press.

23. Paull, A., J.S. Trier, M.D. Dalton, R.C. Camp, P. Loeb, and R.K. Goyal. "The histologic spectrum of Barrett's esophagus." N Engl J Med 295 (1976) 476-480.

24. Berquist, T.H., N.G. Nolan, H.C. Carlson and
D.H. Stephens. "Diagnosis of Barrett's esophagus by pertechnetate
scintigraphy." Mayo Clin Proc 48 (1973) 276-279.

25. Fisher, R.S., et al. "Anti-reflux surgery for symptomatic gastric esophageal reflux: mechanism of action." Am J Dig
Dis 23 (1978) 152.

26. Texter, E.C. "Fluorocinematography." Curr Gastro-
enterol 9 (1961) 983-1001.

27. Wolf, B.S. and M.T. Khilnani. "Progress in gastrointestinal radiology." Gastroenterology 51 (1966) 542-559.

28. Ismail-Beigi, F., P.F. Horton, and C.F. Pope. "Histological consequences of gastroesophageal reflux in man." Gastroenterology 58 (1970) 163-174.

29. Kobayashi, S. and T. Kasugai. "Endoscopic and biopsy
criteria for the diagnosis of esophagitis with a fiberoptic eso-
phagoscope." Am J Dig Dis 19 (1974) 345-352.

30. Pope, C.E. "A dynamic test of sphicter strength: its
application to the lower esophageal sphincter." Gastroenterology
52 (1967) 779-786.

31. Winans, C.S. and L.D. Harris. "Quantitation of lower
esophageal sphincter competence." Gastroenterology 52 (1967)
773-778.

32. Conway, J.J., et al. "Radionuclide evaluation of gastroesophageal reflux in children." J Nucl Med 20 (1979) 680.

33. Heyman, S., et al. "The radionuclide detection of
gastroesophageal reflux and aspiration in children." J Nucl Med
20 (1979) 680.

34. Bushkin, F.L., et al. "Post-operative alkaline reflux
gastrititis." Surg Gyn Obst 138 (1972) 933-938.

35. Duplessis, D.J. "Alkaline reflux gastritis." S Afr
Med J 42 (1968) 134-136.

36. Mackman, S., K. Lemmer and J. Morrissey. "Post-operative gastritis and esophagitis." Amer J Surg 121 (1971) 694-697.

37. Scudamore, "Bile reflux gastritis." Amer J Gast 60
(1973) 9-22.

38. Toye, D. and J. Williams. "Post-gastrectomy bile vomiting." Lancet 2 (1965) 524-526.

39. Capper, W.M. "Factors in the pathogenesis of gastric ulcer." Ann Roy Coll Surg Eng 40 (1967) 21-35.

40. Delaney, J.P., J.W.B. Cheng, and B.A. Butler, et. al. "Gastric ulcer and regurgitation gastritis." Gut 11 (1970) 715-719.

41. Duplessis, D.J. "Pathogenesis of gastric ulceration." Lancet 1 (1965) 974-978.

42. Fisher, R.S. and S. Cohen. "Pyloric sphincter dysfunction in patients with gastric ulcer." New Engl J Med 288 (1973) 273-276.

43. Rhodes, J., D.E. Barnardo, and S.F. Phillips, et al. "Increased reflux of bile into the stomach in patients with gastric ulcer." Gastroenterology 57 (1969) 241-252.

44. Gillison, A. "The significance of bile in reflux esophagitis." Surg Gyn Obst 134 (1972) 419-424.

45. Kaye, M.D. and P. Showalter. "Pyloric incompetence in reflux esophagitis." Clin Res 20 (1972) 733.

46. Moffat, R.C. and E.M. Berkas. "Bile esophagitis." Arch Surg 91 (1965) 963-966.

47. Windsor, C.W.D. "Gastroesophageal reflux after partial gastrectomy." Brit Med J 2 (1967) 1233-1234.

48. Johnson, A.G. "Pyloric function and gallstone dyspepsia." Brit J Surg 50 (1972) 450-454.

49. Capper, W.M., Buckler, T.J. and J.V. Kilby, et al. "Gallstones, gastric secretion and flatulent dyspepsia." Lancet 1 (1967) 413-415.

50. Snedecor, G.W. and W.C. Cochran. "Statistical Methods." Sixth Edition, Ames, Iowa State University Press, 1967.

51. Beaumont, W. "Experiments and observations on the gastric juice and the physiology of digestion." Plattsburg, Allen, 1833.

52. Hunt, J.N. and W.R. Spurrell. "The pattern of emptying of the human stomach." J Physiol (London) 113 (1951) 157-168.

534

53. George, J.D. "New clinical method for measuring the rate of gastric emptying: The double sampling test method." Gut 9 (1968) 237-242.

54. Malagelada, J.R., G.F. Longstreth, W.H.J. Summerskill and V.L.W. Go. "Measurement of gastric functions during digestion of ordinary solid meals in man." Gastroenterology 70 (1976) 203-210.

55. Malagelada, J.R. "Quantification of gastric solid-liquid discrimination during digestion of ordinary meals." Gastroenterology 72 (1977) 1265-1267.

56. Fordtran, J.S., and J.H. Walsh. "Gastric acid secretion rate and buffer content of the stomach after eating: Results in normal subjects and in patients with duodenal ulcer." J Clin Invest 52 (1973) 645-657.

57. Horton, R.E., F.G.M. Ross and G.H. Darling. "Determination of the emptying-time of the stomach by use of enteric coated barium granules." Brit Med J 1 (1965) 1537-1539.

58. Pendergrass, E.P., I.S. Ravdin, C.G. Johnston and P.J. Hodes. "Studies of the small intestine. II The effect of food and various pathologic states on gastric emptying and the small intestinal pattern." Radiology 26 (1936 (651-662.

59. Heading, R.C., P. Tothill, G.P. McLoughlin and D.J.C. Shearman. "Gastric emptying rate measurement in man: A double isotope scanning technique for simultaneous study of liquid and solid components of a meal." Gastroenterology 71 (1976) 45-50.

60. Benmair, Y., F. Dreyfuss, B. Fishel, E.H. Frei and G. Gilat. "Study of gastric emptying using a ferro-magnetic tracer." Gastroenterology 73 (1977) 1041-1045.

61. Fordtran, J.S. "Acid secretion in paptic ulcer." In Gastrointestinal Disease. M.H. Sleisenger, J.S. Fordtran, eds. W.B. Saunders Co., Philadelphia, pp 174-188, 1973.

62. Scarpello, J.H.B., D.C. Barber, R.V. Hague, D.R. Cullen, and G.E. Sladen. "Gastric emptying of solid meals in diabetes." Brit Med J 2 (1976) 671-673.

63. Griffith, G.H., G.M. Owen, H. Campbell, and R. Shields. "Gastric emptying in health and in gastroduodenal disease" Gastroenterology 54 (1968) 1-7.

64. Malagelada, J.R., G.F. Longstreth, T.B. Deering, W.H.J. Summerskill, and V.L.W. Go. "Gastric secretion and emptying after ordinary meals in duodenal ulcer." Gastroenterology 73 (1977) 989-994.

65. Chaudhuri, T.K. "Use of Tc-99m-DTPA for measuring gastric emptying time." J Nuclear Med 15 (1974) 319-395.

66. Code, C.F. and H.C. Carlson. "Motor activity of the stomach." In. Handbook of Physiology, Section 6, Alimentary Canal, Vol. IV, CF Code, eds., American Physiological Society, Washington, DC, pp 1903-1916, 1968.

67. Carlson, H.C., C.F. Code, and R.A. Nelson. "Motor activity of the canine gastroduodenal junction: A cineadiographic, pressure, and electric study." Amer J Digestive Dis 11 (1966) 155-172.

68. Bass, P., C.F. Code and E.H. Lambert. "Electrical activity of the gastroduodenal junction." Amer J Physiol 201 (1961) 587-592.

69. Cannon, W.B., and C.W. Lieb. "The receptive relaxation of the stomach." Amer J Physiol 29 (1911) 267-273.

70. Hunt, J.N. and I. McDonald. "The influence of volume on gastric emptying." J Physiol (London) 126 (1954) 459-474.

71. Kwong, N.J., B.H. Brown, G.E. Whittaker, and H.E. Duthie. "Effect of gastrin I, secretin, and cholecystokinin-pancreozimin on the electrical activity, motor activity, and acid output of the stomach in man." Scand J Gastroenterology 7 (1972) 161-170.

72. Thomas, J.E. "Mechanisms and regulation of gastric emptying." Physol Rev 37 (1957) 435-474.

73. Hunt, J.N. "The duodenal regulation of gastric emptying." Gastroentrology 45 (1963) 149-156.

74. Sheiner, H.J. "Progress Report: Gastric emptying tests in man." Gut 16 (1975) 235-247.

75. Hunt, J.N. and W.R. Spurrell. "The pattern of emptying of the human stomach." J Physiol (London) 113 (1951) 157-168.

76. George, J.D. "Gastric acidity and motility." Amer J Digestive Dis 13 (1968) 376-383.

536

77. Meeroff, J.C., V.L.W. Go, and S.F. Phillips. "Gastric emptying of liquids in man: Quantification by duodenal recovery marker." Mayo Clinic Proc 48 (1973) 728-732.

78. Sun, D.C.H., H. Shay, and H.J. Woloshin. "Effect of tricyclamol on gastric emptying and intestinal transit." Amer J Digestive Dis 4 (1959) 282-288.

79. Hopkins, A. "The patterns of gastric emptying: A new view of old results." J Physiol (London) 182 (1966) 144-149.

80. Clarke, R.J. and J. Allexander-Williams. "The effect of preserving antral innervation and of a pyloroplasty on gastric emptying after vagotomy in man. Gut 14 (1973) 300-307.

81. Cobb, J.S., S. Bank, I.N. Marks, and J.H. Louw. "Gastric emptying after vagotomy and pyloroplasty." Amer J Digestive Dis 16 (1971) 207-215.

82. Aylett, P., C. Wastell, and I. Wise. "Gastric secretion and emptying before and after vagotomy and pyloroplasty, with and without continuous infusion of pentagastrin." Amer J Digestive Dis 14 (1969) 256-252.

83. McKelvey, S.T.D. "Gastric incontinence and post-vagotomy diarrhea." Brit J Surgery 57 (1970) 741-747.

84. Smalley, R.V., Malmud, L.S. and W.G.M. Ritchie. "Pre-operative scanning: Evaluation for metastatic disease in carcinoma of the breast, lung, colon, bladder and prostate." Semin in Oncology 7 (1980) 358-369.

85. Eikman, E.A., J.L. Cameron, M. Coleman, T.K. Natarajan, P. Dugal, and H.N. Wagner Jr. "A test for patency of the cystic duct in acute cholecystitis." Ann Int Med 82 (1975) 318-322.

86. Weissman, H.S., M.S. Frank, L.H. Bernstein, and L.M. Freeman. "Rapid and accurate diagnosis of acute cholecystitis with Tc-99m-HIDA cholescintigraphy." Am J Roentgen 132 (1979) 523-528.

87. Rosenthall, L., E.A. Shaffer, and R. Lisbona, et al. "Diagnosis of hepatobiliary disease by Tc-99m-HIDA cholescintigraphy." Radiology 126 (1978) 467-474.

88. Rosenthall, L., C. Fonseca, A. Arzoumanian, M. Hernandez, and D. Greenberg. "Tc-99m-HIDA hepatobiliary imaging following upper abdominal surgery." Radiology 130 (1979) 735-739.

89. Alavi, A., R.W. Dann, S. Baum, and D.N. Biery. "Scinti-graphic detection of acute gastrointestinal bleeding." Radiology 124 (1977) 753-756.

90. Winzelberg, G.G., K.A. McKusick, H.W. Strauss, A.C. Waltman, and A.J. Greenfield. "Evaluation of Gastrointestinal bleeding by red blood cells labeled in vivo with Tc-99m." J Nucl Med 20 (1979) 1080-1086.

91. Winzelberg, G.G., J.W. Froelich, K.A. McKusick, A.C. Waltman, A.J. Greenfield, and H.W. Strauss. "Radionuclide localization of lower gastrointestinal hemorrhage." Radiology 139 (1981) 465-469.

REAL-TIME ULTRASOUND

A. Everette James, Jr.
Arthur C. Fleischer
James Machin
C. Leon Partain
Gadi Horev
Ronald R. Price

Department of Medical Imaging and Radiological Sciences
Vanderbilt University School of Medicine
Nashville, Tennessee

The introduction of gray scale imaging techniques in the early 1970's (1973-1974) remarkably increased the utility of diagnostic ultrasound (1). The ability to portray the internal structure of solid organs and to participate in first order tissue analysis significantly improved the diagnostic information from sonographic studies (2). Lesions could not only be more accurately detected with greater sensitivity but characterizations with patho-anatomical inferences were made possible.

However, structural information provides only a single function analysis of health and diseases. A much more sensitive assessment can be provided by those studies which depict functional information. Thus, the introduction of an imaging modality providing physiological information would represent a significant advance (2-4).

Real-time ultrasound was introduced in the late 1970's and has represented a major advance in assessment of health and disease employing reflected ultrasonic sound waves. Real-time studies not only provide the opportunity to observe physiological motion but also allow almost simultaneous observation of organs and structures from a number of different angles and orientations. In this communication, we intend to discuss the various real-time methods and provide the reader with a general assessment of the virtues and limitations of each. Additionally, we will consider the most interesting and promising technique of pulsed Doppler real-time ultrasound.

REAL-TIME INSTRUMENTATION

A number of classifications and descriptions of real-time ultrasound systems have been offered (5). At the present, we favor subdividing real-time ultrasound (US) equipment into four basic types characterized chiefly by the transducer activation and physical orientation. These descriptors are:

1. Linear sequenced array
2. Phased array with beam steering
3. Phased array of the annular type
4. Mechanical scanner (sector and linear)
   a. "Wobbler" single element
   b. Rotating
5. Single element transducer that moves in linear path.

Differences in transducer design and in the specifics of operation may occur within a single generic type of real-time design, but this classification scheme has proved quite useful. Differences may occur also from the physical orientation of the transducer crystals, the sequence and mode of activation, and the length of the ultrasound path through liquid or the coupling tissue equivalent. Although a few real-time scanners employ analog display, most now employ the digital conversion format. We will discuss real-time instrumentation only as digital scan converter and memory ultrasound technology; a choice quite in keeping with the other descriptions in this text.

Real-time scanning was originally developed to visualize cardiac and associated vascular motion. This was a natural extension of the types of observations commonly employed in M-mode ultrasonography. However, the requirements of transducer design in this specific area of the body were particularly rigorous and other types of instruments were developed to examine other body areas, especially the abdomen and pelvis. Linear array units were reasonably simple and inexpensive to fabricate. For these reasons, they rapidly gained widespread use.

Multi-element linear scanning arrays (Figure 1) are pulsed so as to produce a wave front that is parallel to the transducer face which results in a rectangular field. The "effective" transducer is most often composed of many small crystals that are arranged in a row. The sequence of crystal pulsing is variable depending upon the design. Because the field from a single rather small transducer will diverge rapidly, several transducers may be

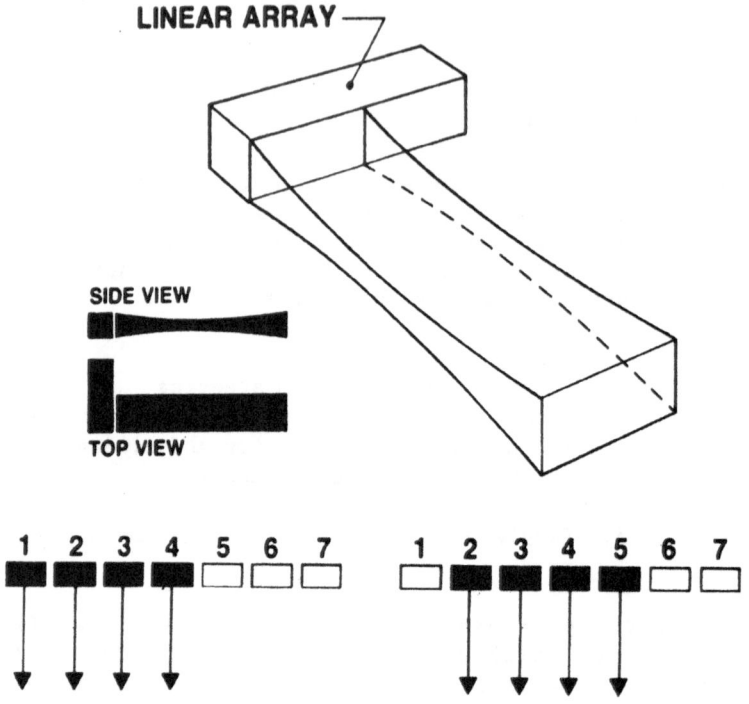

Figure 1. Linear array transducer. (A) Diagrammatic representation of effective beam shape. (B) Diagram demonstrating possible sequence of crystal activities. This sequence can be manipulated electronically to focus the beam, both on sending and receiving the signals.

activated as a group and focussed electronically. In a particular group of crystals, the outer crystals may be pulsed first and the inner crystals delayed. The "field" from that set of transducers can be focussed at some chosen depth depending upon the magnitude of the electronic delays employed. By selectively changing the delay strengths, the focal zone may be scanned through a specified range of depths. Thus, the transmitted signals can be utilized to produce a signal wave front which is optimized at some particular selected depth.

The received signals may also be delayed by a similar chosen set of factors. This selective delay will occur before all the signals are summed or added together. This maneuver has a focussing effect upon the returning ultrasonic sound signals and when coupled with a similar transmission procedure constitutes what is known as a "double focussing" system. One may form a single line scan of a real-time image in the above-described manner. The adjacent scan line is generated by activating another selected group of crystals in a similar manner. Often this adjacent line is generated by shifting a single crystal position along the transducer array. Thus, the same pattern of ultrasound transmission and reception is repeated for another set of crystals and subsequently from all other sets of crystals along the array in a cyclic manner. The resultant effect is that this technique will yield approximately an equal number of scan lines as there are transducer crystals in the array (6).

The type of pulsing and focussing described above improves lateral resolution of the reflected event as well as the sensitivity of the system by increasing the amount of energy in the focal zone. This particular phenomenon is known as constructive interference. The images produced by these systems do not have the distortions which are characteristic of certain other techniques to be discussed subsequently, are in a rectangular format familiar and acceptable to most clinicians, and may be improved by some rather simple and inexpensive engineering principles.

A higher scan line density can be effected by employing more crystals, rescanning using a smaller subgroup of crystals, or by employing electronic steering to sample between previous scan lines. The former method is technically difficult and the engineering expensive. Most often the latter method is chosen. The combined effects of dual focussing and beam steering to increase line density allow present real-time systems to achieve lateral resolution of 1.5 to 2 mm.

Annular phased array transducers may employ oscillating acoustical mirrors to achieve mechanical motion of the ultrasound beam or a subset of transducer signals (Figure 2). In this arrangement, the ultrasound wave is reflected according to the relative angulation of the transducer surface of the annular array with the surface of the mirror. In most machines of this design, a water bath is employed to create an appropriate patient/instrument interface or "coupling."

Certain types of phased array instruments have been constructed that utilize many of the engineering advances which allow a great number of transducers to be contained in a very small space (Figure 3). Recent advances in computer technology will permit this type of physical arrangement. Electronic sequencing of the minute transducers allows the signal to travel into the body tissue as a wave front. This instrumentation is both complex and at present somewhat expensive on a relative basis (7).

542

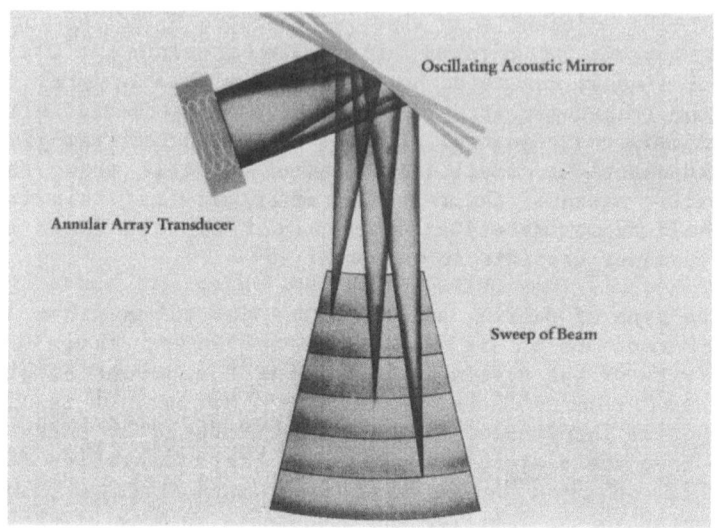

Figure 2. Annular array transducer. Real-time effect is produced by sweeping the beam back and forth by reflecting the focussed beam off a rapidly oscillating acoustic mirror. (Courtesy of SKI).

The mechanical sector real-time scanners have received a great deal of recent interest. These devices have certain inherent advantages. Several types of transducer arrangements have been employed to achieve mechanical motion (Figure 4A,B). A single element linear oscillating transducer may be designed to move in a linear fashion housed in a water bath. An arrangement of this type has been successfully employed in the Microview "small parts" scanner 1). This particular instrument will again be referred to in the subsequent discussion of pulsed Doppler real-time. The pivoted to-and-fro movement of a single transducer may also be used to produce the mechanical motion; this has been termed the "wobbler" technique. Motion of the transducer in this fashion will provide a "pie-shaped" image. Distortion at depth (distance from transducer/patient interface) with this type of instrument has been a significant problem due to memory "drop out".

A very "popular" mechanical sector design has been that of the rotating wheel upon which a number of crystals are located. The crystals are activated at sequenced times during their

1. Picker Corporation, Minor Road, Cleveland, Ohio.

rotation and the transmitted ultrasonic sound beam directed through an aperture in the transducer housing to then pass into the body tissues. The circular motion of the wheel does not appear to have the associated engineering complexity of a number of other designs. The transducer head is small, it is affixed to a drive system that is rather easily "hand held", and its shape and configuration are very readily accommodated by the body surfaces and contours (Figure 5). A pulsed Doppler device can be attached to this type real-time composite transducer without having to alter the structure or configuration significantly. In a more recent design, the same transducer is used for both real-time imaging as well as receiving Doppler signals.

The characteristic differences between cardiac and so-called "body" scanners principally involve those engineering applications that determine the size of the transducer head and the field of view of the image. Phased array instruments with beam steering and many of the mechanical sector transducers produce images with apex angles that are typically between 60 and 90 degrees (Figure 6). This particular format does not present significant problems in cardiac imaging; but the somewhat restricted or "compromised" field of view at the apex of the sector presents problems in imaging superficial structures. An example of a clinical circumstance in which this might prove problematical would be in evaluation of the anterior surface of a solid organ located superficially, such as the liver or the thyroid gland.

Real-time instruments utilizing shared arrays and beam steering produce a "pie shaped" image which often does not allow

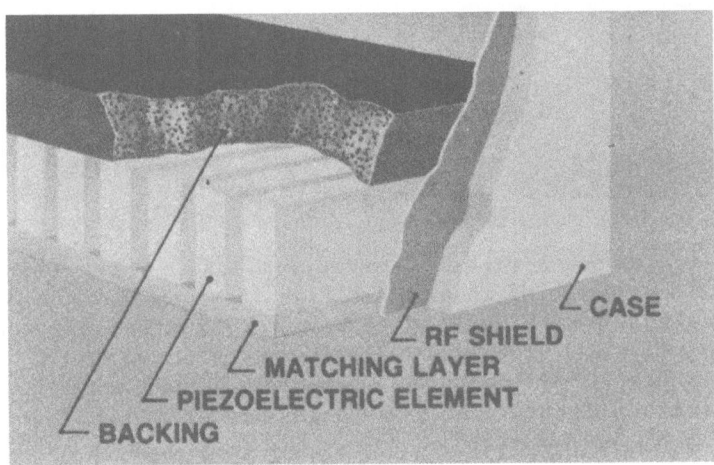

Figure 3. Cross section of multi-element transducer. Current engineering allows packing multiple crystals into a small space.

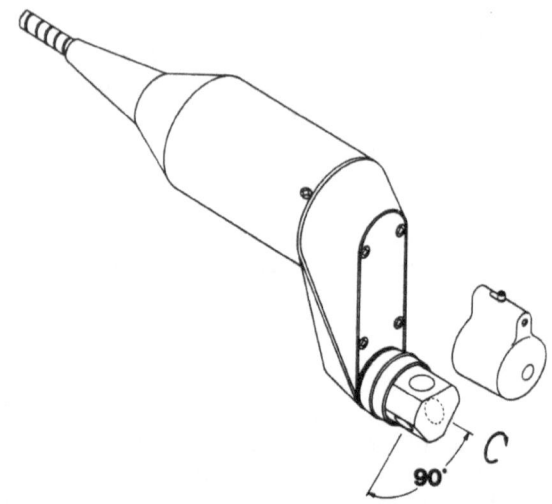

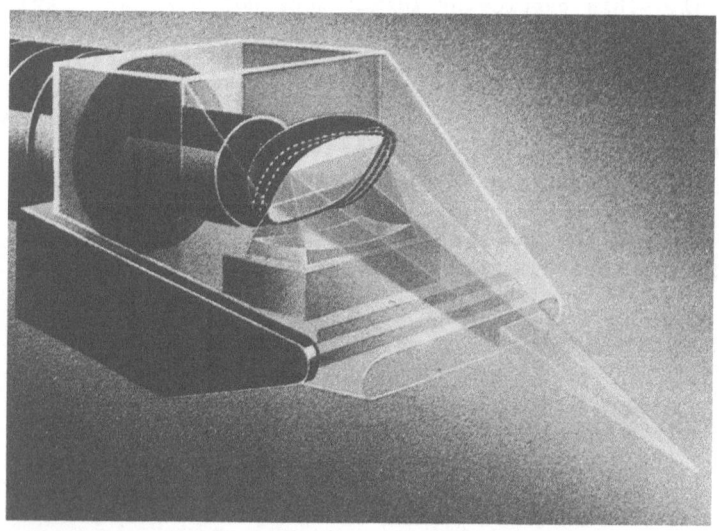

Figure 4. Mechanical sector scanners. (A) Three transducer elements on a rotating wheel allow high frame rates while keeping the scan head small, making this a very versatile scanner. (Courtesy of ATL.) (B) An oscillating acoustic mirror is used to sweep the beam in the "wobbler" mechanical sector scanner. Water bag required in each example for coupling to the patient. (Courtesy of Biodynamics.)

recognition of normal anatomical reference structures. The images also are sufficiently unfamiliar to one's clinical colleagues that credibility and appreciation of the assessment may sometimes be an issue, especially if the images are compared with those of x-ray computed tomography. Because of certain desirable engineering characteristics of phased array devices, instrument manufacturers are continuing to modify and improve transducer design and information recording so that these undesirable features are eliminated. The electronic steering of the phased array methodology has great potential for flexibility of data acquisition.

A general limitation that real-time instrumentation has experienced has been the development of a suitable permanent recording of the data for consultation and archiving. A number of "hard copy" display techniques have been attempted. Videotaping with voice activation allows recording of the orientation, reporting the analysis, and correlating for future clinical reference. The principal limitation of this format is physician viewing time. Digital processing of information storage in all areas of medical imaging will allow not only standardization of image acquisition and display but also data transmission. In addition, the change from analog to digital signal acquisition will permit processing of the images in such manner as to improve recognition by the observer.

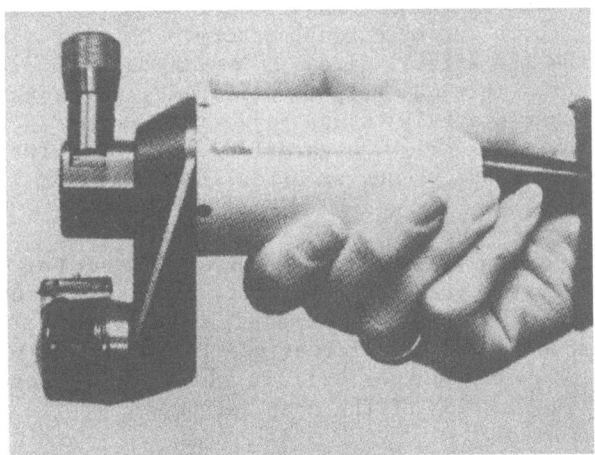

Figure 5. Mechanical sector scanner with pulsed Doppler. This design shows the Doppler transducer attached above the scanner head. This design does not allow simultaneous pulsed Doppler real-time scanning. More recent designs use the same transducer for real-time as well as receiving Doppler signals, allowing simultaneous imgaing. (Courtesy of ATL.)

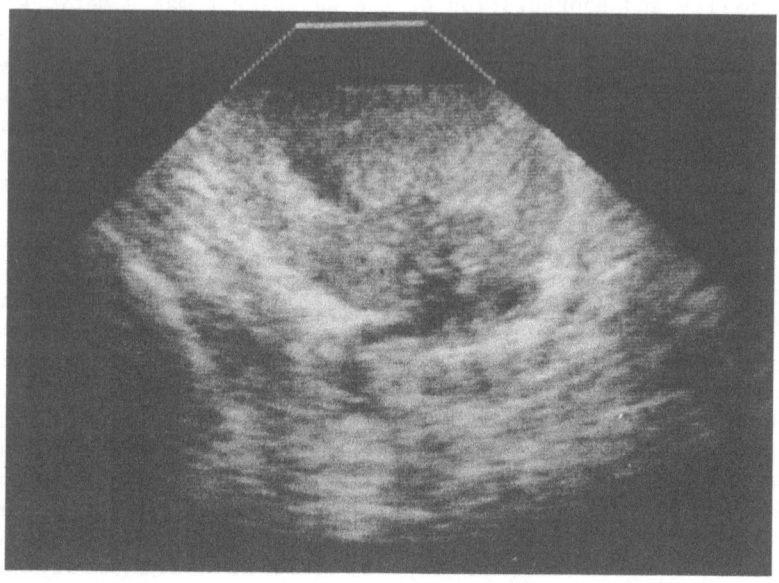

Figure 6. Image from real-time sector scanner is wedge shaped. Imaging deep and shallow structures simultaneously is often not possible with this format. This image of a renal transplant clearly demonstrates the main renal artery. Doppler signals can be obtained from the artery, allowing assessment of flow to the renal transplant. This may help to differentiate rejection from acute tubular necrosis (ATN) since rejection results in diminished renal blood flow, while flow is normal in ATN. Doppler may also be used to detect renal venous or arterial thrombosis.

At the present time, the mechanical sector scanning instruments enjoy the greatest popularity and clinical usefulness. However, fabrication of less expensive delay mechanisms and improved transducer design will continue to expand the utility of phased array systems, and we believe these will represent the real-time instrumentation of the near future.

We have alluded to certain of the advantages of real-time instrumentation in clinical sonographic imaging. The ability to visualize complex human anatomy from a number of different orientations in a very short time interval will add to a more accurate appreciation of the structural characteristics, allow rapid determination of optimum scan planes, and permit the improved identification of normal anatomical structures and their variants. The movement both from involuntary physiological motion and from mechanical motion of human structures will often provide information which can be interpreted in quite meaningful patho-physiological terms. Assessment of vessel wall motion, bowel peristalsis (8), cardiac valve motion and change in cardiac ventricular volume are a few parameters amenable to real-time ultrasound assessment. Because a real-time ultrasound image is viewed continuously and instantaneously, linear structures such as arteries and veins can be examined along their course and caliber assessment for significant distances can be made. The use of ultrasound "contrast media" such as instilled or ingested water and air bubbles in liquid can be used to identify the lumen of both hollow organs and vessels. We have been particularly impressed with the ability of real-time observation of the water installation of stomach and duodenum to evaluate upper abdomen and in the rectum to aid in the identification of normal and abnormal pelvic structures (9). The intentional filling of bladder (urine) and rectum (water enema) may significantly aid in determining the extent of pelvic neoplasms. Likewise, bowel and bladder wall invasion or thickening can be detected by the use of this technique.

Fluid-filled bowel offers a challenge in diagnosis that has been only partly solved by plain film radiographic studies (8,10). The interface between the bowel wall and the intraluminal liquid contents can be readily delineated by ultrasound techniques. The flexibility of real-time imaging makes it particularly useful in this regard. Collections of air in other parts of the bowel can often be avoided by simply changing the position, angulation, or orientation of the transducer with respect to the bowel containing fluid. This maneuver is also useful for viewing inaccessible structures like the pancreas that often lie distal to air/fluid-filled bowel. One can determine the location of an "ultrasonic window" much more easily with the flexible and mobile real-time system than with the static B-mode imaging devices. Additionally, observing the bowel for a few moments will allow determination of whether or not peristalsis is present (8). This may be particularly important in the choice of therapeutic regimen for the fluid-filled bowel.

Abdominal trauma is an important clinical problem. Often the ability to evaluate the integrity of solid organs such as the liver, spleen, and kidney is necessary (10). Free fluid from rupture of a hollow viscous, bleeding from an organ laceration or disruption, or from the presence of a retroperitoneal bleed or hematoma will significantly alter patient management (11). The highly mobile, flexible real-time ultrasound systems will permit these kinds of evaluations in a short time period without patient discomfort or risk.

The incidence of intracranial hemorrhage in premature neonates with minimal clinical findings makes real-time ultrasound clinically efficacious. The real-time ultrasound examination has proven to be of great importance because of the speed, lack of patient discomfort, ability to transport the imaging device into the nursery and examine the neonate in the isolette, and the absence of significant biological implications (12). From these studies, one can detect both intracisternal, intraventricular and subependymal hemorrhage as well as the development of hydrocephalus (13,14). Real-time ultrasound has revolutionized this evaluation process and has largely replaced x-ray computed tomography as the procedure of choice for this assessment.

Abdominal masses and renal abnormalities in neonates and infants have also proven to be easily assessed by real-time ultrasound studies. Again, the circumstances of bringing the imaging device to the patient where life support instrumentation may be required has been shown to be of rather fundamental importance and favors greatly the use of this methodology. Certain radiographic and nuclear medicine procedures have been replaced by ultrasound studies performed using real-time instrumentation.

Thus, real-time instrumentation has received almost immediate general acceptance (7). We would predict that in a few years the virtues of this form of instrumentation will gain more widespread use and acceptance despite competition provided by such promising and important techniques as digital radiography and nuclear magnetic resonance, which are also discussed in this symposium.

REAL-TIME PULSED DOPPLER ULTRASOUND

The measurement of volumetric blood flow is of fundamental importance in the assessment of tissue perfusion as a reflection of tissue viability (15). At present, no noninvasive method has been developed and successfully employed to determine volumetric blood flow in the clinical circumstance.

In general, to measure volumetric blood flow by ultrasound one must independently measure the area of the blood vessel cross-section (usually in cm^2) and the average flow velocity (in cm/sec). Sonographic Doppler techniques have concentrated upon the detection and measurement of flow velocity (16).

In this discussion, we will only consider the principles of the Doppler phenomenon in a summary fashion, leaving the reader an opportunity to review the chapter by Wells (17) as well as other detailed articles on this subject (6,18,19). The Doppler signal results from a rather fundamental principal of the effect of a moving structure upon an impinging ultrasonic sound wave. A moving structure will cause a reflected or backscattered ultrasound signal frequency to be shifted up or down by an amount

proportional to the interface velocity acting upon the sound beam
axis expressed as:

$$\pm \, \Delta f = \frac{2Vf_o}{c} \, Cos \, \theta \tag{1}$$

The relation of the received frequency (f_r) compared to the
original is expressed as:

$$\underline{+} \, \Delta f = f_o - f_r \tag{2}$$

When the impinging sound passes into a blood vessel, the moving
red cells will shift the backscattered energy frequency
proportional to their velocity. Blood flow disturbances secondary
to anatomic defects such as stenotic vessels, plaques, or
partially occluded valves or lumina can be detected by noting
differences in the frequency spectrum of the Doppler signal.

Moving blood will gain kinetic energy as it accelerates
through the narrowing in a lumen whether it is in a vessel or
heart valve. Once the blood passes a point of narrowing into a
region of larger caliber, the velocity will decrease. The energy
will be given up in the form of turbulence or eddies and
vortices.

Continuous wave Doppler instruments have been used for this
type of assessment, but they lack both adequate range and suffer
from ambiguities in localization. One of the more practical means
to improve localization of returning signals to a Doppler
instrument is to pulse the source and add a range to the
receiver.

A pulsed Doppler system employs different principles than
those employed by a pulsed echo instrument. A pulsed Doppler
system excites the transmitting transducer at a precise and known
frequency. Thus, when the echo returns it can be compared to that
of the original transmitted burst to determine the Doppler shift
(Figure 7A,B). In practice, we detect the Doppler shift at
selected points along the ultrasound beam over the depth set by
the pulse repetition rate.

A pulsed Doppler system alone will not provide sufficient
information regarding the origin of the reflected echo (shift).
Thus, we combine it with a real-time echo system (Figure 8). This
"duplex system" has the capability of recording both the Doppler
shift and the vessel image from which the recording is made
(Figure 9) (20).

Although we have emphasized the imaging aspect of a duplex
system, in certain circumstances one may be able to detect an

550

abnormality that is not well visualized. The so-called "soft plaques" have an acoustical impedence that approximates that of blood. However, the vessel wall image on the echo system will not be the same as that depicted by the Doppler vessel lumen image. The sensitivity in this clinical circumstance has yet to be determined.

Quantification of the physiological significance of vascular lesions by ultrasound study has been considered one of the potential virtues of this form of inquiry. When blood moving in a vessel lumen encounters a sudden reduction in the area of the lumen, there will be an acceleration in velocity. The physical reason for this phenomenon is the requirement to maintain a constant flow rate through the compromised vessel area. The kinetic energy is stored in the moving blood and as soon as the vessel lumen enlarges, it will be released and the velocity reduced. When the energy is released, flow disturbances occur which produce flow fluctuations in the flow velocity about the average velocity over the area of the vessel lumen. The magnitude

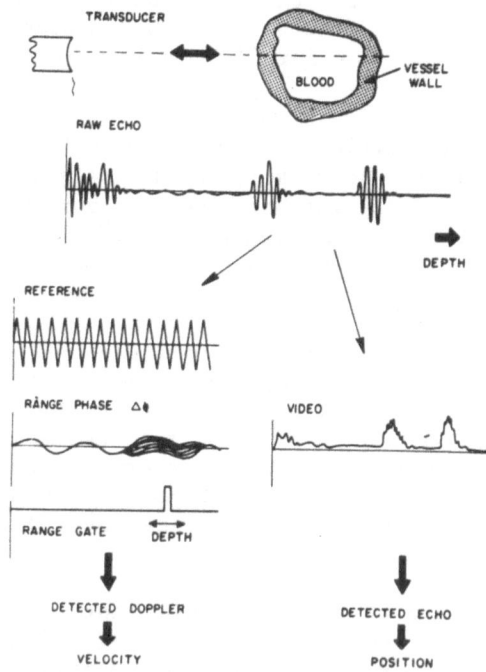

Figure 7A. Schematic of pulsed Doppler. By determining change in frequency of returning signal compared to transmitted signal, velocity of blood flow can be determined. By use of a range gate, only selected depths are detected. (Reprinted from Radiologic Clinics of North America, Vol. 14, 1980, with permission.)

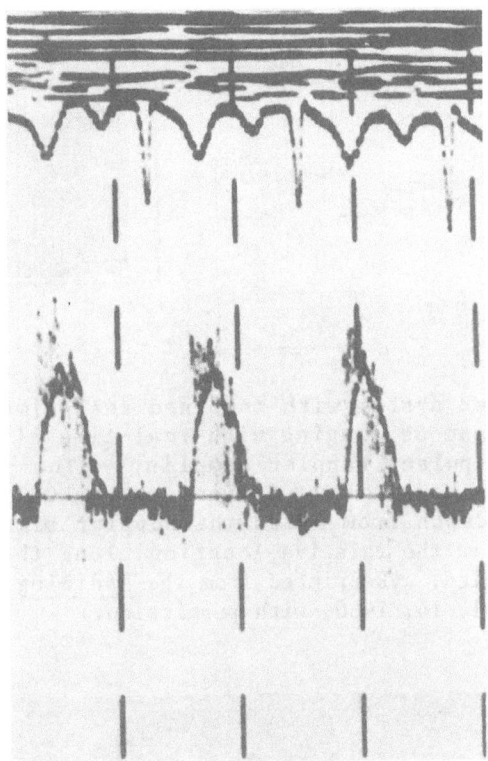

Figure 7B. Normal Doppler tracing. Vertical dashed lines represent timing marks. Simultaneous EKG trace is above the Doppler frequency shift curve. A normal tracing is characterized by a rapid upslope in systole followed by a general downslope until the next systole. (Courtesy of Lincoln Burland, M.D.)

of the turbulent intensity is inversely related to the degree of occlusion. By monitoring the width of the Doppler shift (Δf), one may determine the magnitude of the fluctuation of the velocity. Methods and parameters for a mathematical and quantitative analysis of this type study have been developed (15). Some groups have advocated using a combination of a velocity ratio and an assessment of fractional broadening. They believe that a set of blood flow parameters in combination with image data employed for orientation will provide the best approach to determine vascular occlusion.

Combined real-time and Doppler imaging may prove useful for evaluating a number of clinical areas including:

1. Renal blood flow in native as well as transplanted kidneys (refer to Figure 6)

552

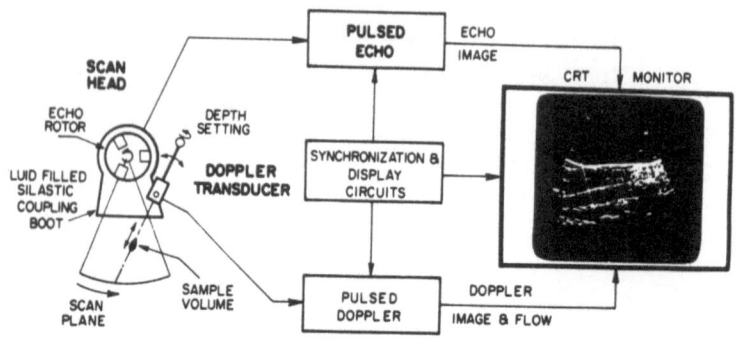

Figure 8. Duplex system with combined real-time and pulsed Doppler. Simultaneous imaging with real-time allows accurate orientation for pulsed Doppler sampling. The vessel to be measured is imaged and a cursor is used on the CRT to determine accurately the depth from which the Doppler signal is to be recorded as well as the relative location along the axis of the vessel to be sampled. (Reprinted from the Radiologic Clinics of North America, Vol. 14, 1980, with permission.)

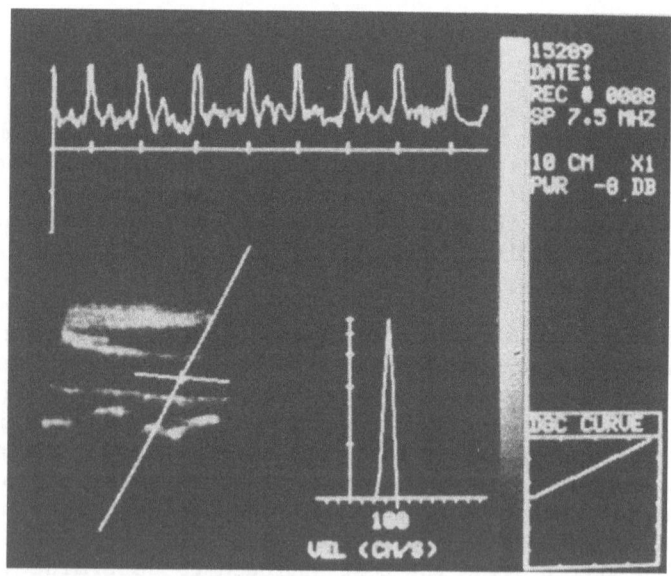

Figure 9. Normal common carotid real-time image and Doppler recording. Cursor marks the point from which the flow velocity is measured within the common carotid artery. (Courtesy of Lincoln Berland, M.D.)

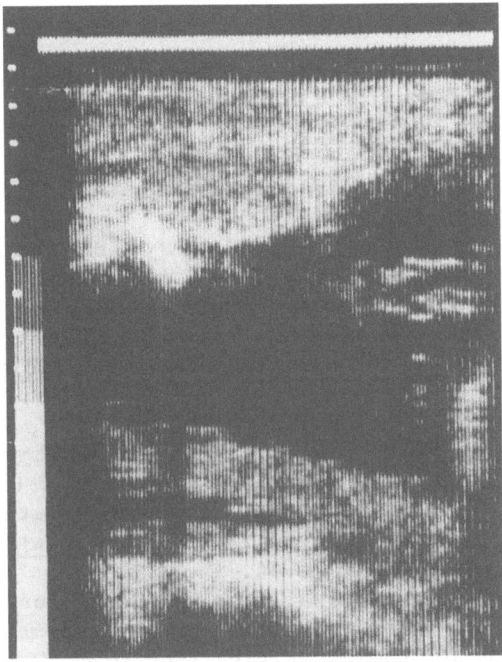

Figure 10. Real-time scanning of the long axis of the umbilical cord demonstrates the umbilical vein and two umbilical arteries. Range gated pulsed Doppler signals can be obtained from the umbilical cord which correlate with relative blood flow. Blood flow determinations may have potential applications in assessing the growth retarded fetus.

2. Umbilical blood flow in intrauterine growth retardation (Figure 10)
3. Portal vein blood flow in the presence of portal hypertension
4. Blood flow in IVC in right heart failure
5. Patent ductus arteriosus
6. Flow gradients across cardiac valves.

In summary, real-time pulsed Doppler ultrasound is a method that appears to offer a safe, relatively inexpensive method of diagnostic inquiry. In this symposium, many alternative imaging techniques are discussed. How the information obtained by real-time pulsed Doppler will compare with that obtained by digital radiology, positron emission tomography, or nuclear magnetic resonance should be determined by greater clinical experience and appropriately designed efficacy studies.

554

REFERENCES

1. Carson, P.L. "Grey-scale ultrasound: Understanding an innovation in imaging to speed realization of its potential." Applied Radiology 6 (1977) 185-189.
2. Linzer, M. and P.N.T. Wells. Report on the symposium. NBS Special Publication No. 525. (Washington, D.C.: U.S. Government Printing Office, 1979) 3-9.
3. Fleischer, A.C. and A.E. James, Jr. Introduction to Diagnostic Sonography (New York: John Wiley & Sons, Inc., 1980).
4. Fields, S. and F. Dunn. "Correlation of echographic visualizability of tissue with biological composition and physiological state." Journal of the Acoustical Society of America 54 (1973) 809.
5. James, A.E., Jr., Goddard, J., Price, R.R., Jones, T. and R.L. Powis. "Advances in instrument design and image recording." Radiologic Clinics of North America 18 (1980) 3-20.
6. Wells, P.N.T. "Real-Time Scanning Systems," in New Techniques and Instrumentation in Ultrasonography (New York: Churchill Livingstone, 1980) 69-84.
7. James, A.E., Jr., Fleischer, A.C., Jones, T.B., et al. "Ultrasound: Certain Considerations of Equipment Usage," in The Physical Basis of Medical Imaging (New York: Appleton-Century-Crofts, 1981).
8. Fleischer, A.C., Muhletaler, C.A. and A.E. James, Jr. "Sonographic assessment of the bowel wall." American Journal of Roentgenology 136 (1981) 887-891.
9. Peterson, L. and P. Cooperberg. "Ultrasound demonstration of lesions of the gastrointestinal tract." Gastrointestinal Radiology 3 (1978) 303-306.
10. McCort, J.J. The Acute Abdomen: Radiographic Examination in Blunt Abdominal Trauma (Philadelphia: Saunders, 1966).
11. Heller, R.M., Coulam, C.M., Allen, J.H., et al. "Diagnostic imaging in pediatric emergencies." Southern Medical Journal 73 (1980) 844-849.
12. Fleischer, A.C., Hutchison, A.A., Allen, J.H., Stahlman, M.T., Meacham, W.F. and A.E. James, Jr. "The role of sonography and the radiologist-ultrasonologist in the detection and follow-up of intracranial hemorrhage in the preterm neonate." Radiology 139 (1981) 733-736.
13. James, A.E., Flor, W.J., Novak, G.R., et al. "The ultrastructural basis of periventricular edema: Preliminary studies." Radiology 135 (1980) 747-750.
14. Fleischer, A., Hutchison, A., and S. Kirchner. "Cranial real-time sonography in the preterm neonate." Diagnostic Imaging 3 (1981) 20-31.
15. Baker, D.W. "Application of pulsed Doppler techniques." Radiologic Clinics of North America 18 (1980) 79-103.

16. Woodcock, J.P. and R. Skidmore. "Principles and Applications of Doppler Ultrasound," in New Techniques and Instrumentation in Ultrasonography (New York: Churchill Livingstone, 1980) 166-185.

17. Wells, P.N.T. "Pulse-echo methods," in Biomedical Ultrasonics (New York: Academic Press, 1977) 228-248.

18. Strandness, D.E., Jr. and D.S. Sumner. "Applications of ultrasound to the study of arteriosclerosis obliterans." Angiography 26 (1975) 187.

19. Coulam, C.M., Erickson, J.J., Rollo, F.D. and A.E. James, Jr. The Physical Basis of Medical Imaging (New York: Appleton-Century-Crofts, 1981).

20. Eyer, M.K., Brandestini, M.A., Phillips, D.J. and D.W. Baker. "Color digital echo-Doppler image presentation." Ultrasound in Medicine and Biology 7 (1981) 21-31.

COMPARISON OF DIFFERENT IMAGING TECHNIQUES FOR THE PREDICTION AND IMAGING OF PATIENTS WITH ABDOMINAL, PELVIC OR THYROID DISEASE

DR. V. RALPH McCREADY

Director, Department of Nuclear Medicine and
Ultrasound, Royal Marsden Hospital, Sutton, Surrey,
U.K.

INTRODUCTION

This paper aims to define exactly what information is
produced by radionuclide, ultrasound and CT scanning in the
various diseases affecting the thyroid, liver, pancreas, kidneys
and pelvic organs. The advantages and limitations of the
different types of non invasive investigations will be stressed.
At times there has been less emphasis on the actual contribution
made by these tests, the choice depending more upon availability
and their relative cost. However now that the tests are becoming
more generally available and that personnel with increased
experience are on hand to carry them out, there is a need for a
more careful evaluation of the actual information obtainable from
a particular test and how far this information can be used to
give a definite diagnosis.

GENERAL COMMENTS

To anyone outside the diagnostic imaging field and even to
some of those within the specialty the choice of a particular
test or order of tests can be quite difficult. It is hoped that
by presenting in some detail the actual information derived from
each type of non invasive investigation, the referring physician
or surgeon will be in a better position to judge the relative
merits of the different tests.

CT scanning, ultrasound and radioisotope imaging use
different physical principles to achieve the end image. For this
reason it should be obvious that the tests are likely to be

complementary and that their relative value in diagnosing a pathological abnormality will differ in different parts of the body. Plain X-rays make use of the fact that X radiation is attenuated strongly by high atomic weight elements. Thus bones show up best against soft tissue and soft tissue shows up best against air. Plain X-rays are best for showing up bony abnormalities, lesions in the chest and calcium (indicating chronic lesions) in the abdomen. CT scanning also makes use of X-rays but the images are more related to electron density. This is low in the case of fat and higher in the case of all the other soft tissues making up the organs. Thus CT scans show the outlines of organs particularly well. The images presented are usually in cross section which is advantageous in showing the relations of the organs to each other and in demonstrating the spread of a disease from one organ to another. However the sections are relatively thin and to get a complete picture a large number of sequential slices is required. In a patient with definite signs of a disease the radiation hazard is probably of little importance but the apparatus employed is expensive and the tests are still fairly time consuming. CT scans have their limitations. When compared area for area with ultrasound imaging the detail is relatively poor particularly when examining soft tissues. Of course such statements have to be qualified by the fact that if more time and radiation is employed a higher resolution can be achieved. There is however a limiting factor in that most space occupying lesions with the exception of water and fat do not have a marked difference in electron density from normal tissues and therefore the diagnosis of space occupying lesions can be difficult. The problem in finding a suitable agent to increase the contrast in the tumour and therefore the smallest lesion detectable is the same as is found in developing a tumour localising agent for radioisotope imaging.

Ultrasound imaging relies on the difference of elasticity between the different tissues. The greatest difference found within the body is between soft tissue and fluid. The end image is the result of ultrasound wave scattering and reflection. The combination of both yields the best pictures in situations where there is blood, water or bile present in the lesion. The outlines of organs are not so well displayed in this type of investigation and gas and air form an impenetrable barrier to ultrasound waves. Thus it will never be possible to produce the same pretty cross sections that are possible with CT scanning. However unlike CT scanning it is possible to see very small vessels and the internal structure of the liver, spleen, pancreas, kidney and uterus by using suitable acoustic windows. There are hopes that the analysis of the echo pattern in normal and abnormal situations using a computer and mathematical techniques will help to make the diagnosis of abnormalities more objective. At least to the eye the internal pattern seen in many abnormalities is little different from that of the rest of the normal surrounding tissue. Thus although the resolution is high there must be quite a few abnormalities which are not detected by ultrasound even under the best conditions. It is also worth noting that although many of the examinations are carried out by the doctor, the amount of time spent in post processing the scans is very much smaller than that done in CT scanning. It is worth considering that when comparing tests the end result of CT scanning when seen by the referring physician has been processed by a doctor who has decided what is abnormal and then sets out to display this "abnormality" to its best advantage. There is a definite need for more objective diagnosis when using both CT and ultrasound.

Radioisotope imaging usually displays normal physiology. Abnormalities are seen in general as non radioactive cold lesions. Because the contrast between the normal area and abnormal area is generally low the minimum detectable lesion is usually quite large. The alternative situation where there is concentration of a radio-nuclide in an abnormality such as in functioning carcinoma of the thyroid demonstrates how specific and detailed this approach would be if radiopharmaceuticals which concentrated in particular diseases could be developed. After many frustrating years there are now signs that this may be happening, for example the use of monoclonal antibodies and the use of labelled precursors to adrenal hormones. Also the development of emission tomography together with the labelling of physiological compounds with positron emitters still yields the possibility of demonstrating in-vivo imaging by physiological changes. So far the best results have been limited to the brain but these are very exciting. Since it is difficult to generalise when comparing the three main non-invasive techniques it is more valuable to examine a limited number of organs in more detail to show the relative advantages and limitations of each technique.

THE THYROID

The thyroid provides the best example of the use of radio-isotope imaging to reflect physiological function. Radioisotope techniques are used in three main situations namely thyrotoxicosis, the diagnosis of lumps in the neck, functioning thyroid carcinoma.

Thyrotoxicosis

Radioimmunoassay of thyroid hormones form the usual basis for the laboratory diagnosis of thyrotoxicosis. Radionuclide imaging is valuable in demonstrating focal autonomous function prior to possible surgery while ultrasound imaging can help produce volume measurements of the thyroid gland. These measurements can then be used to calculate the appropriate dose of radioactivity required for patients having therapy doses of radioiodine.

Masses in the Neck

With an incidence of carcinoma of 1 in 10 in single nodules of the thyroid there is an argument for elective surgery rather than awaiting the results of a variety of non invasive tests. However in many cases it is more appropriate to adopt a conservative approach and non invasive imaging can help in eliminating at least some of the possible diagnoses.

Most abnormalities in the thyroid are seen as non radio-active areas. In general the size, position and shape of the cold area is of little help in making a differential diagnosis. The use of other radionuclides which concentrate in tumours of the thyroid also have been of little use in helping to confirm or exclude malignancy. Such non functioning lesions can range from cysts and tumours to areas of haemorrhage or thyroiditis.

Ultrasound is useful in detecting fluid filled areas and in particular cysts can be diagnosed as well defined areas without internal echoes and which demonstrate through transmission of the sound waves (Fig. 1). Ultrasound imaging is of less value in differentiating between the various causes of solid lesions. A well defined area with uniform moderate echoes is more likely to be benign than malignant whereas a large area with reduced echoes is more likely to be malignant than benign.

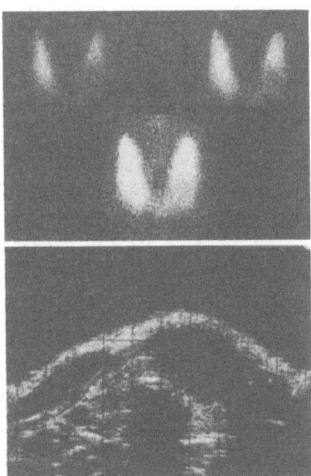

Fig. 1. This patient shows a useful combination of ultrasound and isotope imaging. He presented with a sudden swelling in the left lobe of the thyroid gland. A suspected haemorrhage was confirmed by the low/no echo area in the ultrasound examination. The right lobe is normal in both examinations.

560

Plain X-rays can still help in the differential diagnosis of masses in the neck. The lesions are often better seen on xero radiography which edge enhances opaque areas. This test is especially sensitive for the detection of calcification, differentiating between amorphous material in benign adenomas and shell-like calcification in long standing cysts.

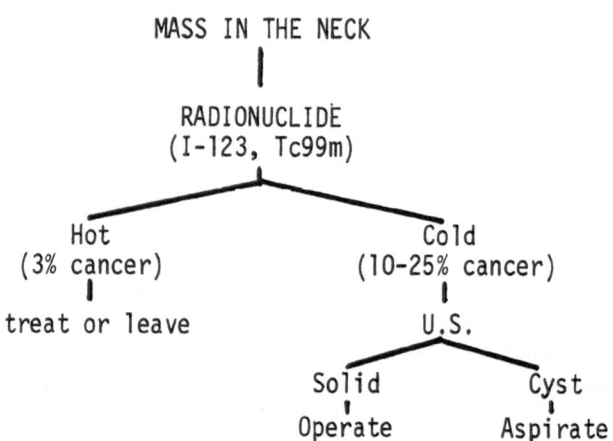

Fig. 2

There is little information in the literature on the accuracy of the various tests. From physical analysis it is · probably of the order of 1 cm at best. However figures are not yet available for the relative sensitivity of the various tests.

Differentiated Thyroid Carcinoma

This is probably the only situation where a radionuclide concentrates in a carcinoma. In these cases the radioiodine can be given in large doses to treat the lesion as well as display its distribution throughout the body. The usual pattern is to give an ablation dose of approximately 80 mCi to ablate all the normal residual thyroid tissue. Following this successive therapy doses concentrate in the papillary or follicular carcinoma of the thyroid. Radioisotope imaging can then display the location of the metastases together with an indication of their level of concentration of the radionuclide. As the carcinoma converts the iodine into hormone,measurement of the hormone levels in the blood is also of value in determining the total amount of functioning carcinoma. When the patient is thought to be cured plain X-rays of the chest can be used to complement follow up studies with smaller doses of radioiodine together with X-rays of the skeleton and bone scintigrams where appropriate. Thyro-globulin measurements are currently showing promise of being an even more sensitive indicator of the presence of residual thyroid normal or carcinomatous tissue.

THE LIVER - FOCAL DISEASE

The detection of space occupying lesions in the liver in both benign and malignant disease remains difficult in spite of the recent advances in non invasive imaging. For this organ ultrasound, radioisotope imaging and CT scanning all have their particular advantages and disadvantages.

Isotope imaging is carried out with a radioactively labelled colloid which concentrates in the reticulo-endothelial system. Space occupying lesions are seen as non radioactive areas which for physics reasons limit the size of the minimum detectable lesion. Recently developed radioisotope emission tomography improves the situation somewhat but does not overcome the problem of normal variations mimicking the presence of disease. The isotope image gives little information other than the presence or absence of disease. Attempts at using radionuclides for differential diagnosis either by dynamic imaging or static imaging have proved relatively fruitless.

Ultrasound imaging has higher inherent resolution and also the ability to distinguish between fluid and solid areas in the liver. Thus with careful imaging a higher sensitivity is achieved than is possible with radioisotope approaches. However not all lesions show a pattern which is different from normal tissue nor do they always have an outline separating normal and abnormal areas. In general the appearances on an ultrasound image are those one would expect with cysts showing up as clear non echogenic areas with through transmission. Abscesses can show similar features but tend to be more ragged and have some echo structure within the involved area (Fig. 3).

Solid lesions show a wide variation of echo intensity and pattern. Metastases are generally multiple often with low level echo patterns. Lesions with increased echoes are often associated with the gut (Fig. 4). Primary liver carcinoma can present with a wide variety of appearances, none of which are specific for this disease. In such situations Gallium isotope scans can help a little by indicating those areas that are growing.

Lesions seen on ultrasound imaging can also be seen on CT scanning but with perhaps slightly more difficulty. CT scanning is not limited by the problems that affect ultrasound, namely overlying gas and bony structures but in general the detail seen on ultrasound images exceeds those found on most CT scans.

562

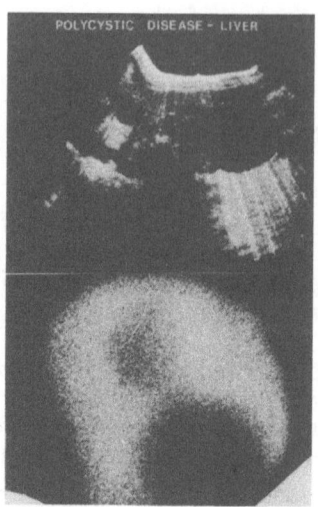

Fig. 3. An ultrasound longitudinal scan (upper) and isotope scan (lower) of a liver involved by polycystic disease. Note the well defined anechoic regions with through transmission on the ultrasound scan.

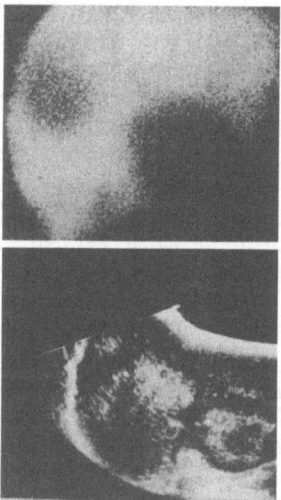

Fig. 4. Ultrasound (lower) and isotope scans (upper) showing lesions that would pass for cysts in the isotope scan but on ultrasound scanning show a high level echo pattern. The appearances suggest secondaries from a gut neoplasm.

Both techniques can be used to facilitate percutaneous biopsy techniques. This is especially so when using ultrasound with real time imaging.

Choice of Tests

Ideally the choice of tests should depend on their relative accuracies. However it is difficult to get figures for sensitivity and specificity especially when one considers that the yardstick against which non invasive tests are compared is particularly unreliable. Laparotomy and biopsy close to the time of scanning have yielded variable results, while autopsies rarely are carried out in patients where there is minimal disease. It is in this situation where non invasive tests could be most useful and where good measurements of sensitivity are needed. Figures that are available show that there is relatively little difference in sensitivity between radioisotope, ultrasound and CT imaging. The latter two are of course of more value because of the ability to help in the differential diagnosis.

Thus taking all factors into consideration most diagnosticians seem to agree that the first test should be radio-nuclide image, followed by an ultrasound scan and then a CT scan if necessary. Equivocal areas where a hepatoma is suspected can be investigated with a Gallium 67 scan (Fig. 5).

LIVER - DIFFUSE DISEASE

By definition diffuse disease is usually due to a collection of physically small abnormalities. Thus it would be unlikely that imaging techniques can detect these directly.

The poor resolution of radioisotope imaging reduces its value in detecting small diffuse abnormalities. However the overall hepatic cell function can often be reduced resulting in colloid being taken up in the spleen or bone marrow. This overspill uptake is a good indirect measure of abnormal liver function but it does not usually help in making a differential diagnosis (Fig. 6).

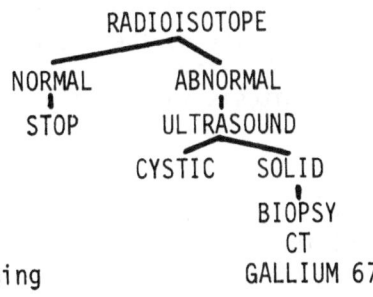

Fig. 5. Liver Imaging

564

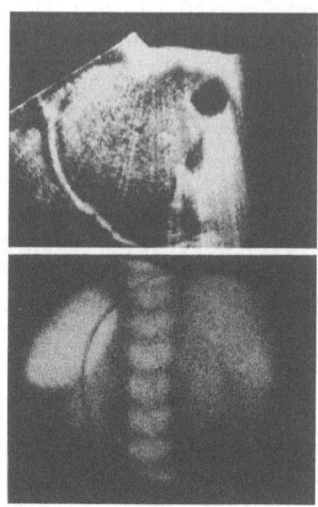

Fig. 6. Ultrasound (upper) and isotope images (lower) in a
patient with liver cirrhosis. The ultrasound image shows the gall
bladder, ascites near the diaphragm and increased attenuation.
The isotope scintigram shows the uneven liver colloid uptake,
increased activity in the spleen and overspill to the bone marrow.

Ultrasound can detect smaller metastases than would be
visible by radioisotope imaging but it is only possible when they
are multiple. They can otherwise be confused with vascular areas
although this confusion may be resolved in due course by using
Doppler techniques. A uniform increased high echo pattern is
usually specific of diffuse liver disease. On the other hand
normal pattern does not exclude it. It is difficult to differentiate between diseases such as cirrhosis and fatty degeneration on
the ultrasound appearances alone.

CT scanning can show the alteration of the outline of the
organ, non uniform attenuation, and such specific signs as the
alteration in the ratios of diameters of the various lobes.
Patients with fatty infiltration and haemochromatosis show
associated changes in the density of the liver and this is best
measured by CT numbers. With fatty infiltration the density is
reduced while in haemochromatosis the density is increased.

Choice of Tests

Isotope imaging gives the best indication of disordered liver
function and the size of the organ. CT scanning is best at
demonstrating the outline of the organ and therefore indirectly

helps in the differential diagnosis particularly of cirrhosis. It
is of unique value in diagnosing and following up haemochromatosis
and is valuable also in fatty infiltration. Ultrasound is
probably the best method of finding small diffusely spread
metastases. A high echo pattern with increased attenuation is
almost always associated with fatty infiltration or cirrhosis.
The difficulty in confirming a hepatoma in diffuse cirrhosis
remains. Gallium 67 scanning can be of great value but a negative
scan does not exclude the possibility of a carcinoma.

BILIARY SYSTEM IMAGING

As in renal diagnostic studies it is important to decide on
whether functional or morphological information is required. For
morphological studies ultrasound gives the best resolution and
detailed information whereas for demonstrating function such as
duct patency radionuclide tests are best.

Several radiopharmaceuticals are now available for imaging
biliary system function. Iminodiacetic acid labelled with
Technetium 99m gives both high sensitivity and good resolution.
When given intravenously the common bile duct is imaged within
10 minutes, the gall bladder within 30 and following this activity
can be seen in the small gut having passed down the biliary system.
Patients with obstruction show delayed excretion while patients
with longstanding liver disease show reduced concentration and
excretion. These tests are best in situations where gall bladder
function and estimates of duct patency (especially postoperative)
are required.

Ultrasound is valuable in demonstrating the size, shape and
position of the gall bladder. The presence or absence of stones
can be easily detected by their acoustic shadow. The intrahepatic
ducts and common bile duct can be visualised especially when they
are dilated following an obstruction (Fig. 7).

CT scanning can show the same features as would be found on
ultrasound scans. They are shown in a transverse plane rather
than in the sagittal plane. The features are perhaps less obvious
on CT scans but on the other hand it is possible to show the
pancreas, liver and duct system as well as the vessels in a single
plane.

The three main clinical situations which present for
evaluation by these non-invasive tests include acute cholecystitis,
chronic cholecystitis and patients presenting with jaundice.

566

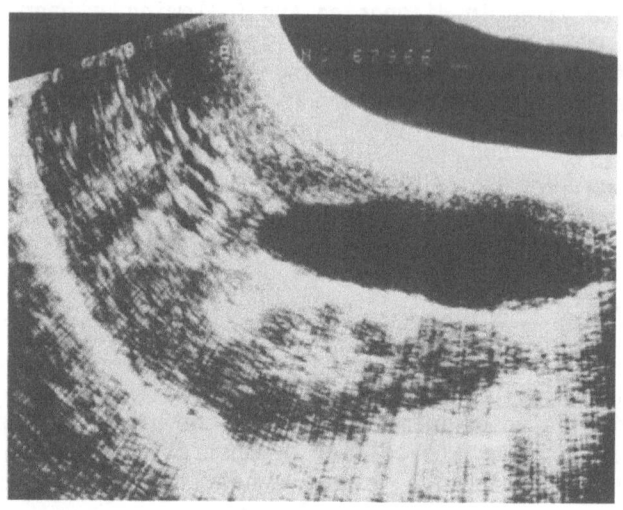

Fig. 7. A longitudinal ultrasound of a liver showing a dilated gall bladder with a little sludge and dilated intra-hepatic ducts in a patient who presented with jaundice.

Cholecystitis

In patients with acute cholecystitis the almost 100% incidence of obstruction of the cystic duct results in non visualisation of the gall bladder following the injection of Technetium labelled HIDA. This technique is highly accurate, false positives being virtually absent. In patients with chronic cholecystitis most will have had an oral cholecystogram before presenting for other non invasive investigations. HIDA chole-scintigraphy will sometimes image the gall bladder when oral cholecystography is negative. A computer and a gamma camera dynamic series can be used to evaluate the ability of the gall bladder to contract. Ultrasound is valuable in detecting the presence of gall stones and gall bladder wall thickening. In patients where no calculi have been found and the oral chole-cystogram is negative a Technetium 99m HIDA study is valuable in demonstrating gall bladder function to exclude chronic chole-cystitis (Fig. 8).

Jaundice

In patients presenting with jaundice the first test is undoubtedly ultrasound. Using ultrasound the liver can be evaluated for the presence or absence of metastases. The bile

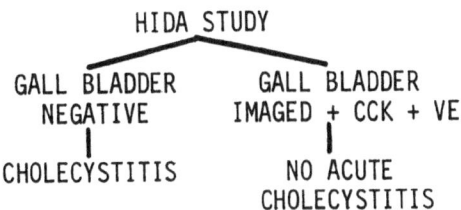

Fig. 8. Acute cholecystitis

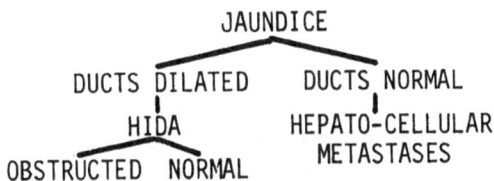

Fig. 9. Jaundice

ducts can be examined for dilatation and the gall bladder imaged
to detect the presence of stones. The pancreas can also be
imaged to exclude a carcinoma or pancreatitis as the cause of the
biliary obstruction. Using ultrasound alone the site of
obstruction can be assessed in about 50% or more of cases (Fig.9).

PANCREAS

The diagnosis of pancreatic abnormalities remains one of the
more difficult problems in non invasive diagnosis as well as in
general medicine. Although the earlier diagnosis of pancreatic
carcinoma probably would make little difference to survival
nevertheless the problem of the differential diagnosis between
carcinoma and pancreatitis is an area where progress would greatly
help the patient. Recent advances in non invasive diagnosis of
pancreatic abnormalities have included investigations using radioisotope, ultrasound and computerised axial tomographic imaging.

In isotope imaging uptake of seleno methionine in the pancreas
accurately reflects pancreatic function and this can easily be
imaged using subtraction scanning techniques. However the test
seems to be rather too sensitive with most abdominal abnormalities
producing abnormal or absent pancreatic concentration of the
labelled enzyme. In this situation it is rarely possible to
diagnose the presence of a space occupying lesion nor is it
usually possible to localise even benign disease to the pancreas.
Attempts to improve the situation using new instrumentation or
radiopharmaceuticals such as emission tomography or Carbon 11

568

labelled compounds has not really increased the chances of this approach giving a better differential diagnosis. However lack of uptake in the pancreas does confirm the suspicion of abdominal disease and in this sense a normal pancreas isotope scan is valuable in excluding disease with a high degree of confidence.

Ultrasound now has a firm place in the non invasive diagnosis of pancreas disease. Features which can be deduced from the ultrasound examination are the size of the pancreas, focal changes in echo pattern, the presence or absence of calcium and the presence or absence of fluid. Unfortunately many of the features seen in ultrasound imaging are common to carcinoma, acute and chronic pancreatitis. With a clinical history the interpretations of the scans can be more valuable. In terms of detecting an abnormality of the pancreas the sensitivity of the test is high and in spite of what has been said above in some hands the operator has been able to differentiate between cancer and pancreatitis in 75% of patients. An overall accuracy rate of the order of 94% has been achieved in detecting pancreatic disease (Fig. 10).

The features seen on CT scanning of the pancreas are similar to those found by ultrasound and include enlargement, changes in shape, duct dilatation, calcium, alteration in density and specific for CT scanning the loss of fat planes. CT scanning does not suffer with the problems found in ultrasound due to gas and

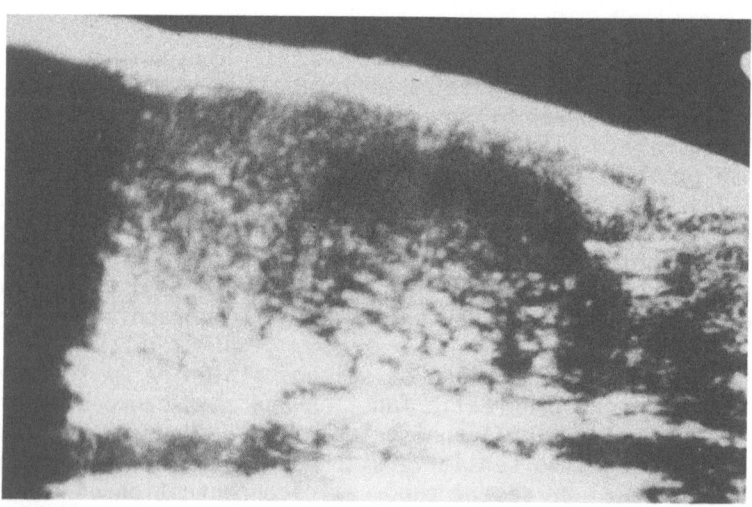

Fig. 10. An ultrasound longitudinal scan showing a large carcinoma of the pancreas below the liver and anterior to the inferior vena cava.

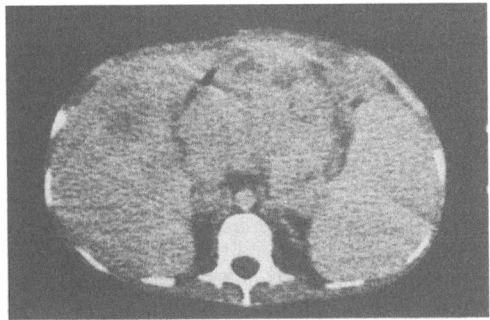

Fig. 11. A carcinoma of the pancreas with hepatic secondaries demonstrated on a CT scan.

other artefacts. The presence or absence of calcium is best seen on the plain X-ray. One sign specific to CT scanning is the loss of the fat plane in carcinoma or pancreatitis (Fig. 11).

Choice of Test

In choosing between the tests it is obvious that ultrasound is quick, available and cost effective. However for pancreatic scanning as opposed to other organs considerable skill is required and it must be appreciated that in up to 20% of patients it is not possible to get an acoustic window. As with radioisotope imaging a normal ultrasound image is usually correct. In an abnormal situation the CT scan gives more information since it provides a cross section of all the surrounding organs. It is therefore usual to start with ultrasound and perhaps use a radioisotope image to confirm normality. If a cyst or mass is seen this can be biopsied under ultrasound control. In patients with more complicated problems a CT scan is indicated and in patients with chronic pancreatitis a CT scan may be the most efficient first test looking for small calcifications, atrophy, fibrosis, pancreatic duct dilatation and pseudocysts (Fig. 12).

```
                    ULTRASOUND
                   /          \
        GAS                      NO GAS
         |                         |
        ISOTOPES                  TUMOUR
        ERCP                      CYSTS
        or                        GALL BLADDER
        CT                        BILE DUCTS
                                  LIVER METS.
```

Fig. 12. Pancreas Imaging

KIDNEY

In examining the kidney it is important to distinguish between the necessity for a test of renal function and a test of renal morphology. It is still traditional to start the investigation of the kidney with a plain X-ray looking for the renal outline, the presence or absence of calcium and the presence of other masses in the abdomen.

Radioisotope imaging is more valuable in detecting abnormalities of renal function. It is usual to screen a patient with a measure of total glomerular filtration using an in vitro method. Following this individual renal function can be traced using preferably labelled hippuran but more usually Tc99m labelled DTPA. The advantage of the latter is the higher count rate but the test may not give as clearly defined results as those using hippuran. While a simple time activity curve is quite valuable a more analytical approach using renal transit can help in differentiating between disorders of renal function and delayed transit due to obstruction. In some cases a DMSA scan is valuable in outlining the kidney from the morphological point of view. While poor at showing space occupying lesions it is valuable in finding an elusive kidney with minimum radiation and trauma to the patient (Fig. 13).

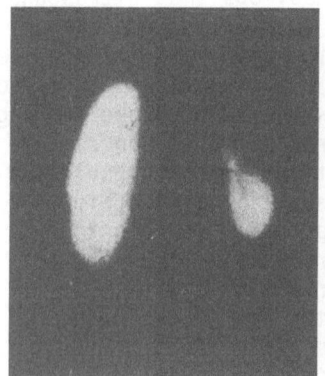 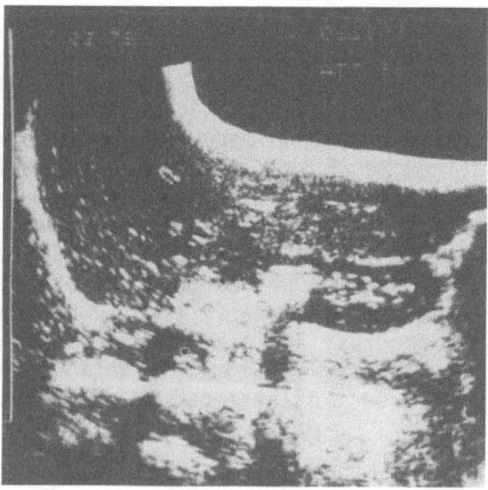

Fig. 13. A DMSA scan taken following a right heminephrectomy. A pyrexia of unknown origin was explained by a high echo area in the upper part of the renal bed throwing a gas acoustic shadow posteriorly. This was due to gas in an inflammatory collection.

Ultrasound imaging is quick, safe and atraumatic. It also can be used to measure renal size but is best at showing the presence or absence of fluid. From this can be deduced the presence of cysts, hydronephrosis and the thickness of the renal cortex. Tumours are seen with a variable pattern but the differential diagnosis is usually quite obvious.

As in other situations CT scanning is valuable in showing the total cross section. Although it is limited to one cross section of the patient per slice it can show all the features found in ultrasound together with the spread of disease to the areas around the kidney.

Choice of Test

Thus for the measurement of renal function radioisotope methods are recommended and will give much better results than the more usually employed intravenous pyelogram (IVP). For morphological diagnosis it is usual to commence with a plain X-ray and often with an IVP in spite of the fact that ultrasound will give most of the information found by the IVP with less preparation and effort on the part of the patient. In cases of carcinoma of the kidney a CT scan is more useful to show the size of the tumour (Fig. 14).

PELVIS

All three non invasive imaging modalities have been used in assessing pelvic disease. Perhaps they are of less value in this area since most lesions are more easily accessible by physical examination than elsewhere in the abdomen.

Tumour localising pharmaceuticals have been of less value in detecting primary disease and spread in the abdomen than in the chest. Gallium 67 has problems due to bowel excretion and retention in the rectal area. [111]In Bleomycin is excreted through the kidneys and there is less confusion between abnormalities and normal physiological excretion. It is also thought to be of more

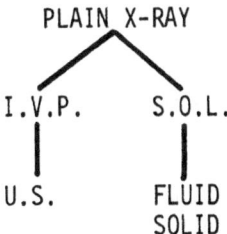

Fig. 14. Renal Imaging

value in squamous carcinoma. However overall radioisotope imaging is little used for imaging the lower abdomen.

Ultrasound imaging has been used extensively in assessing pelvic abnormalities. The examination is facilitated by having a full bladder. This displaces the bowel upwards revealing the lateral pelvic walls and rectal areas. As elsewhere the ultrasonographer looks for alteration in the outlines of the organs, in this case the uterus and the bladder and the presence of areas with unusual echo patterns.

Using these techniques it is possible to image and locate ovarian and uterine tumours as well as demonstrate and stage bladder tumours. However apart from obvious invasion of surrounding tissues it is usually difficult to differentiate between benign and malignant lesions (Fig. 15).

A good success rate in preoperative detection of malignant ovarian neoplasm with figures of 97% sensitivity and 84% accuracy in differential diagnosis is being reported. Postoperatively also ultrasound has proved valuable in the follow up of this disease with accuracy of 84% correlation with laparotomy being found. The detection of peritoneal spread has proved more difficult with only about one-third of involved cases being detected.

CT imaging has been reported to be of less value in the pelvis than elsewhere. Essentially the same information is produced as is found with ultrasound but the detail of ultrasound is lacking. As with ultrasound a full bladder is essential since fluid in the small bowel causes confusion with space occupying lesions. The fat planes help to outline the seminal vesicles in the male more clearly than with ultrasound. Pelvic lipomatosis is

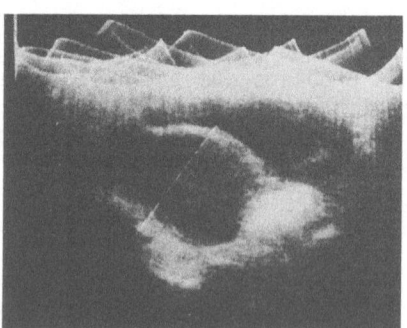

Fig. 15. An ultrasound examination of the pelvis showing a large mass posterior to the bladder. This was a malignant ovarian neoplasm.

a rare condition which is better shown by CT. CT is particularly valuable for patients who require radiotherapy treatment plans. The cross sectional presentation is ideal and of course the computer capabilities of the device can be harnassed to compute the dose rates at each point allowing for tissue attenuation.

CONCLUSION

It is hoped that this presentation has illustrated the need for closer integration of the non invasive imaging modalities. The problem of differential diagnosis remains. However current research shows promise that tissue characterisation in ultrasound or attenuation values in CT coupled with the morphological appearances may help produce more accurate diagnoses than were possible previously.

FURTHER READING

Ultrasound in Tumour Diagnosis, Hill C.R., McCready V.R., Cosgrove D.O., Eds., Pitman Medical, England, 1978

The Role of Radionuclide Imaging in Relation to Other Organ Imaging Modalities: Thyroid, Liver (Biliary System), Pancreas, Bone and Bone Marrow, Medical Radioisotope Scintigraphy, IAEA Vienna (Proceedings Symposium on Medical Radioisotope Scintigraphy, Heidelberg, 1980)

UTILIZATION OF SPECIAL COMPUTERIZED TOMOGRAPHY AND NUCLEAR MEDI-
CINE TECHNIQUES FOR QUALITY CONTROL AND FOR THE OPTIMIZATION OF
COMBINED PRECISION CHEMOTHERAPY AND PRECISION RADIATION THERAPY

Albert L. Wiley, Jr., M.D., Ph.D., George W. Wirtanen,
M.D., and I-Chu Chien, M.S.
Departments of Human Oncology and Radiology, Universi-
ty of Wisconsin Center for Health Sciences, Madison,
Wisconsin 53792

ABSTRACT

We have previously reported the use of a combination of precision (selective, intra-arterial) chemotherapy and precision radiotherapy for advanced pancreatic, biliary tract, and sarcoma-
tous malignancies. There were some remarkable responses, but
also a few poor responses and even some morbidity. Accordingly,
we are attempting to develop methods of pre-selecting those patients whose tumors are likely to respond to such therapy, as
well as methods for improving the therapeutic ratio by the rational optimization of combined therapy. Specifically, clinical tumor
blood flow characteristics (which we monitor with nuclear medicine techniques) may provide useful criteria for such selection.
Also, we qualitatively evaluate the drug distribution or exposure
space with specialized color-coded computerized tomography images,
which demonstrate spatially dependent enhancement of intra-arterial contrast in tumor and in adjacent normal tissues. Such clinical data, we suggest could improve the quality control aspects
of intra-arterial chemotherapy administration, as well as the
possibility of achievement of a significant therapeutic ratio by
the integration of precision chemotherapy and precision radiation
therapy.

INTRODUCTION

Numerous laboratory and some clinical studies suggest that
the potential of combined chemotherapy-radiation therapy to improve survival rates for patients with advanced cancers is real;

and the clinical investigation of such combined therapy, therefore, seems appropriate. Furthermore, the clinical use of combined therapy is practical and cost effective, inasmuch as exces-
sively expensive or exotic equipment is not required. Thus, if a
real therapeutic ratio is ever clinically demonstrated with some
form of combined therapy, the United States health care system
could readily and quickly deliver such therapy to large populations through existing community hospitals. This report describes
our attempts to achieve an improved therapeutic ratio with a
particular form of combined therapy. But, we suggest that the
concepts developed and technologies used could also be applied to
other general forms of combined therapy investigations (such as
hyperthermia with drugs).

Currently, the main factor retarding the development of a
significant therapeutic ratio with combined therapy seems to be
the lack of a clinical, "ideal" radiation potentiating drug which
could be given orally or intravenously and which would concentrate primarily within tumor cells, and yet minimally in normal cells.
Consequently, any beneficial effects on the therapeutic ratio
with clinical trials with combined therapy have been inconclusive.
As an example, even when there has been a suggestion of improvement in local control and survival (such as the University of
Wisconsin experience with radiation and systemic 5-FU in advanced
head/neck cancer), morbidity and some complications have made the
regimen less attractive.[1,2] At this time, it seems unlikely
that such "ideal" drugs will be available in the near future.
But, there are presently available radiosensitizing and radiopotentiating drugs, and rational clinical investigation of the optimization of the combination of existing drugs and radiation
seems appropriate.

We propose the following thoughts (as a system analysis type
of approach) to the optimization of combined chemotherapy-radio-
therapy.

1)   As we have previously suggested[3,4] significant
        thought and effort should be made to develop precision
        delivery of drugs with the actual "tailoring" of the
        high concentrations of drug exposure to the tumor volume,
        while simultaneously minimizing exposure to the surround-
        ing normal tissues. In the past this has been difficult
        to achieve, primarily because there has been poor tech-
        nology for the in vivo, clinical monitoring of drug dis-
        tributions. (For example, one common method has been
        biopsy and analysis of the specimen; but this is inva-
        sive and subject to significant interpretation difficul-
        ties due to tumor heterogeneities.) Now, however, (with
        the development of positron-labeled drugs and emission
        computerized tomography, nuclear magnetic resonance

scanning, and special techniques of transverse axial
computerized tomography) non-invasive, in vivo clinical
monitoring of the drug distribution space is becoming
possible. When the capability for such monitoring is
further developed, we suggest that the delivery of precision drug therapy can be achieved and optimized. As
examples, we will describe some of our preliminary efforts to use nuclear medicine and computerized tomography techniques for monitoring, and subsequent adjustment
of intra-arterial drug delivery into tumor specific arteries.

2)   We suggest that precision delivery of the radiation
therapy is also an essential feature in attempting to
optimize combined chemotherapy-radiation therapy. And,
we have reported the use and development of electron arc
therapy and magnetically modified electron radiation distributions as probably the most practical mode of deli-
vering precision, cost effective radiation therapy to
the large and unevenly distributed cancer patient populations[5,6] seen in the United States health care system.

3)   Accordingly, in order for "precisely tailored" drug
distributions and "precisely tailored" radiation distributions to be effective, they must also be spatially
combined in a fashion dictated by the individual patient's
normal and tumor anatomy - i.e., the drug distribution
space, the radiation distribution, and the details of
the patient's tumor and normal tissue boundaries must
all simultaneously be well defined spatially, expressed
in the same format, and referenced to a common coordinate system. (We emphasize that appropriate "in vivo"
adjustments in these respective distributions can be
carried out only when both the drug and radiation distributions are monitored, described and analyzed in a common coordinate system - and preferably expressed in the
transverse axial format.) With appropriate development
of the currently available technologies of computerized
tomography and nuclear medicine, we can hope for a more
optimal spatial integration of drug and radiation distributions in the future.*

*We recognize that much more information than the drug exposure
space is important for true optimization of drugs and radiation
(either ionizing or hyperthermic) - i.e., the drug delivery and
exposure space is only one of the important factors, in addition
to the drug extraction and metabolism parameters, but the precise
delivery of the drug primarily to the tumor volume seems to us to
be an important first step in optimization of drugs with radiation.

In this report we will discuss some of the currently available technologies, techniques, and quality control procedures that we have employed in our clinical investigative efforts to optimize combined intra-arterial chemotherapy and radiation therapy.

MATERIALS AND METHODS

Intra-arterial Catheter Placement Techniques

In pilot studies and protocols with combined intra-arterial drugs and radiation, we have treated advanced and unresectable tumors with techniques previously described.[7] Briefly, small (1.7 mm O.D.) polyethylene catheters, using the transbrachial artery approach, were inserted into tumor specific arteries under fluoroscopic monitoring. These catheters may remain in-place for chronic, continuous drug infusion from weeks to months. There have been few major complications and acceptable morbidity in over 4,000 catheter placements done in the University of Wisconsin Division of Radiation Oncology.

Nuclear Medicine Techniques

All radiopharmaceuticals in this study were given through the intra-arterial catheter. For assessment of the catheter location-specific perfusion space, and the detection and quantitation of arterio-venous shunts in the tumor, 2-3 mCi of ^{99m}Tc macroaggregated human serum albumin (New England Nuclear) in a 3 cm^3 volume of normal saline was slowly injected, followed by a 10 cm^3 flush with normal saline. Immediately thereafter, activity data in the desired region were accumulated and stored with Nuclear Chicago or General Electric scintillation camera heads (medium energy parallel hole collimators), interfaced to the disk of a Digital Equipment Corporation PDP-11/40 computer system. The "Gamma 11" software system provided for the necessary mathematical operations on the stored data (i.e., background subtraction, "region of interest" analysis and the generation of time-activity curves for each "region of interest").

For further assessment of the drug perfusion space and for relative assessment of regional blood flow, three millicuries of ^{133}Xe (General Electric Radiopharmaceuticals) in 3 cm^3 of normal saline was "pulse" injected and promptly flushed with 10 cm^3 normal saline. The same equipment and techniques described above were used for data accumulation and analysis, except that a low energy collimator head was used. Regional perfusion images (generally in the coronal projection) and regional blood flow values in tumor and surrounding normal tissue were calculated essential-

ly as described by others,[8,9] except that we use a locally developed software program (TUMFLO)[10] for statistical curve fitting of the region specific time-activity data. (A partician coefficient of 1.0 for ^{133}Xe was assumed.)

Computerized Tomography Techniques

Computerized tomography scans are done on an EMI 5005 scanner, with a 13 mm slice thickness. The slice location is generally referenced to some scout film landmark (such as a vertebra).
As an attempt to monitor (in the transverse axial format) vascular tumor boundaries and the consequent drug exposure space, we
developed a procedure called an "arterial infusion CT scan". Our
"arterial infusion CT scan" consists of the concurrent, slow
(approximately 20 cc/min) infusion of RENO-DIP, 14% iodine (approximately 300 cc) into a tumor specific artery, during the CT scan.
This slow infusion rate better approximates the physiological
blood flow rate than does conventional angiography and, consequently, the artifacts of the contrast distribution ordinarily
seen with the usual high pressure, high flow rates of conventional angiography are not present. Thus, the image obtained more
accurately reflects the drug distribution produced in our protocols of slow, chronic intra-arterial infusion. Also, the "infusion CT" images provide a means of monitoring contrast distributions (i.e., drug exposure space) in the transverse axial format,
which we suggest is a special and unique requirement for tumor
specific tailoring of the drug distribution with tumor specific
tailoring of the radiation distribution. The transverse axial
format is preferable for monitoring the drug exposure space (i.e.,
contrast distribution) since the radiation distribution for treatment planning is usually calculated and presented in the transverse axial format and radiation oncologists are more accustomed
to such presentation.

Our radiation therapy-dedicated DeAnza PDP-11/34 image analysis system creates useful, specialized displays and CT number
analysis capability on the above described "arterial infusion CT
scans" (which are accumulated by our EMI 5005 scanner and stored
on 9 track magnetic tape for subsequent analysis on the system).
Locally developed software for the system provides for rapid
pixel-pixel subtractions of "no contrast" from "contrast" scans
and for "search and grouping" routines and for boundary defining
algorithms. These capabilities enable the generation of color-
coded CT images with concurrent explicit definition and presentation of both anatomical and contrast distribution boundaries. The
software program is relatively fast and, therefore, has the clinical utility of giving rapid feedback to the clinician of a
color-coded, concentration dependent, contrast distribution image
overlaying well defined anatomical and tumor boundaries (all in
the transverse axial format). Only with convenience and utility

(i.e., rapid, explicit and convenient feedback of the image) are such monitoring techniques likely to be utilized by busy clinicians.

RESULTS

In this communication we present examples of our efforts to use special techniques of computerized tomography and nuclear medicine for clinical monitoring of A-V shunts, regional tumor blood flow, and drug exposure space. The feedback of such data to the clinician should facilitate his optimization of combined therapy by enhancing the rational integration of drugs and radiation. The results of these efforts can probably be best summarized by specific reference to the data in the form of specialized images, which are presented and discussed in the following figures.

580

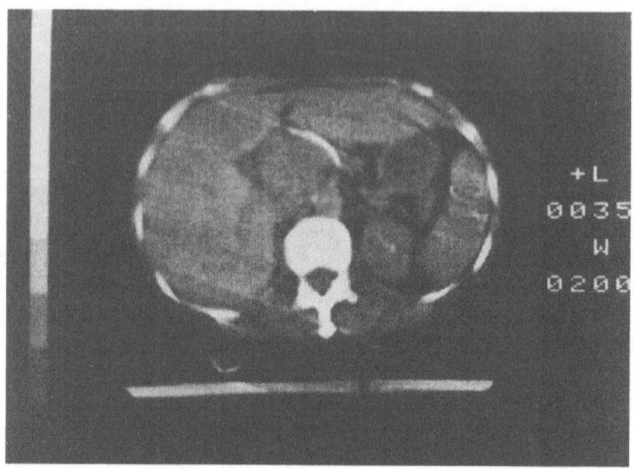

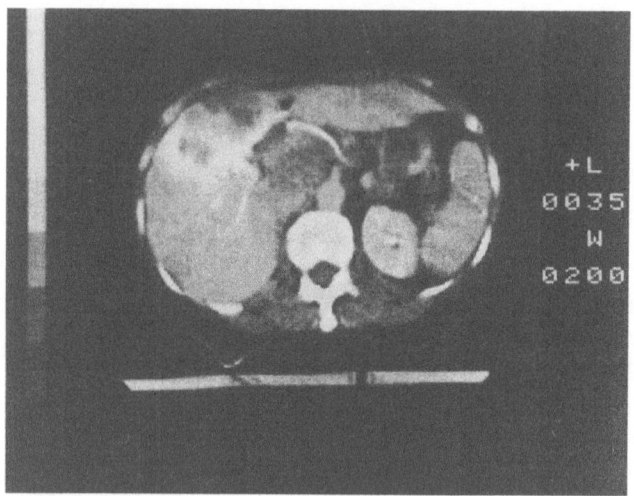

FIGURE 1: (TOP)   A CT scan taken through the mid-liver of a
                    patient with a primary tumor in the head of
pancreas, prior to contrast infusion into the hepatic artery. Note
the contrast filled catheter and that there is no definite visualization of hepatic metastasis.

         (BOTTOM)   A CT scan taken through the same section as
                    above, except that this scan was taken during
the infusion of contrast into the hepatic artery. Now the presence
of numerous discrete regions of hypovascularity and hypervascularity, consistent with hepatic metastasis is well documented. Such

explicit definition of tumor boundaries and the drug exposure
space are generally not seen by conventional arteriography and CT
techniques. Also, presentation of these parameters in the transverse axial format facilitates integration of this information on
the drug exposure space with radiation therapy treatment planning.

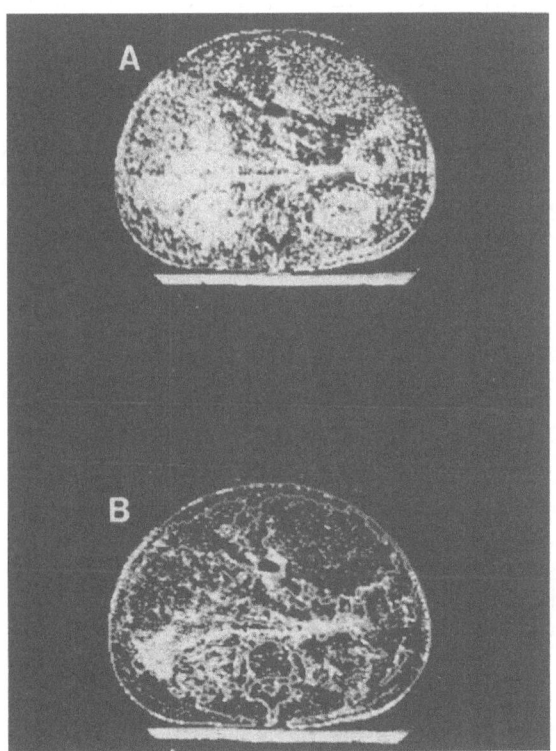

FIGURE 2: A) **CT image** obtained by subtracting a "background",
non-infused image from the same arterial contrast
infused image. Note that the contrast distribution overlays normal and tumor tissue defined boundaries such that the contrast
distribution can be explicitly related to anatomical boundaries.
For this image the threshold setting for CT number is "10" in our
DeAnza defined settings which range from "0" to "255".

B) As a means of accessing relative variations of contrast concentration (which should be related to the
spatial variations of drug concentration) within specified anatomical boundaries, the threshold setting for the DeAnza CT number may
be changed. In this figure the threshold has been increased from
"10" to "20". As an example of this procedure this image indicates
a higher concentration of contrast in the posterior right lobe of
the liver, as well as in a linear structure (probably the splenic

582

vein). Note that both kidneys also have dense clusters of "CT numbers" larger than the threshold of "20". (The image printed here unfortunately is not in color, and therefore fails to adequately demonstrate the explicit definition of color-coded anatomical boundaries with respect to contrast distribution. For example, if a tumor centered coordinate system were assigned to this transverse axial image (which simultaneously displays anatomy and the drug exposure space, represented by contrast), then a tumor-tailored radiation distribution could be precisely spatially integrated with some radiation-enhancing drugs, such as actinomycin-D. We believe that only with such data and images (where radiation, drug, and anatomical data are reduced to the same frame of reference) is a real therapeutic ratio with combined therapy likely to be achieved by clinicians.

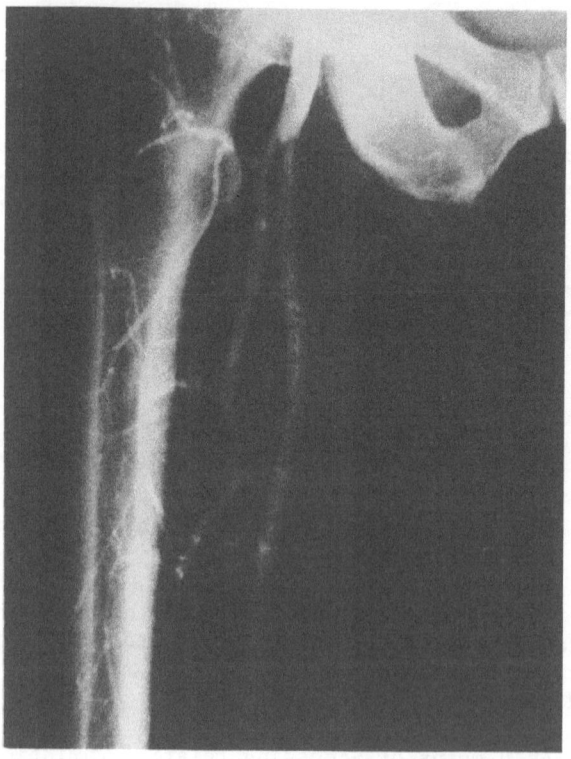

FIGURE 3: Femoral artery arteriogram of thigh containing lipo-
           sarcoma. There is poor demonstration of the tumor,
due to poor tumor vascularity. This tumor was treated with a
combination of concurrent intra-arterial actinomycin-D and
radiation therapy.

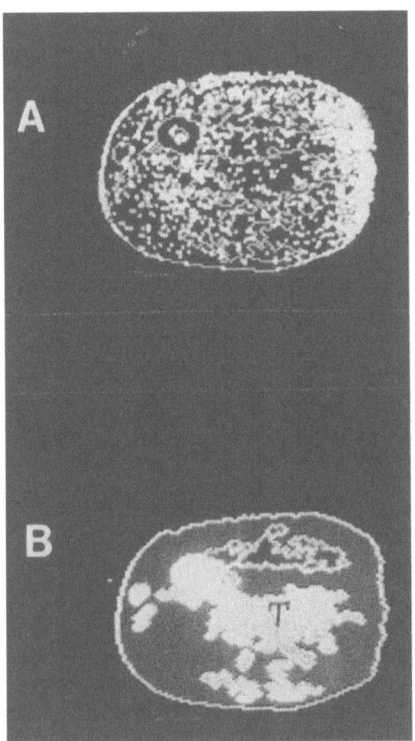

FIGURE 4: A) "Subtraction CT infusion scan" through the thigh
            sarcoma of Fig. 3 (obtained in the same manner as
the scans in Fig. 2). The contrast distribution is concentrated
primarily at the medial skin and subcutaneous areas, rather than
in the mid-thigh region of known liposarcoma. This image is consistent with poor perfusion of the deep tumor by the intra-arterial drug (actinomycin-D), which correlates well with relatively
poor clinical tumor response and the enhanced skin reaction observed following the therapy. Further development of these
studies may help to prospectively decide whether to treat with
or without the drug infusion.

           B) CT scan through the thigh containing liposarcoma
            (Fig. 3). Note the region of low CT number con-
sistent with liposarcoma, in the mid-thigh. For better demonstration of regions of approximate iso-CT number, the various
CT number regions are "grouped" and color-coded for more explicit
demonstration of these regions. Here, a tumor region of approximate iso-CT number is labeled by "T". This type of image facilitates tumor boundary identification, which is very helpful in
treatment planning.

584

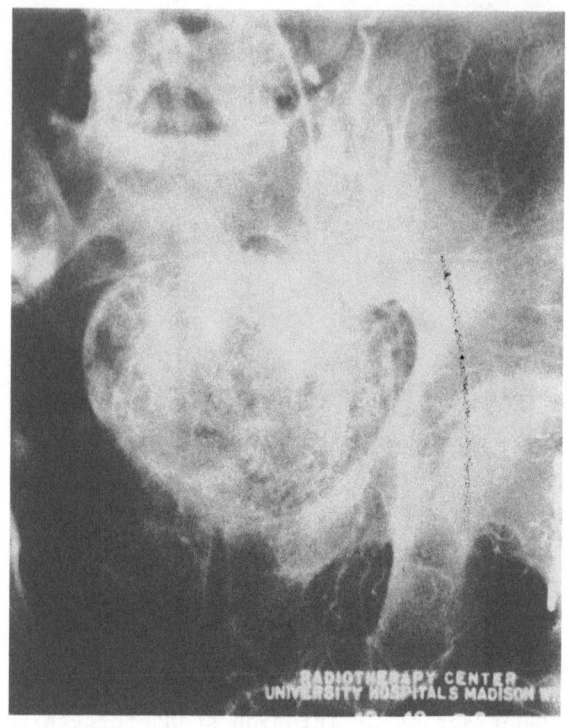

FIGURE 5: Hypogastric arteriogram of a large hemangiosarcoma
occupying most of the left and mid-pelvis.

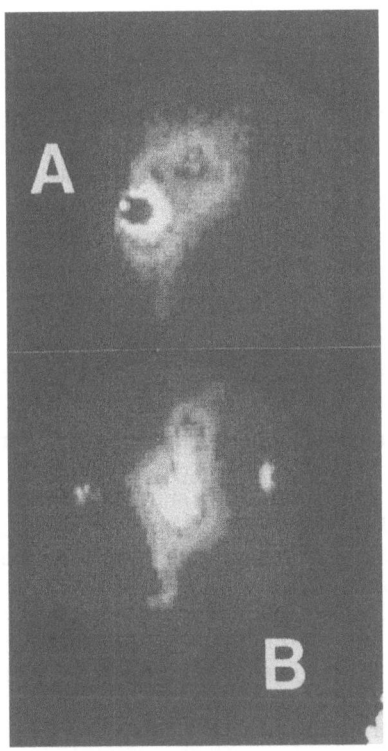

FIGURE 6: A) ^{99m}Tc macroaggregated albumin perfusion scan obtained by injecting into the same hypogastric
artery catheter shown in Fig. 4. Note relatively uniform perfusion of the tumor with this particular catheter position. The
"bull's eye" type appearance in the viewers' left portion of the
image is probably the localization of the ^{99m}Tc MAA in perivesi-
cular capillaries, with the inner area of"zero"activity being
urine inside the bladder. Furthermore, as a means of detecting
and subsequently quantitating arterio-venous shunts in the tumor,
the lungs were also monitored following the intra-arterial injection of the ^{99m}Tc MAA and were noted to have approximately 30%
of the total activity, indicating the presence of arterio-venous
shunts in this tumor.[1]

B) Intra-arterially administered ^{133}Xe scan of the
same tumor shown in "A". Also demonstrating good
tumor perfusion with minimal perfusion of extra-tumor tissues.
"Regions of interest" were selected for monitoring ^{133}Xe washout
throughout the tumor for generation of time-activity curves and
subsequent regional blood flow calculations. Regional variations
of blood flow in this tumor were 27, 25, 27, and 15 cm^3/min./100
gm. of tissue[1]), confirming relatively homogeneous tumor blood
flow throughout the tumor. Consistent with these scan results,
this patient had an excellent tumor response, and no significant
side effects to the therapy (intra-arterial actinomycin-D and
radiation) and is now 3 yr. NED.

DISCUSSION

For optimization of combined chemotherapy-radiation therapy,
we suggest that accurate, three-dimensional data on the individual patient's tumor and normal tissue boundaries, and the subsequent "tumor-tailored", delivery of both radiation and drug distributions is required. Clearly, the "in vivo" monitoring of the
drug exposure space and certain quality control measures (such as
the selection of patients whose tumors are likely to respond to
such therapy and the selection of the best catheter position for
tumor perfusion) are also essential. We have presented examples
of how we utilize presently available techniques from computerized
tomography and nuclear medicine to meet some drug distribution
monitoring and quality control requirements. It is our opinion
that the optimization and integration of these combined therapy
modalities will be facilitated only if an effort is made to monitor and reduce all anatomical data and data on the drug exposure
space to the transverse axial format. Such data monitoring is
now clearly possible with the present technologies of computerized tomography and emission computerized tomography and allows for
the presentation of all such data in the same coordinate system,
where chemically enhanced and modified radiation isodose distributions can be generated.[11]

---

1. The above nuclear medicine studies were done with single photon radiopharmaceuticals and conventional gamma camera equipment
which routinely presents images in the coronal format. The accumulation and presentation of the data in this format has only
qualitative value; but the transverse axial accumulation and presentation is likely to be more quantatively accurate and useful
in integrating it with CT data. Our future studies will primarily
utilize positron-labeled radiopharmaceuticals that will be monitored by our recently acquired ORTEC-ECAT scanner and displayed
in the transverse axial format.

As quality control procedures for selecting tumors which are likely to respond to our combined therapy protocols, information regarding the presence, absence and degree of arterio-venous shunts and the relative uniformity of tumor blood flow may be of assistance. For example, with more experience in the correlation of such data as shown in Fig. 2, 3, 4, 5, and 6 with the tumor and normal tissue response to therapy, we should be able to develop some criteria for improving patient selection for this therapy and/or for appropriate adjusting of treatment techniques, so as to minimize complications. Also, as an example of how the type of studies presented in this paper may help to optimize combined therapy, we noted in one patient some increase in regional tumor blood flow (with ^{133}Xe studies) following a fractionated course of radiation; which may suggest that for some clinical tumors, the drug distribution in some clinical tumors might be improved if the drug infusion is given following a course of fractionated radiation.

Since 1965 the University of Wisconsin Hospital has had a major interest in the use of combined intra-arterial drugs and radiation therapy for advanced and unresectable bone and soft tissue sarcomas, renal, head and neck, and more recently upper gastrointestinal (primarily pancreas) malignancies.[11,12,13,14] Our conclusions from these studies are that long term, often dramatic local tumor controls are possible, and some unresectable tumors have become resectable; so the regimen seems to have real value for some patients. A detailed understanding of the regional blood flow and subsequent drug distribution-concentration space in the individual patient's tumor could further improve the usefulness of the regimen. Thus far, we have only discussed the spatial and drug concentration-distribution dependent factors in the optimization of drugs and radiation. There is also a time dependent factor in optimization which we have previously addressed,[4] i.e., the time at which the radiation is given with respect to the timing of a radiosensitizing or radiopotentiating drug has a significant effect on the therapeutic ratio.

The studies presented are examples of the potential usefulness of computerized tomography and nuclear medicine techniques and of some of our efforts to develop space-time dependent optimization of a particular form of combined therapy. But we further suggest that the problems and questions raised, and the technologies and techniques demonstrated, may also have direct application to optimization attempts with other forms of combined therapy (such as hyperthermia combined with drugs).

588

REFERENCES

1. Lo, T.C.M., Wiley, A.L.,Jr., Gollin, F.F., Ansfield, F.J.,
    Brandenburg, J.H., Davis, H., Johnson, R.O. and Ramirez, G.:
    "Combined radiation therapy and 5-fluorouracil for advanced
    squamous cell carcinoma of the oral cavity and oropharynx: A
    randomized study". AM. J. ROENTGENOL. 126:229-235, 1976.

2. Gollin, F.F., Ansfield, F.J., Brandenburg, J.H., Ramirez, G.,
    and Vermund, H.: Combined therapy in advanced head and neck
    cancer. A randomized study". AM. J. ROENTGENOL. 114:83,1972.

3. Wiley, A.L.,Jr., Wirtanen, G.W., Holden, J.E., and Polcyn,R.E.:
    "Utilization of a selective tumor artery catheterization tech-
    nique for the intra-arterial delivery of chemotherapeutic
    agents and radiopharmaceuticals in a combined chemotherapy-
    radiotherapy clinical research program". RADIOBIOLOGY, RE-
    SEARCH AND RADIOTHERAPY, Vol. 1, International Atomic Energy
    Agency, Publication No. ISBN 92-0-010377-4, Vienna, pp. 389-
    412, 1977.

4. Wiley, A.L.,Jr., Brandenburg, J.H., Ramirez, G., Johnson,R.O.,
    Lieberman, L., and Vermund, H.: "Treatment of advanced squa-
    mous cell carcinoma of the base of tongue with combined radia-
    tion therapy and 5-fluoouracil - Optimization with ^{18}F-5-FU".
    ACTA RADIOL. (THER.)18:235-243, 1979.

5. Paliwal, B.R., Wiley, A.L.,Jr., Wessels, B.W., and Choi, M.
    C.: "Magnetic modification of electron beam dose distribu-
    tions in inhomogeneous media". MED. PHYS. 5(5):404-408,1978.

6. Paliwal, B.R., and Wiley, A.L.,Jr.: "Modification of electron
    beam dose distributions using a magnetic field". ACTA RADIOL.
    (THER.)18:57-64, 1979.

7. Wirtanen, G.W.: "Percutaneous transbrachial artery infusion
    catheter techniques". AM. J. ROENTGENOL. 17:696-700, 1976.

8. Wagner, H.N.,Jr.: "Regional blood flow measurements with
    ^{85}Kr and ^{133}Xe". Dynamic Clinical Studies with Radioisotopes,
    U.S. AEC SYMPOSIUM Series 3:189-212, 1968.

9. Cannon, P.J., Dell, R.B., and Dwyer, E.M.,Jr.: "Measurement
    of regional myocardial perfusion in man with ^{133}Xe and a scin-
    tillation camera". J. CLIN. INVEST. 51:964-977, 1972.

10. Madsen, M., Wiley, A.L.,Jr., Polcyn, R.E., and Nickles, J.R.:
    "Regional blood flow in tumors". ABSTRACT. Radiological
    Society of North America, Nov. 1978.

589

11. Wiley, A.L.,Jr., Wirtanen, G.W., Wu, J.P., Jaeschke, W.,
    Ansfield, F.J., Ramirez, G., and Davis, H.L.: "The treatment
    of osteogenic sarcoma with combined intra-arterial actinomy-
    cin-D and radiotherapy". ANN. CLIN. RES. 6:330-337, 1974.

12. Wiley, A.L.,Jr., Wirtanen, G.W., Joo, P., Ansfield, F.J.,
    Ramirez, G., Davis, H., and Vermund, H.: "Clinical and
    theoretical aspects of the treatment of retroperitoneal malig-
    nancy with combined intra-arterial actinomycin-D and radio-
    therapy". CANCER 36:107-122, 1975.

13. Wiley, A.L.,Jr., Wirtanen, G.W., Ansfield, F., and Ramirez,G.:
    "Combined intra-arterial actinomycin-D and radiation therapy
    for surgically unresectable hypernephroma". J. UROL. 114:
    198-210, 1975.

14. Wiley, A.L.,Jr., Wirtanen, G.W., Davis, T.E., Ramirez, G.,
    Davis, H.L., Carbone, P.P., Wolberg, W.H., Johnson, R.O.,
    and Crowley, J.J.: "Preliminary results on the treatment of
    unresectable pancreatic carcinoma with a combination of pre-
    cision (intra-arterial) chemotherapy and precision radiation
    therapy. PANCREATIC CANCER: NEW DIRECTIONS IN THERAPY
    MANAGEMENT, Masson Publishing Co., New York, pp. 97-106, 1981.

(Supported in part by the National Cancer Institute, Wisconsin
Clinical Cancer Center Grant CA-19278-06.)

SINGLE PHOTON EMISSION COMPUTED TOMOGRAPHY AND ALBUMIN COLLOID IMAGING OF THE LIVER

Barbara Y. Croft, C. D. Teates, and Janice C. Honeyman

Division of Medical Imaging, Box 486, University of Virginia, Charlottesville, Virginia 22908

ABSTRACT

A single photon emission computed tomography (ECT) system using the GE 400T Anger camera with 37 PM tubes and the SPETS software has been installed in our clinical laboratory. It has been used in the study of liver imaging with Tc-99m albumin colloid and other agents.

The object of the study is to define what improvement in liver diagnosis might be made using ECT. The new information ECT gives access to is cine of the rotating liver and transverse, coronal, and sagittal sections of the liver. The significant problems in ECT imaging are statistics and resolution, scattering, patient movement, gamma ray attenuation, and artifacts introduced in the data acquisition and processing.

Patients were injected with 3-4 mCi (ca 120 MBq) of colloid; five standard liver-spleen views and a 64-image ECT study were acquired. The ECT images were acquired either in a circle of the radius of the longer transverse axis of the patient or in an ellipse to match the patient contour. Studies were corrected for the attentuation of the Tc-99m gamma rays by tissue.

A series of normal and abnormal patients have been studied and the data analyzed. The significant change in the technique of ECT imaging is the elliptical motion of the camera head which allows a better approximation of the patient contour and improves the spatial resolution of the images.

1. INTRODUCTION

In this paper, we shall report the results of studies of the conditions for single photon emission tomographic (ECT) liver imaging. It was felt that ECT resolution was being compromised by the distance between the collimator face and the patient surface, especially in the front and back. A method was developed for easily repositioning the camera to alleviate this problem. Several factors, including the importance of the parallel head, the Anger camera Tc-99m window width, the importance of the flood field uniformity correction, and the importance of minimizing the distance between the collimator face and the patient surface, have been addressed. The studies included phantom and point source imaging and patient imaging.

2. MATERIALS & METHODS

The patients were those who presented themselves to the Nuclear Medicine Laboratory for liver imaging. The experimental radiopharmaceutical, Tc-99m albumin colloid 1), was discussed with each patient. Those who elected to sign the consent form were injected with 3 mCi ± 10% (112 MBq) of the albumin colloid. Those who did not sign were injected with 3 mCi ± 10% (112MBq) of Tc-99m sulfur colloid 2). The patients were not specially selected for tomographic imaging; however those imaged did have to be able to lie still for 22 minutes, to move their arms over their heads, and to have a liver-spleen image which fit in the field of view.

The GE 400T 3) large field of view tomographic Anger camera acquired five routine static projections, anterior, posterior, right and left laterals, and left anterior oblique, with 800K to 1M cts per image. The patients were imaged supine on the special GE table. The low energy high resolution collimator and a 20% Tc-99m window were used routinely, as was the uniformity correction. When these views were completed, the patient was repositioned for tomographic imaging. The table was raised or lowered to place the patient's liver on the axis of rotation. The SPETS 4) (1) acquisition software, running on a PDP 11/34 computer 5), with Gamma 11-FB, was initialized. Sources were positioned around the patient for the attenuation correction measurement according to the computer instructions. Data were usually acquired at 64 angles for 20 secs/angle. The anterior image had approximately 140K cts, with lower counts/image usually acquired in other angular positions around the patient.

1. Microlite™, New England Nuclear, Billerica, MA
2. Syncor International Corp., Sylmar, CA
3. General Electric Medical Systems Division, Milwaukee, WI
4. Nuclear Diagnostic AB, Stockholm, Sweden
5. Digital Equipment Corporation, Maynard, MA

The SPETS software was used to perform filtered back projection of the data to create tomographic images. A hard filter, Shepp-Logan, was employed in the back projection. The images were a nominal 1.2 cm thick, corrected for attenuation using the linear algorithm and an attenuation coefficient of 0.14 cm^{-1}. The images were viewed using Gamma-11 software routines. For hard copy reproduction of patient liver images, the interpolative routine IT2, which smooths and doubles the image size, was used. Hard copies were created on film with the Illinois Imaging Electronics formatter 6) and Kodak NMB film. Hard copies were made of the transverse images; coronal and sagittal sections were sometimes created and photographed. Raw data were archived on magnetic tape. Rotating liver cines were created for physician viewing.

Point sources were imaged using the same camera, hardware and software. The Alderson liver phantom, with its 3cm lesion in place in the right lobe was filled with 3.5 mCi (131 MBq) of Tc-99m, laid on the imaging table, and imaged at a time per angle which would give approximately the same counts per image as our patients, so that images could be compared. The Tc-99m window of the Anger camera was varied from 20% to 15% in some experiments.

A special leveling bar was fashioned which allowed the technologist to reposition the camera close to the patient during the data acquisition. The bar keeps the camera face parallel to the axis of rotation. In addition, since the camera moves longitudinally on the arc of a circle, the table has to be repositioned on its track to compensate for head movement. The SPETS software allows the acquisition to be stopped and restarted, so this maneuver need not be performed while the camera is being indexed to its next angular position. When the leveling bar was used, it was attached before the start of data acquisition and the collimator face brought close to the patient. As the camera indexed, the technologist would stop acquisition when necessary, raise (or lower) the camera head to be close to the patient again, reposition the table and restart the acquisition. Use of the bar by a trained technologist adds only a few minutes to the examination.

3. RESULTS

A point source experiment was performed to assure ourselves that it is necessary to keep the head of the camera parallel to the axis of rotation. Figure 1 shows the result of imaging two point sources with a parallel head and with the head angled 2.5° from parallel. When all the acquired frames are added together,

---

6. Illinois Imaging Electronics, Addison, IL

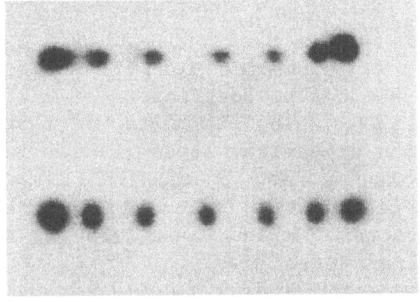
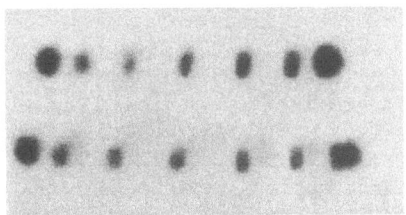

Figure 1. This is an image of the sum of images of two point sources acquired at 16 angles with the collimator face parallel to the axis of rotation.
Figure 2. This is an image of the sum of images of two point sources acquired at 16 angles with the collimator face 2.5° from parallel to the axis of rotation. Note the ellipse.

the sources should appear on a line. If the head is angled, the image of the sum of the acquired frames appear on an ellipse or crown with the closer portions brighter and in better focus (Figure 2). The further the source is from the axis of rotation, the larger and more obvious will the ellipse be. When these images are used for reconstruction, the angled head gives a broader FWHM than the parallel head. This is one effect which is less of a problem at the center of the field than on the edge.

The phantom results, shown in table I, are quite striking. The narrowing of the Tc-99m window and the use of the leveling bar to reposition the camera head close to the object allow for great improvements in contrast (Figures 3,4,5). In addition, Figure 6 shows the image of the phantom uncorrected for flood field uniformity. Note the ring artifacts. These seem to be caused by the pattern of the tubes in the uncorrected field; the PM tubes appear in a hexagonal pattern in the uncorrected flood. The effect of a less sensitive camera area is to create a cold circle on a transverse section (3). This suggests the necessity of using the uniformity correction for tomography.

TABLE I
Contrast of 3 cm lesion in the liver phantom on transverse section

Experimental Conditions	Tc-99m Window	Contrast
Without UC*	20%	0.40
With UC	20	0.44
With UC & leveling bar	20	0.62
With UC	15	0.65
With UC & leveling bar	15	0.71
* Uniformity Correction		

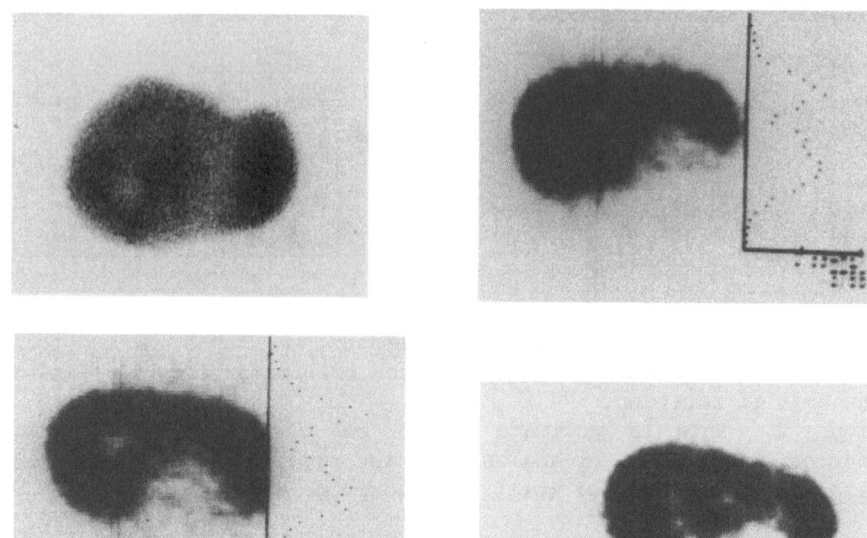

Figure 3 (upper left). This is the anterior image of the liver phantom with a 15% Tc-99m window and a 3 cm lesion.
Figure 4 (upper right). This is a transverse section of the liver phantom imaged in Figure 3. Note the lesion contrast.
Figure 5 (lower left). This is a transverse section of the liver phantom imaged with a 15% window, a 3 cm lesion, and the leveling bar used to allow the camera to come close to the phantom. The scale shows the counts across the lesion.
Figure 6 (lower right). This is a transverse section of the liver phantom imaged with a 20% window and no uniformity correction. Note the circular artifacts.

Three patients of the 19 thus far imaged will be discussed below to illustrate the use of the instrument and its refinements. The emission tomograms are compared to transmission tomograms.

Case 1: A 57 y.o. white woman presented with recurrent breast cancer and chest wall tumor. A chest transmission tomogram (TCT) was acquired and processed by our body scanner 7). The liver was imaged at the start of the examination and was normal. Five months later she was imaged with Tc-99m sulfur colloid and emission tomography (ECT) was performed and was also read as normal. The transverse sections are compared (Figures 7-12).

---

7. Delta 2020, Technicare, Solon, OH

Case 1. Normal liver examination. ECT and TCT compared.
Figure 7 (upper left). Liver-spleen transverse ECT.
Figure 8 (upper right). Transverse TCT at the same level.
Figure 9 (middle left). Transverse ECT.
Figure 10 (middle right). Transverse TCT at same level.
Figure 11 (lower left). Transverse ECT.
Figure 12 (lower right). Transverse TCT at the same level.

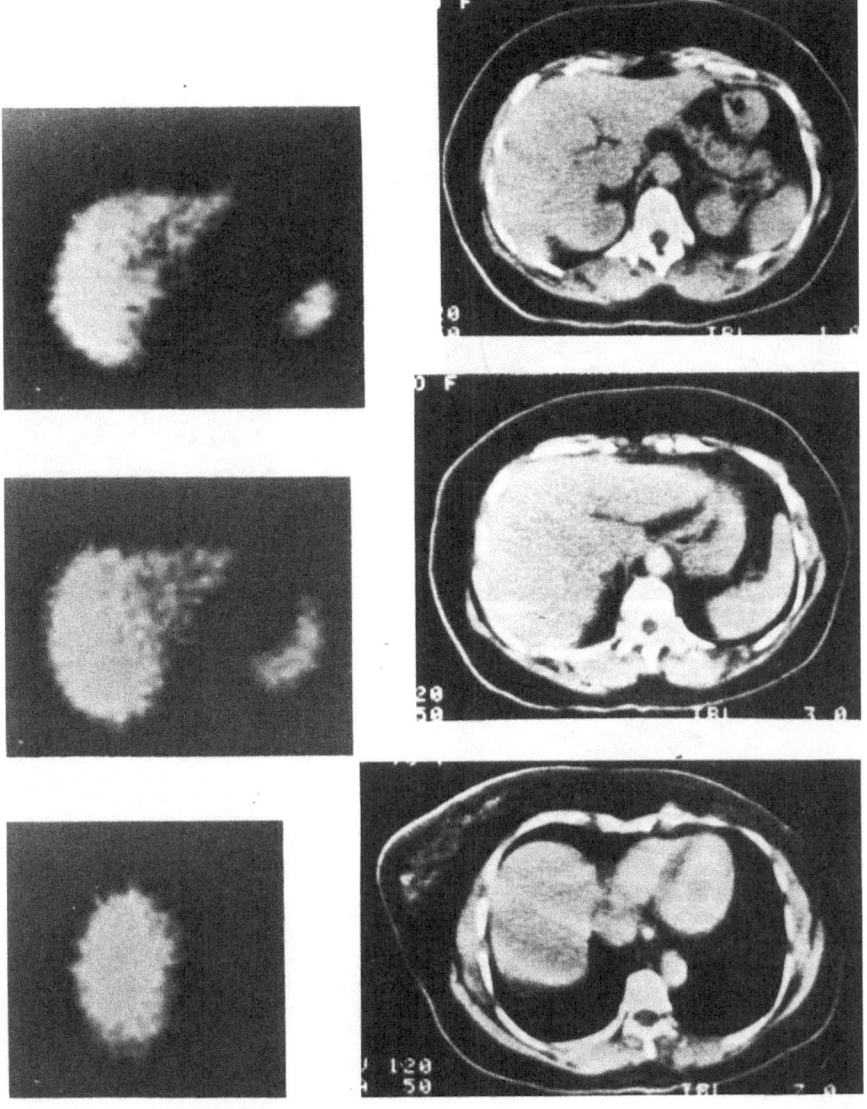

596

Case 2: Case 2 is a 53 y.o. white woman with carcinoma of the
colon treated with 5FU. She had been imaged at another hospital
where the lesions were noted 31 months before the ECT. She had
several liver scans over the interval in which progression and
regression of liver lesions were noted. Eighteen months prior to
the ECT study, she had abdominal TCT showing several lesions. The
patient was injected with 3.3 mCi (124 MBq) of Tc-99m albumin
colloid and imaged. The two sets of transverse tomographic images
are compared (Figures 13-20). Her lesions have changed in the
intervening months, probably because of therapy and her disease.

Case 2. Metastatic colon carcinoma. ECT and TCT comparison.
Figure 13 (upper left). Transverse TCT. Note gall bladder
shadow. All TCT was 18 mo. prior to ECT.
Figure 14 (upper right). Transverse ECT at same level.
Figure 15 (middle left). Transverse TCT. Note posterior lesion.
Figure 16 (middle right).Transverse ECT. The lesion has regressed.
Figure 17 (lower left). Transverse TCT.
Figure 18 (lower right).Transverse ECT. Note progression of
lesions. The spleen is overflowed to show liver detail.

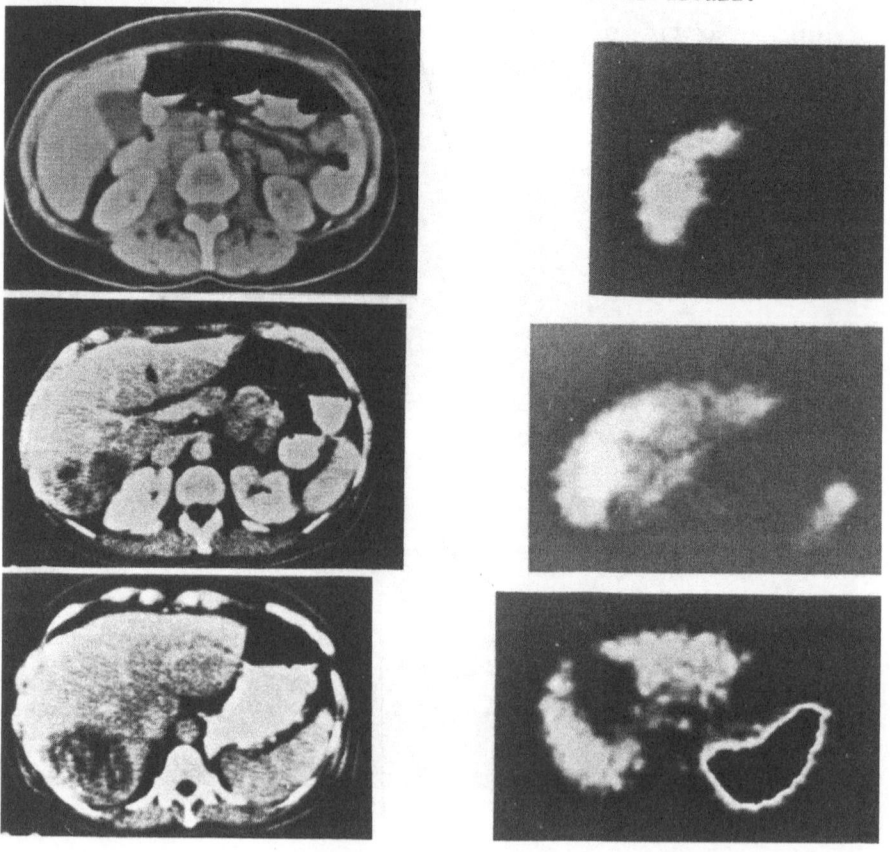

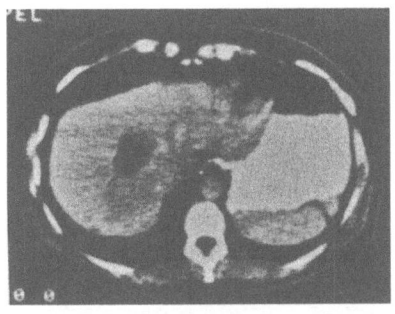 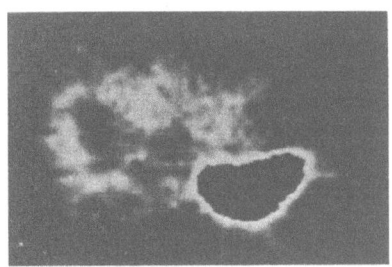

Case 2 (continued). Metastatic carcinoma of the colon.
Figure 19 (left). Transverse TCT.
Figure 20 (right). Transverse ECT. The lesions are separate and
have progressed.

Case 3: Case 3 is a 46 y.o. white woman with glomerulonephritis
and a cold thyroid nodule who presented most recently with a fever
of unknown origin. She had a gallium scan consistent with
glomerulonephritis on which decreased uptake in the posterior part
of the liver was noted. On a sonogram performed immediately
afterward, a large liver lesion was visualized and the diagnosis
of hemangioma was entertained. Three days later she was injected
with 3.2 mCi (120 MBq) of Tc-99m albumin colloid and imaged. The
one-second colloid vascular sequence showed an area of decreased
vascularity but raised questions about hypervascularity in the
upper pole. The posterior view showed a large defect in the right
lobe of the liver. ECT was performed, again showing the cold
areas (Figure 21).

The next day the patient was returned to the nuclear medicine
laboratory, injected with 15.1 mCi (566 MBq) of Tc-99m tagged to
red blood cells in vivo. A one-second vascular sequence was made,
showing a large avascular lesion which began to fill in the later
images of the sequence. On the early and late static images, the
lesion was noted to have filled with radioactivity, leaving some
photon deficient areas: this is again characteristic of a
cavernous hemangioma. The ECT images make the lesions plain
(Figure 23). Two days later the patient had a TCT study with
contrast, with the same findings (Figures 22, 24). An aortogram
was also performed, in an attempt to resolve questions concerning
the blood supply to the hemangioma, because surgery might be
possible. This question was unresolved.

4. DISCUSSION

The experiments tell us that although there is a great deal
of scattering in the body (4) and interference in the

598

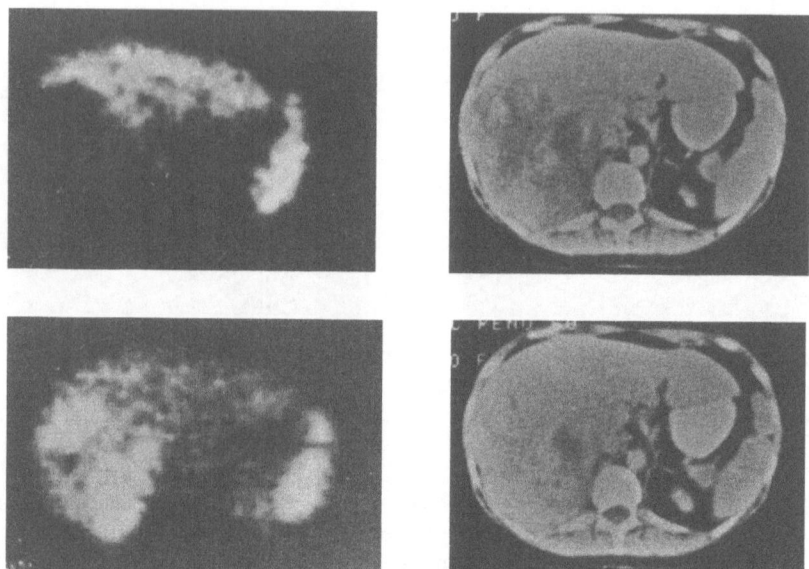

Case 3. Cavernous hemangioma of the liver.
Figure 21 (upper left). Albumin colloid ECT transverse section of the liver and spleen. Note the large filling defects in the posterior of the right lobe.
Figure 22 (upper right). TCT without vascular contrast. Note corresponding defect in liver.
Figure 23 (lower left). Labeled red cell ECT transverse section of the liver, about 2 hr post injection. The lesion has filled.
Figure 24 (lower right). TCT with vascular contrast, 6 min after injection. Defect fills with contrast.

reconstruction of photon deficient images, it is still worth all of our efforts to improve resolution. The particular maneuvers of this paper are narrowing the Tc-99m window and positioning the collimator face as close as possible to the patient to take advantage of the collimator's resolution while being sure to keep the head parallel to the axis of rotation. The movement of the camera in an ellipse rather than circle around the patient does not alter the back projected images, so long as the collimator face is parallel to the axis of rotation and the patient is in the same location in the matrix. As for patient liver imaging, other studies have confirmed the efficacy of the technique (2). Our numbers cannot do that, so we have chosen case material to illustrate the utility of the technique, especially in an institution where nuclear medicine and body TCT cooperate closely. The images are of comparable sizes and can even be overlaid.

Gamma emission imaging of the liver does have special problems: the thickness and shape of the organ make visualization of deep lesions difficult, and respiratory and other motion limit reliable resolution to 2-3 cm. ECT definitely can be helpful in overcoming the first problem but cannot be of any special utility for the second. Since the motion is more complex than simple translation (4), it is hard to see how any technique other than carefully instructed breathholding or gating could be helpful. Computer center-of-mass or autocorrelation maneuvers cannot be of much use in a deformable plastic organ.

This study has prompted us to make some suggestions for improvements to the imaging equipment and computer programs used for ECT. These suggestions apply to all the instruments currently in use:

1. Automate the camera-head repositioning: sense the patient position; move the head automatically and connect the table to the head angle measurer so the table moves automatically when the camera head moves.

2. Change the shielding of the head so that it will allow the edge of the active area of the collimator to be close to the edge of the camera head. This would make patient anatomy (shoulders, hips, etc) much less of a problem.

3. Tailor the table even more to the conditions of the examination. Far too often the table is the widest point of the ellipse. Perhaps a table with a "waist" would allow the camera to be closer to the patient in the laterals. Tables must be constructed to have a low coefficient of absorption, strength, and flexibility. Within these confines, perhaps by supporting both ends during scanning, it should be possible to get the camera head close to the patient.

4. The computer programs, which are very flexible, should allow the patient images to be corrected for lengthwise motion. Patients will translate themselves up and down the table, especially as the restraints interfere with setting the camera close to the patient. Alternatively this problem could be solved during imaging by having the camera track the patient as he is being imaged and move the table in response to patient motion.

5. Become very aware of the degradation of the image that even apparently small errors in Anger camera imaging or camera motion could cause.

600

REFERENCES

1. Larsson, Stig A. "Gamma Camera Emission Tomography." Acta Radiologica Supplementum 363 (1980), pp 1-75.

2. Israelsson, A., Lagergren, C., Larsson, S., and Lundell, G. "Detection of space occupying lesions of the liver and spleen: A comparison of emission computer reconstructive tomography and conventional gamma camera scintigraphy." Proceedings of a Symposium on Clinical Use of Emission Tomography Using Single Photon Radiopharmaceuticals, March 1980, to be published by the Bureau of Radiological Health, FDA, USDHHS, 1981, pp 171-176.

3. Shepp, L.A. and Stein, J.A. "Simpulated reconstruction artifacts in computerized x-ray tomography." Reconstruction Tomography in Diagnostic Radiology and Nuclear Medicine. Michel M. Ter-Pogossian, et al, eds (Baltimore: University Park Press, 1977), pp 33-48.

4. Line, B.R., Jones, A.E., Carter, P.A., and Johnston, G.S. " Effect of respiration and patient position on liver-spleen scans determined by multi-gated image analysis." Functional Mapping of Organ Systems and Other Computer Topics, Peter D. Esser, ed (New York: Society of Nuclear Medicine, 1981), pp 65-81.

AUTOMATIC ANALYSIS OF DIAGNOSTIC FEATURES FROM DIGITIZED RADIO-COLLOID LIVER IMAGES

E.A. Eikman, V.K. Jain, G.A. Mack, J.A. Madden, M. Lotz

University of South Florida and the James A. Haley
Veterans Administration Hospital, Tampa, Florida

ABSTRACT

In radiocolloid liver imaging, increased liver mass, and
patchiness of the radiocolloid image are difficult for the physician to evaluate subjectively. We devised an automatic, computer-
assisted method that aids in objective measurement and interpretation of these two image features, and summarize our methods in
this paper. Our estimate of liver mass, and a texture index of
image patchiness designated T2:D2, are calculated from a pre-
processed gamma camera image of the right lateral projection of
the liver. At the operating point of liver mass estimate >2.0 kg
or T2:D2 > 0.54, the specificity was > 0.95 and sensitivity 0.5 for
detection of liver disease in a population of male patients with
independent histologic liver diagnoses or normal volunteers.

This developmental approach is potentially adaptable to other
digital images.

INTRODUCTION

Radiocolloid liver imaging is widely used as an aid in diagnosis and management of liver diseases. Reported false positive
or false negative rates average about 20% under a variety of
experimental conditions, with a wide range of accuracy among
observers applying subjective criteria. (1-4) The variable
accuracy of the physician's subjective interpretation of liver
images is an important diagnostic limitation. Objective means of
quantifying important liver image features should improve the
diagnostic value of liver scintigraphy.

We focused our work on liver image features that are especially difficult to assess subjectively: liver image patchiness and liver mass.

We describe in this paper some details of the methods we have used for analysis. A report of details of clinical results and comparison with human observers is in preparation.

METHODS

Overall approach

Our image analysis approach is diagrammed in Figure I. All steps shown in the solid rectangles are carried out automatically, without operator intervention except to initiate a processing command.

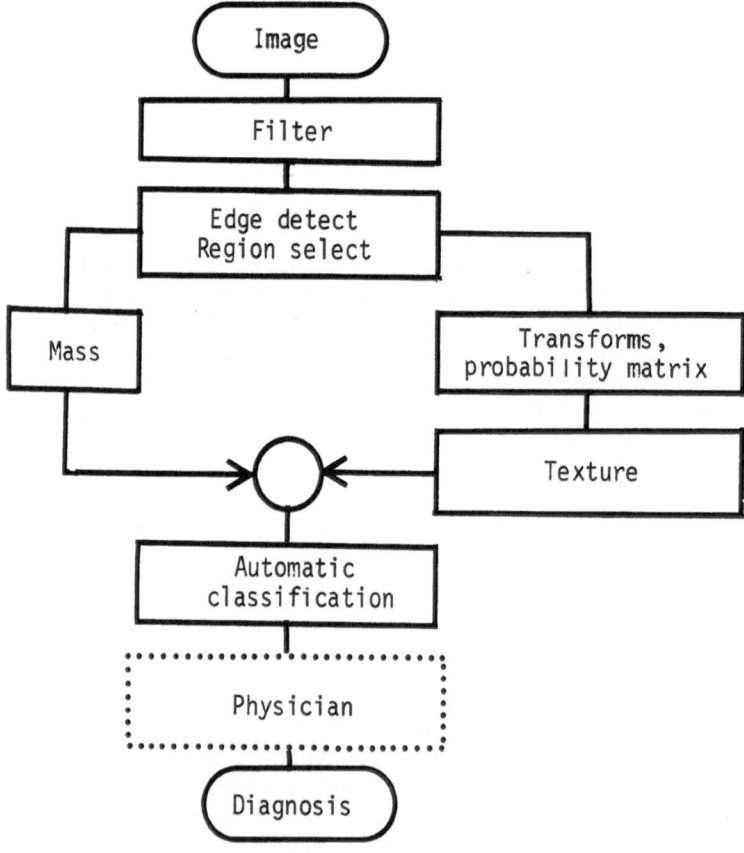

Fig. I   An approach to image analysis.

Image production

Gamma images of the right lateral projection of the liver were acquired 15-30 min after i.v. injection of 2-4 mCi of Tc-99m sulfur colloid in the supine patient. A gamma camera with a high-resolution parallel-hole collimator was used to construct a 400,000-count image, using a 20% window centered over the 140-keV photopeak. On each day of imaging, a 2-million-count image of a Tc-99m uniform pool source was obtained to detect changes in uniformity and sensitivity of the detector and to provide an image-size reference. The analog position signals were digitized with a Searle 100 MHz Wilkinson-type analog to digital converter, and acquired in computer memory as a 64 x 64 matrix. Each matrix unit corresponds to a 4 mm x 4 mm region (5).

Low pass filter

The digital filter used is a nine-point weighted-average filter computed in the spatial domain:

$$g(x,y) = \sum_{k=-1}^{1} \sum_{m=-1}^{1} w(k,m)\, g(x-k,y-m) \tag{1}$$

$$w(k,m) = \begin{array}{ccc} .08 & .08 & .08 \\ .08 & .36 & .08 \\ .08 & .08 & .08 \end{array} \tag{2}$$

More than 99.5% of the image energy is confined to the low frequency region, (6), $\{ |f_x| \lesssim 6f_1, |f_y| \lesssim 6f_1 \}$ where $f_1 = 1/64\Delta$ mm^{-1}; $\Delta = 4$mm. The filter (2) has a frequency characteristic $H(f_x,f_y)$ given by:

$$\begin{aligned} H(f_x,f_y) &= H(f_x)H(f_y) \\ &= (0.6+0.566 \cos \pi f_x \Delta)(0.6+0.566 \cos \pi f_y \Delta) \end{aligned} \tag{3}$$

If we denote $H(f_x=0)$ as H_o, then:
$$H(f_x = 6f_1)/H_o = 0.98$$

The gain within the image frequencies is between 1 and
$$H(6f_1,6f_1) = (0.98)^2 = 0.96$$

Thus, for practical purposes the liver image remains undistorted by use of this filter. Assuming the image noise generated by the statistical nature of the radioactive decay process to be a completely uncorrelated spatial process, it can be shown that the variance of the noise decreases to 0.19 of its original variance by use of the filter described in equations (1) and (2).

Edge detection, region of interest selections

An edge-shaping operator was applied to the filtered data to accentuate the boundaries. Each image pixel, $f(x,y)$, was replaced with:

$$f(x,y) = \begin{cases} f(x,y) \left[\dfrac{f(x,y)}{T}\right]^4, & \text{for } f(x,y) < T \\ T, & \text{for } f(x,y) \geq T \end{cases}$$

where T is 25% of the maximum pixel count in the image, or 150, whichever is smaller.

A 25-point smoothed Laplacian operator was applied:

0	-1	-1	-1	0
-1	2	1	2	-1
-1	1	0	1	-1
-1	2	1	2	-1
0	-1	-1	-1	0

Each pixel was replaced by a summation over the nearest-neighbor pixels using these coefficients. The Laplacian operator gives a measure of the curvature with respect to the x-y plane for any point in the image. Maximum curvature occurs where the slope of radioactivity is changing most rapidly.

The resulting matrix was partitioned into sixteen 8 x 32 submatrices, and a maximum Laplacian was found for each row in each of the partitions (9). An adaptive count threshold was determined for each partition by computing the average of the pixel counts at the Laplacian maxima. All image points below the threshold for the partition were set to zero.

The image area was computed from the number of nonzero pixels and normalized to a reference area defined by the field of view.

Liver Mass Estimation

Liver weights found at autopsy were used to derive an index of liver mass, using the automatically measured area of the right lateral projection of the liver (8). Figure 2 shows the basis for derivation of this index.

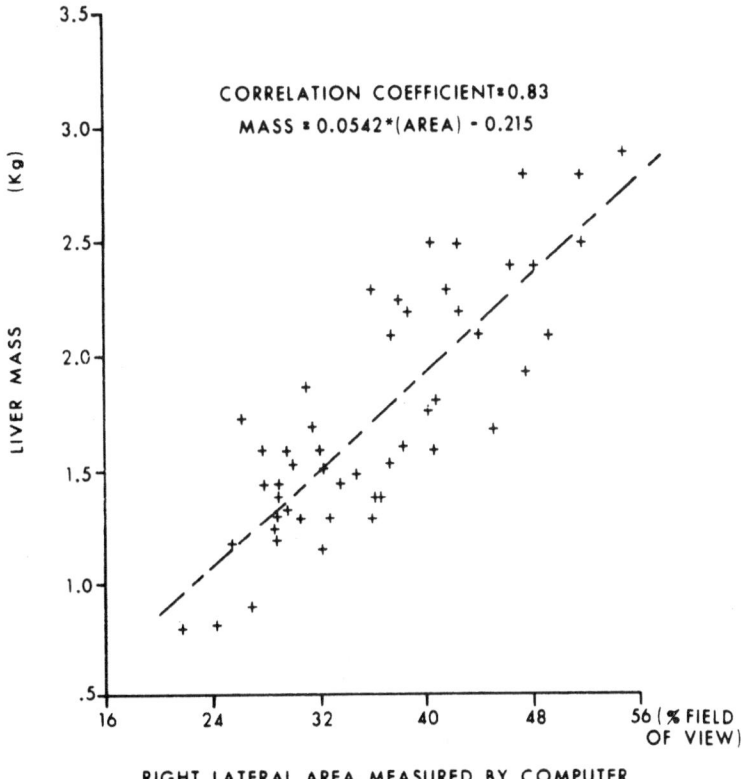

Fig. 2   Liver mass at autopsy, and liver area as determined automatically on a processed image, using 10 inch field of view gamma camera.

Texture Measurement

Gray level transformation. After the preprocessing operations
a 64-level cumulative histogram is calculated from the resulting
image. From the histogram, eight equally likely radioactivity
count intervals are identified. The image is normalized by
transforming it into this eight level domain. Since the filter
used severely attenuates the spatial frequencies due to counting
statistics, the transformed image more accurately represents
true differences in radioactivity.

Feature extraction. Feature extraction was completed by a
series of computational steps which produced spatial-dependence
probability matrices (SP matrices) (7,8), and texture indices.
The SP matrices are defined as follows:

Consider two image matrix elements as shown in Fig. 3. We
designate the pair (D,θ) as the vector displacement. Let their
radioactivity levels be denoted as A_1 and A_2.

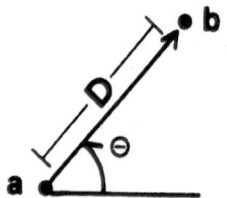

Fig. 3   Matrix element pair with vector displacement (D,θ)

Then, by p(i,j | D,θ) we denote the probability with which the
radioactivity level at one matrix element equals i and at the
other matrix element it equals j while the pair has a vector
displacement (D,θ). To state this more precisely, let:

> M(D,θ) = Number of matrix element pairs with vector
> displacement (D,θ) in the entire image, or
> region of interest, for which the first
> element has a radioactivity level A_1 = i
> and the second element has a radioactivity
> level A_2 = j.

In terms of the above definitions, we can state

$$p(i,j \mid D,\theta) = \frac{P\ \{i,j \mid D,\theta)}{M(D,\theta)}$$

The expression p(i,j/D,θ) denotes the probability with which the
intensity at pixel a - i, and the intensity at pixel b = j, given
the vector separation (D,θ).

The texture of an image is the characteristic repetition of
unit patterns in the image. We have used texture measurements
to extract the overall patchiness or inhomogeneity of radionuclide
uptake.

To measure the patchiness or inhomogeneity of the liver, a
modified algorithm is then used to compare the radioactivity of
each pixel of the liver image matrix with the radioactivity of
its neighbors. For the current work we used the texture index
T2, a measure of squared differences over the image.

One satisfactory texture measure T2 is defined by

$$T2 = \sum_{i,j=1}^{n} (1-j)^2\ p(i,j \mid D,\theta)$$

where n is the number of gray levels used in the transformed
image. In particular, T2D2 denotes the above measure with D=2
pixels.

Diagnostic Application

A preliminary analysis of the diagnostic efficacy of liver
mass estimation was performed in a population of 112 males with
independent diagnoses. The population included 15 patients with
histological evidence of tumor in the liver, 63 with histological
evidence of diffuse liver disease, and 34 normals. In patients
with an automatically estimated mass > 2.6 kg, the probability

608

of liver disease was > 0.95, the specificity > 0.96 and the sensitivity 0.33. Figure 4 shows the distribution of these patients, using a Parzen density estimate (10).

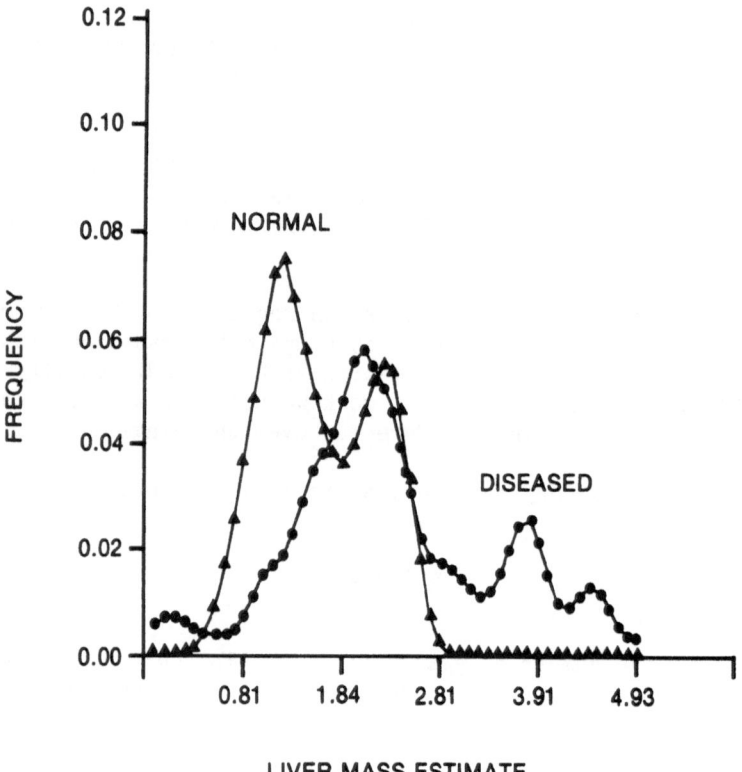

Fig. 4   Distribution of liver masses among patients and normal volunteers

Our population does not contain enough persons with very large body surface areas to provide a basis for correcting the mass criterion for the larger liver masses that are normal in patients with very large livers. By omitting persons with a body surface area of greater than $2m^2$, an operating point of 2.0 kg yields similar accuracy, and reduces the population by a single normal individual.

Using the texture index T2:D2 at an operating point of T2:D2 $\geq$ 19, the probability of liver disease was > 0.95, the specificity > 0.98, and sensitivity 0.2.

When we use both the mass criteria and the texture criteria for liver disease, the sensitivity of the combined methods are improved to about 0.5, and, with specificity > 0.95.

Discussion

In this work, we describe the basis for objective, quantitative indices that enable the physician to establish reproducible diagnostic thresholds to aid in the diagnosis of disease from radiocolloid liver images. In the diagnostic application illustrated, high specificity was achieved with moderate sensitivity. The choice of this operating point is appropriate when false positive results are undesirable, as in many screening applications, or when other independent image features or diagnostic tests are available to increase sensitivity. The diagnostic criteria reported here may be dependent on the test population, as well as on the imaging equipment utilized.

In related work, we are comparing computer diagnostic reliability with that of physician observers. The approach that we report here appears to be superior to physician observers in the population we have tested so far (11). This new method will probably be most effective when used by physicians as an element in a comprehensive diagnostic approach.

The development of tomographic imaging techniques, and the improving anatomic resolution of nuclear and other imaging techniques will aid in extension of this approach to additional imaging problems, both with nuclear and other imaging modalities.

Acknowledgments

This research was aided by Grant ROI GM22890 from the National Institutes of Health, and the Medical Research Service of the Veterans Administration. We thank Michael Courey, Shirley Conway, Ignace Przekop, and Lee Ann Zavosky for technical assistance. We thank Sarah Connelly for aid in portions of this work.

610

REFERENCES

1. Poulose, K.P., R.C. Reba, F.H. DeLand, et al. "Role of liver scanning in the preoperative evaluation of patients with cancer." Br Med J 4 (1969) 585-587.

2. Lin S., C.M. Mansfield, S. Kramer, et al. "Liver scanning in patients with suspected or proven cancer." Am J Roentgenol Radium Ther Nucl Med 108 (1970) 98-101.

3. Ludbrook J., A.H. Slavotinek, and P.M. Ronai. "Observer error in reporting on liver scans for space-occupying lesions." Gastroenterology 62 (1972) 1013-1019.

4. Nishiyama H., J.T. Lewis, A.B. Ashare, et al. "Interpretation of radionuclide liver images: do training and experience make a difference?" J Nucl Med 16 (1975) 11-16.

5. Eikman, E.A., G.A. Mack, V.K. Jain, et al. "Computer-assisted liver mass estimation from radiocolloid gamma-camera images." J Nucl Med 20 (1979) 144-148.

6. Jain, V.K., E.A. Eikman, D.L. Flower, et al. "A Method for Computer Analysis of Texture in Radionuclide Liver Images." Proceedings of the San Diego Biomedical Symposium (1975) 167-173.

7. Haralick, R.M., K. Shanmugam and I. Dinstein. "Textural features for image classification." IEEE Trans. on Systems, Man and Cybernetics. SMC-3(6) (1973) 610-621.

8. Hayes, K.C., Jr., A.N. Shah and A. Rosenfeld. "Texture coarseness: further experiments." IEEE Trans. on Systems, Man and Cybernetics. SMC-4(5) (1974) 467-472.

9. Jain, V.K., G.A. Mack, J.A. Madden, et al. "A texture vector approach to detect focal defects in radionuclide liver images." Proceedings San Diego Biomedical Symposium (1976) 203-206.

10. Meisel W.S. "Computer-oriented approaches to pattern recognition." New York: Academic press (1972)

11. Eikman, E.A., G.A. Mack, V.K. Jain, et al. "Computer-assisted diagnosis of liver disease." J Nucl Med 22 (1981) P87.

INTERVENTIONAL ULTRASOUND

Robert M. Allen, M.D.

The Fairfax Hospital, Department of Radiology

In this workshop there will be a discussion of interventional ultrasound techniques involving cyst puncture, needle aspiration, and biopsy of masses, drainage of abscesses in various locations, antegrade renal studies, and percutaneous nephrostomies. Case presentations of these procedures will demonstrate their usefulness and methodology in every day hospital in-patient and out-patient settings.

Ultrasound has been useful for several decades for evaluation of masses, primarily to separate cysts from solid or mixed type masses. It was a natural progression, therefore, that aspiration of cysts was the first widespread interventional percutaneous technique using ultrasound. From those early days about a decade ago to the present day it has gradually become a misnomer to call the ultrasound suite a noninvasive diagnostic laboratory as was common in some areas. After cyst puncture gained acceptance, ultrasound guided biopsies and more sophisticated drainage procedures followed.

Ultrasound guidance during percutaneous needle insertions has some advantages over alternative methods. Using the versatility of the articulated scanning arm, the cyst or mass to be punctured can be rapidly evaluated in multiple planes without mechanical limitation. While the ultrasound characteristics are analyzed, the simplest, safest approach may be selected avoiding organs and structures unrelated to the puncture, and thus reducing discomfort and complications. The progress of the needle may be monitored during insertion by a realtime unit if needed and the tip of the needle may be seen within a cyst or fluid filled structure with an A-mode scope. Following the puncture procedure, the field may be re-examined immediately to confirm the results of drainage procedures and search for complications. The most common complication is hemorrhage which is seen as a new echo-free space, but even hemorrhage is not very frequent and not reported as serious. The last, but not least, advantages of ultrasound are the low cost and great physical flexibility of the ultrasound equipment. This equipment is widely available because it is cheap compared to CAT scanners and even high quality radiographic-fluoroscopic units. A good real-time scanner costs less than a standard R-F unit and one-tenth as much as a body CT unit. In addition, the unit requires no special installation, no special leaded room, and frequently no special wiring. While virtually all of these units come on wheels to move about the room in which they are used, some are also truly portable and are built to be moved around the hospital to the patient.

Alternative methods of percutaneous needle puncture are blind puncture, radiographic or fluoroscopic assisted puncture and CT guided puncture. Blind puncture is only satisfactory in superficial palpable masses. R-F guidance is desirable when the injection of contrast is contemplated such as in transhepatic intraductal biliary manipulations or in the biopsy of small pathologic lymph nodes still opacified following lymphography. This method frequently results in considerable radiation to the patient and physician. Biplane fluoroscopy is preferred but is only available in a few large institutions. CT guided puncture is necessary if the lesion cannot be visualized by ultrasound because of its small size or location. It is a time consuming procedure using extremely expensive equipment which is not always available. The approaches are frequently awkward and limited to coronal planes because the scanning arc has physical limitations. Except where it is truly indicated, the CT biopsy is a substitution of expensive and sophisticated equipment for more reasonable approaches.

There are several considerations when preparing for a needle aspiration. Preliminary scanning is necessary to select an approach while avoiding unnecessary puncture of other organs, the bowel, the pleura, or obvious vascular structures. Puncture of the pancreas, retroperitoneal lymph nodes or other retroperitoneal structures using a ventral approach traverses the bowel without complication by using a small #23g (0.7 mm diameter) needle. These needles are actually smaller than those used to suture bowel. Selecting the size and length of the needle is, therefore, dictated by the depth of the mass and the intervening tissues in the needle path. Cyst drainage is accomplished with small bore needles while core biopsies of kidney often call for a 16 or 18 gauge needle. While aspiration of cells from hard tumors is usually successful with very small guage needles, softer lymphomatous tissue may require a larger bore to obtain the larger clumps of cells necessary for accurate diagnosis. Therefore the type of mass punctured

also influences the bore of the needle. Selection of the transducer is very subjective, depending on the ultrasound equipment
used and the physician's preference. Most often, the Grey scale
scanning arm transducer that is used in the preliminary scanning
is all that is needed. The electronic measuring cursor is used to
determine the angle of insertion as well as the depth of the
puncture needed. Real-time sector or linear array transducers
may also be used. Special biopsy transducers are available to
guide the needle during insertion while the mass is in view in
A-mode or M-mode display. These transducers usually have a central
guide hole or slot through which the needle is inserted; the slot
type allows the transducer to be moved away without disturbing
the needle. Various transducers with parallel needle insertion
devices are also offered by some manufacturers for their own
instruments. The physician is able to choose the method with which
he is most comfortable to accommodate the clinical and anatomic
setting at hand.

After the planning and preparation process, there are only a
few precautions to performing the puncture. Most important is to
be aware of any defect in the blood clotting mechanism or any other
tendency to hemorrhage. With special care, the procedure may still
be performed but a clotting defect should be corrected ahead of
time if possible. One does not knowingly needle Echinococcal cysts
or aneurysms. Pheochromocytomas have been known to cause rapid
increase in blood pressure when disturbed so that the proper medication to control blood pressure should be at hand if a supra-renal
mass is being approached.

After the needle approach has been determined and the appropriate site selected, the skin is prepped and anesthetized. A
small nick in the skin with a pointed scalpel blade allows easier
insertion of the needle and results in a better "feel" of the
tissues as the needle passes through. The needle is then inserted
to a predetermined depth using a needle stop if necessary. Often,
the needle must be inserted one or two cm. farther than measured
because a cyst wall may invaginate before it is punctured and a
movable mass or organ may be displaced away by the needle tip before
it is entered. When a cyst is punctured, the needle tip is seen
on the A-mode scope as a spike in the fluid filled cavity and the
fluid can then be aspirated. If an aspiration biopsy is being
performed, the stylet is removed from the needle and short jabbing
insertions are then made within the mass while suction is applied
with the syringe. The suction is then released and the needle is
withdrawn. The cells or core will remain in the needle. The
specimen is then blown or flushed onto a slide or into a specimen
bottle. When the aspiration has been completed, the patient is
rescanned. If a cyst were evacuated, the extent of drainage can
be evaluated. The injection site is also examined for hemorrhage
at this time. Since most hematomas arise slowly, examination in

12-24 hours would be more useful in this regard, if clinically indicated. The patient should be comfortable at the completion of the procedure, and if much pain occurs, a complication should be considered.

When a specimen has been obtained for laboratory examination, it must be properly cared for. The local pathology laboratory will probably have their own procedure to follow, but in general, the specimen must be protected from air drying by immersion in alcohol or saline. If slide smears are drawn, they may be air dried or immersed in alcohol immediately, at the preference of the pathologist. After the specimen has been examined under a microscope and has been determined to be satisfactory, the needling procedure may be terminated.

Now this general approach to ultrasound guided needle aspiration may be varied to accommodate different diagnostic and therapeutic purposes depending on the organ and anatomic space involved. In the kidney, cyst aspiration has already been discussed. It is well known that many of these cysts will recur and some may continue to enlarge. Permanent obliteration of cysts has been brought about by the injection of various substances but none of these has been widely accepted. Recently, the injection of alcohol into cysts has been shown to prevent recurrence and may be the answer to this problem. An infected cyst may be drained, cultured, and flushed with the appropriate antibiotic with good results. Renal biopsy of the lower pole cortex is performed with a variety of larger needles, usually 16 gauge, to obtain a core biopsy. Drainage of the renal pelvis is useful in urinary obstruction for treatment as well as for the diagnosis of the site and nature of the obstruction. The needle is inserted into the lower half of the kidney from a slightly lateral approach so that it passes through the cortex first before entering the pelvis, avoiding not only large vessels but also the possibility of tearing the unprotected free wall of the renal pelvis. Contrast is then injected to demonstrate the site of the obstruction which may be at the ureteropelvic junction or further down the ureter. Stones may be manipulated and stints may be inserted across obstructing tumors or periureteral fibrosis. Following a guidewire exchange and dilatation of the track, a #8 French pigtail catheter may be inserted for longterm drainage. At the skin surface, a Molnar button which has been passed over the catheter is sutured to the skin stabilizing the catheter while protecting the skin surface.

In the liver, small bore #22 or #23 French "skinny" needles are used whenever possible to avoid lacerations and hematomas. Core biopsies with larger needles result in hematomas of 2-4 cm. in diameter and some bile leak into the abdomen but when these procedures are not followed by ultrasound or CAT scan examinations, these complications usually resolve unnoticed. If a small needle aspiration reveals an abscess, a #8 or #12 trochar driven drain may be inserted through a nick in the skin parallel to the diagnostic needle. It is then driven to a predetermined depth into the abscess for drainage. The pleural space should be avoided as it should in all liver punctures, so that there will be no spread of bile or infection to the pleural space and no pneumothorax. If an abscess is deep within the liver, instead of inserting a large trochar, trauma to the liver may be lessened by inserting a #19 needle. When it is confirmed to be within the abscess by aspiration of pus, a guidewire may be passed to lead a #8 French pigtail or straight catheter into the abscess. Contrast can be injected later to confirm the placement of the catheter in the abscess cavity and this may be repeated periodically to follow resolution of the abscess.

Pancreatic masses are usually located in the head or body of the organ and can only expand anteriorly toward the ventral abdominal wall because it is the path of least resistance. Therefore, these masses actually are often very superficial and are approached directly through the epigastrium. A #22 or #23 "skinny" needle is used for biopsy so that puncture of the colon or stomach will not result in leakage. We have used the Madayag needle for the last several years in pancreatic biopsies occasionally obtaining a core biopsy rather than just a simple aspiration of cells despite its small bore. Drainage of pseudocysts and pancreatic abscesses have been widely reported in the literature and are successful using the previously described principles. We have not had any experience in this area because pseudocysts have been treated by open surgery in our hospital.

Intra-abdominal and pelvic tumors of other organs and spaces may be biopsied using the guidelines already discussed. Intra-peritoneal or retroperitoneal masses are approached by the shortest skin-tumor distance also. Retroperitoneal tumors and lymphadenopathy frequently occur in patients with a previous history of malignancy and the pathologist is able to determine whether the process is the same or different. The accuracy of pathologic diagnosis of pelvic tumors is at least 75%, depending on the type of specimen obtained and the experience of the microscopist with this type of biopsy. Abdominal abscesses can be located and drained by needle aspiration or by catheter drainage over a longer period of time. At the same time, a culture and sensitivity can determine the appropriate antibiotic for systemic treatment. The only recurring abscess in our series was in a retained ureter three years after a nephrectomy. The patient had been on dialysis for years because of polycystic kidneys which led to the nephrectomy. The abscess recurred because it was later found to be within a retained ureter which communicated with the bladder and was, therefore, a sinus tract capable of re-infection.

616

Both in the discussion here and in the cases presented, ultrasound has been shown to be a superior aid in the diagnosis and drainage of fluid filled spaces and the biopsy of solid masses in the abdomen and pelvis. Because it is accurate, available, convenient and versatile, it is unsurpassed for general use in these procedures.

REFERENCES

1. Goldberg BB, Pollack HM: Ultrasonic aspiration biopsy techniques. J Clin Ultrasound 4:141, 1976

2. Goldberg BB, Pollack HM, Kellerman E: Ultrasonic localization for renal biopsy. Radiology 115:167, 1975

3. Holm HH, Rasmussen SN, Kristensen JK: Ultrasonically guided percutaneous puncture technique. J Clin Ultrasound 1:27, 1973

4. Kline TS, Neal HS: Needle aspiration biopsy: A critical appraisal. JAMA 239:36, 1978

5. Pederson JF, Cowan DF, Kvist J, et al: Ultrasonically-guided percutaneous nephrostomy. Radiology 119:429, 1976

6. Smith EH, Bartrum RJ: Ultrasonically guided percutaneous aspiration of abscesses. Am J Roentgenol 122:308, 1974

7. Smith EH, Bartrum Jr RJ, Chang YC, et al: Ultrasonically guided percutaneous aspiration biopsy of the pancreas. Radiology 112:737, 1974

*Part X: Cost-Effective and Cost-Benefit Assessment of New High
           Technology Procedures*

DIAGNOSTIC IMAGING IN DEVELOPING COUNTRIES

N. T. Racoveanu, M.D.

Chief, Radiation Medicine Unit,
World Health Organization, Geneva

1 INTRODUCTION

An important component of modern health care, that of diagnostic imaging, comprising radiodiagnostic and nuclear medicine,
faces severe constraints in the developing world. The aim of this
paper is to review these constraints, to stress the effects seen
on the qualitative and quantitative results of the diagnostic imaging systems, and to outline some of the solutions which could be
envisaged to correct and improve the actual situation.

The developing world comprises approximately 140 countries
with a population of about 2.9 billion as compared with that of
approximately 1.3 billion in industrial countries.

Historically speaking, diagnostic imaging services in the
developing world have followed the patterns of the industrialized
world with a lapse in time which varies from place to place. As
an example, the Barnard Institute of Radiology, in Madras (India),
was established during the first decade of this century, while in
other areas of the developing world, particularly in Africa, radiodiagnostic services became a reality only 15-20 years ago. Nuclear
medicine services are still in a more primitive stage and less than
50% of the countries in the developing world have nuclear medicine
facilities.

Many factors have influenced the historical development of
diagnostic imaging facilities in the countries of concern and
cannot be easily differentiated from those which constitute the

TABLE 1   RATIO POPULATION/X-RAY MACHINES IN FIVE WHO REGIONS

Number of Countries and Mill. Population for each Category of Coverage

Population per 1 x-ray machine	AFRO		AMRO		EMRO		SEARO		WPRO		TOTAL	
	No. of countr.	mill. people	No. of countr.	mill. people	No. of countr.	mill. people	No. of countr.	mill. people	No. of countr.	mill. people	No. of countr.	mill. people
Less than 50 000	3	1.5	28	171.0	10	34.8	1	1.5	8	56.5	50	265.3
50-100 000	3	17.3	4	2.2	7	80.7	1	620.0	1	2.8	16	723.0
More than 100 000	11	69.3	3	9.9	6	126.4	3	58.2	0	0	23	263.8
Total	17	88.1	35	183.1	23	241.9	5	679.7	9	59.3	89	1252.1

TABLE 2   RATIO POPULATION/DIAGNOSTIC RADIOLOGIST IN FIVE WHO REGIONS

Number of Countries and Mill. Population for each Category of Coverage

Population per 1 radiologist	AFRO		AMRO		EMRO		SEARO		WPRO		TOTAL	
	No. of countr.	mill. people	No. of countr.	mill. people	No. of countr.	mill. people	No. of countr.	mill. people	No. of countr.	mill. people	No. of countr.	mill. people
Less than 100 000	2	1.0	15	166.1	3	12.8	1	1.5	2	0.2	23	181.6
100-500 000	0	0	8	16.1	6	87.1	0	0	2	36.5	16	159.7
More than 500 000	14	143.1	3	14.6	8	143.5	3	58.6	1	2.9	29	362.7
Total	16	144.1	26	196.8	17	243.4	4	60.1	5	39.6	68	684.0

TABLE 3   RATIO POPULATION/MEDICAL RADIOLOGICAL TECHNICIAN IN FIVE WHO REGIONS

Population per 1 medical radiological technician	Number of Countries and Mill. Population for each Category of Coverage											
	AFRO		AMRO		EMRO		SEARO		WPRO		TOTAL	
	No. of countr.	mill. people	No. of countr.	mill. people	No. of countr.	mill. people	No. of countr.	mill. people	No. of countr.	mill. people	No. of countr.	mill. people
Less than 50 000	4	8.0	22	178.1	4	15.6	1	1.5	6	39.8	37	243.0
50-250 000	4	36.0	6	19.1	7	165.6	2	639.8	0	0	19	860.5
More than 250 000	9	114.3	0	0	6	52.5	2	93.7	0	0	17	260.5
Total	17	158.3	28	197.2	17	233.7	5	735.0	6	39.8	73	1364.0

actual constraints faced by such countries. It is, therefore, worth beginning with a thorough analysis of these constraints.

2 CONSTRAINTS FACED BY DIAGNOSTIC IMAGING SERVICES IN DEVELOPING COUNTRIES

The major results of the factors analysed here are of a quantitative and qualitative nature, expressed simply as:

a) lower number of diagnostic imaging procedures performed per patient attending the health care facilities; and

b) poorer quality of diagnostic imaging procedures performed.

Both can influence patient management and consequently the total efficacy/efficiency of the health care system in the countries involved. The principal factors responsible for such results are:

2.1 Ratio of Diagnostic Imaging Equipment and of Specialized Personnel to Population

Available data are mostly incomplete and unreliable, and the figures given in tables 1, 2 and 3 should therefore be considered only as an indication of the actual situation (1). The tables present figures referring to radiodiagnostic services; similar data on nuclear medicine are not shown as the Register prepared by IAEA in 1974 is outdated (2).

Table 1, analysing the ratio population/x-ray machine in 89 developing countries, representing 1.25 billion population, shows that only 50 countries, with 0.26 billion people, have 1 x-ray machine for less than 50 000 people, which is the ratio considered to be acceptable. The rest, 0.99 billion people, of the 39 countries are either poorly (1 machine for 50-100 000 people) or very poorly (1 machine for more than 100 000 people) covered.

The radiological personnel (radiologists and radiographers) present ratios which are even worse than the x-ray machines, as given in Tables 2 and 3. It is known that a number of African countries have no specialist radiologists and that in South-East Asia, 1 radiologist often serves 1-1.5 million people.

Extrapolating from the figures given in tables 1-3, the actual coverage with diagnostic radiology can be described as follows:

very poor for approximately 1.6 billion people
poor for approximately 1.2 billion people
acceptable and good for approximately 1.4 billion people

2.2 Uneven Distribution of Diagnostic Imaging Facilities

The ratio of x-ray machine/population gives only a very incomplete picture of the current availability of radiological equipment for the population of a given country. Most of the diagnostic imaging facilities are concentrated in big cities, leaving large areas of rural and suburban population with no or very low coverage.

In order to have an x-ray examination, the people of underserved areas have to travel long distances, and spend a significant amount of time and money. The uneven distribution is also responsible for the over-crowded services at university and other big hospitals, where the number of examinations performed is very high in comparison with some small medical institutions, where radiological facilties are often under-used.

Table 4 shows the number of examinations and films per year in radiodiagnostic departments in some developing and industrial countries. The figures were obtained from a random sample of university and teaching hospitals and demonstrate that the number of x-ray examinations is by no means much lower in the developing countries than in industrial ones. The only difference is that in the latter the procedures practised at the university hospitals are only a small fraction of the entire number of x-ray examinations, while in developing countries these represent the majority of such examinations. At the same time, in industrial countries a much higher percentage of specialized procedures are performed at this level, while in developing areas, this percentage is low - the most sophisticated radiodiagnostic departments performing a great number of basic x-ray examinations which do not require the available equipment and technical skill.

Table 5 gives further essential data; the number of examination and films per radiologist per year. While radiologists in industria countries are examining 2 500 to 6 000 patients per year, or 8-15 000 films, the radiologist in the developing country has to examine 11 000 to 20 000 patients per year or more than 25-40 000 films. This pressure of work is the consequence of the poor coverage of the population as well as the uneven distribution of

TABLE 4   WORKLOAD AND NUMBER OF RADIOLOGISTS IN VARIOUS
RADIOLOGICAL DEPARTMENTS THROUGHOUT THE WORLD

Institution	Workload per Year			
	No.patients examined	No.films exposed	No.exams with contrast or fluor.	No. of radio- logists
Barnard Institute, Madras, India	136,500	251,800	10,385	10
Kenyatta Hospital, Nairobi, Kenya	90,874.	232,185	7,138	3
Connaught Hospital, Freetown, S.L.	37,420	56,120	-	2
Mulago Hospital, Kampala, Uganda	21,008	39,553	2,463	1
Siriraj Hospital, Bangkok, Thailand	130,000	-	19,525	-
Dacca Med. College, Dacca, Bangladesh	56,200	-	-	-
General Hospital, Rangoon, Burma	67,000	-	-	-
General Hospital, Colombo, S. Lanka	125,000	-	-	-
King Edward Hospital, Bombay, India	~100,000	-	-	-
McMaster University, Hamilton, Canada	53,802	149,477	29%	-
Bristol University, Bristol, U.K.	156,367	391,000	26,644	18+8
Strahlen Institute, Tübingen, FRG	74,728	256,728	72,489	29
Abt. Radiol., Aachen, FRG	47,000	127,000	38,000	6+6
Inst. Radiol., Bern, Switzerland	74,484	219,952	67,882	22
Glostrup Hospital, Copenhagen, Denmark	94,492	290,783	22,907	-
Utrecht Hospital, Utrecht, Netherlands	82,500	~400,000	13,500	31
Inst. Radiol., Genoa. Italy	29,426	108,500	2,960	10

TABLE 5   NUMBER OF PATIENTS, FILMS EXAMINED AND SPECIAL
EXAMINATIONS PERFORMED PER YEAR BY ONE RADIOLOGIST

Institution	One Radiologist has to Examine per Year		
	No. patients	No. films	contrast media and fluoroscopic exams
Barnard Institute, Madras, India	13,500	25,180	1,040
Kenyatta Hospital, Nairobi, Kenya	11,360	29,023	900
Connaught Hospital, Freetown, S.L.	18,710	28,060	-
Mulago Hospital, Kampala, Uganda	21,008	39,553	2,463
Bristol University, Bristol, U.K.	6,014	15,040	1,024
Strahlen Institute, Tübingen, FRG	2,576	8,852	2,499
Abt. Radiol., Aachen, FRG	3,916	10,583	3,166
Inst. Radiol., Bern, Switzerland	3,385	9,996	3,085
Utrecht Hospital, Utrecht, Netherlands	2,661	12,900	435
Inst. Radiol., Genoa, Italy	2,942	10,850	296

radiological facilities throughout the country.

It is obvious that a radiologist who has to examine two or three times more patients during a given time assisted by less qualified auxiliary staff, and with equipment which very often does not perform at its full capacity, will produce diagnostic information of lower quality. Unfortunately, objective data to prove this assertion are not available at present.

2.3 Number of Diagnostic Imaging Procedures per 1000 People per Year

Data obtained by WHO for UNSCEAR; new report as well as examples taken from the UNSCEAR 1977 Report, are shown in Figure 1. All data refer to radiodiagnostic examinations and at least two conclusions can be drawn. First, a big difference is seen in the number of x-ray examinations between industrial and developing countries; this difference is of 5 to 10 fold. Second, there is a similar difference in the number of examinations within urban and rural areas in the developing countries themselves (see Brazil, Kenya), stressing once again the effect of the uneven distribution of radiological facilities.

A better understanding of the number of x-ray examinations per 1000 population per year, which may be optimal for the health care of a given population, can be obtained from the population age structure, hospital morbidity and estimated number of x-ray examinations performed at present, as presented in Figure 2. Data presented pertain to three different categories of countries with respect to age and morbidity structure.

Considering the role played by x-ray examinations in various types of diseases and for various age groups, it is not difficult to understand that Canada, with a much older population and a higher prevalence of chronic and degenerative diseases, would need a larger number of x-ray exams/1000 people/year than Burma, which has a considerably younger population and a higher prevalence of infections and parasitic diseases, and where x-ray examinations are not always essential. Even recognizing this fact, we still cannot accept that an order of magnitude should exist between the two countries. If we regard the quite similar frequency of diseases of the respiratory tract and accidents + violence in the two countries mentioned, it can be assumed that while Canada benefits from adequate x-ray facilities, allowing all patients in need to have the requested examinations, in Burma, where the facilities are limited in number, many patients are unable to obtain the required investigations.

626

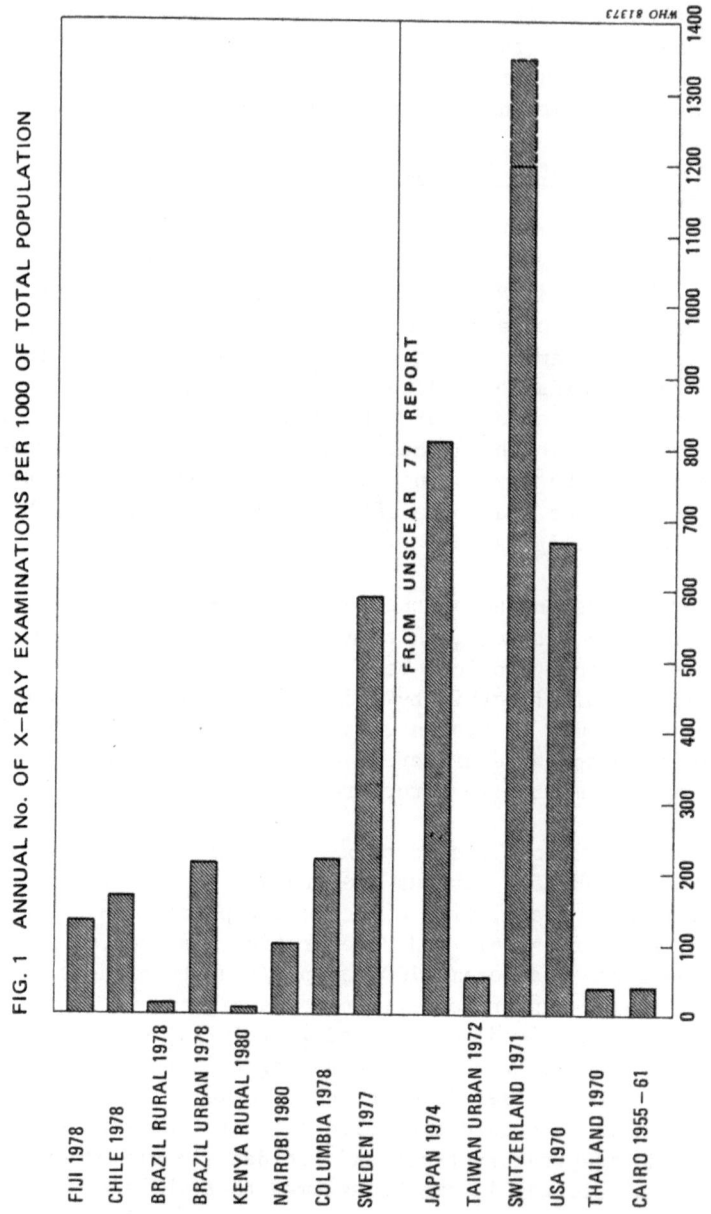

FIG. 1 ANNUAL No. OF X—RAY EXAMINATIONS PER 1000 OF TOTAL POPULATION

FROM UNSCEAR 77 REPORT

WHO 81373

FIG. 2 DISTRIBUTION OF POPULATION BY AGE GROUP AND HOSPITAL MORBIDITY PATTERN

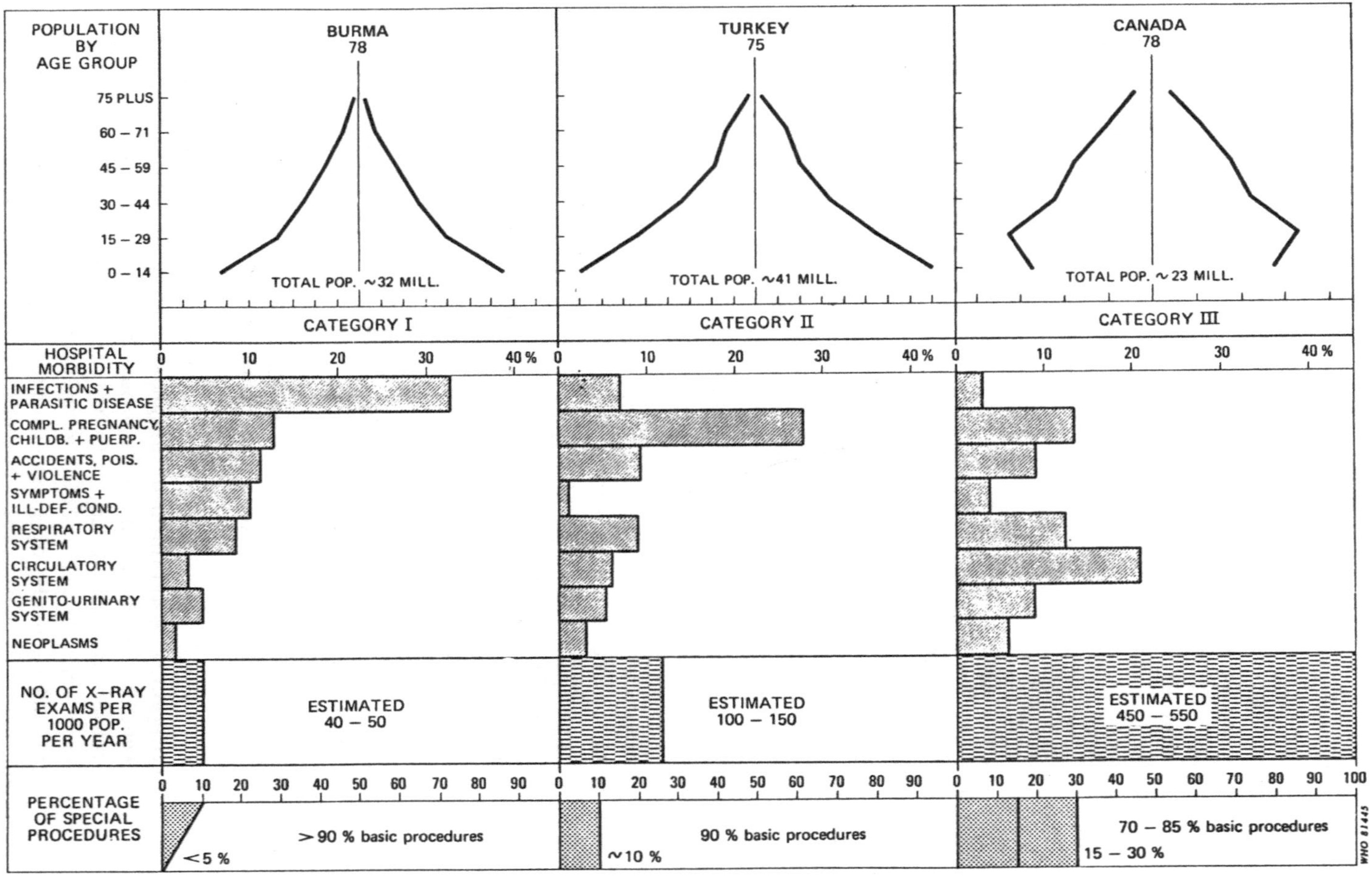

2.4 Adequacy of the Equipment for Diagnostic Imaging

One of the prerequisites in producing diagnostic quality images is the necessity for equipment which functions within the accepted limits. Diagnostic imaging equipment is designed and constructed in industrial countries, and only a few exceptions to this rule are seen. Most of the industrial countries do not face problems of difficult climatic conditions (heat, humidity, cold, dust, etc.), of unreliable power supply (frequent power cuts, drops in voltage, change in frequency, high impedance lines, etc,), or of biological agents (insects, moulds, rodents, etc.) that could damage the equipment.

At the same time, there are wide differences between industrial and developing countries in salary scales, employment policies and total economic approaches and systems. For reasons related to high personnel costs, the designers of medical equipment have a tendency to reduce to a minimum the manpower involved in equipment handling, resulting in a high degree of automation.

These two factors of inappropriate design for local climatic and power supply conditions and increasing automation, make most of the equipment available on the market unsuitable for large use in developing countries.

The situation is made even worse by the haphazard supply policy of countries which accept donations from very diverse sources; sometimes purchasing the cheapest equipment offered, irrespective of its performance or, on the contrary, the most expensive and advanced for which neither the service nor the expertise for its proper use exist. Many examples of this have been seen by the writer when visiting countries in the Middle-East, Africa and South-East Asia. A few will be described here:

- purchase of x-ray machines which are too low powered to be able to undertake all the examinations requested;

- machines with a high degree of automation therefore susceptible to frequent breakdowns which cannot be repaired by local engineers;

- incorrect installation of diagnostic imaging equipment frequently with an inadequate power line (high impedance), which constitutes a major factor for under-exposure and causes erratic functioning of air conditioning due to power cuts and exposure of gamma cameras, computers, and similar equipment to unsuitable temperatures, humidity, etc;

- inadequate protection of sensitive parts of the equipment (image amplifiers, scintillation crystals of nuclear medicine equipment) permit the climatic factors to affect performance;

- too great a variety of types and brands of equipment preventing the adequate provision of spare parts and supplies of recording materials (films, recording paper, etc.).

These are just a few examples intended to illustrate the problem of unsuitable equipment.

2.5 Maintenance, Repair and Testing of Equipment

These factors constitute a critical element of equipment performance and are neglected in most of the developing countries. Neither the normal daily care, which should be undertaken by the equipment operator, nor the periodic maintenance, which needs the presence of an engineer or technician, are normally carried out in most of the departments in the developing world. In the absence of such maintenance programmes, small faults in equipment which are not detected and corrected in time, result in the occurrence of a total breakdown. It is only at this time that a service engineer is called in.

Depending on local circumstances (availability of funds, location of service engineer, availability of spare parts, etc.) the equipment can be non-functional for a period varying from a few days to many years! A considerable number of such machines are never repaired and become obsolete after only a short time, without any consideration for the investment made and the respective lack of return.

It can be stated that in most of the developing world the highest proportion of the cost of a diagnostic imaging procedure results from the amortizement of the capital cost of the equipment and the cost of films and chemicals, radiopharmaceuticals or contrast media, while that of manpower (personnel operating the equipment) and of patient hospitalization, is only a minor part of this total, as shown in Table 6.

Another important link in equipment care, which is missing in the circumstances outlined above, is that of testing and calibrating which should be undertaken on installation, after repair, and at intervals. This is not routinely done, even in industrial countries, as was demonstrated at the workshops organized by WHO and the Federal Republic of Germany on Quality Assurance in Diagnostic Radiology (3) and Nuclear Medicine (4).

TABLE 6   ESTIMATION OF COSTS OF AN AVERAGE RADIOGRAPHIC EXAMINATION
IN INDUSTRIAL AND DEVELOPING COUNTRIES

1. Cost of Machine   US$ 100,000

   no. exams/year   6,000
   average life span   10y = 60,000 exams
   cost/exam   US$ 1.7

2. Cost of Films
   and Chemicals   US$ 1.5/exam

3. Cost of Personnel &
   Hospital Overheads

   Industrial Country   Developing Country
                              $ $ $ $
   radiol. 1½/6000 ex.x 50,000=75,000   0.75/6000 x 2,000=1,500
   radiogr.1/6000 ex. x 25,000=25,000   1.0/6000 x 1,200=1,200
   eng. 0.05/6000 ex. x 40,000= 2,000   0.01/6000 x 1,800=   1.8
   hospital overheads /year   =20,000   =1,000

	US$	%	US$	%
cost/exam. - machine	1.7	(7.2)	1.70	(44.5)
- films, chemicals	1.5	(6.4)	1.50	(39.3)
- personnel	17.0	(72.4)	0.45	(11.7)
- hospital	3.3	(14.0)	0.17	(4.5)
Total cost/exam	23.5	(100.0)	3.82	(100.0)

TABLE 7   DECREASE IN NUMBER OF PATIENTS X-RAYED

Year	Number of Patients X-rayed		
	Hospital	Private Cases	Total
1975	37,107	6,847	43,454
1976	49,016	14,926	63,942
1977	53,996	17,262	71,254
1978	47,757	14,681	62,432
1979	42,980	10,820	53,800
1980	40,914	15,288	56,202

X-ray machines with untested/uncalibrated kV, mA meters, timers, etc. as a cause of non-diagnostic quality images, have been found by studies carried out in the USA, UK, Australia (4, 5, 6, 7). This situation is much more common in the developing world from which, unfortunately, not much reliable data is available. It is also valid for nuclear medicine equipment, for which testing and calibration is also essential. A few studies have been conducted by the IAEA in a number of countries in South-East Asia and Latin America and their results should soon be compiled. WHO is also planning an international intercomparison of diagnostic images obtained with gamma cameras, which will start in Europe and be gradually expanded to include the developing countries.

2.6 Image Detectors and Image Recording Equipment

Two major aspects will be reviewed under this subject:

a)   the sensitivity of the image detectors and of the image recording equipment;

b)   the availability of image recording material.

It was already pointed out in 2.4 that inadequate protection and care of sensitive parts of the image detectors, such as intensifying screens, fluoroscopic screens, image amplifiers used in fluoroscopy, crystals used in scanners or gamma camera, can reduce or destroy their performances and therefore interfere with the quality of the diagnostic image obtained. It has been proved, for instance, that rare earth screens are sensitive to hot and humid climates which favor mold growth on the screen and that detectors such as caesium iodide or sodium iodide, etc. are highly sensitive to humidity, high temperature, or sudden changes in temperature. Therefore image amplifiers used in x-ray machines and detectors used in nuclear medicine equipment (scanners, gamma camera), need particular care in countries where such climatic conditions prevail. A considerable number of image amplifiers in developing countries lose their sensitivity two to three years after installation.

Even the simple screen used for direct fluoroscopy, unprotected against direct day- or fluorescent light gradually decreases its sensitivity, requiring higher exposure for production of the same amount of light photons.

The foregoing are all current causes of non-diagnostic quality of images in countries where there are difficult climatic conditions and a lack of special care of image detectors.

Decrease in sensitivity of image recording material, and in particular of radiologic films, is due to the storage and transport under unsuitable conditions (extremes of temperature, humidity, presence of chemical vapours, etc.) and of processing under incorrect conditions (temperature, time, concentration of chemicals). A test, made by the writer, on films obtained from the central store of one Middle-East country, showed an average background fog density of 0.8, which stresses the importance of suitable storage conditions for films.

In a number of developing countries, the availability of films has become a real problem during the last few years. The increased price of silver, which has been reflected in the price of films, has seriously reduced the quantity of films which can be afforded by countries in which the total health expenditure is situated between less than 1 to 10 US$ per inhabitant/year. As a result films are in very short supply in such areas and the number of x-ray examinations is decreasing. The figures given in Table 7 were obtained from a radiology department of a medical college in one of the South-East Asian countries.

Some small countries in Africa, Latin America and Pacific areas are facing difficulties in obtaining films because the small quantities ordered are not interesting for the suppliers, particularly if the delivery has to be divided into quarterly batches. At the same time, the prices charged by some local dealers in developing countries are much higher than those of the producer, which represents another burden.

Silver recovery, which can represent a possibility of decreasing the price of films and reintroducing silver into circulation, is applied in only very few developing countries.

The problem of film prices and their related shortage is gradually becoming one of the major factors which could prevent the balanced development of radiology to cover underserved population in the developing world. No solutions are available which could be used on a wide scale and this problem which is critical for the further progress and coverage by radiological services of the world's population requires the urgent attention and support of the scientific community.

2.7 Circulation, Storage and Retrieval of Diagnostic Imaging Information

The utility of diagnostic imaging techniques depends on the diagnostic information obtained reaching the physician who has

referred the patient in sufficient time to be used for his diagnostic and treatment decision. It is also important that such
information be properly stored and retrieved when necessary for
appropriate follow-up of the patient, for teaching and other
similar purposes. This entire process of circulation, storage and
retrieval of the diagnostic information, needs an adequate infra-
structure and trained personnel. Departments where more than
100 000 patients are examined each year require a more reliable
system than the simple manual handling of the information. A study
performed in Nairobi (8), with regard to the storage and retrieval
of the radiodiagnostic information, found that approximately 24.5%
of diagnostic information stored in previous years was not retriev-
able by normal procedures.

It is clear that departments with a high workload will have a
much larger problem of storage and retrieval, as well as of mis-
labelling, which may often lead to film retake. Adequate structures
and facilities for the circulation, storage and retrieval of diagnostic information are demanding in terms of personnel and equipment, particularly in departments with a very heavy workload, and
may involve the use of computers, as is already the case in
industrial countries.

The major factors responsible for the difficulties seen in
diagnostic imaging departments in developing countries have been
reviewed: in summary the following conclusions can be drawn:

i)   the average patient in developing countries receives only
     1/2 to 1/10 the number of x-ray investigations performed in
     industrial countries, and probably a figure which is an order
     of magnitude lower for the nuclear medicine investigations;

ii) the quantity of diagnostic information obtained per surface of
     film (or g of silver) used cannot be estimated properly
     because of lack of specific data. On the one hand, the more
     advanced cases with easily seen lesions are probably reaching
     the diagnostic imaging departments in developing countries,
     while in industrial countries these facilities are largely
     used for all kind of patients, some of whom are in stages
     where the diagnostic information is not so evident. On the
     other hand, due to a number of factors such as pressure of
     work, poor quality of image, insufficient experience and/or
     training, a fair amount of significant diagnostic information
     could be missed, thus decreasing the efficacy of diagnostic
     imaging procedures;

iii) the quality of the diagnostic image obtained seems, on average, to be poorer in developing than in industrial countries due to a number of factors related to: poor equipment performance, decreased sensitivity of image detectors and recording media, and other similar objective factors, to which the subjective ones related to human behaviour and conscientiousness could be added. Again it should be mentioned that objective evidence is not available to enable the presentation of solid data on the difference in image quality between the two categories of countries considered here;

iv) There is a very obvious difference in cost of diagnostic imaging procedures between the two categories of countries considered. In industrial countries, 73% of the cost is represented by the salaries of the personnel, approximately 14% by the administrative costs of the hospital, and less than 14% only by the equipment amortizement, films and chemicals. In the developing countries, however, the equipment amortizement represents approximately 45%, the films and chemicals 39%, the salaries of personnel less than 12% only and the administrative charges of the hospital approximately 4%. This essential difference should be taken into consideration when measures to improve the diagnostic imaging procedures in developing countries are taken.

3 SUGGESTED SOLUTIONS TO THE PRESENT CONSTRAINTS FACED BY DIAGNOSTI IMAGING SERVICES IN DEVELOPING COUNTRIES

The complex picture given of the present situation of diagnosti imaging services in a large part of the world emphasizes that finding solutions leading to an improvement is neither easy nor simple. They will have to take into account both the quantitative and the qualitative aspects of the diagnostic imaging services and the personnel. They must be socially acceptable, and take into consideration the economic aspects, the real priorities within the healtl care system, the availability of personnel, etc.

WHO has concentrated its activities in the field of Radiation Medicine during the last few years on two major targets, namely:

i) better coverage of the population with radiation medicine services (radiodiagnosis, radiotherapy, nuclear medicine);

ii) better use of such services within national health systems, which includes quality assurance and efficacy/efficiency of utilization.

3.1 Improvement of the Ratio of Imaging Equipment and Specialized Personnel to the Population

Diagnostic imaging services must be planned carefully in order to give an even coverage of the whole population. When reviewing the situation of the services present in all developing countries, it can be seen that of the three levels usually recognized, the Specialized Radiological Service (SRS), which represents the most developed type and is located at university hospitals or specialized medical institutions, is available in a majority of developing countries and is of an acceptable standard in terms of equipment and staff. The General Purpose Radiological Service (GPRS), which represents the intermediate level, located in a provincial hospital and able to perform most of the investigations, is at present in a less favourable situation both in terms of equipment and staffing. The lowest echelon, the Basic Radiological Service (BRS), located in small rural or suburban hospitals, health centres, etc., equipped with a simple x-ray machine, and designed to perform only basic x-ray examinations, is the least developed unit in the whole radiological network. This explains the current emphasis placed by WHO on the BRS as a solution for improving coverage with radio-diagnostic services. The BRS concept (9, 10) covers both equip-ment (11) and the training component (12, 13), and is meant to increase the number of radiological facilities at the periphery of health care system. This would result in:

a) the local medical units, with additional diagnostic facilities, being able to serve better the patients and reduce the number of cases referred to other hospitals, with a corresponding increase in their acceptance and credibility by the local population;

b) a reduction in the time and money spent by people previously obliged to travel sometimes long distances for the examination, as well as in the delay in diagnosis caused by this;

c) a lessening in the overcrowding of radiological services of referral hospitals, with a consequent improvement in the quality of work and the handling of a higher percentage of the less simple cases, which need the competence and technology existing at this level (4).

In order to get the BRS accepted as a solution in the largest possible area of the world it is essential to have:

a) an x-ray machine which can produce all types of basic radio-graphs and which can work from power lines with great fluctuations, or even in the absence of electricity. At the same time the machine should be easy to operate and to maintain, with systems for breakdown detection. The technical specifications of such a machine have been prepared by the WHO BRS Advisory Group (15) and equipment meeting these is now under construction by a number of x-ray manufacturers;

ii) a training package for the operator of the BRS machine and for the general practitioner who will use the radiographs, in order to improve his/her diagnostic decision. The first part of this training package has already been prepared and the second is under preparation.

It has to be mentioned here that the BRS solution will increase the number of films used in developing countries and that valid alternatives to the present film supply problem will have to be found.

3.2 Designing Adequate Equipment and Premises for Diagnostic Imaging Services in Developing Countries

The BRS will be a solution for only some of the constraints on diagnostic imaging services in developing countries. Those related to the lack of suitability of the equipment existing at the GPRS and SRS levels, as well as to all nuclear medicine equipment, will remain. In tackling these problems efforts should be directed towards the design of more suitable equipment and premises. The IAEA started work in this direction some years ago, designing equipment for use in nuclear medicine units. Similar efforts have been made by a few institutions in the countries concerned and the Bhabha Atomic Research Centre (BARC - Trombay, India) represents a positive example.

Technical solutions to the following factors have to be considered in the design of suitable equipment.

a) power supply - frequent voltage changes of greater than ±15%, with simultaneous variations in frequency; consideration should also be given to energy-saving systems, which can render the equipment more energy efficient;

b) climatic conditions - and the presence of biological agents which can damage the equipment;

c) robust mechanical construction to withstand operation by less skilled personnel;

d) no high degree of automation or unnecessary sophistication because the cost of the personnel operating the equipment is low, and the sophistication introduces additional reasons for breakdown and increases the cost;

e) simple maintenance and easy detection of faulty parts - which can be achieved in particular by modular construction;

f) availability of spare parts for a period of at least equivalent to the average lifespan of the equipment;

g) availability of materials used for image recording, processing, etc;

h) possibilities that the equipment, or at least part of it, can be constructed in the developing countries.

Not only the equipment but also the premises in which it is to be installed need to be suitable and care has to be taken to achieve:

i) maximum natural protection from climatic conditions, without excessive use of energy (air conditioning, etc.);

ii) appropriate circulation of the patients and personnel;

iii) flexible utilization of rooms with possibilities for further expansion of the service;

iv) the required radiation protection, without excessive structural shielding, which can increase the cost of the building.

As industrial countries have at present reached a high degree of coverage with fully equipped diagnostic imaging services, it would seem worthwhile for scientists and techologists involved in the design of radiological and nuclear medicine equipment and of buildings in which such equipment could be installed, to devote part of their work to the design of services for developing countries. As mentioned above, this would not be simple and may require more expertise than foreseen. For example the mistakes made in the design of a number of hospitals recently built in the oil rich countries of the Gulf area need to be thoroughly studied to ensure that they are not repeated.

3.3 Improving the Policy for Equipment Purchase, Maintenance, Repair and Testing

Very few developing countries have an equipment purchasing policy. If such policies had existed and had been thoroughly implemented, the manufacturers of medical equipment would have been obliged to design and construct suitable equipment for the developing countries long ago.

The aims of a rational policy for equipment purchase should be:

i)   to accept only types of equipment which are suitable in terms of running costs, installation, utilization, etc;

ii) to purchase only the number or amount which is needed and therefore can be properly used;

iii) to consider the need for spare parts, service contracts, and all supply items which need to be regularly replaced;

iv) to supervise the distribution of equipment in order to obtain a homogenous coverage of the territory;

v)   to establish and supervise a network of workshops for equipment maintenance and repair, as well as the testing/calibration activities.

It is evident that the equipment purchasing policy is the prerogative of the national health authorities and that coordinated efforts should be made at the international level to assist them, not only by offering recommendations and guidance, but also with unbiased technical reports on the performance of equipment available on the international market.

The maintenance and repair of equipment is another essential activity requiring promotion in the developing countries. Routine maintenance, fault finding and testing should be taught to all equipment operators and become a compulsory element of their job description. Workshops for maintenance should be established in all developing countries for the periodic checking of equipment and for repair when a fault occurs. WHO has already started technical cooperation with a number of Member States in this field including:

-    the establishment of workshops where maintenance and repair can be undertaken together with in-service training of technicians;

- the establishment of training centres at the inter-country or inter-regional level, where more advanced training than that mentioned above can be carried out.

Equipment testing and calibration is an important part of the quality assurance programme which should be widely introduced in all countries, as already recommended by the two workshops organized in 1980 by WHO and the Government of the Federal Republic of Germany.

3.4 Improve the Policy of Purchase, Storage and Transportation of Radiological Films, Radiopharmaceuticals, etc.

This constitutes another key factor in the improvement of diagnostic imaging. The film quality suffers in most of the developing countries because of unsuitable storage, transportation and processing. A correct policy to avoid most of the present difficulties should start with the purchase of films and radio-pharmaceuticals and be flexible enough to accommodate specific needs which may appear suddenly and also assure that the films and radio-pharmaceuticals are regularly received. Another important factor is that of customs clearance, which needs to be simplified to avoid the long delays at present occurring. The third critical factor is the storage of films and radiopharmaceuticals at the central and local levels, and where suitable environmental conditions should be ensured. This also applies to transportation from the stores to the users. Any disruption in supply and too lengthy storage at the user's end, where the conditions cannot be controlled, should be avoided.

The fourth critical factor is the utilization of the films and radiopharmaceuticals, which cannot be discussed at length here. Procedures for developing films at much higher temperatures than the normal 18-22°C are now available for manual processing. These should be made available to all countries where climatic conditions render such processing compulsory. WHO, has to include action in this field in its future activities.

Simple techniques to test the quality of radiopharmaceuticals should be developed and made available to all users, and the programme on quality assurance in nuclear medicine includes this aspect.

The fifth critical factor is the particular care which has to be applied to image detectors in areas with difficult climatic conditions. The procedures for preventing each type of detector from losing its sensitivity or introducing false images (artifacts) have to be thoroughly studied, standardized and disseminated to all specialists concerned. Such procedures should also form part of the training programme of equipment operators.

3.5 Research for Alternatives to Film Image Recording in Diagnostic Radiology Applicable to Developing Countries

This represents an area of great interest for the future of diagnostic radiology in developing countries. The alternatives to be considered will not be discussed here since they are not easy to forecast at the present time. Those currently offered (xerography, electronic image reconstruction, non silver films) seem to be unsuitable for the conditions described throughout this paper. It should be stressed once again, however, that they are of great importance if radiology is to be widely used for the health care of the world's population.

3.6 Improvement of the Storage, Retrieval and Circulation of the Diagnostic Image Data

This constitutes another factor which should be given consideration.

Designing appropriate systems to be applied to various levels of health care for the circulation, storage and retrieval of data, is another area in need of attention. WHO should obtain the cooperation of specialists working in various countries and at various levels of health care in this type of applied research to find adequate solutions which can then be made widely available.

3.7 Appropriate Training of Specialists for Diagnostic Imaging Services in Developing Countries

This aspect was not analysed in the first part of this paper, although a considerable number of the constraints mentioned there originate from the way in which the specialists from developing countries were, and continue to be, trained. Most are trained abroad in industrial countries as there are only a few places where radiologists, nuclear medicine specialists, medical physicists, etc. can be trained in developing countries (few countries in Latin America, 1-2 in Africa, 1-2 in the Middle-East, 3 in South-East Asia, etc.).

The training is at present strongly biased by the conditions relevant to diagnostic imaging services in industrial countries and, as a result, the specialists formed attempt to recreate such conditions in their native country, if they return. This is the major reason for the building up of a relatively high proportion of quite advanced diagnostic imaging services in big cities, and particularly in the capitals. At the same time, the selection of equipment is also made under the influence of the training centre and not after a realistic appraisal of the problems needing to be solved.

The curricula for the training of radiologists and nuclear medicine specialists for developing countries will have to place much greater emphasis on:

i) the specific pathology of the areas where the trainee will be working - as reflected in the particular diagnostic imaging technique he/she will be using (radiology, nuclear medicine);

ii) the role of the diagnostic imaging technique in the diagnostic and therapeutic decision process;

iii) the appropriate equipment and premises with which the specialist would be able to work well given the local conditions (economic, climatic, maintenance, etc.);

iv) the type of personnel he/she has to train to assist with the work (radiographers, technicians for maintenance, etc.);

v) the quality assurance technology which should form an intrinsic part of the routine activities.

Attention needs to be given to the training of medical physicists, who today have only a very minor involvement in diagnostic imaging activities in developing countries.

The third category of personnel for which a careful reorientation of training is needed is that of medical radiological technician (MRT) or radiographer. Training facilities for this category exist today in a number of developing countries, but the programme is neither sufficiently practical nor adapted to the specific conditions outlined in this paper. Very little is taught on equipment maintenance, testing and calibration, fault finding, and quality control. These subjects will have to be introduced together with a really practical training. No radiographer should be allowed to qualify before performing a specified number of diagnostic quality radiographs for each major radiographic position.

642

An attempt has been made to analyze here the present constraints on diagnostic imaging activities in developing countries, together with solutions which could be envisaged to improve the situation. It is evident that such solutions will require extensive international cooperation and imaginative efforts to mobilize all the scientific, technical and financial resources needed for their broad implementation.

References

1. Brederhoff, J. and N.T. Racoveanu. "Radiology in the Developing World." Paper presented at the XV International Congress of Radiology, Brussels (June-July 1981).

2. "Register of Medical Radioisotope Units"(Preliminary Edition). A technical document issued by the International Atomic Energy Agency, Vienna. IAEA-167 (1974) 335 p.

3. Workshop on Quality Assurance in Diagnostic Radiology jointly organized by WHO, Geneva, Institute for Radiation Hygiene, Federal Health Office, and Gesellschaft für Strahlen- und Umweltforschung, mbH, München, Nueherberg, Federal Republic of Germany (20-24 October 1980) (in press).

4. "Quality Assurance in Nuclear Medicine." Report of the International Meeting organized by WHO, Geneva in collaboration with Institute of Nuclear Medicine, German Cancer Research Centre, Heidelberg, Institute of Radiation Hygiene, Federal Health Office and Gesellschaft für Strahlen- und Umweltforschung mbH, München, Neuherberg, Federal Republic of Germany, Heidelberg (17-21 November 1980) (in press).

5. Trout, E.D. et al. "Analysis of the Rejection Rate of Chest Radiographs Obtained During the Coal Mine Black Lung Program." Radiology 109 (1973) 25-27.

6. Berry, J. and R. Oliver. "Spoilt Films in X-Ray Departments and Radiation Exposure to the Public from Medical Radiology." British Journal of Radiology 49 (1976) 475-476.

7. McKinlay, A. and B. McCauley. "Spoilt Films in X-Ray Departments." British Journal of Radiology 50 (1977) 233-234.

8. Whittaker, L. "Efficacy/Efficiency Studies," Project No. 14 (unpublished) (1979) (personal communication).

9. Racoveanu, N.T. "The Basic Radiological System: A Concept for Better Coverage with Diagnostic Radiology of the World Population." Newsletter of the ISR, vol. 8, No. 2 (1979) 9-10.

10. Racoveanu, N.T. "Diagnostic Radiology in Rural Hospitals or Health Centres." Report of the First Consultation on Radiology in Africa, Nairobi, Kenya (25-28 November 1980) 33-53.

11. Holm, T. "Experiences with a BRS WHO Unit." Paper presented at the XV International Congress of Radiology, Brussels (June-July 1981).

12. Palmer, P.E.S. "The Basic Radiological System." Report on the First Consultation on Radiology in Africa, Nairobi, Kenya (25-28 November 1980) 23-32.

13. Palmer, P.E.S. "BRS Manuals on Radiological Techniques and Diagnostics." Paper presented at the XV International Congress of Radiology, Brussels (June-July 1981).

14. Racoveanu, N.T. "Toward a Basic Radiological Service." WHO Forum (in press).

15. "Technical Specifications for the X-Ray Apparatus to be Used in a Basic Radiological System." WHO Offset document RAD/81.2 (1981) 4 p.

TECHNOLOGY AND THE STATE: THE EMERGENCY OF HEALTH CARE RATIONING

JEAN DE KERVASDOUE, JEAN FRANCOIS LACRONIQUE, JOHN R. KIMBERLY

One has only to travel from Hong Kong to New York or from
Buenos Aires to Moscow to appreciate the power of technology as. a
force for standardization in contemporary life. Similarities in
architecture, in mass transit facilities, and in department store
wares are visible reminders that technology transcends political
ideology. Public discussions of nuclear arms limitations are
psychological reminders of the unforeseeable anarchistic and
irreversible nature of much technological development.

In this paper we examine the role of technology and the
"technological network" in health care, identifying and discuss-
ing many questions about the contributions of technology to life
and health, questions which are particularly troublesome because
they often invoke considerations of morality and economics simultaneously. The questions, though difficult, are real, and
responding to them with sensible, reasoned policy is one of the
challenges for health policymakers in the coming years.

The Technological Network

Our perspective on our subject is broader than some. We are
impressed by the pervasiveness of interconnectedness in health
care technology. In strict definitional terms, the French definition of technology differs slightly from its Anglo-Saxon
equivalent. The Larousse dictionary makes an explicit reference
to industry and its processes, while Webster's defines the word
as the totality of means employed to procure for man the objects
necessary for his subsistence and comfort. "Technology" is an
extension of the word "technique." Anything which uses or
involves technical intervention can be called technological. In

the area of health, consideration of technology should not be limited to the instruments and techniques used by doctors. It extends to the entire spectrum of the work of health care professionals from the use of the telephone to computer programing. Technology in health care also means documentation and modern methods in pedagogy and promotion. It includes the vast field of prostheses and instruments which change the lives of handicapped people. Modern services are included, as is genetic engineering for industrial purposes, because knowledge about the interaction between living organisms and their evironments is beginning to be explained by technological processes (genetic recombination). Technology thus comprises a whole network of sciences which are increasingly interdependent. Modern biology, for example, would not exist without optics, computer science, and solid physics.

A modern hospital is a particularly dense concentration of the technological network. Although the network is more dispersed in what we call private practice, a general practitioner is dependent upon pharmacists, radiologists, and laboratories, which assist his diagnosis and prescribed treatment.

The interdependent character of technology in health care makes evaluation difficult. The example of a new X-ray machine illustrates the problem well. It is certainly possible to evaluate the quality and cost of the prints it makes in comparison with those already on the market. But the real question is whether the machine can produce new information. Then it must be determined if this additional information is useful, if applicable therapies exist, and if trained personnel are available. To evaluate the machine fully, one must refer to its necessary complements.

The notion of a "network" allows us to describe the source of future developments. Innovations have essentially two sources. They may come from the linear development of a single concept or from the conjunction of two previously independent branches of technology which creates new uses and further developments. The former is illustrated by the modern stethoscope, which differs only slightly from Laennec's first model although it is made of material unknown in the 19th century. Telecommunications are descendents of the telephone and the computer. Their proper applications go well beyond the domain of their parent technologies.

What can we expect from this network with regard to the health sector? Can it be controlled? What sort of choices confront us in the coming years? These questions are addressed in the following pages.

The End of Empiricism

Since the beginning of this century, life expectancy in
Western societies has increased considerably while morbidity
rates have declined. At birth, life expectancy for men is 70
years and for women 76 years. In fact, infant mortality has
decreased considerably also. The most common illnesses are
chronic diseases affecting the elderly.

Technology has contributed measurably to this evolution.
Vaccines and antibiotics have made redundant most hospital beds
intended for infectious illnesses. Yellow fever has almost dis-
appeared. Diabetics can live. But in certain areas little progress has been made. There are no cures for numerous cardiovascular and cerebrovascular illnesses as well as most cancers. Few
major discoveries have been made in the last 20 years, and many
of those that have been announced and heavily publicized, such as
interferon, have not lived up to expectations.

The case of interferon is instructive. Many articles were
written about this "miracle protein" before conclusive laboratory
results were available. The actual substance tested was often
impure, control groups were inappropriate, and dosages varied
widely from test to test. In addition little was known about how
it functioned on the molecular level, nor was it certain whether
patients had differential sensitivities to this drug. However,
the wave of publicity created great expectations in the absence
of empirical evidence.

This is not an exceptional case. There have been other
examples of what can be called "expectation inflation." At the
beginning of this century, no effective treatment for cancer
existed. The first positive results of radiation treatment in
certain cases of skin cancer have been extended today to other
tumors, even when effectiveness has not been demonstrated. Today
it is not unlikely that a particular cancer therapy regimen is
used as much because it is codified and priced as becasue it is
effective. It is difficult to avoid becoming caught up in the
wave of increased expectations; the only control, albeit imperfect, is the ethics of scientists.

For most of us, however, the gaps between promise and performance do not destroy our hopes. We must accept the inevitable
side effects of effectiveness; technology has its risks. If it
cures, it can also injure or even kill, particularly where there
is negligence, lack of scientific knowledge, or imperfect
training of medical personnel.

Technology in health is expensive, not so much because of equipment costs, but because of the need for qualified personnel. They are thus the origins of a "prescribed" demand by practitioners, which poses the problem of their justification, and validation of their widespread use on the basis of scientific methods.

Technical Innovation, Cause or Product of Increased Health Care Costs?

To a large extent, technical innovations are statistically linked with growing consumption of medical services, and these with growing costs. When the components of medical care are analyzed, it is evident that the sector showing the most rapid increases in cost are those in which technical advances have recently emerged. Thus, in France, in the area of outpatient services, laboratory tests and radiology have expanded rapidly, with respective annual growth rates of 22% and 7.6% while traditional medical acts such as house calls and group consultations have progressed slowly. In the United States, total domestic shipments of X-ray apparatus and electromedical devices increased at an annual rate of approximately 24 percent between 1972 and 1977.

This evolution is most visible in the public hospital sector in France because this is the privileged domain of high-technology therapy. The growing role of technical services in hospital care is illustrated by the growth of radiological acts and laboratory tests per admission for all categories of hospitals (table 1). Private practice also reflects the role of innovation. In France, radiology accounted for 12.6% of medical activity in private practice in 1959. In 1976 the figure was 20.2%. Technical progress as measured in consumption of technical procedures accounts for about 2/3 of the increase in volume of medical acts independent of price increases.

Table 1

Public General Hospitals (France)

Year	Number of "Z" *		Number of "B" **	
	By Admission	By Day	By Admission	By Day
1965	22.48	1.0	250	7.8
1970	30.59	1.7	298	16.4
1973	37.54	2.4	394	25.1

Annual Growth Rate in Percentage

1965-1973	6.6	11.6	12.6	16.7
1970-1973	7.1	12.2	9.8	15.2

* - X-ray procedures are evaluated according to "Z". The more complex a procedure, the higher its "Z" number.

** - Biological tests are evaluated according to a "B" number.

The causal relation between accelerating technical progress and growing expenses is difficult to determine. Increasing costs can be linked to technological advances in many cases, but in a few instances, costs for individual treatments are reduced. For policy purposes, the direction of causality is of fundamental importance. If one accepts the innovation-push hypothesis, efforts to improve productivity in the health care system should be aimed at qualitative control, requiring judgments about the future potential of an innovation in the earliest stages of its development.

The alternative hypothesis explains technical innovation as the response of human genius to legitimate needs. In this view, only excessive use and consumption should be criticized. The eventual control of use would be wholly quantitative; the nature of technical innovation would not be questioned, only its long-term effect. Although these two hypotheses theoretically are not mutually exclusive, differences in the casual priority they assign to innovation and the resulting differences in implications for health policy effectively force a choice between them.

The Justification of Technical Progress

Technical progress and care quality

The introduction of a technical innovation is normally justified on the basis of an improvement in the quality of services rendered by the health care system. Although it is a classic opposition to set off the notion of qualitative evaluation (subjective) against quantitative measurement (objective), it is possible to analyze the marginal benefits of technical progress by breaking down the notion of quality into five components, each objectively measurable:

--technical efficacy (better diagnosis, more effective treatment)

--security

--cost factor

--comfort (respect for the patient, speed and painlessness of care)

--accessibilty

Each of these factors must be evaluated on different scales and can be analyzed separately. But the overall evaluation of an innovation can be thought of as a complex function of these five independent variables.

Technical Efficacy

Efficacy can be evaluated in terms of decreased mortality, morbidity, and illness rates. Recent examples of technological advances that would rate highly on this dimension include:

--The use of chemotherapy in treating hematosarcomas. What was a mortal illness 10 years ago is now usually curable.

--Artificial prostheses (hip joints in particular) which have transformed prognosis of traumatic and rheumatoid pathology for the elderly.

--Intensive care facilities which can sustain vital functions. Progress here has even led to charges of overuse (artificially prolonging life).

It must be noted here that scientific evaluation procedures for new therapies are generally applied only to innovations in medication, and not to advances in medical instruments. Several explanations are usually advanced to account for this fact:

--Controlled therapeutic tests would be difficult to organize for instruments because of problems in random selection and the composition of test groups.

--Progress is more tangible in the area of instrumentation than in that of medication. Strict experimental protocol is not yet needed here; whereas in the domain of medication we are dealing with active molecules where only marginal improvement over existing projects can be expected.

In our opinion, these are questionable arguments which are
themselves not based on objective criteria. We must also point
out the total lack of methods for determining the efficacy of
organizational innovations.

Cost Factors

Many innovations have brought about a reduction in unit
costs for treatment. The development of simple tests and instruments (chemically reactive paper tests, enzyme analyses, etc.)
exemplifies automation of numerous analytic techniques in biology.

We must consider, however, that at least in France the substitution of a new technique for an old one is progressive and
that for a certain time the new technique can be very profitable
because the tests performed are reimbursed according to the
existing procedures classification.

In the case of laboratory equipment, this factor has played
an undeniable role in the rapid diffusion of new techniques.
Ease of use and a reduction in unit tests, both consequences of
automation, are also incentive factors which explain the rapid
growth of consumption in this sector. We should also mention in
this regard the development of home usage of renal dialysis
machines. Unit treatment costs have been reduced by 50%.

Comfort and Security

Innovations may seek to minimize the following accidents and
inconveniences which treatment can create for the patient and
those around him:

> --accidents and therapy

> --pain

> --waiting

> --violation of privacy

> --side effects on family or social life

The increased current effort to develop "noninvasive" techniques is an example of how such an aim can supersede the technical efficacy of treatment. The following recent innovations are
examples of this trend:

> --electrocardiography

--isotope scintography

--echo-tomography, echo-cardiography (ultra-sound)

--thermography

--computerized axial tomography (C.A.T. scanning)

These examples all have in common a relative innocuousness. These tests may be repeated without risk and are usually based on automated techniques which makes them simple to use. These two features are particularly favorable because they free us from traditional inhibiting factors in the diffusion of technical innovations and training of highly skilled personnel.

One consequence of this is rapid expansion of the applications of these techniques, a phenomenon especially visible in the case of C.A.T. scanners. Another almost caricatural example of this trend is the widespread use of thermography. It is generally accepted that this technique is of practically no diagnostic benefit except in the confirmation of breast cancer, a condition which can be precisely diagnosed by histology.

Accessibility

In France and the US, the development of home care and "day hospitals" permits easy access to quality treatment and avoids traditional hospitalization in the future. Improvements in tele-communications (such as information retrieval, optimal organization of hospital consultations, and long-distance consultation) will move us in the direction of better access to health care systems. The result is sure to be an increase in demand. Unless substitution effect can be achieved by reducing the capacity of present health care facilties, we can expect an increase in consumption generated by the addition of new services to preexisting ones.

Overall, then, any improvement in one of the above-mentioned variables, even if it doesn't affect the technical efficacy of the system, can be considered as a contribution to the quality of care. As long as there are positive results in one area, it can be argued that general improvement has been made even if the introduction of an innovation causes a drop in performance in another variable. This is the case, for example, with certain pain-relieving therapies in terminal cancers, where a gain in comfort is sometimes achieved against a decrease in life expectancy. On the other hand, the higher risks of a difficult operation are sometimes preferred in hopes of a more effective cure.

If one accepts this reasoning and the existance of

substitutions within the notion of "quality of treatment," a
classic formula taken from the economics of goods and services
can be applied. A demand function can be constructed in which
the traditional variable "price" (whose variations determine consumption) will be successively replaced by the variables "risk,"
"pain," (or comfort) and difficulty of access. Intuitively we
see that an improvement in these factors is capable of increasing
demand. This dynamic is well-illustrated by any empirical observations which show an increase in consumption of technical procedures.

Addition and Substitution of Techniques

Diffusion is not identical from one technique to the next.
In some cases the new technique is efficacious, simple to apply,
and inexpensive. It thus diffuses rapidly. Frequently, however,
the new technique is complex and requires new equipment and a
trained medical staff. It is expensive and its effectiveness is
not apparent at the time of its introduction, but rather must be
determined by studies over several years.

The place of innovation in the arsenal of diagnostic methods
and therapies will then be usually integrated into the treatment
process as supplemental element. The marginal cost will not be
taken into account (it will rarely be budgeted) and it will only
be a question of the marginal benefit, however small this may be.
It will be studied (theses, articles, demonstrations, etc.)
because it shows the different "actors" of the health care system
in another light, different from the normal market relationship
where supply and demand are equalized.

A most striking example of a new technology added to the
market is the case of vascular X-ray examinations, angiography.
The radiological technique for exploring arteries is several
decades old; it is also dangerous, costly, and painful. The
necessary equipment is very expensive (about 500,000 francs or
$90,000). The norm in France is one such apparaturs per million
inhabitants. The appearance of the scanner and echo-tomography
in France around 1975 should have drastically altered the
treatment situation since these two techniques permit a reduction
in vascular radiography. However, an evaluation of the years
following its appearance shows that in reality vascular X-ray
installations have maintained a steady level of activity during
this time. Nowhere was a significant reduction in the number of
anteriographies observed. On the contrary, authorizations for
the purchase of vascular X-ray machines are relatively easy to
obtain while scanners are difficult to obtain.

Perhaps in the coming year technology will contribute notably to cost reductions in certain diagnostic examinations or

certain therapies. It is, however, unrealistic to expect the kinds of overall reductions in costs in health that are generally associated with technical progress in other sectors, where increased productivity means falling prices.

The C.A.T. scanner is a case in point, and its history is intriguing. The initial idea was not new but had never been exploited in the United States, where it had been discovered. The inventors, a neurologist and a physicist, never succeeded in interesting either doctors or Americal industry in the idea.

A British engineer, G. Hounsfield, and a firm, EMI, however, took up the idea and succeeded in construction in 1967 an instrument capable of producing section images of objects (tomographies) far superior to those produced by conventional radiological techniques. In 1976 an apparatus for medical use derived from this principle was constructed with the aid of the British Health Ministry. The first prototype was installed in the Atkinson Morley Hospital in London in October 1971.

Clinical experiments quickly demonstrated the potential of the machine, particularly in the diagnosis of brain tumors. The first international publication appeared in 1972. In June 1973 the first two commerically functioning units were installed in the Mayo Clinic and the Massachusetts General Hospital and were an immediate success. Siemens and Ohio Nuclear brought out machines in 1974. By the end of 1975, there were 20 builders, the largest being EMI (Great Britain), Pfizer, and Ohio Nuclear (US).

In August 1976, 328 machines were functioning in the United States, and by 1978, more than 1200. There is now a ratio of one machine per 250,000 inhabitants, of which 2/3 are "head only" and the rest "full body" machines. The highest concentrations are in Florida and California.

According to most authorities, this is an excessive concentration, even if 80% of these machines are located in large university hospitals. They argue that these machines are expensive to buy and also very expensive to operate. The proponents of the technology point to three essential advantages it offers:

--The scanner is a "noninvasive" apparatus and extensive delays in diagnosis can thus be avoided or reduced in duration.

--The scanner replaces other tests (angiography, encephalographs) which are more costly and dangerous.

--By improving precision in diagnoses, the scanner can

reduce expenses for certain unnecessary therapies which are
dangerous and always expensive.

These are all valid arguments, but an analysis of the
machine after a number of years of experience indicates that the
scanner is certainly not an "economical" instrument.
Justification for its use is above all medical. In other words,
it improves the conditions of the patient being examined (reduced
waiting time, risk, and discomfort), while raising the level of
technical precision in diagnosis.

Such qualities are without doubt sufficient to establish the
scanner as a valuable technical advance. But in addition to its
pure "technical" interest, the scanner is also a prestige instrument, which makes it a symbol of the art equipment. It is thus
very attractive to the doctor as well as to the public. It is
also a relatively simple instrument to use.

For all of these reasons, the scanner can easily become a
high-demand item, whose only present limiting factor is "medical
judgment." But can doctors really use "judgment" in this domain?
Is this new demand justified? Does it lead to an improvement in
the general quality of medical care?

These three questions are basic to the general problem of
technical progress in medicine. In effect, by its own technical
progress it imposes a special burden on the populace, which as a
result has the right to demand a limit on the expenses which it
supports.

What will be the basis for these justifications? Will the
criterion be diagnostic efficiency of the apparatus or survival
rates of patients? The example of the scanner is particularly
interesting since it illustrates the clear opposition between
these two aspects. It is undeniable that the new technique has
completely changed X-ray diagnosis in all intracranial pathology
and considerably improved pelvic exploration.

On the other hand, how can we fail to observe that little
progress has been made in the treatment of brain and pancreas
tumors and most secondary metastases in the last ten years?
Because the medical profession places as much value on the "diagnostic" as on the "therapeutic" states of its activity, it is
virtually incapable of judging the "ultimate" effectiveness of a
particular technique. Such questions involve thought processes
which are by and large foreign.

An entirely different problem is that of the geographical
distribution of equipment. Given that a certain technique is
medically useful, how many machines are necessary to satisfy

needs and where should they be located? In France, for example,
the "optimal" norm has been defined as one scanner per million
inhabitants according to the directives of the "carte sanitaire,"
which governs the distribution of "heavy" equipment designed for
medical use. Yet no one can really say at this time if the
French norms conform more to needs than the American "fait accom-
pli." The economic justification for the "norm" is that it
locates control at the level of supply instead of at the level of
demand. But how does or should one judge the reasonableness of
this justification? This brief discussion of the scanner example
illustrates many of the difficult questions of social philosophy
and policy that must be addressed as new medical technologies are
developed and begin to diffuse.

3. Technology Under Surveillance

Can technology be controlled in its development as it is in
its applications?

Few today would seriously propose a moratorium on technological research. Many advances are still to be made, and
developments which encourage fundamental hopes for society are
not likely to be stifled. Progress is the issue and with it, the
will to better the human condition. Even if desirable, a
moratorium would be virtually impossible to carry out. No
country, however powerful it may be, has a monopoly on research
in this domain. If any one country halted production of a particular technology, it would run the risk of ensuing economic
difficulties. What that country did not make another would, and
there would be strong pressure to import new products. The arms
race continues despite the dangers and economic hardships it
causes the nations who participate in it. How realistic is it
then to expect a halt in the race for medical progress, a race
which is generally considered to have beneficial human consequences?

On the other hand, the demand of patients and doctors for
ever more costly new techniques, techniques whose benefits do not
always match purchase and operations costs, seems virtually
limitless. Given that moratoriums on research are unlikely and
that demand for new technology is likely to remain strong, what
policy options are available? Two alternatives deserve comment:
(1) evaluating the quality of techniques as they appear and
developing only the best (this is the aim of technological evaluation), or (2) orienting research towards those areas where
need is greatest and where potential benefits are largest.

What can be expected from these two alternatives?

Testing Medical Techniques

Technological evaluations should strive, on the one hand, to verify the actual performance of a techique, and on the other hand, to pass judgment on its total effect, the advantages and inconveniences it causes the individual and society. Evaluation methods of this sort have long been used in the biomedical field, particularly in the area of pharmaceutical products where the development and commercial exploitation of new drugs is circumscribed by legislation and a complex controlling apparatus.

Until recently, the instruments and apparatus used in medicine have been much less rigorously controlled, although as with drugs, they may have harmful as well as beneficial effects. New initiatives in evaluation methods are thus chiefly concerned with instrument technology, and specific methodology must be developed to deal with the particular aspects of this field.

The procedure manual of the Office of Technology Assessment (OTA), created in 1973 by the US Congress, defined four evaluation criteria:

1 - The expected benefit, even if multiple, must be identified and measurable.

2 - The field of medical application of the new technique must be rigorously defined.

3 - The evaluation must be made in reference to a given population.

4 - Application conditions must be precise.

There is, of course, no such thing as an abstract evaluation whose objectivity would satisfy all. At a certain point it is always necessary to make a vain judgment, to ponder advantages and inconveniences. For example, effectiveness and safety standards will differ for each technology. Effectiveness is defined in terms of benefits; whereas safety is expressed in terms of acceptable risk. Often measured separately, the qualities are, however, often interdependent. A classic example of the interrelation between effectiveness and safety is the case of mammography or the systematic detection of breast cancer. The potential benefits of this technique are derived from a test which itself submits the patient to an appreciable risk. The benefit and risk factors can not thus be considered separately, and indeed, the study panel on breast cancer detection of the National Institutes of Health recommended that this technique not be used systematically on women under the age of 50. Each doctor is of course free to interpret this ruling in his daily practice.

Many cases are less simple than this one. For example, two methods for treating chronic renal failure exist, transplantation and dialysis machines. Dialysis treatment is more expensive, and life expectancy of a patient so treated is less than for the case of transplants. However, there is an appreciable risk involved in the operation. The transplant patient thus has a longer average life expectancy, but at the same time a higher short-term mortality risk in the six months following his operation. Which is, from his point of view, the best choice, assuming he has a choice, which is not always the case? The answer varies from individual to individual even though, collectively speaking, transplantation seems better because it is less costly and more effective.

In addition to these difficulties in principle, there are methodological problems.

1. Side Effects

When the effectiveness of a method is measured, the number of beneficial effects is usually limited. On the contrary, the search for undesirable and unexpected side effects cannot be limited to the area of specific investigation. Surveillance of harmful effects is usually more complex and expensive than the simple measuring of benefits.

2. Number of People Concerned

A technology is considered effective if it affects a large enough number of beneficiaries. On the contrary, the risks involved in the use of a technology should be considered even if they concern only a small proportion of patients. A comparison of risk and benefits for a medical technique will depend to a large extent on a necessarily objective appreciation of the importance of the problem for the concerned population.

3. Delay in Cause and Effect

The beneficial effects of a medical technique are usually noticed before the adverse and harmful effects, thus making long-term evaluation necessary. And in the case of certain diagnostic and therapeutic methods, this delay can reach even the level of a generation; e.g., the thalidomide case or diethylstilbestrol.

Finally, as in the case of renal failure treatment, the different parties view the situation very differently primarily because the collective financing of health costs causes each individual to be involved in an infinity of individual choices. The patient whose choice is a key element in the system is

especially sensitive to considerations of effectiveness, comfort,
and security. Often the collective level disparities in equipment and access to care seem unjust to him, and he has a tendency
to accept technology as a guarantee of quality. Health professionals are familiar with this outlook, and they often seek to
satisfy the constant demand for technical progress. This phenomenon explains the rapid deployment of scanner equipment in the
United States, an illustration of the popular adage "We have to
keep up with the Joneses."

The attitude of agencies whose responsibility is to
reimburse costs for medical procedures linked to technical
advances is sometimes characterized as retrograde and restric-
tive. But one needs to understand that they cannot always pay
for everything for everyone.

The Emotional Component

The specter of limiting availability raises emotional issues
around freedom of choice for the patient, equality of access to
quality treatment, and the potentially life-saving benefits of
certain techniques. Indeed, the foundations of free enterprise
in a free society enter the debate. On the other hand, the
motives of those raising these issues can be questioned, and sus-
picions can be voiced about the competence and professional
ethics of doctors. A conflict often ensues, especially since we
are dealing with emotional issues. The subject of technical progress is extraordinarily difficult to treat dispassionately. The
arguments advanced by the two factions are often buttressed by
statistical "evidence" carefully chosen to support their point of
view.

The situation is further complicated by the fact that judgment about the intrinsic value of a technique, its utility and
necessity, are not adequate. Its use must also be evaluated.

When a technology is placed on the market, its evaluators no
longer control it, and it is not always certain to be used judi-
ciously. We can draw an analogy with traffic lights. Any technique has a green-light zone for which it has been proven useful.
It also has a red-light zone where technique is useless and noth-
ing is gained by employing it. But it also has a yellow zone
which can be very large. In this zone either the effectiveness
has not been proven with certainty, or its use is mitigated by
inconvenience. In this case, it could be used when conventional
treatment fails. In our opinion, the size of this intermediate
zone explains the difference in practice from one country to
another or from one region to another or from one doctor to
another in the same country. In the absence of a yellow zone, it

would be hard to explain why states which have technologically comparable systems of health do not have the same norms and practices. But they certainly do not, as is illustrated by the fact that at the beginning of the 1970s the US citizen was 38 times more likely than a Swede to undergo a coronary bypass.

A priori evaluation is not sufficient; practices must be controlled and comparisons made between different ideal standards and actual concrete utilization. This is the whole idea behind health care quality evaluations. But this entails a change in the nature of evaluation. It is no longer simply a matter of examining an isolated technique. The way in which individuals or even medical teams use the technique becomes a matter for serious attention. This shift raises the visibility of individual performance substantially, and is not likely to be warmly embraced by the medical profession.

Despite the complexity of the methods necessary for this type of evaluation, their development is apparent today, especially in the United States. However, the effect of these measures on health expenditures is not clear for the immediate future. We think it justified to see that, in the long run, these measures will not stop cost increases and that they perhaps favor it. In the near and distant future, these measures will probably eliminate a number of abuses such as unnecessary operations and examinations. But the proof of ineffectiveness here must be overwhelming to actually stop a practice. However, clinical proof is not always easy to find because of the methodological limitations which doctors and social science researchers must contend with. And when in doubt one follows Wildavsky's dictum:

"You can always do something."

But there is no reason to assume that there will be a reduction in costs as practice approaches the norms desired by the clinical specialist. The norms will be applied in all cases and in all hospitals. A different norm for rural hospitals as opposed to university hospitals is inconceivable. This would go against egalitarian principles, and such a proposition would not be politically viable. The consequences of this will be an impetus for development of subspecialties and heavy equipment in medium-sized cities. In effect, if the criterion for results in the health system is technical medical performance, it is easy to show that subspecialists of a technique who are familiar with the use of heavy equipment are more effective. But the measure of efficacy is of course produced by the subspecialties. In evaluating doctors, we adopt that ideology. What counts is the doctor-patient relationship and not the health of individuals living in society. The quality control system, as it is conceived in the United States and as it tends to develop in Western European countries, is not a measure of the overall efficacy of the medical system and its impact on the health of the population; it is a measure of the efficacy of medicine, formulated by doctors with their instruments of measure. This is certainly not without interest for the patient and even for the public. They can better organize medical expenditures since they control the functions of production. But medicine has other functions than technology. And despite great progress it is still in its infancy in many areas where needs go unmet.

Evaluation is not useless. It is difficult, restricted, and often biased, but it gives a necessary guarantee to consumers. It reduces abuses, and defines what is known and what is not, all very important services. We would even say that the development of technological evaluation and quality control of treatment are the major innovations of the last 10 years in the area of health policy and that their consequences will be felt in the coming years. However, these methods are not a panacea, and it must be noted that they do not suffice by themselves to control the development of technology and still less to limit health care cost.

Science Policy

Given the difficulty of controlling the utilization of a technique once it has been introduced, an alternative would be to orient research so that only potentially useful techniques are developed.

But are we searching in areas where there are problems, or do we continue to find in areas where there are solutions? The answer to this question constitutes, in our opinion, a preliminary to all scientific policy. If we work in areas where there are solutions and where the development of knowledge will eventually allow us to solve problems which are not necessarily the most socially important ones, then science policy will simply be a matter of financing research and guaranteeing the autonomy of researchers. This is certainly not an insignificant role, but one of limited importance. If, on the other hand, we search in areas where problems exist, science policy will become an instrument of choice in the economic and social development of nations and, in our case, of health policy.

It thus seems important to examine how this question has been answered. One could argue that such examination is unnecessary, for we need only observe the evolution of science policies in Western countries to conclude that these policies seem to have become an element of general policy after a long period of isolation from economic circumstances. In effect, science policy seems to be increasingly subordinated to general economic strategies, to employment policies, and to regional government policies, whereas in its beginnings it was relatively independent of these contingencies.

Science policy was created at the demand of men of science, but these scientists from the beginning conceived of their participation in policy planning as an evil necessary to their research. In certain instances, the attitude has become decidely noncooperative or even hostile. Although they are used to accepting the means accorded them to carry out their work, they have accepted with great difficulty the notion of controlling agencies outside of their own community. In less than 30 years, they have gone from near total freedom to an ever more restricted and controlled freedom.

An analysis of the texts on biomedical research taken from different national plans in France clearly shows this evolution. In the Second Plan one reads:

"Experience has shown, especially in the case of medicine, that the most productive means of research is to leave initiative absolutely in the hands of researchers as well as the choice and means of their research programs. Profitable applications usually arise in unpredictable fashion from pure research. It is the role of governing bodies of research to assure them this liberty."

This is a way of saying that although research structures can be planned, their subjects and methods certainly cannot be and should be left entirely to the researcher's initiative.

In the Seventh Plan (1970-1975), the language changed dramatically. "Priority objectives" such as the biology of the brain were invoked. The socioeconomic importance of each subject was studied, and certain themes such as "the functional organization of the neuron" were indicated for development.

A long road has been traveled between these two plans, and we can distinguish three phases in this evolution of science policy since the war.

The first phase had its origins in the evolution of the amount of funds necessary for research. When a laboratory and a few instruments were no longer sufficient scientists were led to demand subsidies from the state. To justify these demands, they alluded to the importance or even the necessity of their work in obtaining certain technical "payoffs" in the fields of defense and the economy. It goes without saying that once the size of

the "pie" had been defined, they were the only masters of its
pieces. The text from the second plan is very characteristic of
the first phase.

The second phase proceeds naturally from the first. In
effect governments believed the scientists' argument according to
which scientific research was the driving force behind military
independence and social and economic development. This belief
was based on a premature generalization derived from a few cases
(the atomic bomb, the transistor, etc.). It was no longer only a
question of defining the pieces of the pie to be shared, but
also, and above all, the respective size of these pieces.

The third phase dawned with the recognition by governments
that not only did science have a social impact, but also that
science could be used to attain certain objectives. The guiding
principle of scientific research was no longer the simple desire
to solve theoretical problems or to further our understanding of
nature. It had also become a search for solutions to economic,
political, and social problems. A significant event of this
third phase appeared in the American political scene after
President Nixon's "war on cancer," and the resultant National
Cancer Act met with, if not defeat, at least an unending struggle
without spectacular victories. In 1971, Nixon had declared "the
time has come for the same type of concentrated effort which
smashed the atom and brought man to the moon to be oriented
towards the conquest of this terrible disease. Let us make the
national commitment to attain this objective." The analogy here
was simple; if we can send a man to the moon, we should be able
to find a cure for cancer. But, in the words of a scientist at
the time: "Could we send a man to the moon if we didn't know
Newton's Laws?" It seems not. We do not know if cancer is a
single disease of cellular malfunction or if it is more than a
hundred distinct diseases which occur in four general forms. Ten
years after the unprecedented effort, the answer to this fundamental question has not been found.

This intrinsic difficulty led Lewis Thomas to conclude that,
in research policy, there are only two approaches. The first is
a direct approach which can be used when there is a 90% chance
for success. This was the case, for example, in the struggle
against polio. After it had been established that the disease
was caused by a virus with three types of antigens, it was only a
matter of determining if a vaccine based on a dead or active
virus would be the most effective. The types of possible solutions were thus known, as were the means to this end. This is
not always the case. In most instances there is no analogy or
model to base research on.

The potential solutions are unknown, and here Thomas advises us to "measure the quality of work by the degree of surprises it produces," that is to say by the difficulties between the expected results, the common sense of the scientific community at a given moment, and emperical results which challenge this common sense. In brief, surprise is the mark of success. Thus it is not easy to orient research, and its results are not always foreseeable.

Similarly, in a comparative study of cancer and respiratory disease research in France, Jean de Kervasdoue has shown that the needs of the population based on morbidity and mortality statistics had a negligible role in the relative importance accorded to these two fields of research. The evolution of research in these two disciplines was primarily influenced by the evolution of scientific paradigms on one hand and by institutions on the other.

For example, the Pastorien paradigm was a dominant influence, not only in the research and discovery of the tuberculosis bacillus, but also in the development and implementation of different prophylactic methods. The demonstration of the utility of the paradigm made it possible to maintain and strengthen a number of social hygiene measures despite resistance to these frequently unpopular prophylactic policies.

The influence of institutions is also certain. Either the institution assures communication between different disciplines, all of which profit from the experience, or it prevents or restricts such contacts.

During the 20th century in France, several governments responded to growing social pressure and individual demands for a solution to cancer. They aided in the creation of specialized research institutes for cancer where the scientific tradition could develop. Since cancer was designated as a high-priority problem, large sums of money were set aside for research in this area.

This attracted researchers who might not have come simply out of interest in the problem to be solved. There was a social demand which scientists could easily satisfy, all the more so since clinical application was still far in the future. However, it is not certain that this situation, which is ongoing, will produce the desired result—the rapid discovery of a therapeutic solution for cancer.

The mechanisms which explain quantitative and qualitative differences between two close domains of research depend on numerous factors. Among these, the objective definition of the problems plays only a small role. The pressure of certain groups, the existence of institutions, and chance happenings can aid or restrain diversify or restrict the evolution of research. Having said this, although one can argue that the meager diversity of French researh in lung disease limits its originality, one cannot argue that greater diversity will necessarily result in systematic solutions to the problems considered. One can search where there are problems, but one is not certain to find solutions.

It must not be inferred from these preceding arguments that science policy is without effect. For example, the state must compensate for industry's tendency to finance only what will be profitable in the near term. This practice is not always consistent with a reduction in social costs. The state must also create openings and points of contact between complementary disciplines, but here they are dealing with the unforeseeable. Technology will not be controlled by science policy because discoveries are difficult to predict and because no single country has a monopoly on knowledge.

Industrial competition and secrecy are the norm today; whereas 20 years ago, an atmosphere of openness, universalism, and the desire to increase knowledge and benefit mankind was more characteristic of the scientific community. The desire to maintain employment, to balance the trade deficit, and to export takes precedence today. To export, a nation must produce, and high-technology items with diverse applications, especially in the biomedical domain, are particularly attractive products.

France has tried to develop a national industry in medical technology although this sector had been heavily dominated by foreign industry. This is also why biotechnology was chosen in France as a priority sector to receive aid for technical and scientific development. But even if this policy succeeds, control will be difficult to exercise. Business will in all likelihood invoke the following argument:

"If you want us to penetrate foreign markets, we must first grow domestically. You, the representatives of the state, must let us sell the technology which we develop."

Managerial methods which will by themselves control and organize health care systems do not yet exist. Only a global approach can attain this. In our view, the most viable option is rationing, rationing which is based, above all, on political and ethical criteria. Russel's recent study of the diffusion of new technologies points in this direction. She concluded that it is no longer reasonable to expect societies to pay for technologies which offer the promise of saving the life of one person. Simple economics, then, dictate the need for a more global view, a frame of reference to arbitrate among various interests.

Certain countries such as Great Britain are better equipped
than others to move into this new phase. Others must change profoundly the organization of their health care systems. This is
the case for France and the United States. But before considering the countries separately, we must return to the principle of rationing, its necessity and its consequences.

The word is likely to scandalize. In France it evokes for
older people the period of the Second World War, ration tickets,
long lines, the black market, etc. To say that rationing is the
future seems paradoxical or even funny, or that one has a dark
sense of humor. It does not seem a serious possibility. And yet
it is the simple consequence of two phenomena.

We treated at length the first: the growth of technological
innovations ever more numerous and costly in a field where consu-
mer appetite seems insatiable and where manufacturers have no
personal interest in limiting costs. The second is the fact that
values and laws exist in western societies which make it unthink-
able to let the health sector be governed entirely by the dynamics of the market. The inequities which would result would be
unacceptable for most people in those societies.

Some form of social security will continue to exist. It
cannot, however, continue to pay for everything indefinitely. We
have seen that the evolution of prevention as well as technology,
even if they achieve notable gains especially in the coming
years, will not significantly reduce spiraling health costs.
This will be the prime point of conflict among different professional and political groups.

To limit cost increases, a global framework must be defined,
and the criteria of definition can only be "political" in the
most noble sense of the term. The synthesis must be based first
on moral values which take into consideration economic, sociolo-
gical, and technological factors. Cost restrictions lead necessarily to rationing. Rationing itself, however, raises important
moral questions that would need a specific treatment.

NEW AND EMERGING HEALTH CARE TECHNOLOGIES: ASSESSING EFFICACY,
SAFETY, AND COSTS

Seymour Perry, M.D.

Department of Health and Human Services,
Public Health Service, Office of Health
Research, Statistics,and Technology, National
Center for Health Care Technology

This NATO Advanced Studies Institute on Diagnostic Imaging
in Medicine has dealt with a variety of innovative techniques for
peering into the human body. The ability to inspect that organism
and to use these images as important information is one of the
great success stories of modern technology. The implications for
patient care in the future are enormous.

Considerations of the uses and limits of the images produced
by these remarkable techniques, however, raise issues and questions
which are vital to physicians, patients, third-party payers, and
policy makers. The issues and questions concern the safety and
efficacy of these technologies and their descendent technologies
as well as their cost to both the patient and to society. These
are some of the broad and often difficult concerns which the
National Center for Health Care Technology was established to
address.

In this discussion, I will briefly describe the process by
which the Center has attempted to surface and to answer these
questions. Although the Center will probably not survive the
present Administration's budget cutting activities, it represents
a unique and unprecedented effort in medicine -- an effort aimed
at coping with some of the complex issues and problems which
have been engendered by the remarkable medical innovations we
have witnessed in the last two decades.

From my admittedly biased perspective, formal, neutral, and ongoing assessments of medical technologies are essential if technological innovation is to be fostered and promoted.

The National Center for Health Care Technology was authorized by the U.S. Congress to assess health care technologies and coordinate these activities within the Department of Health and Human Services. The law (P.L.95-623) which created the Center in late 1978 defines health care technology broadly to include any means to prevent, diagnose, or treat disease or promote health. Furthermore, it calls for evaluation not only for safety and efficacy, but also for the social, ethical, and economic implications of technologies. Thus, the mission of the Center is to sponsor assessments of health care technologies; provide advice on the appropriate use of new and existing technologies, including recommendations on coverage under Medicare; and to fund research related to health care technology assessment.

In carrying out its mandate, the Center attempts to develop evaluative information about health care technologies useful to decision makers in the public and private sectors, including providers of health care services; agencies with reimbursement, regulatory, health planning or related responsibilities; and, the public.

In order to carry out this broad mission, the Center has emphasized the role of medical professional societies, experts in and out of the government, industry, and others. The Center looks primarily to the private sector as the appropriate locus to assume responsibility for performing the evaluations and for developing the recommendations. The Extramural Research Program of the Center is aimed at gathering primary and secondary data so as to foster evaluations based on scientific evidence. Openness and broad participation by all those with relevant interests are encouraged.

It is important to emphasize that the programs of the Center are not intended by the Congress to prescribe or regulate the practice of medicine. Rather, its goal is to provide the medical community and others with the best current and most accurate information to assist those involved in health care delivery in carrying out their responsibilites. Hence my earlier comment about the uniqueness of the Center in the Federal Government.

HISTORICAL PERSPECTIVES: Diagnosis by Biologic Imaging

An historical perspective is a vital element in assessing any health care technology. This is particularly true because the health care system, as we know it, evolved with little available technology, certainly in terms of devices. "The medical care system was not designed to deliver cost-effective technology to patients. Instead, technology has gradually crept into practice with little or no rational planning."(1) Therefore, awareness of some historical factors which contributed to the present situation becomes all the more important in determining what the future may bring.

The ability of physicians to examine the architecture of internal organs during life, approaching the ease and clarity after death, has increased in an exponential fashion since the early seventeenth century. The importance of the internal environment and, more importantly, physicians' desire to inspect it has been a constant theme in the development of the medical sciences.

Sounds emanating from within the human body were among the earliest parameters having diagnostic importance. Hippocrates was the first to describe the basic aspect of auscultation in his de morbis: "You shall know by this that the chest contains water and not pus, if in applying the ear during a certain time on the side, you perceive a noise like that of boiling vinegar."(2)

After Hippocrates, physicians largely ignored the ideas suggested by this passage, but reported occasionally on the generation of sounds by organs within the body.(3) Observations and classification of external signs of disease and discovery of the internal intricacies of the human body after death commanded the attention of medical men for many centuries, although the anatomical basis of disease was not easily or quickly established.

Reiser comments in his excellent book, Medicine and the Reign of Technology, that "in the seventeenth century, the physician principally used verbal and visual techniques to make a diagnosis. He listened to the patient's description of his symptoms, and observed his appearance and that of his body fluids. In the eighteenth century, the physician began to use manual techniques. Morgagni and his successors dissected the dead body to find pathological lesions left by disease, which they correlated with symptoms the patient had described. Arenbrugger introduced percussion, and the manipulation of the living body to find signs of disease, whose traces might later be visible at autopsy. Together, Morgagni and Arenbrugger and their followers prepared the way for the introduction of tools to aid in diagnostics."(4)

In 1819, a young French physician, Laennec, published his description of a new technique, "mediate auscultation," which made it possible for the physician to detect pulmonary disease in living patients by studying the character of the sounds emanating from the chest. Importantly, Laennec described a device by which to perform this diagnostic procedure, the

stethoscope. The stethoscope enabled physicians to acquire
information about the status and functions of organs in the chest
previously unavailable in the living patient and in some instances,
not obtainable even at autopsy. The ambition to learn more
inspired inventions which allowed physicians to penetrate the
exterior surface and to peer within various portions of the body.

The first of these instruments with which the physician
could glimpse the internal structure of the body was the ophthalmoscope developed in 1850 by a German physician and scientist,
Von Helmholtz. The ophthalmoscope was the first device ever
employed for diagnostic purposes by which the interior parts of
a living body could be studied. It is, in no small way, the
direct predecessor, by slightly more than one hundred years, of
the most innovative applications of X-ray technology, positron
emission tomography, ultrasonics, and the various technologies
which have been discussed in this forum.

Development of instrumentation to aid the physician in
"seeing" into the living body has proceeded at a rapidly increasing rate since then. Close on the heels of the ophthalmoscope
was Czermack's description of the laryngoscope in 1857. Then,
significantly, Roentgen's discovery and subsequent medical
application of the X-ray in 1895 gave the physician not only a
view of the interior of the body but that view was captured on
film--the patient needed to be present for examination only, and
later the X-ray picture could be studied and compared with other
X-rays. The low cost of the machine and the simplicity of the
process helped lead to its rapid spread and to modifications of
the process, e.g., ingestion of bismuth to explore the gastrointestinal tract from end to end.(5) As Banta has stated, "of all
the instruments of visual diagnosis, the X-ray produced the most
significant changes in the methods physicians used to evaluate
illness. This machine challenged the value of touching, listening
to, and talking to the patient in the diagnosis of disease. The
X-ray was so widely accepted that when reports that X-rays could
destroy organic life and produce damage to the skin began to
appear by 1900, these harmful effects were minimized by many
physicians. They confidently asserted that X-ray injury was
unusual and was produced principally by unskilled use."(6)

Increasingly sophisticated X-ray devices and techniques
were developed and rapidly put into use in the twentieth century,
each improvement greatly enhancing the physician's ability to use
visual images in the diagnostic process. Then, in 1963, Cormack
reported in the Journal of Applied Physics the concept of
computerized axial tomography (CT). He described the idea of
"making measurements of the X-ray transmission along lines
parallel to a large number of different directions so as to obtain
a sequence of X-ray transmission profiles."(7) He suggested that

his results were relevant to the field of radiology, but
practical application was thought technically infeasible in
part because, at the time, computers were very large devices.
As we know, it was about a decade before the first clinically
useful CT head scanner was developed by Hounsfield followed
shortly thereafter by the whole body scanner.

It is clear that the development of imaging technologies
in medicine has been the focus of the the imagination, talent,
and resources of generations of medical investigators and, most
innovative industrial groups in and out of the health field. It
is fair to say that no other area of medical technology has come
so far, so fast, and with such dramatic results. It is also
fair to say that the uses and limitations of these technologies
have raised many issues concerning safety, efficacy, economics
and ethics. These issues have lead to serious and significant
external restraints, at least in the United States, as never
before in the development, diffusion, and use in practice of
technologic innovations.

As an aside, it is interesting to remember that unanticipated
problems accompanying technological innovations are not new. For
example, one of the earliest technologists in the U.S., Benjamin
Franklin, was concerned over the danger of poisoning from the
lead used in the distilling apparatus to make rum and from drinking
water collected off lead coated roofs. In the nineteenth century
there were anxieties about steamboat transport. High pressure
steam engines often exploded because wrought-iron shells were used
with cast iron heads having different coefficients of expansion.(8)
So the present day issues and problems associated with new technologies are not unique although they may be unprecedented in total
number. It is on these questions and issues of efficacy, safety,
and cost which I would now like to focus, as well as to describe
the efforts and perspectives of the National Center for Health
Care Technology.

ASSESSING EFFICACY, SAFETY, AND COSTS

These unprecedented innovations in diagnostics and the issues
surrounding their application leave the conscientious practitioner
in want of much information. The problem is greatly compounded
because developments in most of these areas come with remarkable
rapidity, and, in diagnostic imaging, simultaneously across a
broad front. The non-expert practitioner needs the most current
information, particularly concerning safety and effectiveness; and
the information should be communicated to him in an understandable
form.

Technology assessment is a new and evolving process and
when it comes to the evaluation of health care technologies,

none of the approaches used thus far is free from fault. It was the view of our National Council that an electric approach should be utilized; that different methods are required to evaluate technologies depending on the questions and problems they pose. Methods might range from full assessments utilizing existing data and prospective studies to evaluations where existing data sources only are examined.

The Center and the Council have devoted a good deal of effort to the process of assessment as well as to the selection of technologies for assessment. Criteria for assigning priorities to candidate topics have been developed, but it became clear shortly after this effort was initiated that any given criterion might have a different significance depending on the stage of development of the technology at issue.(9) Accordingly, development was divided into three categories:

Emerging Technologies - Those at the stage of applied research before clinical trials are completed but likely to be used in the practice of medicine within five years.

New Technologies - Those which have passed the stage of clinical trials but are not yet widely disseminated throughout the health care system.

Old or Existing Technologies - Those technologies currently in use.

The following criteria for setting priorities among technologies for assessment vary according to these categories.

Emerging Technologies

Potential benefit. Special attention should be given to those technologies in the emerging phase that appear most promising with encouragement of more rapid progress in these areas.

Unusual safety or health questions. There should be particular concern with public health and safety regarding the probability of adverse effects of an emerging technology rather than with risks to the individual at this stage of development.

Other issues relevant to emerging technologies include the perception of serious ethical issues and the potential for wide utilization.

672

New Technologies

As with emerging technologies, the highest priority should
be given to potential benefit. Consideration should also be
given to the complexity of a new technology and to its users.

Potential ease of diffusion. Technologies likely to diffuse
rapidly because of simplicity, low unit cost, or replacement of a
more expensive or cumbersome technology should be given a higher
priority than complex technologies likely to have restricted use.
Safety must also be an important consideration in this category.

Old or Existing Technologies

From time to time there may appear a newly recognized safety
concern over an existing technology either because the technology
is being used more often or because new knowledge becomes
available. For example, it has become evident in recent years
that the risks associated with certain X-rays may outweigh the
potential benefit. This may be the case with dental radiographs
at least in the light of widely held impressions in the U.S. that
they are being overused. A technology assessment forum on dental
radiology recently sponsored by the Center concluded that routine
radiographs for dental caries are not appropriate in the absence
of clinical indications.(10)

The more widespread the use of a technology and the higher
its unit cost, the greater its overall economic impact, and thus,
the greater is the need for review including a study of its cost-
effectiveness.

With respect to emerging technologies and to only a slightly
lesser extent to new technologies, it is important to raise a
cautionary note when it comes to technology assessment. It is to
be emphasized that only in unusual circumstances would a technology
in the "emerging phase" become a candidate for a full-blown
technology assessment. By definition, an emerging technology is
one which is evolving so that an assessment done at a point in
time in that evolution might be worthless, misleading, or harmful.
Unusual circumstances in which an assessment at this stage might
be useful would include surfacing of serious ethical, legal, or
other issues. On the other hand, evaluations for safety and
efficacy while development is underway would likely be of little
value since refinements in the technology might drastically alter
the results within a very brief period of time. If an evaluation
is undertaken for some other reason, the results can only be
considered tentative. However, even with that qualification, an
adverse conclusion may have lasting adverse effects.

The Center is responsible for two types of evaluations: (1) assessments of "high priority" technologies and (2) evaluations provided for the Health Care Financing Administration for its use in making coverage decisions.

(1) Assessment of "High Priority" Technologies

With advice of the National Council on Health Care Technology, the Center sponsors broad assessments of technologies which, by virtue of the fact they are used widely, are of major economic cost, or raise significant issues of safety, efficacy, ethics, or legal implications are considered worthy of special attention. The Council has identified a number of such technologies including, among others, coronary artery bypass surgery, dental radiology, cesarian delivery, end-stage renal disease, and hip/knee replacement. Coronary artery bypass surgery (11), dental radiology, and cesarian delivery (12) have recently been subjected to assessments.

(2) Evaluations for Medicare

These assessments which focus on safety and effectiveness are performed at the request of Medicare. Issues such as cost and cost-effectiveness are not addressed since Medicare coverage decisions must by law take into account only whether a technology is "reasonable and necessary". The process employed by the Center in providing these assessments emphasizes the role of the private sector, particularly that of the professional medical societies and industry, and has been described elsewhere.(13) As of this writing, the Center has provided Medicare with approximately seventy-five such evaluations. These studies are published regularly in the Journal of the American Medical Association.

CONCLUSION

Innovations in diagnostic imaging are at the leading edge of the remarkable progress in medicine that we have witnessed in recent years. Like other innovations they have brought with them complex problems and issues concerned not only with safety and efficacy but with costs, cost-effectiveness, and other societal issues. With time, issues of safety and efficacy are usually resolved and often costs are eventually reduced. However, we are not permitted the luxury of waiting for long periods of time because of both concerns over undue risks and costs to patients and because society is demanding an acceleration of the normal process of evaluation. We must deal with the problem now; the task is to balance the competing aims of developing safe and truly effective diagnostic technologies and the costs that society is willing to pay. It is essential that we succeed in this task for, if we fail, inevitably there will be generated a public perception that the medical and scientific communities and the health care industry are unwilling or unable to assume this responsibility and that it should be assigned to others.

The Center has made a start in technology assessment. In my view, formal efforts in technology assessment are essential. This is particularly true during this era when we are witnessing enormous developments on a broad front.

Health care costs are increasing in all countries in part due to technological innovations. There are many who say that these costs have not been reflected in improved care so that it is incumbent on the professions involved in health care to be diligent about dissipating health care dollars. Research must not be impaired but (1) funds for health care should not be utilized for research purposes unless there is a deliberate policy to do so and (2) it is wasteful, and indeed dishonest and unethical, to utilize unproven and experimental technologies in routine practice (either by the generalist or the specialist) and to charge for the application of such technologies.

As appropriate we should assess the state-of-the-art so that what is known and what is not known at a given point in time is clearly delineated for all who have need for such information--the practicing community, third-party payers, policy makers and not least, the public.

Although the Center may disappear, it is gratifying that some sectors of organized medicine in the U.S. are initiating technology assessments, and in Europe, the European Medical Research Councils and the World Health Organization are also beginning such activities.

REFERENCES

1. Banta, David; et al. Toward Rational Technology in Medicine (Springer Publishing Company, New York, 1981), 21.

2. Laennec, R.T.H. A Treatise on the Diseases of the Chest... 2nd Edition, Translation by John Forbes, T. & G. Underwood London, 1821. (Reprinted by Macmillian, Hafner Press, New York, 1962), 23.

3. Reiser, Stanley. Medicine and the Reign of Technology (Cambridge University Press, Cambridge, 1978), 23.

4. IBID, 22.

5. Banta, David; et al. Toward Rational Technology in Medicine (Springer Publishing Company, New York, 1981), 25.

6. IBID, 25.

7. Ledley, Robert. "Computerized Tomography: A Progress Report," Computers in Health Care (Society for Computer Medicine, 1978), 131.

8. Florman, Samuel. "Living with Technology: Tradeoffs in Paradise," Technology Review, August/September, 1981, 24.

9. Procedures, Priorities and Policy for Assessment of Health Care Technology (National Center for Health Care Technology, Department of Health and Human Services, 1980).

10. Dental Radiology: A Summary of Recommendations from the Technology Assessment Forum, National Center for Health Care Technology, Journal of the American Dental Association, 1981, 423.

11. Report from NCHCT: Coronary Artery Bypass Surgery, NCHCT Technology Assessment Forum, Journal of the American Medical Association, 1981, 1645.

12. Cesarean Childbirth, National Institutes of Health Consensus Development Conference Summary, 1980, 3.

13. Perry, Seymour, and Eliastam, Michael. The National Center for Health Care Technology, Journal of the American Medical Association, 1981, 2510.

The assistance of Mr. Lawrence Deyton in preparing this paper is acknowledged with deep appreciation.

Part XI: Meeting Overview and Images of the Future

IMAGES OF THE FUTURE

Henry N. Wagner, Jr., M.D.

Professor of Medicine, Radiology and Environmental
Health Sciences, The Johns Hopkins Medical Institutions,
Baltimore, Maryland 21205-2179

More than any other branch of medicine, nuclear medicine
teaches us that structure and function are but two aspects of the
same thing. In biological systems what we call structures are
slow processes of long duration. What we call functions are fast
processes of short duration. Nuclear images are symbolic representations of the patterns and changes in the spatial and temporal
distribution of the chemical substances that make up our bodies.
Until now, our major concepts of disease have been based on the
discipline of gross pathology, which provides a limited sort of
information analogous to that obtained from an archeological exca-
vation.

Nuclear images are not limited to static patterns, but are
also concerned with time, and are presented either as a cinematic
display of serial static images or as a "functional image", first
described in 1969 (1). In such images, regional function is portrayed by representing in the images the rate of change in regional
concentrations of radioactive tracers rather than simply the quantities of the tracers in various parts of the body.

The new imaging modalities--nuclear imaging, digital radiography, ultrasonography and nuclear magnetic resonance imaging--
permit us to visualize the structure and function of the human body
during life in ways that at times surpass the perception of pathol-
ogists at the autopsy table or surgeons at the operating table.
The physiological and biochemical orientation of nuclear medicine
is becoming more clear, as is our ability to discern abnormalities
at an earlier stage, even before structural changes have occurred.

THE CYCLOTRON

An important stimulus to the biochemical orientation of nuclear medicine is the biomedical cyclotron. Ernest Lawrence,
inventor of the world's first cyclotron in 1931, saw its potential
in biology and medicine. His fourth machine, described in 1939 as
"the medical cyclotron of the Crocker Radiation Laboratory", was
dedicated to this purpose. Carbon-11, fluorine-18, nitrogen-13
and oxygen-15 are among the most promising of the biologically
important nuclides with short physical half-lives and must be produced at or near the site of their use. Although the most important radioactive tracer in biological research is reactor-produced
carbon-14, this nuclide has three disadvantages: (1) Its long half-
life of over 5000 years precludes its use in human in vivo tracer
studies unless the nuclide is excreted rapidly, as in tests where
$^{14}CO_2$ is released in the breath. (2) Its long half-life precludes
repeated studies. (3) It decays with the emission of soft beta
particles which cannot be localized within the body to permit
studies of regional biochemistry and physiology.

Carbon-11 does not have these limitations. Its half-life is
20.4 minutes; it decays by emitting 0.972 MeV positrons with emission of annihilation radiation that can be detected at great distances from the site of emission by two or more detectors in coincidence to permit precise spatial localization. The short half-
life limits its use to compounds that can be labeled rapidly and
to experiments in which the tracer is followed for only a short
period of time. Fortunately, talented synthetic organic chemists
with increasing interest in nuclear medicine have developed fast
syntheses, many of which have been automated. Ter-Pogossian and
I predicted in 1966: "The importance of carbon in biology is so
great that there seems to be little doubt that ^{11}C can be used in
many studies that have been impossible before."

Carbon-11 was used as a radioactive tracer in biological experiments even before the discovery of carbon-14. A large number
of organic compounds, including acetic acid, lactic acid, succinic
and fumaric acids were studied after labeling with ^{11}C in the
1930's and 1940's.

Carbon-11 is usually produced and in some studies used in the
form of carbon monoxide, carbon dioxide or cyanide, which are used
as precursors of several labeled compounds.

Carbon-11 can be prepared by bombarding nitrogen gas with
protons via the $^{14}N(p,\alpha)$ ^{11}C nuclear reaction. The nitrogen target
yields primarily ^{11}CO and $^{11}CO_2$ when high purity nitrogen is bom-
barded and $H^{11}CN$ when 5% hydrogen is mixed with the N_2. An example
of the direct use of the produced nuclide is the labeling of red
blood cells with carbon monoxide.

Oxygen-15 decays with a half-life of 122 seconds, emitting 1.726 MeV positrons. It is prepared by bombarding nitrogen with deuterons by the $^{14}N(d,n)^{15}O$ nuclear reaction. The target material used is air circulating continuously in the cyclotron beam. It is used to measure regional oxidation as well as in the form of CO, CO_2 and H_2O.

POSITRON EMISSION TOMOGRAPHY

Until the development of tomographic imaging, planar imaging devices such as Anger scintillation cameras produced two-dimensional images of the three-dimensional distribution of a radioactive tracer within the body. The sensitivity of the device decreases with distance and activity in front and back of the regions of interest all contribute to the production of a distorted image of the true distribution of the radioactive tracer. Prior to tomography, quantification was limited by the distorting effect of planar imaging and only relative activity could be assessed. The two greatest contributions of positron emission tomography are better chemistry and better quantification. More precise quantification is possible when the radioactive tracer emits a positron during the process of radioactive decay. The emitted positron combines with an electron and the two particles are mutually annihilated with the emission of two gamma rays traveling in opposite directions. These gamma rays travel from the inside to the outside of the patient's body and are detected by hundreds of crystal scintillation detectors surrounding the body. Spatial localization is obtained by the fact that gamma rays detected simultaneously by any pair of detectors represent activity located somewhere along the line joining the two detectors. A mathematical algorithm, called "filtered back-projection," is used by a computer to reconstruct an image of the sites where positrons interacted with electrons within the regions being examined by the array of detectors.

Positron-emission tomography (PET) not only improves quantification by restricting the region of interest to a given slice through the body, but also is well suited for measurement of the important positron-emitting nuclides, carbon, nitrogen, oxygen and fluorine.

REGIONAL GLUCOSE METABOLISM

An essential first step in many studies is measurement of the rate at which a radioactive tracer is delivered to the various parts of an organ after intravenous injection. One approach to measurement of regional cerebral blood flow is to image the distribution of water labeled with oxygen-15 that results from the con-

tinuous inhalation of ^{15}O-carbon dioxide. The short half-life of
2 1/2 minutes requires an imaging device that has the ability to
measure very fast counting rates. Other tracers used to measure
regional blood flow are nitrogen-13 ammonia and carbon-11 butanol.
Using 15 MeV protons, about 150 mCi of ^{11}C can be produced per
microamp of current in the cyclotron. Small hospital cyclotrons
with currents around 50 microamps can produce as much as 7-8 Ci
of ^{11}C activity.

Among the most important studies are those in which regional
cerebral glucose metabolism is measured using either ^{18}F or ^{11}C
deoxyglucose (3). The method most widely used to produce ^{18}F involves the bombardment of neon-20 with deuterons according to the
$^{20}Ne(d,\alpha)^{18}F$ nuclear reaction. Fluorine gas is produced, is used
to fluorinate 3,4,6-tri-o-acetyl-D-glucal which is hydrolyzed and
purified to yield 2-^{18}F-deoxyglucose. At UCLA two preparations
of 15-25 mCi are routinely prepared semi-automatically with 95%
purity and less than 1 mR radiation exposure to the chemists.
This synthesis was developed by Ido and his associates at Brookhaven National Laboratory (4). More recently Elmaleh in Boston and
Tewson in Houston and their coworkers have described syntheses
based on $H^{18}F$ rather than F_2 gas. Reivich, Kuhl, Wolf and associates performed the first positron-emission tomographic studies of
the brain in man with 2-^{18}FDG in 1979 (5). Their studies were
based on the now-classical method of Sokoloff who used ^{14}C deoxyglucose and autoradiography to measure local cerebral glucose
metabolism in animals (6).

Phelps and Huang extended Sokoloff's model to account for slow
dephosphorylation of 2-^{18}FDG-6-phosphate (7). The latter compound
is formed when 2-F-deoxyglucose is transported into brain cells
and subsequently serves as a substrate of the enzyme hexokinase
to form 2-FDG-6-phosphate. Subsequent metabolism then occurs at
a slow rate permitting multi-view and multi-plane imaging with
positron-emission tomographic devices.

Fluorine-18 has a half-life of 109.7 minutes and decays by
positron emission. It is not only a useful label for deoxyglucose
but also for drugs, such as narcotics, that are bound by specific
receptors in the brain.

An example of the use of a positron-emitting tracer study in
clinical neurology is in the selection of patients for surgery in
treatment of focal epilepsy. In 1980 Kuhl et al described the
finding of localized regions of diminished ^{18}F-deoxyglucose metabolism at the sites of origin of epileptic seizures in patients
with temporal lobe seizures. Surgical removal of the seizure
focus resulted in marked relief of seizures in previously untreat-
able patients. Deoxyglucose metabolism has also been found to be
deranged in patients with stroke, senile dementia and Huntington's
disease.

Di Chiro (1981) has evidence that measurement of regional metabolism of cerebral tumors might provide a non-invasive assessment of their malignancy. Initial correlations of metabolic activity with biopsy assessment of the degree of malignancy have been good.

SENSORY ACTIVATION

One of the most fundamental questions in biology is the mechanism by which physical and chemical processes within the brain determine behavior. Related questions are how the external world is represented in the brain, and whether anything recognizable in the biology of the brain is relatable to thought and/or language.

It is now well established that sensory stimulation, such as sound, sight and touch activate electrical activity with the brain and that such stimuli also increase cerebral blood flow and metabolism in specific regions of the brain. Focal increases in cerebral blood flow during voluntary movement of the hand occurred in the region of the contralateral post-central gyrus. These can now be measured in man with ^{18}F deoxyglucose.

It is well-established that certain behavior patterns are associated with well-defined areas of the brain. The question is whether we can identify them by measuring their biochemical activity. Until now much of the information that we have about localization of function comes from the study of patients with brain tumors or cerebrovascular disease, from ablation or electrical stimulation experiments. For example, stimulation of the brainstem and contiguous areas can elicit reactions of defense, flight and hunger; stimulation of various regions of the cortex can yield visual and auditory reactions, among others. The most fundamental question remains: can we identify biochemical reactions associated with consciousness? Can we identify biochemical reactions related to thinking, recalling, perceiving and deciding?

Localization of mental activity in the brain--which we now take to be common knowledge--was not always accepted. For example, Aristotle believed that the physical seat of mental activity was the heart rather than the brain.

Perhaps someday it will be possible to write a book entitled "Elements of Psychochemistry", analogous to Gustav Theodor Fechner' book in 1860, called "Elements of Psychophysics".

682

NEURORECEPTORS

One of the most important uses of radioactive tracers has been to reveal the existence of substances on cell membranes or within all types of cells that bind endogenous molecules or exogenous drugs with a high affinity. Most of our knowledge has been derived from in vitro studies, usually based on the use of tritiated ligands, but the use of gamma or positron-emitting radionuclides has made possible the extension of these studies to living human beings. Essential to the receptor concept is that the binding of the ligand by the receptor elicits a physiological or pharmacological response.

In the case of drugs, agonist activity is not related solely to the binding affinity of the ligand for the receptor, but also to an efficacy factor characteristic of a given agonist. On the other hand, antagonist activity can be closely related to binding affinity alone.

A major role of radiolabeled ligands is to permit demonstration of saturability, by providing labeled substances of high specific activity as well as high affinity.

One of the characteristics of the use of positron-emitting, short-lived radionuclides is that, at least in theory, they can be prepared at high specific activities.

It is now clear that neurotransmission involving receptors is important for the normal functioning of the nervous system. Positron-emission tomography can help us to measure the location and biochemical activity of these "recognition" sites as well as the relationship between affinity and the physiological/pharmacological action, i.e., we can assess the functional "relevance" of the binding phenomenon. In essence, what we search for are regional biochemical correlates of psychological phenomena and neuropsychiatric disorders. Such correlates would not only be expected to have an important effect on conceptualization of disease processes, but also could be of value in assessment of the effects of therapeutic drugs. Such studies could extend the type of relationship that Creese and others reported for anti-psychotic drugs, that is, that the inhibition of ^{3}H-haloperidol to dopamine receptors in calf brain correlated with the clinical effectiveness of these drugs.

Attention is being directed to the four major biogenic amines: dopamine, norepinephrine, epinephrine and serotonin. All four are integrated to affect normal behavior and possibly psychiatric disorders, such as depression, and neurological disorders, such as Parkinson's disease. For example, abnormal motor activity can be produced in animals by injection of dopamine into the substia nigra and striatum of animals, and destruction of nigra-striatal pathways has been found in patients with Parkinson's disease. It has been postulated, but not proved, that the meso-limbic dopaminergic pathway is involved in schizophrenia.

One type of problem that might be solved at least in part by assessment of the activity of dopamine receptors is related to the treatment of Parkinsonian patients with L-dopa. Although many patients are helped, longterm treatment can lead to dementia and declining effectiveness. Other related disorders that may involve the extrapyramidal system are Huntington's disease and torsion dystonia.

OPIATE RECEPTORS

The existence of an opiate receptor was proven in 1973 by the in vitro binding studies of Pert and Snyder (8), Simon et al, and Terenius. Kuhar et al then showed that there were marked regional differences in the localization of opiate receptors in rat, monkey and human brain (9). In some studies ^{3}H-diprenorphine was used to map the distribution of opiate receptors by autoradiography. These receptors were found in anatomical regions involved with physiological processes affected clinically by opiates. For example, a high density of opiate receptors was found in the substantia gelatinosa of the spinal cord, an area known to be involved in the sensation of pain. Areas of the brain involving pain such as the intralaminar nuclei of the thalamus were also found to have high densities of opiate receptors. One part of the limbic system, the amygdala, was found to have the highest concentration of opiate receptors in the brain, which may be related to the euphoria-inducing effects of these drugs.

In addition to binding opiate drugs, opiate receptors bind the two natural opiates, β endorphin, found in enormous concentrations in the pituitary but in low concentrations in the brain, and enkephalin, which is found at levels 10 times as high as β endorphin in the brain.

Autoradiography of tritiated neuroreceptor ligands led to the localization of opiate receptor sites in experimental animals. Positron-emission tomography makes it possible, at least in theory, to localize these in living human beings and determine whether regional abnormalities in the affinity of the receptors occur in certain diseases. Problems that remain to be addressed include:
(1) Choice of the best neuroreceptor ligand to be labeled.
(2) Synthesis of a labeled ligand of adequate affinity and specific activity. (3) Determination of the optimum times at which to measure regional activities after ligand administration.
(4) Quantification of ligand distributions within various regions of the brain by positron-emission tomography. (5) Correction for

684

non-specific binding. (6) Validation studies in animals and normal human beings. (7) Clinical studies.

To date we have synthesized 14 compounds that bind to opiate receptors and can be labeled with fluorine-18. Our plan is to inject a radiotracer ligand that has a high affinity for the opiate receptor and a slow rate of dissociation of the ligand after binding. Affinity constants are of the order of 10^9 or 10^{10} M^{-1}. The subsequent rate of clearance from receptor sites after uptake depends on the dissociation rate constant observed in equilibration experiments but also on receptor concentrations and the phenomenon of "rebinding" of the radiotracer after it dissociates into the synaptic cleft. The amount of radioligand that can be administered by intravenous injection is limited by the saturability of the receptors and by possible pharmacologic actions. If the administered dose continues to be increased, the specific/non-specific binding ratio decreases.

DOPAMINE RECEPTORS

^{3}H-spiperone, a radioligand antagonist of dopamine receptors, has an affinity constant for binding to the dopamine receptor of 1 to 2 x 10^{10} M^{-1}. When injected into rats, binding in the region of the caudate nucleus is much more avid than in the cerebellum which contains low concentration of dopamine receptors (10). At one hour after intravenous injection, the binding ratio is 6:1, becoming 12:1 after 24 hours.

^{3}H-spiperone is not specifically bound by the dopamine receptor, but also binds to serotonin, an alpha-adrenergic receptor, and to a fourth binding site not yet characterized. When the administered dose exceeds 50 μg/kg, the striatal/cerebellar ratio decreases as the receptors become saturated. The uptake ratios of spiperone labeled with ^{11}C or ^{18}F of high specific activity remains to be determined. To date we have prepared a whole series of spiperone and benperidol analogs and have studied their in vitro and in vivo binding. With spiperone itself, at a dose of 10 μg/kg in the rat, approximately 15% of the striatal dopamine receptors are occupied. With extrapolation of animal data to human beings, we can calculate that about 11,400 counts can be accumulated per 1 x 1 cm volume element in the caudate nucleus compared to 1,900 counts in the cerebellum, both accumulated over a 15-minute period. Thus it seems that in vivo tomographic studies in man are feasible. As yet, however, this has not been accomplished, since our cyclotron and positron-emission tomography device have just begun to operate.

THE FUTURE

The production of these and other positron-emitting radio-nuclides has resulted in as many as 60 cyclotrons worldwide dedicated to nuclear medicine research. Automated radiosyntheses are used to produce useful labeled molecules on a regular basis. The operation of the cyclotrons themselves is also highly automated. Limited studies can be performed even if a cyclotron is not available. Important positron generator systems include germanium-68 → gallium-68; strontium-82 → copper-68; xenon-122 → iodine-122, and iron-52 → manganese-52m. Of course, none of these can be used to study glucose metabolism.

An increasing number of papers on positron-emission tomography are being presented at national and international scientific meetings. Many deal with a quantitative assessment of regional cerebral blood volume and flow or regional metabolism, using labeled deoxyglucose or oxygen. Several groups, including ours, are attempting to map the distribution of neuroreceptors in normal persons and patients with neurological or psychological disorders. Special emphasis is being directed toward opiate and dopamine receptors.

RELATIONSHIP TO OTHER TYPES OF IMAGING

Several important advances in medical imaging are developing simultaneously, i.e., positron-emission tomography, single photon emission tomography, digital radiography, nuclear magnetic resonance imaging, and ultrasonography. While it is impossible to predict the future with certainty, perhaps it is safe to make certain assumptions as we go forward:

(1) Regulatory and bureaucratic delays and increasing perception of the risk of radiation are likely to slow scientific and clinical progress unless they can be counteracted.

(2) Simultaneously advancing technologies will compete for financial resources.

(3) Chemistry, physiology and pharmacology are likely to continue their striking advances, e.g., in brain chemistry.

(4) The images of ultrasonography may become of unacceptable quality in the future, and be replaced by nuclear magnetic resonance imaging.

(5) If the information is of great value, expensive technology will continue to be developed, perhaps related to the fact that only about 5% of total hospital costs are attributable to diagnostic procedures, including imaging and laboratory tests. The greatest cost-saving lies in better treatment.

(6) Positron-emission tomography holds the greatest promise for providing chemical information, but at great expense and relative complexity.

686

(7) Nuclear magnetic resonance holds the greatest promise in providing structural information, again at high cost and complexity.
(8) Anatomical information is likely to reach a plateau soon.
(9) Positron-emission tomography is likely to have its greatest impact on the conceptualization of disease processes, by permitting direct evidence of chemical dysfunction. Perhaps its most closely allied science will be pharmacology.

REFERENCES

1. Kaihara, S., T.K. Natarajan, C.D. Maynard and H.N. Wagner, Jr. "Construction of a functional image from spatially localized rate constants obtained from serial camera and rectilinear scanner data." Radiology 93 (1969) 1345-1348.
2. Ter-Pogossian, M.M. and H.N. Wagner, Jr. "A new look at the cyclotron for making short-lived isotopes." Nucleonics 24 (1966) 50-56.
3. Phelps, M. "Positron computed tomography studies of cerebral glucose metabolism in man: theory and application in nuclear medicine." Seminars in Nuclear Medicine 9 (1981) 32-49.
4. Ido, T., C.N. Wan, V. Casella, et al. "Labeled 2-deoxy-D-glucose analogs. ^{18}F-labeled 2-deoxy-2-fluoro-D-glucose, 2-deoxy-2-fluoro-D-mannose and ^{14}C-2-deoxy-12-fluoro-D-glucose." Journal of Labelled Compounds and Radiopharmaceuticals 24 (1978) 174-183.
5. Reivich, M., D. Kuhl, A. Wolf, et al. "The (^{18}F) fluoro-deoxyglucose method for the measurement of local cerebral glucose utilization in man." Circulation Research 44 (1979) 127-137.
6. Sokoloff, L., M. Reivich, C. Kennedy, et al. "The (^{14}C) deoxyglucose method for the measurement of local cerebral glucose method for the measurement of local cerebral glucose utilization: theory, procedure and normal values in the conscious and anesthetized albino rat." Journal of Neurochemistry 28 (1977) 897-916.
7. Phelps, M.E., S.C. Huang, E.J. Hoffman, et al. "Tomographic measurement of local cerebral glucose metabolic rate in humans with (F-18) 2-fluoro-2-deoxy-D-glucose. Validation of method." Annals of Neurology 6 (1979) 371-388.
8. Pert, C.B. and S.H. Snyder. "Opiate receptor: demonstration in nervous tissue." Science 179 (1973) 1011.
9. Kuhar, M.J. "Opiate receptors: some anatomical and physiological aspects." Annals of the New York Academy of Sciences 311 (1978) 35.
10. Kuhar, M.J. "Histochemical localization of neurotransmitter receptors," in H.I. Yamamura, S.J. Enna and M.J. Kuhar, eds., Neurotransmitter Receptor Binding 1978 (Raven Press, New York).

11. Creese, I. "Receptor binding as a primary drug screening device," in H.I. Yamamura, S.J. Enna and M.J. Kuhar, eds., Neurotransmitter Receptor Binding 1978 (Raven Press, New York).

688

698

SPEAKERS/PARTICIPANTS LIST OF ADDRESSES

Professor W. E. Adam
Abt Radiologie III
Nuklearmedizin Steinhovelstrasse 9
D-7900
Ulm, Germany

Philip O. Alderson, M.D.
Columbia Presbyterian Hospital
Nuclear Medicine Division
622 West 168th Street
New York, N.Y. 10032
U.S.A.

Dr. Robert Allemand
Laboratoire d'Electronique et de
 Technoilogie de l'Informatique
Avenue Des Martyrs
85X
38041 Grenoble Cedex
France

Robert Allen, M.D.
Department of Radiology
Fairfax Hospital
Fairfax, Va.
U.S.A.

Joseph Alter, M.D.
155 E. 76th Street
New York, N.Y. 10021
U.S.A.

G. J. Arink, Ph.D.
N.V. Philips Medical Systems
Eindhoven, The Netherlands

J.C. Baron, M.D.
Service Hospitalier
Frederic Joliot
Department de Biologique
Commissarai a L'Energie Atomique
91406 Orsay
France

Alfred John Bedford, M.D.
USAF Hospital
Box 59
APO New York 09220

Walter Bencivelli, M.D.
CNR Institute of Clinical Physiology
c/o Universita di Pisa Via Savi
8 - 56100 Pisa
Italia

Anna Benini, Ph.D.
Servizio di Fisica
Sànitaria
Ospedale Maggiore
I43100 Parma
Italia

Herman Bieber, Ph.D.
Exxon Corporation
Box 45
Linden, N.J.   07036
U.S.A.

Prof. J. Ch. Bolomey
Professor at Paris-Sud University
Laboratoire des Signaux & Systems
Ecole Superieure d'Electricite
Plateau du Moulon
91190 GIF-FUS-YVETTE
France

A. Bertrand Brill, M.D.
Medical Department
Brookhaven National Laboratory
Upton, N.Y.   11973
U.S.A.

Thomas F. Budinger, M.D., Ph.D.
Donner Laboratory & Dept. of Electrical
 Engineering & Computer Sciences
University of California
Berkeley, Ca.   94720
U.S.A.

Maj. Anna K. Chacko, M.D.
Maj. USAMC
P.O. Box 126
Tripler Army Medical Center
Honolulu, Hawaii   96859
U.S.A.

Antonio Chiesa, M.D.
Department of Radiology
University Hospital
37134 Verona
Italia

A. M. Coblentz, Ph.D.
Laboratoire d'Anthropologie
 et d'Ecologie Humaine
Universite Paris V .
45 rue des Saints-Peres
75270 - Paris Cedex 06
France

C. Constantinides, M.D.
Alexandra University Hospital
Vas.Sophias Ave. and K. Lourou Str.
Athens 611 Greece

Durval Campos Costa, M.D.
R. Falcao 686
4300 Porto
Portugal

Barbara Y. Croft, Ph.D.
Dept. of Radiology, Box 170
University of Virginia
Charlottesville, Va.   22908
U.S.A.

Mr. Harold Davidson
Office of the Director of Army Research
Department of the Army
Washington, D.C.   20310
U.S.A.

Arthur Lima de Bastos
Macieïra de Sarnes
S. Joao da Madeira
Portugal

A. de Carvalho, M.D.
Rontgenafdeling R
Arhus Kommunehospital
8000 Arhus C - Danmark

Jean de Kervasdoue, Ph.D.
Directeur, Des Hopitaux
Ministere de la Sante
8 Avenue de Segur
75007 Paris
France

Alessandro Del Maschio
Istituto di Radiogia
Polichniani, 2
35100 Padova
Italia

Jean-Pierre D'Haenens, Ph.D.
38240 Meylan
77 Avenue de Graisivaudan
Grenoble, France

Alessandro Distanti, M.D.
CNR Institute of Clinical Physiology
c/o Universita di Pisa via Savi
8 - 56100 Pisa
Italia

Luigi Donato, M.D.
CNR Institute of Clinical Physiology
c/o Universita di Pisa via Savi
8 - 56100 Pisa
Italia

Edward A. Eikman, M.D.
Section of Nuclear Medicine
Veterans Administration Hospital
13000 North 30th Street
Tampa, Fla.   33612
U.S.A.

David R. Elmaleh, Ph.D.
128 Pleasant Street
Brookline, Ma.   02146
U.S.A.

Giampiero Feltrin
Via Lodi 32
Vicenza (C.P.36100)
Italia

Prof. Cesare Fieschi
3ª Cattedra di Clinica Neurologica
Viale dell'Universita, 30 - 00185 Roma
Italia

Robert E. Foy, Jr., M.D.
Radiation Services, P.A.
Coffee General Hospital
400 North Edwards Street
Enterprise, Al.   36330
U.S.A.

Fernando Godinho
Av. Raimba D. Amelia
18-3º Esq.
1600 Lisboa

David J. Goodenough, Ph.D.
The George Washington University Medical Center
Division of Radiation Physics
The Warwick Bldg.
2300 K Street, N.W.
Washington, D.C.   20037
U.S.A.

Eugene M. Grivsky, D.Sc.
4407 Eastwood Court
Fairfax, Va.   22032
U.S.A.

Riccardo Guzzardi, Ph.D.
Consiglio Nazionale Delle Ricerche
CNR Institute of Clinical Physiology
c/o Universita di Pisa Via Savi
8 - 56100 Pisa
Italia

Austin B. Harrelson, M.D.
1805 Monument Avenue, Suite 106
Richmond, Va.   23220
U.S.A.

Thomas C. Hill, M.D.
Department of Radiology - Nuclear Medicine Division
New England Deaconess Hospital
185 Pilgrim Road
Boston, Mass.   02215
U.S.A.

Fritz W. Hofmann, Ph.D.
Siemens AG
UB Med
127 Heukestrasse
Erlangen, West Germany

Shlomo Hoory, Ph.D.
3E Mill Drive (1F)
Great Neck, N.Y. 11021
U.S.A.

J. Jerome Hopperstad, M.D.
3132 Minnehaha Crt.
Wayzata, Mn. 55391
U.S.A.

A. Everett James, Jr., Sc.M., J.D., M.D.
Department of Radiology
Vanderbilt University Hospital
Nashville, Tn. 37232
U.S.A.

Yerassimos Kekkeris, M.D.
University of Thrace
Ghair of Automatic Control Systems
Xanthi - Greece

Remy Klaus, Ph.D.
Companie Generale de Radiologie
13th Square Max Hymans
75741 Paris Cedex 15
France

Lawrence E. Larsen, M.D.
Chief, Microwave Research
Walter Reed Army Institute of Research
Washington, D.C. 20012
U.S.A.

Niels A. Lassen, M.D.
Bispebjerg Hospital
Bispebjerg Bakke 23
2400 Kobenhavn NV
Denmark

R. D. Lele, M.D.
Chief Physician and Chief of Nuclear Medicine
Jaslok Hospital & Research Center
Bombay 400026
India

George S. Lerman, M.D.
Kent Radiology Associates
640 S. State Street
Dover, Delaware 19901
U.S.A.

J.W. Ludwig, M.D., Ph.D.
St. Antonius Ziekenhuis
Jan van Scorelstraat 2, Utrecht
The Netherlands

Col. Robert Lull, M.D.
Chief, Nuclear Medicine Service
Letterman Army Medical Center
P.O. Box 272
Presidio San Francisco, Ca. 94129
U.S.A.

Leon S. Malmud, M.D.
Temple University Hospital
Section of Nuclear Medicine
3401 N. Broad Street
Philadelphia, Pa. 19140
U.S.A.

Victor R. McCready, M.Sc.
Royal Marsden Hospital
Department of Nuclear Medicine
Sutton, Surrey, United Kingdom

Maria A. Mourao
R. de Bitaraes, 68
4100 Porto
Portugal

Peter Muto
56 v. Posillipo
80123 Naples
Italia

Thomas O'Beirne, M.D.
93 Highfield Park
Dundru, Dublin
Ireland

Seymour Perry, M.D.
Director, National Center for Health
 Care Technology
Assistant Surgeon General
Department of Health & Human Services
Parklawn Bldg., Rm. 17A29
5600 Fishers Lane
Rockville, Md. 20857
U.S.A.

M. Pistolesi, M.D.
CNR Institute of Clinical Physiology
c/o Universia di Pisa Via Savi
8 - 56100 Pisa
Italia

Carlo Poy, M.D.
Medico Chirurgo
Specialista in Radiologia Medica
Consulente in Radiopatologia e Radioprotezione
20147 Milano
Via S. Saint Bon, 7
Italia

Brian R. Pullan, Ph.D.
University of Manchester
Department of Medical Biophysics
Stopford Building
Oxford Road
Manchester M13 9PT
United Kingdom

N.T. Racoveanu, M.D.
Chief Medical Officer
Radiation Medicine
World Health Organization
1211 Geneva 27
Switzerland

Maj. Gen. Garrison Rapmund, M.D.
CDR/USAMRDC
Fort Dietrick
Frederick, Md. 21701
U.S.A.

Richard C. Reba, M.D.
Division of Nuclear Medicine
George Washington University Hospital
901 Twenty-Third Street, N.W.
Washington, D.C. 20037
U.S.A.

Prof. Dr. Fevzi Renda
Director, Dept. of Nuclear Medicine
Ankara Medical School
6/4 Tahran Caddessi
Kavaklidere
Ankara, Turkey

Erik L. Ritman, Ph.D.
Head, Biodynamic Research Unit
Mayo Clinic and Foundation
Rochester, Minnesota 55901
U.S.A.

Walter L. Robb, Ph.D.
Vice-President & General Manager
Medical Systems Division
General Electric Company
P.O. Box 414
Milwaukee, Wi. 53201
U.S.A.

Giuseppe Roberti, M.D.
Istituto di Fisica Sperimentale
Della
Universita di Napoli
80138 Napoli
Via Antonio Tari, 3
Italia

S. David Rockoff, M.D.
Department of Radiology
The George Washington University Hospital
901 Twenty-Third Street, N.W.
Washington, D.C. 20037
U.S.A.

Lloyd Salisbury
10138 Crestwood Road
Kensington, Md. 20795
U.S.A.

Marco Salvatore, M.D.
Nuclear Medicine Department
National Cancer Institute
Pascole Foundation
Naples 80100
Italia

A. M. Santolicandro, M.D.
CNR Institute of Clinical Physiology
c/o Universita di Pisa Via Savi
8 - 56100 Pisa
Italia

Alton R. Sharpe,Jr., M.D.
Medical College of Virginia
Virginia Commonwealth University
MCV Station
Box 1
Richmond, Va. 23298
U.S.A.

Stephen H. Sherman, M.D.
2037 Windy Hill Road
Allentown, Pa. 18103
U.S.A.

Michel M. Ter-Pogossian, Ph.D.
Department of Radiology
Washington University School of Medicine
510 South Kingshighway
St. Louis, Mo. 63110
U.S.A.

A. Todd-Pokropek, Ph.D.
Department Medical Physics
University College Hospital
Medical School
London, United Kingdom

Jacqueline Vignaud, M.D.
Professor of Radiology
Fondation Ophtalmologique
25 a 29, Rue Manin
75940 Paris Cedex 19
France

Henry N. Wagner, Jr., M.D.
Director, Divisions of Nuclear Medicine
The Johns Hopkins Medical Institutions
615 North Wolfe Street
Baltimore, Md. 21205
U.S.A.

709

Peter N.T. Wells
Department of Medical Physics
Bristol General Hospital
Guinea Street
Bristol BS1 6SY, United Kingdom

Albert L. Wiley, Jr., M.D., Ph.D.
Division of Radiation Oncology
Wisconsin Clinical Cancer Center
600 Highland Avenue
Madison, Wi. 53792
U.S.A.

Col. Philip Winter, M.D.
Department of Defense
Washington, D.C. 20310
U.S.A.